A tailored education experience —

Sherpath book-organized collections

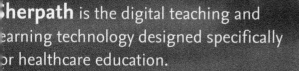

Sherpath is the digital teaching and learning technology designed specifically for healthcare education.

Sherpath book-organized collections offer:

Objective-based, digital lessons, mapped chapter-by-chapter to the textbook, that make it easy to find applicable digital assignment content.

Adaptive quizzing with personalized questions that correlate directly to textbook content.

Teaching materials that align to the text and are organized by chapter for quick and easy access to invaluable class activities and resources.

Elsevier ebooks that provide convenient access to textbook content, even offline.

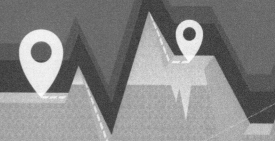

**VISIT
myevolve.us/sherpath**
today to learn more!

21-CS-0280 TM/AF 6/21

CONTENTS

LEADING AND MANAGING IN NURSING

EIGHTH EDITION

PATRICIA S. YODER-WISE, RN,
EdD, NEA-BC, ANEF, FAONL, FAAN
Professor and Dean Emerita
Texas Tech University Health Sciences Center
School of Nursing
Lubbock, Texas

SUSAN SPORTSMAN, PhD, RN,
ANEF, FAAN
Managing Director
Collaborative Momentum Consulting
St. Louis, Missouri

ELSEVIER

Elsevier
3251 Riverport Lane
St. Louis, Missouri 63043

LEADING AND MANAGING IN NURSING, EIGHTH EDITION

ISBN: 978-0-323-79206-6

Notice

Practitioners and researchers must always rely on their own experience and knowledge in evaluating and using any information, methods, compounds or experiments described herein. Because of rapid advances in the medical sciences, in particular, independent verification of diagnoses and drug dosages should be made. To the fullest extent of the law, no responsibility is assumed by Elsevier, authors, editors or contributors for any injury and/or damage to persons or property as a matter of products liability, negligence or otherwise, or from any use or operation of any methods, products, instructions, or ideas contained in the material herein.

Previous editions copyrighted 2019, 2015, 2011, 2007, 2003, 1999, 1995.

International Standard Book Number: 978-0-323-79206-6

Senior Content Strategist: Yvonne Alexopoulos
Senior Content Development Manager: Luke E. Held
Senior Content Development Specialist: Joshua S. Rapplean
Publishing Services Manager: Deepthi Unni
Project Manager: Sindhuraj Thulasingam
Design Direction: Brian Salisbury

Printed in the United States of America.

Last digit is the print number: 9 8 7 6 5 4 3 2 1

Working together
to grow libraries in
developing countries

www.elsevier.com • www.bookaid.org

This book is dedicated to all the nurses who have carried the world through the pandemic from 2020. Some lost their lives; some experienced severe cases of COVID-19; some have what we now term long COVID; all suffered mental and physical exhaustion—at least at times, as did many others. Many were in direct care roles—often substituting for physicians and family–; some were in leadership roles trying to keep up with ever-changing policies; some were in educator roles moving from classrooms to online instruction or from clinical to simulation environments; some were students who are now our practitioners. No matter what role you served in during this time, we thank you for your continued commitment and leadership!

To tomorrow's leaders—we can't wait to see what you will do to continue transforming the nursing profession!
Lead on! ¡Adelente!

EDITORS' MESSAGE TO OUR READERS

Thank you for being a part of *Leading and Managing in Nursing*. We did our best in these hectic times to secure great thinkers and writers to prepare information for you. They have provided general concepts, solid advice, insights based on years of experience and their current best thinking. We all also know that we might alter our thinking on some points, for example, how best to organize the services we provide, based on new data, new technologies, and new thinking. These changes might happen quickly—which is why we consider the top two skills of an effective leader to be listening (with intentionality) and flexibility. If you are someone who likes "to be in charge and plan ahead," you need to rethink how you will thrive in the future. Being in charge in the future is more about clearing the way for great things to happen based on what your team believes is necessary to achieve the mission. And, if you're in an organization that has a 5-year strategic plan, you had best have your own unit or divisional plan that is based on 1 year and that takes into account what you know about the internal and external factors that are likely to be true for the coming year. In other words, thinking long-range has become shorter in terms of the actual plan. The mission should be strong enough to carry the organization for at least 5 years. However, society, the economy, and technology, to name a few factors, change rather rapidly and can dramatically influence what is possible in terms of the actual plan, and those changes can lead to dramatic adjustments in less than 2 or 3 years.

We want you to know the amount of thought we gave some sections and points as we assembled this eighth edition of *Leading and Managing in Nursing*. Here are some examples. In the seventh edition, we titled a chapter *Cultural Diversity and Inclusion in Health Care*. That title now seems inadequate in addressing the issue. We shouldn't simply care about diversity and inclusion, we need to be concerned with the bigger concept of moving toward being a more just organization, thinking more justly about the people with whom we work and those for whom we provide services. Thus, that chapter was renamed *Toward Justice*.

We spent some time discussing whether to adopt the newer word "Latinx" to represent a gender-neutral view of people from a Latino/Latina background. However, we knew from more than one source that many people representative of this group did not like this term. Therefore, you will see Latina/Latino used in the text unless a specific gender is referenced. Similarly, the LGBTQ population has had additional letters added over the years and rather than risk omitting one of the latest, we have chosen to use the LGBTQ+ term to be inclusive of all. These printed words are static. They have to be chosen. In real life, we encourage you to ask people how they might want to be addressed. Just as we see people designate their pronouns below their names in their email signatures as "he/him," "they/their," or "she/her," someone might prefer to be known as a Latinx rather than a Latino—and we won't know unless we ask or validate.

Every chapter mentions a relevant competency, if there is one, from the new Essentials from the American Association of Colleges of Nursing. While these new Competencies are not about leadership per se, they do focus on what a professional nurse is expected to demonstrate as basic competencies to practice in today's world. Five chapters have examples of the new Next-Generation NCLEX® case studies. For students in prelicensure programs, this is an opportunity to practice with some examples of these new testing items on the NGN exam. For the rest of us, this is an opportunity to consider our understanding of the chapter's content and to recall our own experiences of waiting to learn if we had passed the examination or not!

Nursing, as is true of many other fields, has continued to become more complex; and the future suggests that we should anticipate a continued expectation or need for greater learning. We encourage you to do what we do: scour the literature every year to determine what some of the best new practices are in leadership so that you remain current.

The profession's challenges are great and every one of us needs to be part of the solution. Those of us already in the profession eagerly await the answers those of you who will join us soon will bring to help move us ahead as we try to meet the increasing demands of health care for the world's population. We used to talk about the country's population—that is such a narrow view anymore because we truly are a global profession. We cannot continue to "trade" nurses around the world. We are not a commodity. We need to produce more of us. We need to find new ways to organize the services we provide so that we are most efficient in the way we provide care. We need to continue to advocate for our patients and we must advocate for ourselves so that we can be effective in advocating for patients.

Accountability, communication, concern for others, having a purpose—all of these are critical factors to consider as we launch ourselves into our own personal leadership journey, wherever it may lead us.

Lead on! ¡Adelente!

CONTRIBUTORS

Nina Almasy, DNP, RN, CNE
Dean
Health Sciences Division
Austin Community College
Austin, Texas

Joan Benson, MSN, RN-BC, CPN
Director
Clinical Informatics and Practice
Children's Mercy
Kansas City, Missouri

Kristin Katherine Benton, BS (Psychology), BSN, MSN, DNP
Director of Nursing
Texas Board of Nursing
Austin, Texas

Richard G. Booth, RN, PhD
Associate Professor
Arthur Labatt Family School of Nursing
Western University
London, Ontario, Canada

Amy Boothe, DNP, RN, CHSE
Assistant Professor
Traditional Undergraduate Program
Texas Tech University Health Science Center
Lubbock, Texas

Arica Brandford, PhD, JD, MSN, RN
Assistant Professor
School of Nursing
Texas A&M University
Bryan/College Station, Texas

M. Margaret Calacci, MS, CNE, CHSE
Director
Grace Center for Innovation in Nursing
    Education
Edson College of Nursing and Health Innovation
Arizona State University College of Nursing
    and Health Innovation
Phoenix, Arizona

Mary Ellen Clyne, PhD
President and Chief Executive Officer
Administration, Clara Maass Medical Center
Belleville, New Jersey

Jeannette Theresa Crenshaw, DNP, RN, LCCE, IBCLC, NEA-BC, FACCE, FAAN
Professor
School of Nursing
Texas Tech University Health Sciences Center
Lubbock, Texas

Mary Ann Donohue-Ryan, PhD, RN, APN, PMH-CNS, NEA-BC, CPHQ
Executive Leadership Consultant
Department of Nursing Administration
Chilton Medical Center
Atlantic Health System
Pompton Plains, New Jersey

Karen A. Esquibel, PhD, APRN, CPNP-PC
Director of Pediatric Nurse Practitioner Studies
Graduate Program
Texas Tech University Health Sciences Center School of
    Nursing
Lubbock, Texas

Victoria N. Folse, PhD, APRN, PMHCNS-BC, LCPC
Director and Professor
Caroline F. Rupert Endowed Chair of Nursing
School of Nursing
Illinois Wesleyan University
Bloomington, Illinois

Jacqueline Lytle Gonzalez, DNP, APRN, MSN, MBA, NEA-BC, FAAN
Former Senior Vice President/System Chief Nursing
    Officer
Administration
Nicklaus Children's Health System
Miami, Florida
Adjunct Professor
School of Nursing & Health Studies
University of Miami
Coral Gables, Florida

Debra A. Hagler, PhD, RN, ACNS-BC, CNE, CHSE, ANEF, FAAN
Clinical Professor
Edson College of Nursing and Health Innovation
Arizona State University
Phoenix, Arizona

Jenny Horn, DNP, MHA, RN-BC
Senior Director
Clinical Applications & Informatics
Clinical Informatics
Keck Medicine of USC
Kansas City, Missouri

Karren Kowalski, PhD, RN, NEA-BC, ANEF, FAAN
President & CEO
Kowalski & Associates
Larkspur, Colorado

Maureen Murphy-Ruocco, APNC, MSN, CSN, EdM, EdD, DPNAP, SFNAP
Professor Emeritus and Former Associate Dean
Nursing and Education
Felician University
Lodi and Rutherford, New Jersey
Nurse Consultant/Nurse Practitioner
Associate Dean and Professor
School of Nursing and Health Education
Felician University
Lodi, New Jersey

Sylvain Trepanier, DNP, MSN, BSN, RN, CENP, FAONL, FAAN
Chief Nursing Officer
Executive Offices
Providence
Renton, California

Diane Margaret Twedell, DNP, MS, CENP
Nurse Administrator
Provider Relations
Mayo Clinic
Rochester, Minnesota

James Jeffery Watson, DNP, RN, NEA-BC, CNE
Associate Professor
School of Nursing
Texas Tech University Health Sciences Center
Lubbock, Texas

Coleen Wilson, DNP, RN, NEA-BC
Director, Adult Inpatient Nursing
UCLA Health
Santa Monica Medical Center
Santa Monica, California

Margarete L. Zalon, PhD, RN, ACNS-BC, FAAN
Professor, Nursing
University of Scranton
Scranton, Pennsylvania
Director, Health Informatics Program
University of Scranton
Scranton, Pennsylvania

REVIEWERS

Shelley Austin, DNP, MNSc, BSN, ADN, RN
Henderson State University
Arkadelphia, Arkansas

Emerald Bilbrew DNP, MSN, BSN, RN, CMSRN
ADN Nursing Instructor
Fayetteville Technical Community College
Fayetteville, North Carolina

Deborah Birk, PhD, RN, MSN, MHA, NEA-BC
Director of Health Systems and Population Health
Leadership DNP Program & Assistant Professor
Goldfarb School of Nursing at Barnes College of
Nursing
St. Louis, Missouri

Joseph Boney, MSN, RN, NEA-BC
Nursing Lecturer
Rutgers University, School of Nursing
Entry into Practice–Second Degree BS in Nursing
Program
Newark, New Jersey

Stephanie A. Gustman, DNP, RN
Associate Professor and DNP Program Coordinator
Ferris State University
Big Rapids, Michigan

Debra A. Hunt, PhD, FNP-BC, GNP-BC, CNE
Associate Professor
Frontier Nursing University
Versailles, Kentucky

Brian K. Jefferson, DNP, ACNP-BC, FCCM
Acute Care Nurse Practitioner
Hepatobiliary and Pancreatic Surgery
Atrium Health Cabarrus Medical Center
Concord, North Carolina

Alicia Jones, BSN, MSN, RN, FNP-C
Duke University School of Nursing
Marathon Health, LLC
Durham, North Carolina

Wendy Lenon, DNP, MSN, BSN, RN
Associate Professor
Chair, School of Nursing
Ferris State University
Big Rapids, Michigan

Velesha Lera, DNP, FNP-BC, RN-BC
CUNY School of Professional Studies
New York, New York

Donnamarie Lovestrand, RN, MSN, CPAN
Assistant Professor, Nursing Programs
Pennsylvania College of Technology
Williamsport, Pennsylvania

Milena Mardahay, RN, BSN, CGRN
Registered Nurse
University of California, San Francisco
San Francisco, California

Jennifer M. Pierle, MSN, FNP-C, CGRA
Nurse Practitioner
Hendricks Regional Health
Danville, Indiana

Patricia D. Sanders, RN BSN

**Rydell L. Todicheeney, PhD, MBA/HCM, APRN,
PHN, PCCN, ACNS-BC**
Clinical Nurse Specialist
Natividad
Salinas, California

Kathleen A. Ziomek, RN, BSN, MSN, FNP
Daemen University
Amherst, New York

Alyssa Giselle Zwiefelhofer, RN, BSN
Registered Nurse, BSN
Grand Canyon University
Phoenix, Arizona

ACKNOWLDEGEMENTS

Oh that we could say that this book was just the effort of the authors and editors! We thank each of the authors for the work that they did in providing readers with current thinking on complex topics. You, the reader, will find their names and affiliations associated with the chapters they wrote in the Table of Contents. Imagine the amount of effort they exerted in putting that material together for you!

There were almost as many people behind the scenes who made this book possible:

Shelley Burson: Assistant to the Editors and left-brain specialist. Until you have a Shelley in your lives, you don't know what you are missing! Shelley, you know we couldn't do this without you—as we told you many times. THANK YOU!

Yvonne Alexopoulos: Senior Content Strategist and end-run specialist extraordinaire. You have been with L & M for at least four editions—and it shows. Thank you!

Josh Rapplean: Senior Content Development Specialist and juggler of many other roles. This project started out to be such a straight-forward effort and then we had a pandemic that never ended; and we found new ways to work; and you smiled through it all. We really value all you brought to the team! Thank you!

Sindhuraj Thulasingam: Project Manager and survivor of flying emails! When we get "down to the wire," timing gets tight; and we may have bumped into ourselves coming and going a few times; and we made it. Sindhuraj always knew where we were, what was missing, what was done, and what was in development. Thank you!

Robert Wise and **Leonard Keesee**: Husbands Extraordinaire, chief cooks, minimal disruptors, and all-around supporters. We thank you for all you did (or didn't do) that was helpful to our completing this work. We thank you both!

Pat and Susy

The first edition of *Leading and Managing in Nursing* began in a hotel room in New Orleans, Louisiana in January 1990. Darlene Como, the founding publisher of *Leading and Managing*, and I conceptualized a new way of presenting content about leadership and management—one that might engage learners in valuing the importance of roles that support clinical practice. This new approach included personal stories (The Challenge and The Solution), Literature Perspectives, Research Perspectives, synopses, exercises, and boxes of key information. If you had a copy of that first edition and could compare the number of words in it with the number of words in this edition, you would know the field has grown and become far more complex. Nursing has also grown the field of leadership and management research, and so we have many more citations we can share to make this content both theoretical and practical.

We continue to include everything today's nurses need to know about the basics of leading and managing. The changes with each revision of *Leading and Managing* reflect the intensity with which we know how leading and managing influence nurses in direct and indirect caregiving roles, as well as in other aspects of being a professional nurse in a complex, ever-changing, dynamic healthcare environment.

Nurses throughout the profession serve in various leadership roles. Leading and managing are two essential expectations of all professional nurses and become increasingly important throughout one's career. To lead, manage, and follow successfully, nurses must possess not only knowledge and skills but also a caring and compassionate attitude.

This book results from our continued strong belief in the need for a text that focuses in a distinctive way on nursing leadership and management issues—both today and in the future. We continue to find that we are not alone in this belief. This edition incorporates reviewers from both service and education to ensure that the text conveys important and timely information to users as they focus on the critical roles of leading, managing, and following. In addition, we took seriously the various comments offered by both educators and learners.

CONCEPT AND PRACTICE COMBINED

Innovative in both content and presentation, *Leading and Managing in Nursing* merges theory, research, and practical application in key leadership and management areas from direct care situations to clinical team applications to nurse manager issues on a clinical unit. Our overriding concern in this edition remains to create a text that, while well grounded in theory and concept, presents the content in a way that is real. Wherever possible, we use real-world examples from the continuum of today's healthcare settings to illustrate the concepts. Because each chapter contributor synthesizes the designated focus, you will find no lengthy quotations in these chapters. We have made every effort to make the content as engaging, inviting, and interesting as possible. Reflecting our view of the real world of nursing leadership and management today, the following themes pervade the text:

- Every role within nursing has the basic concern for safe, effective care for the people for whom we exist—our clients and patients.
- The focus of healthcare continues to shift from the hospital to the community at a rapid rate.
- People who use health care and the people who comprise the healthcare workforce are increasingly culturally diverse.
- Today, virtually every professional nurse leads, manages, and follows, regardless of title or position.
- Patient, or person, relationships play a central role in the delivery of nursing and healthcare.
- Communication, collaboration, team-building, and other interpersonal skills form the foundation of effective nursing leadership and management.
- Change continues at a rapid pace in healthcare and society in general.

- Change must derive from evidence-based practices wherever possible and from thoughtful innovation when no or limited evidence exists.
- Healthcare delivery is highly dependent on the effectiveness of nurses across roles and settings.

DIVERSITY OF PERSPECTIVES

Contributors are recruited from diverse settings, roles, and geographic areas, enabling us to offer a broad perspective on the critical elements of nursing leadership and management roles. To help bridge the gap often found between nursing education and nursing practice, some contributors were recruited from academia and others from practice settings. This blend not only contributes to the richness of this text but also conveys a sense of oneness in nursing. The historical "gap" between education and service must become a sense of a continuum, not a chasm.

THE READERS

This book is designed for undergraduate learners in nursing leadership and management courses, including those in BSN-completion courses and second-degree programs. In addition, we know that practicing nurses—who had not anticipated formal leadership and management roles in their careers—use this text to capitalize on their own real-life experiences as a way to develop greater understanding about leading and managing and the important role of following. Numerous examples and The Challenge/The Solution in each chapter provide relevance to the real world of nursing.

ORGANIZATION

We have organized this text around issues that are key to the success of professional nurses in today's constantly changing healthcare environment. The content flows from the core concepts (leading, managing, and following; clinical safety; legal considerations; and culture), to knowing yourself (being an effective follower, self-management, conflicts, and power), to knowing the organization (care delivery strategies, staffing), to using your personal and professional skills (technology, delegation, change, and quality), to preparing for the future (personal role transition, self- and career management, and strategic planning).

Because repetition plays a crucial role in how well learners learn and retain new content, some topics appear in more than one chapter and in more than one section. For example, because *problem* behavior is so disruptive, it is addressed in several chapters that focus on conflict, personal/personnel problems, incivility, and self-management. Rather than referring learners to another portion of the text, the key information is provided within the specific chapter.

We also made an effort to express a variety of different views on some topics, as is true in the real world of nursing. This diversity of views in the real world presents a constant challenge to leaders, managers, and followers, who address the critical tasks of creating positive workplaces so that those who provide direct care thrive and continuously improve the patient experience.

DESIGN

The functional full-color design, still distinctive to this text, is used to emphasize and identify the text's many learning strategies, which are featured to enhance learning. Full-color photographs not only add visual interest but also provide visual reinforcement of concepts, such as body language and the changes occurring in contemporary healthcare settings. Figures graphically expand and clarify concepts and activities described in the text.

LEARNING STRATEGIES

The numerous strategies featured in this text are designed both to stimulate learners' interest and to provide constant reinforcement throughout the learning process. Color is used consistently throughout the text to help the reader identify the various chapter elements described in the following sections.

CHAPTER OPENER ELEMENTS

- Objectives articulate the chapter's learning intent, typically at the application level or higher.
- Terms to know are listed and appear in color type in each chapter.
- The Challenge presents a contemporary nurse's real-world concern related to the chapter's focus. It is designed to allow us to "hear" a real-life situation. The Challenge, at the end of the chapter, ends with a question about what you might do in such a situation.

ELEMENTS WITHIN THE CHAPTERS

- Exercises stimulate learners to reason critically about how to apply concepts to the workplace and other real-world situations. They provide experiential reinforcement of key leading, managing, and following skills. Exercises are highlighted within a full-color box and are numbered sequentially within each chapter to facilitate their use as assignments or activities. Each chapter is numbered separately so that learners can focus on the concepts inherent in a specific area and educators can readily use chapters to fit their own sequence of presenting information.
- Research Perspectives and Literature Perspectives illustrate the relevance and applicability of current scholarship to practice. Theory Boxes provide a brief description of relevant theory and key concepts.
- Numbered boxes contain lists, tools such as forms and worksheets, and other information relevant to the chapter.
- The vivid full-color chapter opener photographs and other photographs throughout the text help convey each chapter's key message. Figures and tables also expand concepts presented to facilitate a greater grasp of important materials.

END-OF-CHAPTER ELEMENTS

- The Solution provides an effective method to handle the real-life situations set forth in The Challenge. It contains the response of The Challenge author and ends with a question about how that solution would fit for you.
- Reflections provide learners with the opportunity to reflect on something they've encountered in practice.
- Best Practices identifies a few key ideas that we can carry forward into our practice to be sure we are doing the best we can in relation to the content area discussed in the chapter.

- Tips offer practical guidelines for learners to follow in applying some aspect of the information presented in each chapter.
- References provide the learner with a list of key sources for further reading on topics found in the chapter.
- Next-Generation NCLEX® case studies are included in select chapters to familiarize students with these new testing items for the NGN exam.

COMPLETE TEACHING AND LEARNING PACKAGE

Student Resources

Learning Resources can also be found online through Evolve (http://evolve.elsevier.com/Yoder-Wise/). These resources provide learners with additional tools for learning and include the following assets:

- NCLEX Review Questions
- Sample Résumés

In addition to the text *Leading and Managing in Nursing*, educator resources are provided online through Evolve (http://evolve.elsevier.com/Yoder-Wise/). These resources are designed to help educators present the material in this text and include the following assets:

- NEW! Additional Next-Generation NCLEX® leadership case studies.
- Updated **PowerPoint Slides,** with lecture notes where applicable, are provided for each chapter.
- An updated **ExamView Test Bank** includes answers and a rationale.
- An updated **TEACH for Nurses** ties together the chapter resources for the most effective class presentations, with sections dedicated to objectives, instructor and student chapter resources, teaching strategies, application activities and answers, an in-class case study discussion, and answers to the text Exercise boxes.

CONTENTS

1

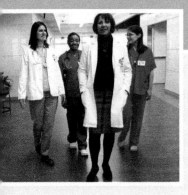

Leading, Managing, and Following

Susan Sportsman and Patricia S. Yoder-Wise

ANTICIPATED LEARNING OUTCOMES

- Demonstrate beginning competence in applying theories tor leadership and management.
- Evaluate leadership and management theories for appropriateness in healthcare today.

- Demonstrate beginning competence in applying concepts of complexity science to healthcare delivery.
- Evaluate the similarities and differences associated with leading, managing, and following.

KEY TERMS

advanced practice registered
   nurse (APRN)
complexity science
Complex Adaptive Science
followership

leadership
leadership theory
management theory
managing
motivation

process of care
quintuple aims
values
vision

THE CHALLENGE

Nursing leaders in long-term care (LTC) facilities face huge challenges in providing safe, compassionate care to their residents. Medically fragile residents, difficulty in maintaining adequate, well-trained staff, and inadequate reimbursement to cover residents' needs all make the lives of the leader—and managers and followers—difficult. As if those problems were not enough, consider the challenge that a newly hired Director of Nursing (DON) in a specific LTC facility faced in the early days of his tenure as Director.

The daughter of a resident who had recently been transferred to the local hospital emergency room because of an untoward change in her condition made an appointment to see the new DON to discuss the negative results of this transfer. As the daughter said, "My poor mother spent 5 hours in the ER and came back here with no change in her condition, except she caught a cold from being in the ER with other sick patients! All the ER doctors did for her was add 3 new drugs to the list of medications she was taking!"

The DON promised to look into the situation and get back to the daughter. As he explored the circumstances of this transfer, he found several systems problems that affected not only this resident but many others in the LTC. Consider the following. The minimum requirement for a physician visit to an LTC facility is a 10- to 30-minute visit

(Continued)

INTRODUCTION

Leadership in nursing has been one of the expectations for new graduates and practicing professionals for decades. It is also one of the recommendations of reports, such as the original *Future of Nursing* report for the Institute of Medicine (now the National Academy of Medicine) (2010). In addition, developing the capacity for leadership is one of the competencies (10-3) identified in the new AACN *Baccalaureate Essentials* (2021).

Why is leadership so important and so expected for all nurses? In part, it is because healthcare is so complex and in part because many people function in illness care, not healthcare. This means that they seek care only when ill and, thus, often have great needs when they interact with healthcare professionals. No matter what we learn (or learned) in school about nursing or leadership, we quickly learn that it isn't enough because nursing and healthcare are complex and change occurs rapidly. The intensity of change between December 2019 and the beginning of 2022 was dramatic and, in some ways, revolutionized the way in which care was delivered and in which every discipline practiced.

Consider the profession of nursing in the context of leadership as a spider web. Every strand is important by itself. It is holding something up or connecting one element to the next. This is similar to the key concepts that underpin leadership. Each is important by itself and connects one element to another. Without each of the elements, some part of the web is insufficient. Yes, we can get by as leaders without certain elements. The questions are why would we want to limit ourselves

and what damage are we doing by not having a full array of what is needed? Just as a spider repeats a pattern in areas where greater strength is needed, so too does nursing leadership. We are repetitive—and deliberately so. That repetitive process is designed to reinforce the leadership process where the greatest challenges occur. Additionally, when a spider web is touched in one spot, the whole web responds. The resilience of the web, unless it is forcefully attacked and damaged, allows it to withstand wind and remain intact to accomplish its mission. Fig. 1.1 illustrates how to consider the interaction of the various concepts affecting nursing leadership.

Nursing is a complex profession in a complex system of healthcare. Nursing roles vary based on setting type and legal expectations from the state board of nursing

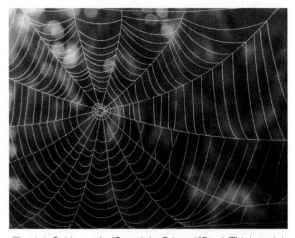

Fig. 1.1 Spider web. (Copyright © jamsi/iStock/Thinkstock.)

and related entities, such as the state department that regulates various aspects of care delivery. Add to those factors professional standards, expected competencies, and future predictions about the potential impact of changes in healthcare delivery on the role of nurses. Being a nurse is an ever-changing, highly challenging responsibility. Why, then, would we want to add specific roles such as leader or manager to such a complex condition? The answer is quite simple—because we work in teams. Whenever that occurs, someone is designated, or emerges, as the leader of the group. Every group has some management functions that must be well executed to be meaningful. If people are not willing to follow in an accountable manner, the team effort is for naught.

In times of chaos, as well as in less hectic environments, nurses often fulfill the roles of leader, manager, and follower on a daily basis. Sometimes, the change occurs without thinking about what role is being enacted at a given time. Leading, managing, and following are not institutionally role-bound concepts. The nurse must lead, manage, and follow within any nursing role, from direct care nurse to chief executive nurse, and do so with fluidity among those roles.

This chapter begins the framing of your professional journey in leading, managing, and following. The chapters that follow add to your development as a professional nurse. Various perspectives on the concepts of leadership, management, and followership are presented. In the end, nurses with leadership, management, and followership abilities will make good clinical decisions; consider the organizational and societal context in decisions; and act as advocates for individuals, families, and groups receiving care.

THE CONTEXT OF LEADING, MANAGING, AND FOLLOWING IN HEALTHCARE

Healthcare occurs almost everywhere. Obviously, it occurs in hospitals, clinics, private practice offices, LTC facilities, schools, and public health services. Less obvious, but equally important, we find businesses that have in-house health services available and large companies (such as CVS and Walmart) offering health services to the public. In part, many of these services first existed to protect the public's health and to address major illnesses—both chronic and acute. Additionally, over the last 30-plus years, the concern about the cost of healthcare at a national level has escalated, resulting in various non-healthcare companies providing ambulatory healthcare services.

In 2008, Berwick and his colleagues developed the Triple Aim as a framework for delivering high-value healthcare in the United States. The Triple Aim was based on three overarching goals: (1) improving the individual experience of care, (2) improving the health of populations, and (3) reducing the per capita cost of healthcare. Achieving the second and third goals contributed to the achievement of the first (Institute for Healthcare Improvement [IHI], 2022). Unfortunately, despite the goals of the Triple Aim initiative, healthcare providers in all disciplines continued to experience significant burnout while dealing with complexity, which reduced the quality of care they provided. Caregiver burnout also led to a shortage of caregivers as experienced providers left their professions.

To address these negative issues, a fourth dimension was added to the Aims (Fig. 1.2) to improve the work life of healthcare providers in all disciplines (Arnetz et al., 2020). As important as the fourth Aim has been, if we think about the work around the Magnet Recognition Program™, we can readily see that the concern about the workplace has been a point for decades (https://www.nursingworld.org/organizational-programs/magnet/magnet-model/).

Since 2009, the healthcare environment has become even more complex. Although the quintuple aims and other quality initiatives have provided leaders with tools

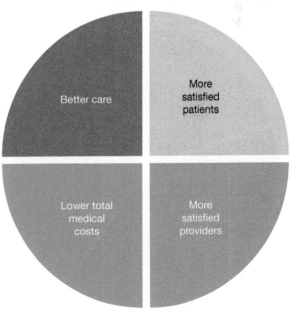

Fig. 1.2 Quadruple Aim.

to improve the patient–provider experience, the healthcare system continues to change from the traditional industrial models of the previous century. The culture in most healthcare organizations today is more ethnically diverse, has an expansive educational chasm (from non–high school graduates to doctorally prepared clinicians), includes multiple generations of workers with varying values and expectations of the workplace, involves extensive use of technology to support all aspects of the organization, and challenges workers and patients with antibiotic-resistant microorganisms and emerging diseases. Certainly, the COVID-19 pandemic beginning in early 2020 has stressed the healthcare system in ways unseen in the last 100 years.

The framework was modified again in 2022 to emphasize the importance of health equity in the overall approach to health care improvement. The authors of the fifth element (Mundy, Cooper, & Mate, 2022) suggest that quality improvement without addressing health equity might not be very satisfactory because disparities remain. As with many other efforts making explicit some aspect of care helps us focus on that aspect in a way that was not present before and may even potentiate other elements in a model. The interaction of these five elements forms a model for improving care that is sustainable.

TABLE 1.1	**Definitions and Interrelatedness of VUCA**
Element	**Definition**
Volatility	Speed of change and fluctuation
Uncertainty	Environment doesn't allow prediction, even through statistics
Complexity	Increased number and variety of interrelated factors
Ambiguity	Difficulty in interpreting situations or inability to draw clear conclusions

Adapted from Kraaijenbrink, J. (2019). Is the world really more VUCA than ever? *Forbes.* January 4, 2019. Retrieved from https://www.forbes.com/sites/jeroenkraaijenbrink/2019/01/04/is-the-world-really-more-vuca-than-ever/?sh=1d159ebb1a64.

Using Complex Adaptive Science to Understand Health Care Today

We have all said, "Wow! I had a CRAZY day!" Often, this frustration comes from dealing with multiple interrelated factors—some seen and some unseen—and dealing with multiple people with multiple perspectives who all have a part to play in resolving the issue. Today, the business industry calls this type of environment or experience *VUCA*—Volatile, Unexpected (or, more commonly, Uncertainty), Complex, and Ambiguous, which implies that there is nothing that we can do to respond to this type of situation (Kraaijenbrink, 2019). Table 1.1 depicts the definitions and interrelatedness of these four concepts:

Although VUCA environments are intimidating, Complex Adaptive Science or Complexity theory, an approach to understanding complex systems, can help us to develop strategies to thrive in VUCA environments. Complex Adaptive Science helps us to understand how complex systems such as healthcare adapt depending on multiple factors within the organization and in the broader environment. The term *complexity* does not refer to the complexity of the decision to be made or to the work environment specifically. Rather, it refers to the way systems adapt and function—where co-creation of ideas and actions unfold in a nonprescriptive manner. Complex Adaptive Science promotes the idea that the world is full of patterns that interact and adapt through relationships. These interactive patterns may be missed when one focuses solely on a single part of a situation. For example, focusing on problems associated with quality care cannot be solved unless staffing patterns, expertise of staff, and the processes of care are also considered.

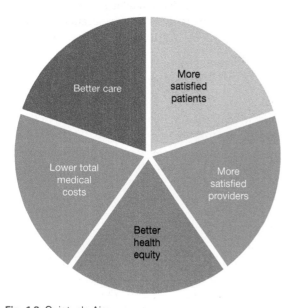

Fig. 1.3 Quintuple Aim.

Stated in nursing terms, nurses care for individual patients who each present a unique challenge. With experience, nurses recognize that patterns of patient behaviors emerge. They learn that certain nursing actions lead to effectively managing pain, engaging family members in end-of-life planning discussions, and addressing a host of other issues. Most healthcare team members are focused on problems and predictable solutions that appear to be linear in nature. However, if we look more deeply at both disease processes and healthcare, we realize that both are an interconnected web of processes and services. Thus, a linear solution may not be feasible, and solutions require adaptations that account for a multitude of factors (Hodiamont et al. 2019).

The complexity of the healthcare system results in chronic clinical and delivery problems, information imbalance (sometimes too much, sometimes not enough), physically and emotionally intense work with little time for reflection (the COVID-19 pandemic is an extreme example of this), increased consumer and regulatory demands, and fatigue from too many cues and reminders!

The goal in a complex adaptive healthcare system when responding to patient and organizational problems is to examine a problem through multiple lenses. A leader in these situations understands that systems are ecological—they restore themselves—and that change can be generated equally from the bottom up, from the top down, or both. Adaptive leaders should recognize that while they may influence overall outcomes, leadership control is neither possible nor desirable.

In these complex environments, information is not a commodity to be controlled by those in charge. Instead, it is intended to be shared with and interpreted by a wide audience—multiple staff, patients, and families—to provide varying interpretations of the same scenario. This strategy results in diverse thinking, which leads to creative problem solving in which multiple individuals may be actively engaged.

Because of this need to use communication widely, relationship building is a central factor in complex adaptive leadership. Poor team communication has been linked to preventable medical errors, high staff turnover rates, and low morale. On the other hand, team members who communicate effectively with each other and feel that their voices are heard are likely to provide safe, high-quality care, be active team members, and stay with the organization over time.

One of the early references regarding the use of Complex Adaptive Science in leading and managing identified four principles that leaders and managers should consider:

1. Leaders must recognize that employees will self-manage into work groups. Rather than exerting control, effective leaders or managers should stimulate creative problem solving.
2. Followers require context to participate effectively in complex circumstances. Understanding the **vision** for the objective to be accomplished allows followers to explore and develop solutions to complex problems preventing the objective from being accomplished.
3. The changing environment requires adaptation. Encouraging this adaptation is where the leader and/or manager can have the most impact.
4. Leaders must address sources of tension and contradiction. Disagreement and tension may be expected as the result of creative problem solving by the group. However, the leader or manager should address this tension so that new alliances may be created that contribute to high-quality outcomes (Haupt, 2003).

Other principles drawn from complexity theory that provide direction for leaders, managers, and followers include the ability to (Anderson & Johnson, 1997):

1. *Identify the "Big Picture," to envision the context of the work beyond the immediate tasks.* The nurse who looks past an individual assignment and comprehends the needs of all units of the hospital, who can focus on the needs of all residents in a long-term care facility, or who can think through the complications of urban emergency department overcrowding is seeing the big picture.
2. *Recognize the dynamic, complex, and interdependent nature of systems*: All things are connected. Patients are connected to families and friends. Together, they are connected to communities and cultures. Communities and cultures make up the fabric of society. The cost of healthcare is linked to local economies, and local businesses are connected to global industries. Identifying and understanding these relationships helps solve problems with full recognition that small decisions can have a large impact.
3. *Use measurable and non-measurable data systems*: We all have a tendency to "see" only what we can measure. Quantitative data are important. On the other hand, if we consider only numbers (e.g., number of patients seen), we might miss a perspective such as lack of engagement in the workplace.

Complex environments make leading, managing, and following increasingly challenging in today's healthcare. The leader must address the needs of the diverse community. Language variations, cultural barriers, and overused electronic communication create opportunities for misunderstanding that could contribute to errors. Followers, managers, and leaders of different generations and values must work together to provide quality care. Although the healthcare environment has many opportunities for making huge strides in improving the quality, what do nurse leaders, managers, and followers need to take advantage of these opportunities?

LEADING, MANAGING, AND FOLLOWING THEORIES

The way nurses lead, manage, and follow has changed over time. Formerly, nurses took direction exclusively from physicians or senior nurses, such as "head" or "charge" nurses. These formal roles still exist in some places; however, the expectation has shifted from a top-down, order-giving model to one in which shared decision-making with collaborative action is the norm. As knowledge has expanded and the array of treatment interventions available to patients has grown, care delivery has moved far beyond what a command-and-control, top-down structure can accommodate in a traditional hierarchical organization.

The theoretical basis for understanding leading, managing, and following originates from multiple disciplines. Early researchers in organization science noted the differences in the ways some organizations operated and suggested that this was due to the leader(s) characteristics or traits. The initial focus of leadership research was on traits of individual leaders rather than characteristics or functioning of the organization. Studies of individual leaders resulted in awareness that some individuals possessed traits that seemed to produce better organizational outcomes. Trait theory, developed from these studies, is still examined as a leadership factor today, even though it holds less influence than some other theories.

LITERATURE PERSPECTIVE

Resource: Begun, J.W., & Jiang, J. (2020). Health care management during COVID-19: Insights from complexity science. Innovation in care delivery. *New England Journal of Medicine Catalyst.* October 9, 2020. https://catalyst.nejm.org/doi/full/10.1056/CAT.20.0541. Accessed, 2021.

A review of experiences of six healthcare organizations during the COVID-19 pandemic was done based on principles from Complexity Adaptive Science. Perhaps no recent experience has demonstrated the unpredictability of the environment as much as the COVID pandemic has. The authors chose six healthcare organizations: (1) a component of a healthcare system, the Department of Surgery at the University of California, San Francisco; (2) an individual hospital, Bichard-Claude Bernard Hospital; (3) healthcare systems, Geisinger Health System, New York City H+H, and Community HealthCare System; and (4) state-wide aggregates of hospitals and a health system (Arizona Surge Line). This review found that the leadership in these organizations had used the following Complex Adaptive Science principles:
1. Use simple rules with a minimum of specification.
2. Build connections and encourage collaboration.
3. Emphasize extensive communication, particularly real-time information.
4. Encourage various views in problem solving.
5. Prepare for surprises.
6. Expect innovation, not damage-mitigation.

Implications for Practice
The consistent mantra of these organizations was "Communicate, Collaborate, and Innovate." This mantra can provide direction for all leaders, managers, and followers to thrive in complex environments.

Researchers in the 1950s and 1960s observed that a leader could be successful in one environment yet not necessarily in another. Situations or activities in the work environment were also found to influence the outcomes. When the setting required reproducible and repetitive tasks, a charismatic leader may be less effective than in an unpredictable or unstructured situation in which the tasks required on-the-spot innovation. Study of the organizational variables resulted in the development of additional theories, including situational/contingency theories that examine variables in the internal and external environments, including the nature of the work itself, worker behavior (individual or group), the predictability or unpredictability of work, and the risks associated with the work. In addition, management theories that address planning, organizing, directing, and controlling aspects of work design were often considered leadership theories. The focus of these theories continued to evolve and often are combined with other theories to guide professionals into evidence-based organizational practices.

Theories that explain the ways in which people are motivated have also been considered as part of leadership theories. These include Maslow's Hierarchy of Needs, Herzberg's Two-Factor Theory, Vroom's Expectancy Theory, and Alderfer's ERG Theory (Existence, Relatedness, and Growth). Attempts at developing theories focusing on followers, such as Leader-Member (LMX), have even been proposed.

Terms such as *leadership theory*, *transformational leadership*, *servant leadership*, *authentic leadership*, *management theory*, and *motivational theory* are interrelated, making it difficult to categorize them in a mutually exclusive manner. In addition, there are theories in other domains that are helpful to leaders, managers, and followers. Some of these theories, such as change, conflict, and economics, individual and group interaction, communication, and social networking, are addressed later in this book.

The Theory Box is organized as an overview of leadership theories, highlighting sets of theoretical works commonly used to demonstrate the variety, approach, and constant evolution of theory development in organizational studies. The complex factors associated with clinical care and organizational functioning explain why no single theory fully addresses the totality of leading, managing, and following.

EXERCISE 1.2 Ponder the leadership theories presented here. Does one seem to make more sense to you than another? Consider, for example, what you were doing the last time you were in the clinical area. Does one theory suggest that you were using it as you enacted your role? Identify one way you can incorporate a leadership theoretical perspective into a daily clinical routine.

THEORY BOX

Leadership Theories

Theory/Contributor	Key Idea	Application to Practice
Trait Theories		
Trait theories were first studied from 1900 to 1950. These theories are sometimes referred to as the Great Man theories, from Aristotle's philosophy extolling the virtue of being "born" with leadership traits. Stogdill (1948) is usually credited as the pioneer in this school of thought.	Leaders have a certain set of physical and emotional characteristics that are crucial for inspiring others toward a common goal. Some theorists believe that traits are innate and cannot be learned; others believe that leadership traits can be developed in each individual.	Self-awareness of traits is useful in self-development (e.g., developing assertiveness) and in seeking employment that matches traits (drive, motivation, integrity, confidence, cognitive ability, and task knowledge).

(Continued)

THEORY BOX — cont'd

Style Theories

Sometimes referred to as *group and exchange* theories of leadership, style theories were derived in the mid-1950s because of the limitations of trait theory. The key contributors to this renowned research were Shartle (1956), Stogdill (1963), and Likert (1987).

Style theories focus on what leaders do in relational and contextual terms. The achievement of satisfactory performance measures requires supervisors to pursue effective relationships with their followers while comprehending the factors in the work environment that influence outcomes.

To understand "style," leaders need to obtain feedback from followers, superiors, and peers, such as through the Managerial Grid Instrument developed by Blake and Mouton (1985). Employee-centered leaders tend to be the leaders most able to achieve effective work environments and productivity.

Situational-Contingency Theories

The situational-contingency theorists emerged in the 1960s through the mid-1970s. These theorists believed that leadership effectiveness depends on the relationship among (1) the leader's task at hand, (2) the leader's interpersonal skills, and (3) the favorableness of the work situation. Examples of theory development with this expanded perspective include Fiedler's (1967) Contingency Model, Vroom and Yetton's (1973) Normative Decision-Making Model, and House and Mitchell's (1974) Path-Goal theory.

Three factors are critical: (1) the degree of trust and respect between and among leaders and followers, (2) the task structure denoting the clarity of goals and the complexity of problems faced, and (3) the position power in terms of where the leader was able to reward followers and exert influence. Consequently, leaders were viewed as able to adapt their style according to the presenting situation. The Vroom-Yetton model was a problem-solving approach to leadership. Path-Goal theory recognized two contingent variables: (1) the personal characteristics of followers and (2) environmental demands. On the basis of these factors, the leader sets forth clear expectations, eliminates obstacles to goal achievements, motivates and rewards staff, and increases opportunities for follower satisfaction based on effective job performance.

The most important implications for leaders are that these theories consider the challenge of a situation and encourage an adaptive leadership style to complement the issue being faced. In other words, nurses must assess each situation and determine appropriate action based on the people involved.

Transformational Theories

Transformational theories arose late in the past century when globalization and other factors caused organizations to fundamentally reestablish themselves. Many of these attempts were failures, but great attention was given to those leaders who effectively transformed structures, human resources, and profitability balanced with quality. Bass (1990), Bennis and Nanus (2007), and Tichy and Devanna (1997) are commonly associated with the study of transformational theory.

Transformational leadership refers to a process whereby the leader attends to the needs and motives of followers so that the interaction raises each to high levels of motivation and morality. The leader is a role model who inspires followers through displayed optimism, provides intellectual stimulation, and encourages follower creativity.

Transformed organizations are responsive to customer needs, are morally and ethically intact, promote employee development, and encourage self-management. Nurse leaders with transformational characteristics experiment with systems redesign, empower staff, create enthusiasm for practice, and promote scholarship of practice at patient side.

THEORY BOX—cont'd

Hierarchy of Needs

Maslow is credited with developing a theory of motivation, first published in 1943.

People are motivated by a hierarchy of human needs, beginning with physiologic needs and then progressing to safety, social, esteem, and self-actualizing needs. In this theory, when the need for food, water, air, and other life-sustaining elements is met, the human spirit reaches out to achieve affiliation with others, which promotes the development of self-esteem, competence, achievement, and creativity. Lower-level needs drive behavior before higher-level needs can be addressed.

When this theory is applied to staff, leaders must be aware that the need for safety and security will override the opportunity to be creative and inventive, such as in promoting job change.

Two-Factor Theory

Herzberg (1991) is credited with developing a two-factor theory of motivation, first published in 1968.

Hygiene factors, such as working conditions, salary, status, and security, motivate workers by meeting safety and security needs and avoiding job dissatisfaction. Motivator factors, such as achievement, recognition, and the satisfaction of the work itself, promote job enrichment by creating job satisfaction.

Organizations need both hygiene and motivator factors to recruit and retain staff. Hygiene factors do not create job satisfaction; they simply must be in place for work to be accomplished. If not, these factors will only serve to dissatisfy staff. Transformational leaders use motivator factors liberally to inspire work performance.

Expectancy Theory

Vroom (1994) is credited with developing the expectancy theory of motivation.

Individuals' perceived needs influence their behavior. In the work setting, this motivated behavior is increased if a person perceives a positive relationship between effort and performance. Motivated behavior is further increased if a positive relationship exists between good performance and outcomes or rewards, particularly when these are valued.

Expectancy is the perceived probability of satisfying a particular need based on experience. Therefore, nurses in leadership roles need to provide specific feedback about positive performance.

In 1969, using empirical research on employee motivation, Clayton Alderfer made adaptations to Maslow's Hierarchy of Needs, collapsing the 5 levels of motivational needs into three core (ERG) needs: (1) existence (basic needs), (2) relatedness needs (social and external esteem), and (3) growth (internal esteem and self-actualization).

Unlike Maslow's theory, ERG needs are not progressive. (For example, with sufficient internal esteem, one may be motivated even if the more basic needs are not met.) Focusing on only one need at a time prevents developing motivational strategies that address the whole person.

Leaders must provide incentives that address the three core needs.

(Continued)

THEORY BOX —cont'd

The Five Practices of Exemplary Leadership, by Kouzes and Posner (2011), is a functional leadership model, which was based on research that asked ordinary people to describe extraordinary leadership experiences when they were at their personal best in leading others. The goal of this research was to find patterns of success.

The patterns Kouzes and Posner found included (1) Model the way, (2) Inspire a shared vision, (3) Challenge the process, (4) Enable others to act, and (5) Encourage the heart.

The authors note that leadership is learned. We must first lead ourselves as a precursor to making a difference as a leader.

The Three Levels of Leadership, by Scouller (2011), is an example of an integrated psychological leadership model that focuses on behaviors of the leader while addressing the leader's inner psychological well-being.

The three domains of leadership in this model are (1) managing self in order to lead, (2) leading the team, and (3) addressing the external environment. This model is illustrated by three overlapping circles representing the leadership domains. The innermost circle, Managing Self Skills, includes vision, integrity, self-awareness, strong commitment, management of time and change, openness to new ideas and learning, technical competencies, social and emotional competencies, and work-life balance. The middle circle of the model involves team building. The relevant skills include developing individuals within the team/organization, executing vision by coaching, mentoring, delegating, placing the right person in the right job, and helping others see their role in the vision. The outermost circle depicts external environment skills. Demonstrating these skills requires being in touch with the external environment, including new plans, programs, and initiatives; anticipating, leading, and adapting to change; networking; and contributing to the good of the society.

The three levels of leadership provide a model for leadership development.

COMPARISON OF LEADING, MANAGING, AND FOLLOWING IN HEALTHCARE

Because of the fluidity with which nurses, regardless of their formal role, move between leading, managing, and following, it may be helpful to distinguish among these areas of competence.

Leadership

Leadership can be defined as the use of individual traits and abilities in relationship with others. The ability to interpret (often rapidly) the environment/context in which a situation is emerging and enter that situation without the use of a predesigned plan is also a leadership skill. Leadership is required when the unknown presents itself, necessitating the use of principles to improve solutions and help others cope, thrive, and function in the situation. In short, leaders tend to influence by inspiring and enabling through advice and counsel (Bradt, 2020).

Gardner's Tasks of Leadership

Gardner (1990) described tasks of leadership in his seminal book, *On Leadership*. These tasks are still applicable today. They include envisioning goals, affirming values, motivating, managing, achieving workable unity, developing trust, explaining, serving as a symbol, representing the group, and renewing. Table 1.2 presents these tasks to demonstrate that leading, managing, and following are relevant for nurses who hold clinical positions, formal management positions, and executive leadership positions. Note that each role represents the interest of the organization, although the focus of attention is different.

Management

Management requires the ability to determine routines and practices that offer structure and stability to others. The manager's focus is to organize, coordinate, and tell others what to do. (Bradt, 2020). The ability to manage is very much aligned with how an organization structures

TABLE 1.2 Gardner's Tasks of Leading/Managing Applied to Practice, Management, and Executive Positions

	BEHAVIORS		
Gardner's Task	Clinical Position	Management Position	Executive Position
Envisioning goals	Visioning patient outcomes for single patient/families; assisting patients in formulating their vision of future well-being	Creating a vision of how systems support patient care objectives, assisting staff in formulating their professional vision of clinical and organizational performance	Visioning community health and organizational outcomes for aggregates of patient populations to which the organization can respond
Affirming values	Assisting the patient/family to articulate personal values in relation to health problems and to appreciate how these values are reflected in health state	Assisting the staff in interpreting organizational values and strengthening staff members' personal values to more closely align with those of the organization	Assisting other organizational leaders in the expression of community and organizational values; interpreting values to the community and staff
Motivating	Relating to and inspiring patients/families to achieve their vision	Relating to and inspiring staff to achieve the mission of the organization and the vision associated with organizational enhancement	Relating to and inspiring management, staff, and community leaders to achieve desired levels of health and well-being and appropriate use of clinical services
Managing	Executing established procedures while considering appropriateness for the individual patient/family	Assisting the staff with planning, priority setting, and decision-making; ensuring that systems work to enhance the staff's ability to meet patient care needs and the objectives of the organization	Assisting other executives and corporate leaders with planning, priority setting, and decision-making; ensuring that human and material resources are available to meet health needs
Achieving workable unity	Assisting patients/families to achieve an optimal, yet realistic, health state and quality of life	Collaborating with staff to achieve optimal team functioning to maximize organizational functioning	Guiding multidisciplinary leaders to achieve optimal organizational functioning to benefit patient care delivery
Developing trust	Maintaining honest, open communication with patients and families; being honest in role performance	Sharing organizational information openly; being honest in role performance	Representing nursing and executive views openly and honestly; being honest in role performance
Explaining	Teaching and interpreting information to promote patient/family functioning and well-being	Providing information to promote organizational functioning and enhanced services	Communicating organizational information to other leaders within the organization and community

Continued

TABLE 1.2 Gardner's Tasks of Leading/Managing Applied to Practice, Management, and Executive Positions—cont'd

	BEHAVIORS		
Gardner's Task	**Clinical Position**	**Management Position**	**Executive Position**
Serving as a symbol	Representing the nursing profession and the values and beliefs of the organization to patients/families	Representing the values and beliefs of the nursing unit to staff, other departments, professional organizations, and the community at large	Representing the values and beliefs of the organization and patient care services to internal and external constituents
Representing the group	Representing nursing and the unit on committees, shared governance councils, and other groups within the organization	Representing nursing on assigned boards, councils, and committees, both internal and external to the organization	Representing the organization and patient care services on assigned boards, councils, committees, and task forces, both internal and external to the organization
Renewing	Providing self-care to maximize one's ability to function as a healthcare team member	Providing self-care to maximize one's ability to function as both a leader and member of the healthcare team	Providing self-care to maximize one's ability to care for patients, families, staff, and the organization served

its key systems and processes to deliver services. In the context of healthcare, a care delivery system is composed of multiple processes necessary to achieve effective patient care. A process of care specifies the desired sequence of steps to achieve clinical standardization, safety, and outcomes. Effective management depends on knowing, adhering to, and improving processes for efficiency and effectiveness. Each person must respect and act on a prescribed role in a process of care. Data-driven outcome measurements provide feedback on the process. Feedback reports provide a basis for improvement programs, which may include coaching and mentoring employees. Rewards for individual and team effectiveness reinforce desired behaviors. Box 1.1 lists Bleich's tasks of management that are essential for effective functioning.

New nurses typically think of management as it relates to either direct patient care or nursing unit management.

You may also be involved in project management. Because nurses are often the end users in the rollout of new care processes, it is important that they are involved in the planning and implementation as well. An example of a situation in which nurses can contribute greatly to overall project success is planning for implementation of a new electronic health record.

BOX 1.1 Bleich's Tasks of Management

1. Identify systems and processes that require responsibility and accountability and specify who owns the process.
2. Verify minimum and optimum standards/specifications and identify roles and individuals responsible to adhere to them.
3. Validate the knowledge, skills, and abilities of available staff engaged in the process; capitalize on strengths; and strengthen areas in need of development.
4. Devise and communicate a comprehensive big-picture plan for the division of work, honoring the complexity and variety of assignments made at an individual level.
5. Eliminate barriers/obstacles to work effectiveness.
6. Measure the equity of workload and use data to support judgments about efficiency and effectiveness.
7. Offer rewards and recognition to individuals and teams.
8. Recommend ways to improve systems and processes.
9. Use a social network to engage others in decision-making and for feedback, when appropriate or relevant.

EXERCISE 1.3 The tasks of management are designed to enact Gardner's tasks of leadership. For example, although the leader may create a culture of trust, the manager offers rewards that reinforce that value. Consider an environment in which you currently work (or worked in the past). Did the roles of a leader and manager illustrate Gardner's tasks? Why or why not? Even if the tasks of the leader(s) and the manager(s) are different, do their behaviors represent a common vision? Why or why not?

Following

Following is a term that is often misinterpreted. Images associated with followers portray passive, uninspired workers waiting for direction. Although that may be accurate for some organizations, following in a high-functioning team is an active, creative role that influences leaders and managers. A healthy definition of *followership* is that each group member contributes optimally in tandem with other group members to achieve clinical or organizational outcomes. All team members are expected to fully participate, using their knowledge, skills, and experience to help deal with complex clinical and organizational issues. In essence, maximal functioning as a team member exemplifies followership. Each person acts together team members with purpose and in a rhythm that addresses the aim at hand. Traits of followers include acting synergistically with others, being enthusiastic and responsible, speaking and acting with principles and integrity, adding value to the work being accomplished, and questioning decisions and directions that are not congruent with the purpose or values of the group. The effective follower is willing to be led, to share time and talents, to create and innovate solutions, to take direction from the manager, and to role model confidence and professionalism. Simultaneously, followers must perform their assigned structured duties, which require critical thinking and decision-making. For example, nurses may demonstrate followership by serving on committees. Even simple activities, such as completing readings and reviewing minutes from previous meetings, are essential for an organization's success. Bleich's tasks associated with followership can be found in Box 1.2

> **BOX 1.2 Bleich's Tasks of Followership**
>
> 1. Demonstrate individual accountability while working within the context of organizational systems and processes; do not alter the process for personal gain or shortcuts.
> 2. Honor and implement care to the standards and specifications required for safe and acceptable care/service.
> 3. Offer knowledge, skills, and abilities to accomplish the task at hand.
> 4. Collaborate with leaders and managers; avoid passive-aggressive or nonassertive responses to work assignment.
> 5. Include evidence-based feedback as part of daily work activities as a self-guide to efficiency and effectiveness and to contribute to outcome measurement.
> 6. Demonstrate accountability to the team effort.
> 7. Take reasonable risks as an antidote for fearing change or unknown circumstances.
> 8. Evaluate the efficiency and effectiveness of systems and processes that affect outcomes of care/service, and advocate for well-designed work.
> 9. Give and receive feedback to others to promote a nurturing and generative culture.

FUTURE IMPLICATIONS

Nurses face the unknown every day. New diseases emerge. For example, the COVID-19 pandemic in 2020 has demonstrated the impact of new disease in ways that healthcare has not been required to address on such a large scale in 100 years. On a more local level, natural disasters such as hurricanes and tornadoes create havoc, leaving many people in need of immediate healthcare and, often, long-term follow-up as a variety of health determinants are highlighted. Even in our individual practice areas, policies and procedures must be adapted to patients' physical and emotional challenges. Each of these situations—and many others like them—requires nurses to step into the unknown, using principles of leadership, management, and followership.

Leadership in uncertain times has been studied in the applied psychology discipline. A review of the literature found that women leaders tend to be preferred over men in crisis situations. Deeper analysis suggests that this preference is related to women's desire to help others as well as the capacity to bounce back from failure more pragmatically than men. Of course, the behavior of men and women are guided by role stereotypes; the behaviors

> **EXERCISE 1.4** Using the definitions for leading, managing, and following noted previously, observe how work is organized in a clinical unit. What situations occurred that could not be predicted? What work followed a routine nature or was driven by protocol? Identify an activity that was driven by principles rather than by formal evidence. Identify an activity that was driven by evidence-based practice or evidence-based organizational practice. Then, notice team functioning. Who led? Who managed? Who followed? Did this happen seamlessly or were there times when there was tension in efforts? Did the roles change depending on the situation? If so, in what way?

RESEARCH PERSPECTIVE

Resource: Sergent, K., & Stajkovic, A. (2020). Women's leadership is associated with fewer deaths during COVID-19 crisis: Quantitative and qualitative analysis of United States governors. *Journal of Applied Psychology, 105*(8), 771–183.

Overview

A review of leadership research in the discipline of Applied Psychology suggests that female leaders tend to be preferred over men during uncertain times. Male leaders tend to focus on solving problems—which, in a stable environment, is appropriate. In contrast, women leaders tend to rely on creativity, intuition, and improvisation, which seems particularly useful to thrive in complex environments. Women are also more likely to communicate widely across their scope of influence, which fosters collaboration among all levels of followers. Such collaboration is consistent with a democratic leadership style, which tends to stimulate diverse ideas, brainstorming, and consensus building.

Sergent and Stajkovic (2020) tested the hypothesis that behaviors of women leaders in time of crisis were more effective that those chosen by men. The researchers implemented a study with both qualitative and quantitative approaches during the 2020 COVID-19 crisis. A total of 251 briefings by the state governors of 38 states regarding the COVID-19 pandemic were analyzed using the Linguistic Inquiry and Word Count software, which included a "feelings" dictionary. The results of the analysis of the briefings of male and female governors were compared. In addition, the number of COVID-19 deaths in each state from January 21 to May 5, 2020 were compared by the gender of the governor.

The results of the analyses of the briefings found that women showed more empathy, focusing on the feelings of others. Quantitatively, those states in which a woman was a governor had a lower COVID-19 death rate during the study period.

Implications for Practice

The researchers suggested that valuing different leadership voices and building a culture of inclusion is important to prepare leaders.

---

required by a crisis can be implemented by any leader who makes an effort to adjust one's behaviors in response to the circumstances (Sergent & Stajkovic, 2020).

Leaders, managers, and followers in healthcare must address the challenges facing our country and provision of care. Access to care, particularly for minority populations, the elderly, and those living in rural areas, continues to be a significant concern. This lack of access is accentuated by the uncertainty regarding the availability of healthcare coverage and the recognition of the health disparities in particular communities. Coupled with these challenges are great opportunities for improving healthcare. Changes in technology and increased innovation, such as the rapid development of vaccines for COVID-19, tell us that all is not lost. With effective leadership, management, and followership, we will be able to meet the challenges.

CONCLUSION

Developing knowledge and skills in leading, managing, and following prepares professional nurses to meet the challenges arising today *and* tomorrow. A more effective and compassionate healthcare system requires well prepared leaders, managers, and followers. Nurses who are competent in enacting each of these roles as opportunities arise can add much to the ongoing improvement of patient care.

Healthcare today is an amalgamation of both traditional and dynamic structures. New theories of leadership will emerge to capture the complexity and globalization of healthcare and changing communication patterns through the influence of the Internet and social media. Professional nurses must be prepared to practice within a system that is both predictable and unpredictable.

Concepts of teamwork and collaborative decision-making are critical in a healthcare environment that is dynamic and ever changing. A nurse has great potential to shape those changes. We do not have to have titles to be leaders; we just have to be living human beings willing to execute our potential. In other words, the synchrony of leading, managing, and following is within each of us.

The collective behaviors that reflect leading, managing, and following enhance each other. All interdisciplinary healthcare providers, including professional nurses, experience situations each day in which they must lead, manage, and follow. Some institutional formal positions, such as nurse manager or charge nurse, require an advanced set of attributes and know-how to establish organizational goals and objectives, oversee human resources, provide staff with performance feedback, facilitate change, and manage conflict to meet patient care and organizational requirements.

THE SOLUTION

Complexity science served as the basis for addressing concerns in this LTC setting. A full-time advanced practice registered nurse (APRN) was employed in the nursing home to work with nursing staff about the importance of recognizing a change in condition, completing an assessment, and obtaining treatment in the nursing home, rather than transferring to the hospital.

Embedding a full-time APRN in the facility resulted in positive outcomes for the residents. The APRN developed relationships with nearly all nursing home staff, no matter their role, and served as an expert clinician and resource. In addition, she volunteered to be on call 24/7 and provided phone support during nonworking hours.

The nursing home was primarily staffed with licensed practical nurses and certified nurse assistants, as is typical of most nursing homes. Education was central to enhancing the clinical skills and decision-making of the nursing staff. Both formal and roving ongoing education was provided as new staff members were hired and new clinical challenges arose. Role modeling by the APRN enhanced clinical reasoning skills when a resident exhibited a condition change. Through early illness recognition, the resident could be treated in a proactive manner at the LTC facility rather than waiting until a significant physical decline occurred that warranted a transfer to the hospital.

Another key feature in the intervention was the use of the Interventions to Reduce Acute Care Transfers (INTERACT) tools. These standardized tools are designed to improve recognition and communication about changes in resident condition. The two main tools used were (1) Stop and Watch and (2) Situation, Background, Assessment, and Recommendation, or SBAR. (Note: The acronym SBAR is slightly different in the INTERACT model.) The Stop and Watch tool is used to report a subtle change in condition. Any person, including those from dietary, housekeeping, and family members, could fill out a Stop and Watch to alert the nurse of a subtle change in resident condition. This allowed those with the most frequent resident interaction to have a means of communicating what might seem a "bit off" or "different" in a resident. The SBAR tool provided a means for documentation of condition change as well as guiding critical thinking about a change in status. Nurses completed the SBAR before contacting a provider. Staff reported feeling more confident and empowered in their job performance.

Management of polypharmacy and reduction of antipsychotic medication was led by the APRN in collaboration with staff physicians. Comprehensive, thoughtful medication reviews were conducted on all residents. The original rate of antipsychotic usage of 30.8% was reduced to 3.3%, all of which were for residents with a diagnosis of bipolar disorder. No antipsychotics have been prescribed for residents with only a psychiatric diagnosis of dementia for more than 3 years. Communication regarding medication management as well as condition change has been enhanced through the use of secure, encrypted electronic communication channels.

Site staff have also been active in the education and implementation of advance directives in the facility as well as in the community. Annually, the center hosts advance directive clinics where staff, residents, families, and community members can fill out an advance directive free of charge. Facility representatives also travel to senior centers within the county to provide education and opportunities to enact an advance directive.

Consistent with complexity science, there was no "magic bullet" that led to the success of the MOQI project at this site. It took a large degree of commitment from staff and providers to be open to a new way of thinking and caring for residents. Care processes and communication channels changed. Monthly quality assurance meetings give actual data demonstrating quality outcomes, which have continued to improve. The change did not occur overnight. It was a gradual change that was nudged and at times pushed by the APRN and the leadership in the home.

Would this be a suitable approach for you? Why?

JoAnn Franklin
Angelita Pritchett

REFLECTIONS

Review your experiences in nursing and healthcare. Think of an example when you have had the opportunity to lead in a challenging situation. When have you been responsible for managing a process? When have you been a follower in correcting a problem?

BEST PRACTICES

Environmental factors often influence the strategies used by leaders. In these circumstances, information sharing, communication, and collaboration are important leadership strategies, particularly in times of uncertainty. As a result, relationship development is a key skill for leaders, managers, and followers. Expanding the relationships within the team encourages diverse thinking (both top down and bottom up), which. in turn, supports effective problem-solving.

TIPS FOR LEADING, MANAGING, AND FOLLOWING

- Use theories of leadership and management to frame complex problems and guide decision-making.
- Recognize that factors on the inside and outside of the organizational environment, including other people, may not be something you can control.
- Situations that are complex or not well understood may require leadership skills.
- Situations that require development of processes may require managerial skills.

REFERENCES

American Association of Colleges of Nursing (AACN). (2021). The essentials: Core competencies for professional nursing education. Retrieved from https://www.aacnnursing.org/Portals/42/AcademicNursing/pdf/Essentials-2021.pdf.

Anderson, V., & Johnson, L. (1997). *Systems thinking basics: From concepts to causal loops.* Waltham, MA: Pegasus Communications.

Arnetz, B., Goetz, C., Arnetz, J., Sudan, S., vonSchagen, J., & Piersma, K. (2020). *Enhancing health care efficiency to achieve the Quadruple Aim: An exploratory study.* NCBI Resources. 13. Retrieved from https://www.ncbi.nlm.nih.gov/pmc/articles/PMC7393915/.

Bass, B. M. (1990). From transactional to transformational leadership: Learning to share the vision. *Organizational Dynamics, 18,* 19–31.

Begun, J. W., & Jiang, J. (2020). Health care management during COVID-19: Insights from complexity science. Innovation in care delivery. *New England Journal of Medicine Catalyst.* October 9, 2020.

Bennis, W. G., & Nanus, B. (2007). *Leaders: The strategies for taking charge* (2nd ed.). New York: Harper Business.

Berwick, D. M., Noland, T. W., & Whittington, J. (2008). The triple aim: Care, health, and cost. *Health Affairs, 27*(3), 759–769. Retrieved from http://www.ihi.org/resources/Pages/Publications/TripleAimCareHealthandCost.aspx.

Blake, R. R., & Mouton, J. S. (1985). *The managerial grid III.* Houston: Gulf Publishing.

Bradt, G. (2020). *The fundamental difference between leading and managing: Influence versus direction.* Retrieved from www.forbes.com/sites/georgebradt/2015/11/24/the-fundamental-difference-between-leading-and-managing-influence-versus-direction/?sh=322883303c73.

Fiedler, F. A. (1967). *A theory of leadership effectiveness.* New York: McGraw-Hill.

Gardner, J. W. (1990). *On leadership.* New York: Free Press.

Haupt, J. (2003). Applying complexity science in practice: Understanding and acting to improve health and healthcare. Plexus Institute, Mayo School of Continuing Medicine Education and the Center of the Study of Healthcare Management, University of Minnesota. https://amee.org/getattachment/AMEE-Initiatives/ESME-Courses/AMEE-ESME-Online-Courses/Leadership-Online/ESME-LME-Resources/Applying-Complexity-Science-to-Health-and-Healthcare.pdf.

Herzberg, F. (1991). One more time: How do you motivate employees? In M. J. Ward, & S. A. Price (Eds.), *Issues in nursing administration: Selected readings.* St. Louis, MO: Mosby.

House, R. J., & Mitchell, T. R. (1974). Path-goal theory of leadership. *Contemporary Business, 3,* 81–98.

Hodiamont, F., Junger, S., Leidl, R., Maier, B. O., Schildmann, E., Bausewein, C. (2019). Understanding complexity—the palliative care situation as a complex adaptive system. *BMC Health Services Research*, *19*(1), 157. https://doi.org/10.1186/s12913-019-3961-0.

Institute for Healthcare Improvement (IHI). (2022). *30 Years of applying quality improvement methods to meet current and future health care challenges*. Retrieved from http://www.ihi.org/about/pages/history.aspx.

Kouzes, J., Posner, B. (2011). The five practices of exemplary leadership (2nd ed.). San Francisco, CA: John Wiley & Sons.

Kraaijenbrink, J. (2019). *Is the world really more VUCA than ever? Forbes*. January 4, 2019. Retrieved from https://www.forbes.com/sites/jeroenkraaijenbrink/2019/01/04/is-the-world-really-more-vuca-than-ever/?sh=1d159ebb1a64.

Likert, R. (1987). New patterns of management. Garland.

Maslow, A. (1943). A theory of human motivation. *Psychological Review*, *50*, 370–396.

Mundy, S., Cooper, L. S., & Mate, K. S. (2022). The quintuple aim for health care improvement a new imperative to advance health equity. *JAMA*, *327*(5), 521–522.

Scouller, J. (2011). *The three levels of leadership: How to develop your leadership presence, knowhow, and skill*. Management Books.

Sergent, K., & Stajkovic, A. (2020). Women's leadership is associated with fewer deaths during the COVID-19 crisis: Qualitative and qualitative analysis of United States governors. *Journal of Applied Psychology*, *105*(8), 771–778.

Shartle, C. L. (1956). *Executive performance and leadership*. Englewood Cliffs, NJ: Prentice Hall.

Stogdill, R. M. (1948). Personal factors associated with leadership: A survey of the literature. *Journal of Psychology*, *25*, 35–71.

Stogdill, R. M. (1963). *Manual for the leader behavior description questionnaire, form XII*. Columbus: The Ohio State University, Bureau of Business Research.

Tichy, N. M., & Devanna, M. A. (1997). *The transformational leader*. New York: John Wiley & Sons.

Vroom, V. H. (1994). *Work and motivation*. New York: John Wiley & Sons.

Vroom, V. H., & Yetton, P. (1973). *Leadership and decision-making*. Pittsburgh, PA: University of Pittsburgh Press.

2

Quality and Safety

Victoria N. Folse

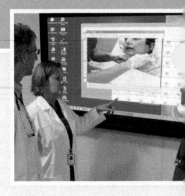

ANTICIPATED LEARNING OUTCOMES

- Incorporate recommendations from key organizations leading patient safety movements in the United States and abroad.
- Integrate clinical safety concepts to promote nurse and patient outcomes.
- Apply quality management principles to clinical situations.
- Use the six steps of the quality improvement process.
- Strengthen roles of leaders, managers, and followers to create a culture of quality and safety.
- Champion diversity, equity, and inclusion to impact quality and safety initiatives.

KEY TERMS

accountability measure
always event
benchmarking
choosing wisely
continuous quality improvement (CQI)
cultural awareness
cultural competency
cultural diversity
cultural sensitivity
culture of safety
DNV-GL
failure mode and effects analysis (FMEA)
hand-off communication
high-reliability organization
near miss

never event
nursing-sensitive indicator
performance improvement (PI)
quality assurance (QA)
quality improvement (QI)
quality management (QM)
risk management
root-cause analysis
sentinel event
situation, background, assessment, recommendation (SBAR)
teach-back
total quality management (TQM)
value-based payment/purchasing

Key Safety and Quality Organizations and Initiatives
Agency for Healthcare Research and Quality (AHRQ)
Institute for Healthcare Improvement (IHI)
International Council of Nurses (ICN)
Magnet Recognition Program®
National Academy of Medicine (NAM; formerly the Institute of Medicine [IOM])
National Quality Forum (NQF)
Quality and Safety Education for Nurses (QSEN)
TeamSTEPPS
The Joint Commission (TJC)

THE CHALLENGE

Efficiency and high quality of care are essential in an emergency department (ED) such as Vanderbilt University Medical Center (VUMC), which sees over 65,000 patients annually. The quality of care provided by VUMC's ED is exceptional. However, at times it can be compromised due to lengthy wait times. Patients often spend 4 or more hours in the waiting room, resulting in many patients leaving without being seen by a medical provider. Sometimes, patients even have to wait outside in the extreme weather.

Patients who spend hours in the waiting room or outside and leave without being seen risk further injury to themselves. A delay in care is also problematic because the triage process does not allow for the provider to place orders and the patient could not receive care until an ED bed was available. The length of stay for patients who are discharged from the ED is also astronomical compared to other academic medical centers. Patients discharged home from the ED are considered noncritical and can leave once laboratory, imaging, and other tests are complete and/or medication is given. Discharging a patient is hindered due to delays in obtaining laboratory specimens and imaging. Keeping noncritical patients in the ED decreases bed availability for sicker, more critical patients and further increases wait times. A need to modify the triage process was identified to decrease wait times and to discharge patients faster.

What would you do if you were this nurse?

Emily Lezcano, RN, BSN
Registered Nurse, Emergency Department, Vanderbilt University Medical Center, Nashville TN

INTRODUCTION

An emphasis on quality and safety is at the core of leading and managing in nursing. Healthcare agencies and health professionals strive to provide the highest-quality, safest, most efficient, and most cost-effective care possible. A commitment to quality and safety should drive staffing and budgeting decisions, personnel policies, information technology, continuing education, and the workplace environment. The philosophy of quality management and the process of quality improvement must shape the entire healthcare culture and provide specific skills and competencies for assessment, measurement, and evaluation of patient care. Nurses perform an essential role in improving healthcare quality and safety and must contribute proactively to a culture of patient safety.

The goal of an organization committed to quality care is a comprehensive, systematic approach that prevents errors or identifies and corrects errors so that adverse events are decreased and safety and quality outcomes are maximized. Leadership must acknowledge safety challenges and allocate resources at the patient care and unit levels to identify and reduce risks. Managers must enhance work environments to support higher-quality care, less patient risk, and more satisfied nurses. Harmful bias and discrimination are pervasive in healthcare and can interfere with the treatment of patients and families. Healthcare professionals and students also experience prejudice and discrimination, sometimes from their patients, that cause harm and negatively impact outcomes. Culturally sensitive leaders provide the opportunity to promote diversity, equity, inclusion, and belonging. Concerns about inequities in healthcare access and delivery require emphasis on how culture impacts care. Inclusion provides a vehicle to improve the quality and safety of healthcare for all while belonging creates engagement and ownership.

INTEGRATION OF QUALITY AND SAFETY IN HEALTHCARE

Healthcare systems that demand quality recognize that survival and competitiveness are built on improved patient outcomes. Success depends on a philosophy that permeates the organization and values a continuous process of improvement. Patient safety and risk management are essential to integrate into broader quality initiatives. The Institute of Medicine (IOM; now the National Academy of Medicine [NAM]) brought the issue of safety and medical errors to the forefront of healthcare awareness in 2000 with its landmark report, *To Err is Human: Building a Safer Health System*. In addition to the NAM, several key organizations, including the Agency for Healthcare Research and

Quality (AHRQ), the National Quality Forum (NQF), the Institute for Healthcare Improvement (IHI), The Joint Commission (TJC), DNV-GL Healthcare, and the Quality and Safety Education for Nurses (QSEN) Institute establish standards for quality and safety in healthcare and in healthcare education. Emphasis on quality and safety inititatives such as QSEN will transform nursing education to prepare practice-ready graduates who apply systems thinking and high reliability principles (Sherwood, 2019). In the prelicensure competencies, for example, teamwork and collaboration clearly relate directly to leading and managing in nursing. Prelicensure students perceive patient-centered care as the most discussed competency and quality improvement as the least reviewed (Cengiz & Yoder, 2020). This chapter is designed to increase quality improvement skills in the classroom, in clinical education, and in simulation. This will, in turn, impact quality and safety in healthcare settings.

CLASSIC REPORTS AND KEY AGENCIES THAT ADVANCE QUALITY AND SAFETY

Multiple reports by key agencies such as the Institute of Medicine (now the National Academy of Medicine) and the Quality and Safety Education for Nurses Institute are reflective of the foundational efforts to focus healthcare on quality, as illustrated in Table 2.1. These reports and related supporting work form the basis for the continued efforts that all healthcare professionals must address to promote safe care.

TABLE 2.1 Major Forces Influencing Patient Safety

Element	Core Relevance	Implications for Leaders and Managers
Reports		
Institute of Medicine (now National Academy of Medicine) Reports	*To Err is Human* (2000): Quantified the role of safety-related errors resulting in patient morbidity and mortality.	Moved safety issues from the incident report level to an integrated patient safety report for the organization. Acknowledged system errors as more common cause of error than individual. Stimulated hospital boards to include reports on quality.
	Crossing the Quality Chasm (2001): Identified the six major aims (safe, effective, patient-centered, timely, efficient, and equitable) for providing quality healthcare.	Moved care from discipline-centric to patient centered. Reinforced the disparities that occur within healthcare, which, in turn, led to a focus on best practices and patient-centered care. Addressed issues such as healing environments, evidence-based care, and transparency, which led to a more holistic environment built on evidence. Provided substantive support for information technology use. Served as impetus for "pay for quality."
	Health Professions Education: A Bridge to Quality (2003): Addressed the issue of silo education among the health professions in basic and continuing education. Identified need to provide patient-centered care, work in interprofessional teams, employ evidence-based practice, apply quality improvement, and utilize informatics.	Attempted to shrink the chasm between education and practice so that interprofessional teams would work more effectively together. Exposed the issue of "silo" education and called for collaborative practice. Increased expectation for participation in lifelong learning.

TABLE 2.1   Major Forces Influencing Patient Safety—cont'd

Element	Core Relevance	Implications for Leaders and Managers
	Keeping Patients Safe: Transforming the Work Environment of Nurses (2004): Identified many past practices that had a negative influence on nurses and, thus, on patients.	Focused on direct care nurses and supported their involvement in decision-making related to their practice. Supported the concept of shared governance. Provided a framework for considering how nurses could determine staffing requirements. Supported public reporting of issues related to unsafe work environments. Moved the Chief Nursing Officer (CNO) into the boardroom as a key spokesperson on safety and quality issues.
	Future of Nursing: Leading Change, Advancing Health (2010): Identified 8 recommendations based on evidence that the profession must attend to, including improving nurse education, ensuring that nurses can practice to the full extent of their education and training, providing opportunities for nurses to assume leadership positions, and improving data collection for policymaking and workforce planning (see Box 2.1).	Created state coalitions focused on improving nursing. Created nursing/community/business partnerships to accomplish the work. Moved the issue of nurses as leaders to a more visible level.
	Future of Nursing: 2020–2030: Charting a Path to Achieve Health Equity (2021): Expanded vision of original *Future of Nursing* publication to charge the profession to create a culture of health, reduce health disparities, and improve the health and well-being of the U.S. population in the 21st century (see Box 2.1).	Increased emphasis on health promotion and health equity. Continued focus on 2010 recommendations to enhance professionalism.
Agencies/Organizations		
Agency for Healthcare Research and Quality (AHRQ)	Federal agency devoted to improving quality, safety, efficiency, and effectiveness. *www.ahrq.gov*	Provides outcomes research sections as resources for nurses. Created resource of TeamSTEPPS and TeamSTEPPS 2.0 *(www.ahrq.gov/teamstepps/index.html)*
International Council of Nurses (ICN)	A federation of more than 130 national nurses' associations, representing millions of nurses worldwide and designed to be the voice of nursing internationally. *www.icn.ch*	Created the Global Nursing Leadership Institute for strategic policy leadership development. Authors an international Code of Ethics for Nurses.
National Quality Forum (NQF)	Membership-based organization related to quality measurement and reporting. *www.nqf.org*	Provides source for Centers for Medicare & Medicaid Services' never events. Serves as resource for Healthcare Facilities Accreditation Program (a CMS-deemed authority that uses the NQF's Safe Practices). Serves as source of nurse-sensitive care standards.

Continued

TABLE 2.1   Major Forces Influencing Patient Safety—cont'd

Element	Core Relevance	Implications for Leaders and Managers
The Joint Commission (TJC)	Not-for-profit organization that accredits healthcare organizations internationally. www.jointcommission.org	Focuses on outcomes that redirected accreditation processes and, thus, nurses' roles within the process. Changed to unannounced visits and, thus, changed the way that organizations prepare for accreditation. Issues annual patient safety goals and sentinel event announcements.
Magnet Recognition Program®	A designation signaling excellence in nursing and obtainment of successful outcomes within healthcare agencies. www.nursingworld.org/organizational-programs/magnet/	Created unified approaches to seek this designation. Redirected focus to outcomes, including data and efforts related to patient safety.
Institute for Healthcare Improvement (IHI)	Independent, not-for-profit organization focused on advancing and sustaining better outcomes in health and healthcare. www.ihi.org	Supports innovation, including rapid-cycle change projects designed to improve care rapidly. Developed a framework built around improvements in safe and reliable care, vitality and teamwork, patient-centered care, and value-added care processes. Adopts a Triple Aim framework to optimize health system performance by simultaneously focusing on three care dimensions: improving the patient experience of care, improving the health of populations, and reducing the per-capita cost of healthcare.
Quality and Safety Education for Nurses (QSEN)	Comprehensive resource, including references and video modules. Defines essential competencies as patient-centered care, teamwork and collaboration, evidence-based practice, quality improvement, safety, and informatics. www.qsen.org	Created knowledge, skills, and attitudes (KSA) for students and graduates related to quality and safety.

Institute of Medicine (now National Academy of Medicine) Seminal Reports on Quality

This safety-focused work began with the report commonly known as *To Err is Human* (IOM, 2000) and rapidly moved to several other reports designed to set aims of healthcare, address how professionals are prepared, and target key areas such as the practice environment. *Crossing the Quality Chasm* (IOM, 2001) identified six aims of providing healthcare, which remain relevant to today's practice. Equally important to safety issues is how professionals are prepared; the report *Health Professions Education: A Bridge to Quality* (IOM, 2003) established expected competencies for all health professions, including a commitment to ongoing learning. Although the individual has accountability to maintain competence and participate in continuing education,

a high-performing organization values and acknowledges learning as a vital element in being effective.

Keeping Patients Safe: Transforming the Work Environment of Nurses (IOM, 2004) was a major impetus behind many changes designed to improve working conditions for nurses. This report identified lack of trust in organizations; lack of readily available resources; and the presence of unsafe equipment, supplies, and practices as contributions to an unsafe work environment. Another report of importance, though not focused directly on patient safety, is *The Future of Nursing* (IOM, 2010). The numerous citations of evidence related to education, scope of practice, and leadership clearly indicate that if the eight recommendations (Box 2.1) were fully implemented, the quality of care, including safety, would be enhanced. Failure

BOX 2.1 The Future of Nursing Recommendations[a]

1. Remove scope-of-practice barriers.
2. Expand opportunities for nurse to lead and diffuse collaborative improvement efforts.
3. Implement nurse residency programs.
4. Increase the proportion of nurses with a baccalaureate degree to 80% by 2020.
5. Double the number of nurses with a doctorate by 2020.
6. Ensure that nurses engage in lifelong learning.
7. Prepare and enable nurses to lead change to advance health.
8. Build an infrastructure for the collection and analysis of interprofessional healthcare workforce data.

Key Priorities[b]

1. Work over the next decade to reduce health disparities and promote equity.
2. Address rising costs through more equitable care delivery.
3. Use technology to maximize reaching vulnerable populations.
4. Prioritize patient- and family-focused care.

[a]From Institute of Medicine (IOM). (2010). *The Future of Nursing: Leading Change, Advancing Health.* Washington, DC: National Academies Press.
[b]From National Academy of Medicine (NAM). (2021). *The Future of Nursing 2020–2030: Charting a Path to Achieve Health Equity.* Washington, DC: National Academies Press.

practices to benefit patients and nurses who do not hold a baccalaureate degree in nursing?

Subsequently, in 2021, NAM issued a second Future of Nursing report called The Future of Nursing 2020–2030: Charting a Path to Achieve Health Equity, which extended the vision.

Next, consider what progress has been made in your state in increasing the educational preparation of registered nurses as you help create a culture of health, reduce health disparities, and improve the health and well-being of the U.S. population. What resources can you access to learn about the population your clinical agency serves and what actions need to be taken to improve health equity?

to improve practice environments, as directed by the IOM reports, may slow progress toward improving patient safety. *The Future of Nursing 2020–2030* (NAM, 2021) advances issues of diversity, equity, and inclusion as central to quality and safety.

EXERCISE 2.1 The IOM, through its report on *The Future of Nursing* (2010), advocated for having at least 80% of the registered nurse population prepared at the baccalaureate level. The rationale provided was based on numerous studies showing that nurses prepared at that or higher levels produced better patient outcomes. Does that recommendation still make sense in today's work environment? Assume that you work in a facility that does not require all nursing staff to hold a bachelor's degree and does not provide support (time off, tuition reimbursement, recognition of educational achievement). How could you advance quality and safety initiatives, including a change in workplace policies and

Agency for Healthcare Research and Quality

The AHRQ is the primary federal agency devoted to improving quality, safety, efficiency, and effectiveness of healthcare (Agency for Healthcare Research and Quality [AHRQ], n.d.).

AHRQ builds a bridge between research and practice and issues reports on evidence-based practices such as preoperative checklists, bundles to prevent central line–associated bloodstream infections, interventions to reduce urinary catheter care infections, hand hygiene, "do not use" abbreviations, barrier precautions to prevent healthcare-associated bloodstream infections, interventions to reduce falls, use of rapid response systems, and simulation exercises in patient safety efforts. The AHRQ's TeamSTEPPS programs are designed to increase attention to safety within healthcare organizations using the five key principles of team structure, communication, leadership, situation monitoring, and mutual support.

The National Quality Forum

The NQF is a membership-based organization designed to develop and implement a national strategy for healthcare quality measurement and reporting. Through its consensus process, the NQF sets standards and endorses measures that allow for quality comparison across metrics such as settings, states, and diagnoses. The NQF then advises the Centers for Medicare & Medicaid Services (CMS) about measures that can be used to determine payment. As a result, the CMS will not pay for certain conditions that result from what might be termed poor practices or events that should not have occurred while a patient was under the care of a healthcare professional.

The Joint Commission (TJC) is a not-for-profit organization that accredits healthcare organizations. Approximately 4,200 U.S. hospitals and another 380 critical access hospitals maintain TJC accreditation. When TJC changed its focus from process to outcomes, it placed more emphasis on patient safety. As a result, TJC issues annual patient safety goals that are setting specific; a list of "do-not-use" terms, symbols, and abbreviations; and sentinel events. All of these efforts are directed toward improving patient safety.

DNV-GL Healthcare is a relatively new accrediting organization in the United States that has extended accreditation to approximately 500 U.S. hospitals. The accreditation programs directly address CMS requirements and the certification programs leverage the guidance and best practices of clinical specialty organizations across healthcare.

The International Council of Nurses (ICN) is a federation of more than 130 national nurses' associations, representing millions of nurses worldwide, which is designed to be the voice of nurses internationally. ICN's emphasis includes providing culturally sensitive care to ensure quality and safety on an international level.

The Magnet Recognition Program® is a national designation to acknowledge nursing excellence, which recognizes quality and safety. Organizations must demonstrate how they provide excellence across five elements: transformational leadership; structural empowerment; exemplary professional practice; new knowledge, innovation, and improvements; and empirical quality results. From initial designation to redesignation, emphasis is placed on empirical quality results. Since its inception in 1994, approximately 576 hospitals in the United States (about 9%) have received Magnet recognition. Hospitals in other countries also have received this designation.

The Institute for Healthcare Improvement (IHI) merged with the National Patient Safety Foundation in May 2017 and is dedicated to rapidly improving care through a variety of mechanisms, including rapid cycle change projects. This rapid change is built on the theory of diffusion (see the Theory Box). Other significant contributions include initiatives entitled Transforming Care at the Bedside (IHI, 2022c) and Triple Aim for Populations (IHI, 2022d). The Triple Aim focused on improving the health of populations, enhancing the experience of care for individuals, and reducing the per capita cost of healthcare. Then, Arnetz et al., (2020) proposed the addition of the fourth aim: to improve the work life of healthcare providers in all disciplines, which is reflective of all of the years of research related to Magnet organizations. In 2022, IHI, added the Quintuple Aim to focus on health equity (Mundy, 2022).

Quality and Safety Education for Nurses (QSEN) Institute has taken a lead role in promoting quality and safety in healthcare. Nurses, including nurse managers and leaders, can not successfully function today without a focus on patient safety. Nurses must be prepared to continuously improve the quality and safety of the workplaces in their healthcare systems, and they must focus on the six competencies identified by QSEN (2020): patient-centered care, teamwork and collaboration, evidence-based practice, quality improvement, safety, and informatics. Quality necessitates maintaining safety in patient care, with a continual focus on clinical excellence from the entire interprofessional team. Patient safety is a key component of quality improvement and clinical governance while the prevention of adverse events is paramount to improved patient outcomes.

THEORY BOX

Theory/Contributor	Key Idea	Application to Practice
Rogers Diffusion of Innovations (2003)	Diffusion is a process of communication about innovation to share information over time and among a group of people. It provides a framework for successfully implementing nonlinear change. More complex change is less likely to be adopted. Early adopters serve as role models.	Shared leadership supports diffusion and adaptation of innovation. Engage key leaders in a change to infuse the energy from early adopters. Using social media platforms in the hospital culture to engage employees communicates changes quickly. New changes are altered while they are being adopted because new evidence or a better idea emerges.

QUALITY MANAGEMENT IN HEALTH CARE

The terms quality management (QM), quality improvement (QI), performance improvement (PI), total quality management (TQM), and continuous quality improvement (CQI) are often used interchangeably in healthcare, and the terminology continues to evolve. Safety goals are often blended with quality programs that include a culture of safety—a blame-free environment encouraging employees to report errors and prevent situations that threaten safety so that quality can be assured. Designation as a high-reliability organization signals healthcare organizations that achieve the highest quality and safety standards through organizational effectiveness, efficiency, customer satisfaction, compliance, organizational culture, and documentation. The push for greater transparency in healthcare costs and outcomes requires nurse leaders to shape a culture of safety and quality (Bliss et al., 2020). To promote a culture of safety, healthcare leaders must cultivate a favorable implementation climate, demonstrate behaviors that support a safety culture, increase compatibility of working conditions with goals of safety interventions, build confidence in systems to address unprofessional behaviors, and respond to evolving needs (McKenzie, 2019).

In this chapter, quality management (QM) refers to an overarching philosophy that defines a healthcare culture emphasizing customer satisfaction, innovation, and employee involvement. Similarly, quality improvement (QI) refers to an ongoing process of innovative improvements, prevention of error, and development of staff used by institutions that adopt the QM philosophy. Nurses maintain a unique role in QM and QI because of the direct patient care provided at the bedside 24 hours a day and because they have an understanding of a patient's day-to-day issues. Nurses are responsible for early-warning monitoring, and they have direct knowledge of patients' conditions and changes. Favorable nurse-to-patient ratios and active engagement of nurses in patient care improvement efforts promote quality and safety of patient care and also positively affect job satisfaction, improving the work environment (Brooks Carthon et al., 2019). Nurse specialty certification and baccalaureate education have consistently been associated with better patient outcomes (Djukic et al., 2019) as have a skill mix that prioritizes registered nurses (RNs) delivering total patient care in high-acuity units (Havaei et al., 2019). Teamwork is compromised if staffing is inadequate, and research confirms that effective teamwork results in safer care (Bragadóttir et al., 2019). The evidence is also clear that inadequate RN staffing (in number and competencies) increases the risk for poor outcomes for patients (Aiken & Sloane, 2020; Wynendaele et al., 2019) and should be an important consideration for quality and safety initiatives. Improving accreditation and organizational policies requiring baccalaureate education for all nurses could close quality and safety education gaps to promote the quality and safety of patient care (Djukic et al., 2019). In 2020 and 2021, nursing experienced a dramatic shift to team nursing as a result of the COVID-19 pandemic. The subsequent shift of nurses from hospitals to travel agencies and nonacute settings (or nonnursing positions) will have an impact on how care is delivered in the foreseeable future.

Benefits of Quality Management

Healthcare systems that use a comprehensive QM program experience many organizational benefits. First, greater efficiency and proactive planning may overcome some of the resource constraints, including limited reimbursement imposed by prospective payment plans and key staff shortages. Second, successful malpractice suits could be reduced with quality care because QM is based on the philosophy that actions should be right the first time and that improvement is always possible. Third, job satisfaction could be enhanced, because QM involves everyone on the improvement team and encourages everyone to contribute. This style of participative management makes employees feel valued as team members who are empowered to make a difference in quality and safety initiatives.

Planning for Quality Management

Interprofessional planning is integral to the quest for quality. Issues are examined from various perspectives using a systematic process. Planning takes time and money; however, the price of poor planning can be very expensive. Costs of inadequate planning might involve correcting a patient care error, resulting in an extended length of stay and added procedures. In turn, this increases the risk of liability for what was originally done, it risks a negative public image, and it magnifies employee frustration, which promotes turnover. The costs of errors and ineffective nursing actions are avoidable. The CMS has developed several initiatives to measure and incentivize quality improvement, including Hospital Value-Based Purchasing (VBP), Hospital-Acquired Condition Reduction Program (HACRP), and Hospital Readmissions Reduction Program (RRP). VBP initiatives have been put in placd in response to escalating healthcare costs and concerns about quality and safety in healthcare, allowing patients to hold providers accountable for costs and service quality. Value-based payment/purchasing programs reward or incentivize high-performing organizations whose outcomes are consistent with quality of care standards and reduce reimbursement for poor performers (Boylan et al., 2019). Thirty-day readmission, for example, is an accountability metric for hospital performance. Thus, hospital leaders are greatly concerned when a patient requires readmission soon after discharge, because this can signal an issue with the care received and can result in the hospital losing money.

Evolution of Quality Management

Nonhealthcare industries have excelled in focusing on process improvement as part of their core operating strategies. Several models for quality improvement exist in healthcare, including Lean Sigma and Six Sigma, Failure Mode and Effects Analysis, and Root Cause Analysis. Numerous business management philosophies have been expanded and modified for use in healthcare organizations. For example, Lean Sigma and Six Sigma, data-driven approaches targeting a nearly error-free environment, empower employees to improve processes and outcomes (Peimbert-García et al., 2020). As healthcare organizations "go lean," nurses are challenged to eliminate unnecessary steps and reduce wasted processes (saving time and money) to improve quality and the patient experience. Lean and Six Sigma management techniques are most effective with improving quality and efficiency in settings in which processes are linear, such as operating rooms, emergency departments, and intensive care units (Peimbert-García et al., 2020). To achieve this, Six Sigma uses a five-step methodology known as *DMAIC,* which stands for *d*efine opportunities, *m*easure performance, *a*nalyze opportunity, improve performance, and *c*ontrol performance to improve existing processes (GoLeanSixSigma, n.d.). Parallels to the nursing process steps of assessment, diagnosis, planning, implementation, and evaluation can be seen in DMAIC and other QI processes.

Different types of quality improvement methodology can be combined to improve outcomes.

In healthcare, emphasis is placed on the areas of patient safety and patient and employee satisfaction. The role of the leader or manager in this TQM method is to enable the team, remove barriers, and instill accountability. One of the most widely used evidence-based teamwork systems to improve communication and teamwork skills to improve patient safety within organizations is the AHRQ Team Strategies and Tools to Enhance Performance and Patient Safety (TeamSTEPPS 2.0). Teamwork is one of the key safety initiatives that can transform a healthcare culture. Team training is modified for primary care office–based teams as well as for nursing homes and other long-term care settings. A customized TeamSTEPPS plan is available to train staff in teamwork skills to work with patients who have difficulty communicating in English (AHRQ, 2018).

Within healthcare systems, QI combines the assessment of *structure* (e.g., adequacy of staffing, effectiveness of computerized charting, or availability of unit-based medication delivery systems), *process* (e.g., timeliness and thoroughness of documentation, adherence to critical pathways or care maps), and *outcome* (e.g., patient falls, hospital-acquired infection rates, or patient and nurse satisfaction) standards. These three factors are usually considered interrelated, and comprehensive QI initiatives actively involve direct care providers to improve quality and safety. The Literature Perspective presents the impact that staffing has on outcomes for patients after cardiac arrest.

Recognizing the relationship between quality patient care and nursing excellence, the American Academy of Nursing undertook an initiative that resulted in the distinction known as *Magnet*®. The American Nurses Credentialing Center (ANCC) created a process called the *Magnet Recognition Program*®, which recognizes healthcare organizations for quality patient care, nursing excellence, and innovations in professional nursing practice. The term *Magnet*® was chosen to describe a hospital that attracts and retains nurses even in times of nursing shortages. Magnet® hospital research has examined the characteristics of hospital systems that impede or facilitate professional practice in nursing and also promote quality patient outcomes. Common organizational characteristics of Magnet® hospitals include structure factors (e.g., decentralized organizational structure, participative management style, and influential nurse

LITERATURE PERSPECTIVE

Resource: Harrison, J. M., Aiken, L. H., Sloane, D. M., Brooks Carthon, J. M., Merchant, R. M., Berg, R. A., & McHugh, M. D. (2019). In hospitals with more nurses who have baccalaureate degrees, better outcomes for patients after cardiac arrest. *Health Affairs, 38*(7), 1087–1094.

Each 10% increase in BSN-prepared nurses results in a 24% increase in surviving to discharge with good cerebral performance after an in-hospital cardiac arrest. Because many new graduates work on units where the patient population is extremely complex and levels of staffing are variable, it is critical to advocate for changes to staffing to favorably influence safety and quality. Higher educational levels and lower nurse-to-patient ratios allow improved surveillance and promote a practice environment with more favorable nurse and patient outcomes.

Implications for Practice

Findings add to the growing body of evidence that supports policies to increase access to baccalaureate-level education and improved hospital staffing. More innovation is needed to facilitate greater access to baccalaureate-level education for RNs. Healthcare systems that preferentially hire BSN-prepared nurses and incentivize RNs to obtain a baccalaureate degree will see improvments in hospital performance metrics. Improving staffing may serve as a leadership strategy that will translate into an improved patient experience and may generate improved reimbursement.

LITERATURE PERSPECTIVE

Resource: Drew, J., & Pandit, M. (2020). Why healthcare leadership should embrace quality improvement. *The British Medical Journal (Quality Improvement Supplement)*, 49–51.

To create a culture of quality and safety in healthcare, changes to leadership and management, including a shift in thinking, are needed. QI depends on engaging and empowering healthcare teams delivering care and equipping them with the tools and skills they need to improve care. To illustrate, the authors describe an experienced nurse explaining a QI project to improve patient flow. The most striking thing was not her description of the project or how it would benefit patients but instead how the QI project made her feel "valued and respected."

Implications for Practice

Embedding QI in any organization requires a new narrative and a more inclusive leadership model that empowers frontline teams and creates a meaningful role for patients so that improvement is aligned to what both staff and patients need and value. Meeting organizational goals for quality and safety requires that incentives to participate must build on a practice environment culture that values employees.

executives) and process factors (e.g., professional autonomy and decision-making, ongoing professional development/education, active QI initiatives). ANCC Magnet®-designated hospitals and other high-reliability organizations in the United States and abroad generally have lower burnout rates, have higher levels of job satisfaction, and provide higher levels of quality care, resulting in greater levels of patient satisfaction (Aiken & Sloane, 2020). The second Literature Perspective presents the importance of leaders and managers cultivating a practice environment that values employees and promotes an effective QI culture.

Quality Management Principles

The combination of QI ideas from theory and research is sometimes referred to as *TQM* or, more simply, *QM*. The basic principles of QM are summarized in Box 2.2 and are developed further in the next section of this chapter.

> ### BOX 2.2   Principles of Quality Management and Quality Improvement
>
> 1. Quality management operates most effectively within a flat, democratic organization structure.
> 2. A shared commitment to quality improvement is essential for organizational success.
> 3. The goal of quality management is to improve systems and processes, not to assign blame.
> 4. Quality improvement focuses on outcomes and relies on data-driven decisions.

Structure

When decisions are made closest to where they have an effect, people are more satisfied, decisions are more practical, and quality is enhanced. Every organization has some form of hierarchy. When decisions are made remotely from the point of implementation, they may be theoretically correct yet cumbersome, impractical, or costly to execute. Flat, democratic organizations promote decisions being made closest to where they will be implemented.

Shared Commitment

Leaders, managers, and followers must be committed to QI. Top-level leaders and managers retain the ultimate responsibility for QM but must involve the entire organization in the QI process. Although some healthcare organizations have achieved significant QI results without system-wide support, total organizational involvement is necessary for a culture transformation. If all members of the healthcare team are to be actively involved in QI, clear delineation of roles within a nonthreatening environment must be established (Table 2.2).

TABLE 2.2 Roles and Responsibilities in a Quality Improvement Plan		
Role of Senior Leader	**Role of Nurse Manager**	**Role of Follower/Staff (e.g., Direct Care Nurse)**
Leads culture transformation.	Is accountable for quality and safety indicator performance within areas of responsibility.	Follows policies, procedures, and protocols to ensure quality and safe patient care.
Sets priorities for house-wide activities, staffing effectiveness, and patient health outcomes.	Communicates performance priorities and targets to staff.	Remains current in the literature on quality and safety specific to nursing.
Builds infrastructure, provides resources, and removes barriers for improvement.	Meets regularly with staff to monitor progress and help with improvement work.	Promotes evidence-based practice standards.
Defines procedures for immediate response to errors involving care, treatment, or services and contains risk.	Uses data to measure effectiveness of improvement.	Communicates with and educates peers immediately if they are observed not following quality and safety standards.
Assesses management and staff knowledge of quality management process regularly, and provides education as needed.	Works with staff to develop and implement action plans for improvement of measures that do not meet target.	Reports quality and safety issues to supervisor/manager.
Implements and monitors systems for internal and external reporting of information.	Provides time for unit staff to participate in quality improvement measures.	Invests in the process by continually asking self, "What makes this indicator important to measure?", "What has been done to improve it?", and "What can I do to improve it?".
Defines and provides support system for staff who have been involved in a sentinel event.	Observes staff directly and coaches as needed.	Participates actively in the quality improvement activities.
Empowers nursing leaders and direct care providers to implement and evaluate improvement efforts.	Consults quality management team (e.g., Six Sigma) or risk management team as appropriate.	Provides insight as a direct care provider.
Removes barriers and ensures that resources are adequate.	Writes and submits to senior leaders periodic action plan, including performance measures and plans for improvement.	Generates ideas for unit quality improvement efforts
Rewards high-performing teams.	Shares information and benchmarks with other units and departments to improve organization's performance.	Serves as role model for other direct care providers.

To work effectively in a democratic, quality-focused corporate environment, nurses and other healthcare workers must accept QM and QI as an integral part of their roles. Nurses have a direct impact on patient safety and healthcare outcomes and must follow evidence-based guidelines to meet nursing-sensitive outcome indicators. Nursing must be recognized and empowered to mobilize performance improvement knowledge and practice measures throughout the organization. When a separate department controls quality activities, healthcare managers and workers often relinquish responsibility and commitment for quality control to these quality specialists. Employees working in an organizational culture that values quality freely make suggestions for improvement and innovation in patient care.

> **EXERCISE 2.2** Reflect on something that can be improved in one of your clinical settings or in your professional practice environment. Define the problem, using as many specific facts as possible. List the advantages to the staff, patients, and agency of improving this problem. Describe several possible solutions to the problem. Decide whom you could contact about these suggestions.

Goal

The goal of QM is to improve the system, not to assign blame. Managers strive to provide a system in which workers can function effectively. To encourage commitment to QI, nurse managers must clearly articulate the organization's mission and goals. All levels of employees, from nursing assistants to hospital administrators, must be educated about QI strategies.

Communication should flow freely within the organization. When healthcare professionals understand each other's roles and can effectively communicate and work together, patients are more likely to receive safe, quality care. Because QM stresses improving the system, detection of employees' errors is not stressed; if errors occur, re-education of staff is emphasized rather than imposition of punitive measures. When patient safety indicators are used to examine hospital performance, the focus of error analysis shifts from the individual provider to the level of the healthcare system. The use of an electronic health record can improve the quality of healthcare by increasing time efficiency and adherence to guidelines as well as reducing medication errors and adverse drug events. Reducing medication errors through improved hand-off communication (e.g., SBAR [*s*ituation, *b*ackground, *a*ssessment, *r*ecommendation]) and increased use of technology (e.g., electronic health record, barcode scanning) is needed to address time pressures, work overload, and conflicting demands of nurses, including unlicensed assistive nursing personnel. Improving the practice environment will favorably affect quality and risk variables in all healthcare settings.

Focus

QI focuses on outcomes. Patient outcomes are statements that describe the results of healthcare. They are specific and measurable and describe patients' behavior. Outcome statements may be based on patients' needs, ethical and legal standards of practice, or other standardized data systems. Healthcare organizations that implement nursing-sensitive performance measures and accountability measures (TJC, 2021a) value nurses and have a strong commitment to patient care quality and workforce sustainability. This commitment is even more critical because the CMS and some private insurers no longer reimburse hospitals for the costs of additional care required for hospital-acquired injuries and reduce reimbursement for preventable complications. Pay-for-performance strategies, including value-based payment, has the potential to reduce negative health outcomes.

Decisions

Decisions must be based on data. The use of statistical tools enables nurse managers to make objective decisions about QI activities. Collecting data without a preconceived idea is critical to making quality decisions. Quality information must be gathered and analyzed without bias before improvement suggestions and recommendations are made.

CUSTOMERS

Customers define quality. Successful organizations measure the factors that are most important to customers and focus their energies on enhancing quality in these areas. As patients become more sophisticated and view themselves as "consumers" who can take their business elsewhere, they want input into treatment decisions. Although typical patients may not be knowledgeable about a specific treatment, they know if they were satisfied with their experience with the healthcare provider.

Every nurse and healthcare agency has internal and external customers. Internal customers are people or units within an organization who receive products or services. A nurse working on a hospital unit could describe patients, nurses on the other shifts, and other hospital departments as internal customers. External customers are people or groups outside the organization who receive products or services. For nurses, these external customers may include patients' families, physicians, managed care organizations, and the community at large. Some customers (e.g., physicians, patient families) could be either internal or external customers depending on the actual care environment. Managers and direct care nurses need to identify their internal and external customers.

EXERCISE 2.3 Nursing leadership students, as well as nurse leaders and managers, need to decide whether their clinical unit is ready for a unit-based QI team. Ask yourself the following questions about the unit or department:

1. Is communication between nurses and other professionals promoted? If so, how?
2. Could the interprofessional communication process be improved in any way? If so, how?
3. Does your system encourage nurses to act as a team? If so, how?
4. Are other disciplines or departments included in team activities? In what manner?
5. Can the team focus be improved in any way? In what ways?

Public reporting of quality and risk data is changing the way customers make decisions about healthcare and is intended to improve care through easily accessed information. Accredited hospitals are required to collect and report data on performance for core quality indicators, called accountability measures, that produce the greatest positive impact on patient outcomes and for which organizations are held to standards of performance (Box 2.3). These data are made publicly available, including by The Joint Commission (TJC, 2021a) and through Hospital Compare (CMS, 2020a). These data allow customers to (1) find information on how well hospitals care for patients with certain medical conditions or surgical procedures, and (2) access patient survey results about the care re-

---

BOX 2.3 Accountability Measures

- Inpatient psychiatric services
- Venous thromboembolism (VTE) care
- Stroke care
- Perinatal care
- Immunization
- Tobacco treatment
- Substance use

---

ceived during a recent hospital stay. This information allows customers to compare the quality of care in more than 4,000 Medicare-certified hospitals. Patient satisfaction information on Hospital Compare is part of the Consumer Assessment of Healthcare Providers and Systems (CAHPS) Hospital Survey, known as *HCAHPS*. HCAHPS is a national, standardized, publicly reported survey of patient perspectives and satisfaction on care they experience during a hospital stay, including communication with physicians, communication with nurses, responsiveness of hospital staff, pain management, communication about medicines, discharge information, cleanliness of the hospital environment, and quietness of the hospital environment (CMS, 2021b). In addition to Hospital Compare, websites for Physician Compare, Nursing Home Compare, and Home Health Compare provide transparency for consumers. Consumer satisfaction with healthcare can also be assessed through the use of questionnaires, interviews, focus group discussions, or observation. Patients' perspectives should be a key component of any QI initiative. However, patients cannot always adequately assess the competence of clinical performance. Therefore, patient feedback and patient satisfaction surveys must serve as only one data source for QI initiatives.

THE QUALITY IMPROVEMENT PROCESS

QI involves continual analysis and evaluation of products and services to prevent errors, improve processes, and to achieve customer satisfaction. As the term suggests, the work of continuous QI never stops, because products and services can always be improved.

The QI process is a structured series of steps designed to plan, implement, and evaluate changes in healthcare

> ## BOX 2.4   Steps in the Quality Improvement Process
>
> 1. Identify needs most important to the consumer of healthcare services.
> 2. Assemble an interprofessional team to review the identified consumer needs and services.
> 3. Collect data to measure the current status of these services.
> 4. Establish measurable outcomes and quality indicators.
> 5. Select and implement a plan to meet the outcomes.
> 6. Collect data to evaluate the implementation of the plan and the achievement of outcomes.

activities. Many models of the QI process exist, including Six Sigma and DMAIC, but most parallel the nursing process and all contain steps similar to those listed in Box 2.4. The six steps can easily be applied to clinical situations. In the following example, staff at a community clinic use the QI process to handle patient complaints about excessive wait times. An example of the process follows:

A community clinic receives a number of complaints from patients about waiting up to 2 hours for scheduled appointments to see a licensed practitioner. The clinic secretary and direct care nurses suggest to the clinic manager that scheduling clinic appointments be investigated by the QI committee, which is composed of the clinic secretary, two clinic nurses, one physician, and one nurse practitioner. The clinic manager agrees to the staff's suggestion and assigns the problem to the QI committee. At their next meeting, the QI committee uses a flowchart to describe the scheduling process from the time a patient calls to make an appointment until the patient sees a physician or nurse practitioner in the examining room. Next, the committee members decide to gather and analyze data about the important parts of the process: the number of calls for appointments, the number of patients seen in a day, the number of cancelled or missed appointments, time intervals of the scheduled appointments, and the average time each patient spends in the waiting room. The committee analyzes the data and concludes that too many appointments are scheduled based on the number of missed appointments. This overbooking often results in long wait times for the patients who do arrive on time. The QI committee also gathers information on clinic wait times from the literature and through interviews with patients and colleagues. A measurable outcome is written: "Patients will wait no longer than 30 minutes to be seen by a licensed practitioner." After a discussion of options, the team recommends that appointments be scheduled at more reasonable intervals, that patients receive notification of appointments by mail and by phone, and that all clinic patients be educated about the importance of keeping scheduled appointments. The committee communicates its suggestions for throughput improvement to the manager and staff and monitors the results of the implementation of their improvement suggestions. Within 3 months, the average waiting room time per patient decreases to 90 minutes and the number of missed patient appointments decreases by 20%. Because the desired outcome has not been met, the QI committee will continue the QI process.

Identify Consumers' Needs

The QI process begins with the selection of a clinical issue for review. Theoretically, any and all aspects of clinical care could be improved through the QI process. However, QI efforts should be concentrated on changes to patient care that will have the greatest effect. To determine which clinical activities are most important, nurse managers or direct care nurses may interview or survey patients about their healthcare experiences or may review unmet quality standards. The results of the research studies in the Research Perspective give direction to promoting a positive practice environment in nursing homes to improve quality and safety.

Assemble a Team

Once an activity is selected for possible improvement, an interprofessional team implements the QI process. QI team members should represent a cross-section of workers who are involved with the problem. To maximize success, team members may need to be educated about their roles before starting the QI process. One effective approach is to use the existing shared governance processes in place. To develop effective unit-based quality councils, the workplace environment must promote teamwork. Some departments within healthcare facilities are more open to change than others.

RESEARCH PERSPECTIVE

Resource: White, E. M., Aiken, L. H., Sloane, D. M., & McHugh, M. D. (2020) Nursing home work environment, care quality, registered nurse burnout and job dissatisfaction. *Geriatric Nursing, 41*(2), 158–164.

The quality of the practice environment has a tremendous impact on nurse and patient outcomes. In nursing homes, patient outcomes, including more pressure ulcers and increased hospitalizations as well as nurse outcomes of job dissatisfaction and burnout, were associated with poor versus good work conditions. Nurses report missed nursing care in nursing homes—including comforting/talking to patients, providing adequate surveillance, patient/family teaching, and care planning—due to inadequate time and resources. Further, nurses who reported burnout were five times more likely to report missed care. Improvement in quality and safety requires an investment in the nurses providing care to nursing home residents, one of the most vulnerable and complex patient populations.

Implications for Practice

Improving the quality of care and patient safety in nursing homes is a critical issue. A strong correlation has been established between nurse practice environments and patient and nurse outcomes. In good practice environments with adequate staffing and resources, patient and nurse outcomes are improved. The effects of nurse practice environments on nurse and patient outcomes—including nurse job satisfaction, burnout, turnover, and reports of quality and safety—have been established across settings and are particularly elevated in nursing homes.

Nurse managers and leaders in nursing homes have several options for improving nurse and patient outcomes, including improving RN staffing, facilitating a positive care environment, promoting nurse engagement in QI processes, and providing better pay and opportunities for advancement. Nursing homes where the practice environment includes investment in development of staff, QM, and supportive leadership are associated with better nurse and patient outcomes. Nurse managers must promote an empowered workplace and support higher-quality care, less patient risk, and more satisfied nurses.

Collect Data

After the interprofessional team forms, the group collects meaningful data to measure the current status of the activity, service, or procedure under review. Various data tools—including flowcharts, line graphs, histograms, Pareto charts, and fishbone diagrams—may be used to analyze and present this information. The use of empirical tools to organize QI data is an essential part of the QI process. Many newly licensed RNs lack formal training in the use of QI tools and lack sufficient knowledge, concepts, and tools required to fully participate in QI initiatives. QI skills of direct care providers are necessary to identify gaps between current care and best practice and to design, implement, test, and evaluate changes through shared governance.

A detailed flowchart is used to describe complex tasks. The flowchart is a data tool that uses boxes and directional arrows to diagram all the steps of a process or procedure in the proper sequence. Sometimes, just diagramming a patient care process in detail reveals gaps and opportunities for improvement. The flowchart in Fig. 2.1 depicts the process of a home health agency receiving a new patient referral.

Line graphs present data by showing the connection among variables. The dependent variable is usually plotted on the vertical scale, and the independent variable is usually plotted on the horizontal scale. In QI, this technique is often used to show the trend of a particular activity over time; the result may be called a *trend chart*. The line graph in Fig. 2.2 illustrates the number of referrals a home health agency receives during a year.

The histogram in Fig. 2.3 illustrates the number of home health referrals that come from five different referral sources during a selected year. A histogram is a bar chart that shows the frequency of events.

A bar chart that identifies the major causes or components of a particular quality control problem is called a *Pareto chart*. It differs from a regular bar graph in that the highest frequencies of occurrence of a factor are designated in the bar at the left, with the other factors appearing in descending order. Used often in QI, the Pareto chart helps the QI team determine priorities, allowing the most significant problem to be addressed first. The Pareto chart in Fig. 2.4 demonstrates that, on a medical-surgical unit over a

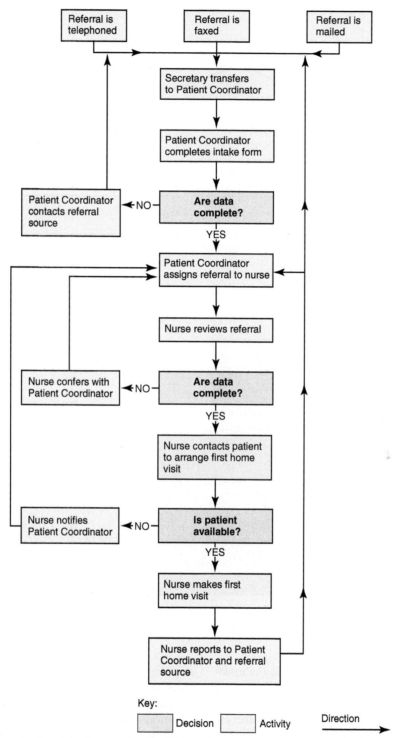

Fig. 2.1 Steps in a flowchart diagramming the process of a new patient referral, starting with the time a home health referral is made and ending with the first home visit.

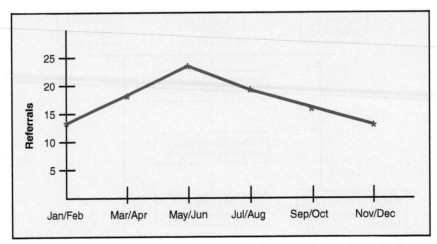

Fig. 2.2 Line graph depicting the number of home health referrals received during 1 year (trend chart).

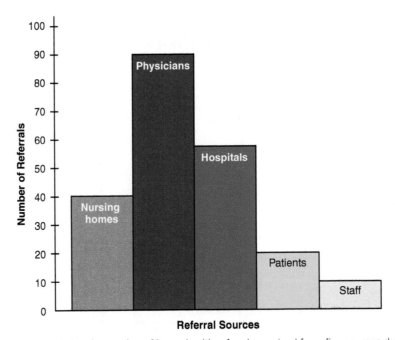

Fig. 2.3 Histogram depicting the number of home health referrals received from five sources during 1 year.

1-month period, omission of vital signs was the most common type of documentation error.

The fishbone diagram is an effective method of summarizing a brainstorming session. A specific problem or outcome is written on the horizontal line. All possible causes of the problem or strategies to meet the outcome are written in a fishbone pattern. Fig. 2.5 uses a fishbone diagram to present possible causes of patients' complaints about extended waits for clinic appointments.

Although QI teams should be able to use these basic statistical tools, analysis that is more complex is sometimes necessary. In this situation, a statistical expert could be included on the QI team or the team may consult a statistician.

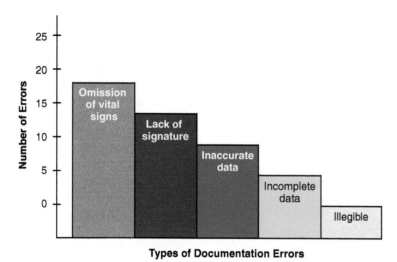

Fig. 2.4 Pareto chart presenting major types of documentation errors that occurred on a medical-surgical unit over a 1-month period.

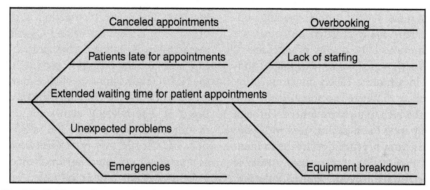

Fig. 2.5 Fishbone diagram showing possible causes of extended wait time for clinic patients.

Establish Outcomes

After analyzing the data, the team next sets a goal for improvement. This goal can be established in a number of ways but always involves a standard of practice and a measurable patient-care outcome or nursing-sensitive outcome. Nursing-sensitive indicators depend on the quantity or quality of nursing care and reflect the structure, process, and outcomes of nursing care. The structure of nursing care is indicated by the supply of nursing staff, the skill level of the nursing staff, and the education and certification of nursing staff. Process indicators measure aspects of nursing care such as assessment, intervention, and RN job satisfaction. Patient outcomes that are determined to be nursing sensitive are those that improve if there is a greater quantity or quality of nursing care (e.g., a decrease in pressure ulcers, falls, intravenous [IV] infiltrations). Some patient outcomes are more highly related to other aspects of institutional care, such as medical decisions and institutional policies (e.g., frequency of primary cesarean sections, cardiac failure) and are not considered nursing sensitive. The interprofessional team should use accepted standards of care and practice whenever possible. Clinical practice guidelines and standards should reflect evidence-based practice and should be updated as new research emerges. Sources that establish these standards include the following:

1. American Nurses Association (ANA) standards of nursing practice
2. State nurse practice acts

3. Accrediting bodies such as TJC or recognition bodies such as the ANCC
4. Governmental bodies such as the AHRQ, the CMS, the Centers for Disease Control and Prevention (CDC) Division of Healthcare Quality Promotion (DHQP), and the National Institute for Occupational Safety and Health (NIOSH)
5. Healthcare advisory groups such as the National Academy of Medicine (formerly known as the Institute of Medicine), the NQF, and QSEN
6. Nationally recognized professional organizations
7. Nursing research/evidence-based, best practice standards
8. Internal policies and procedures
9. Internal or external performance measurement data such as patient satisfaction surveys, employee opinion surveys, safety assessment surveys, and patient or employee rounding

Although individual healthcare organizations may have unique patient needs related to their specific population or environment, many targeted outcomes are similar. One way to evaluate the quality of outcomes is to compare one agency's performance with that of similar organizations. In a process called benchmarking, a widespread search is conducted to identify the best performance against which to measure others. Through this process of comparing the best practices with your practice and process, your organization learns to identify desired standards of quality performance. Available data include all reported hospital-acquired infection rates in other institutions as well as specific data, such as postoperative infection rates in adult surgical intensive care units of similar-size institutions.

However, recent mandates to publicly disclose outcomes, including nosocomial infection rates, highlight potential issues with disclosure of data. Specifically, simply reporting hospital infection rates is not enough to promote hand hygiene practices and may do little to improve outcomes and reduce hospital-acquired infections. Unfortunately, the usefulness of the information from other institutions continues to be hampered by differences in terminology and methodology, including use of present-on-admission data. Information technology plays a vital role in QI by increasing the efficiency of data entry and analysis. A consistent information system that trends high-risk procedures and systematic errors would provide a useful database regarding outcomes of care and resource allocation.

The NQF is designed to standardize measures so that true comparisons can be made.

The National Database of Nursing Quality Indicators (NDNQI) is a national nursing quality measurement program that features nursing-sensitive structure, process, and outcomes measures to monitor relationships between quality indicators and outcomes. The nursing-sensitive quality indicators include hospital-acquired conditions and adverse events subject to the CMS nonpayment rule and provides hospitals with unit-level performance reports, with comparisons with regional, state, and national percentile rankings (Press Ganey, 2020). All indicator data are collected and reported at the nursing unit level, which is valuable for unit-based patient safety and QI initiatives. For example, a report could answer the question, "How is my hospital unit doing relative to the same unit type in peer hospitals?" The NDNQI's nursing-sensitive indicators reflect the structure, process, and outcomes of nursing care. The NDNQI's mission is to aid the nursing provider in patient safety and QI efforts by providing research-based national comparative data on nursing care and the relationship to patient outcomes. Many of the NDNQI indicators are NQF-endorsed measures and are part of the NQF's nursing-sensitive measure set (see Box 2.5). The NDNQI allows additional comparisons of indicators such as nurse job satisfaction, RN education, and certification with adverse patient events such as pressure ulcers, psychiatric patient assaults, and pediatric intravenous infiltration rates. A high-quality work environment, as evidenced by reported job enjoyment and intent to stay, positively affects NDNQI key performance indicators such as patient safety, patient experiences, nurse outcomes, and hospital payment programs. Nursing has been a leader in the information system field by developing standardized nursing classification systems. The availability of standardized nursing data

---

BOX 2.5 Examples of NDNQI Quality Indicators

- Catheter-associated urinary tract infections (CAUTIs)
- Central line–associated bloodstream infections (CLABSIs)
- Patient falls
- Pressure injuries
- Ventilator-associated pneumonia (VAP)
- Ventilator-associated events (VAEs)

enables the study of health problems across populations, settings, and caregivers. Consistent use of standardized language enhances the process of QI and also demonstrates the contributions of nursing to lawmakers, healthcare policy makers, and the public.

Although the NDNQI is nursing specific, the AHRQ (n.d.) reports quality indicators that measure hospital quality and safety performance across disciplines and at the systems level. The AHRQ includes Patient Safety Indicators, a set of hospital-level indicators of safety-related adverse events, as well as Inpatient Quality Indicators and Pediatric Quality Indicators, sets of hospital-level measures of quality for patients.

Three leading nursing classification systems have been identified: The North American Nursing Diagnosis Association International's (NANDA-I) nomenclature (Herdman et al., 2021); the Nursing Intervention Classification (NIC) system (Bulechek et al., 2019); and the Nursing Outcomes Classification (NOC) system (Moorhead et al., 2018). The use of standardized nursing terminologies such as NANDA-I, NIC, and NOC provides a means of collecting and analyzing nursing data and evaluating nursing-sensitive outcomes.

Each classification system focuses on one component of the nursing process. Nursing diagnoses can be labeled using NANDA-I. These diagnosis labels represent clinical judgments about actual or potential health problems. Each diagnosis contains a definition, major and minor defining characteristics, and related factors. Accurate nursing diagnoses guide the selection of nursing interventions to achieve the desired treatment effects, determine nursing-sensitive outcomes, and ensure patient safety (Herdman et al., 2021).

The NIC system consists of interventions that represent both general and specialty nursing practice. Each intervention includes a label, definition, and set of activities that nurses perform to carry it out. For example, pain management is defined and specific activities are listed to alleviate pain or reduce the pain to a level that is acceptable to the patient (Bulechek et al., 2019).

The NOC system consists of outcomes that focus on the patient. It includes patient states, behavior, and perceptions that are sensitive to nursing interventions. Each outcome includes a definition, a five-point scale for rating outcome status over time, and a set of specific indicators to be used in rating the outcomes (Moorhead et al., 2018). Clinical testing for validation and refinement has occurred in various settings. The standardization of

terms continues to develop to reflect current knowledge and changes in nurses' roles and the structure of healthcare systems. The consistency of terms is essential in providing a large database across healthcare settings to predict resource requirements and establish outcomes of care.

Select Plans

Informed by a comprehensive literature review, the team discusses various strategies and plans to meet the new outcome. One plan is selected for implementation, and the process of change begins. Because QM stresses improving the system rather than assigning blame to employees, change strategies emphasize open communication and education of workers affected by the new standard and outcome. QI is impossible without continual education of all managers and followers.

Policies and procedures may need to be written or rewritten during the QI process. Policies should be reviewed frequently and updated so that they reflect best practice standards and do not become barriers to innovation. Communication about the change or improvement is essential (Fig. 2.6).

Evaluate

As the plan is implemented, the team continues to gather and evaluate data to document whether the new outcomes are being met. If an outcome is not met, revisions in the implementation plan are needed. Sometimes, improvement in one part of a system presents new

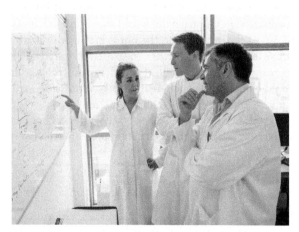

Fig. 2.6 Diagramming a patient-care process in detail can reveal gaps and opportunities for improvement. (Copyright © Wavebreakmedia/iStock/Thinkstock.)

problems. For example, nurses implemented screening for suicide risk in adolescents and adults presenting to the emergency department. A result of this improvement in care was a greatly increased number of referrals for counseling, which overwhelmed the existing hospital and community resources. The interprofessional team may need to reassemble periodically to handle the inevitable obstacles that develop with the implementation of any new process or procedure. Furthermore, individuals outside the organization (external customers) may need to be included in the process. The example that follows also illustrates this idea.

A hospital is implementing a pneumatic tube system to dispense medications. An interprofessional team is assembled to discuss the process from various viewpoints: pharmacy, nursing, pneumatic tube operation managers, aides who take the medications from the pneumatic tube to the patient medication drawers, administrators, and physicians. The tube system is implemented. A nurse on one unit realizes that several patients do not have their morning medications in their medication drawers. The nurse borrows medications from another patient's drawer and orders the rest of the medications "stat" from pharmacy. Other nurses on that unit and other units have the same problem and are taking the same or similar actions. Several problems are occurring—some of the medications are being given late, nurses waste precious time searching other medication drawers, the pharmacy charges extra for the stat medications and is overwhelmed with stat requests, and the situation increases the nurses' frustration level. In some cases, patients suffer because of late administration of medications. QM principles would encourage the nurses to report the problems to the nurse manager or appropriate team member. Further, the patients' charges likely increase the hospital bill. The pneumatic tube team could compile data such as frequency of missing medications, timing of medication orders, and nursing units involved. The problems are analyzed with a system perspective to solve the late medication problem effectively.

> **EXERCISE 2.4** Identify the ethical and moral implications of "borrowing" another patient's medication until it can be replaced by a stat order.

In some organizations, when a change is implemented successfully, the QI team disbands. One of the crucial tasks of the nurse manager is to publicize and reward the success of each QI team. The nurse manager must also evaluate the work of the team and the ability of individual team members to work together effectively.

Some organizations that have used the QM philosophy for several years establish permanent QI teams or committees. These QI teams do not disband after implementing one project or idea. Rather, they may meet regularly to focus on improvements in specific areas of patient care. The use of permanent QI teams or the adoption of a culture driven by QM can provide continuity and prevent duplication of efforts within the quality teams.

QM organizations stress system-level change and the evaluation of outcomes. However, in recent years, the need for process and performance improvement, including individual performance appraisal, has re-emerged within healthcare organizations. Peer review and self-evaluation are performance assessment methods that fit within the QM philosophy.

In addition to using QI to improve overall team performance, any nurse can use the six steps of the QI process to self-evaluate and improve individual performance. For example, a nurse on a medical unit who wants to improve documentation skills might study past entries on patient records; review current institution policies, professional standards, and literature related to documentation; set specific performance improvement goals after consultation with the nurse manager and expert colleagues; devise strategies and a timeline for achieving performance goals; and, after implementing the strategies, review documentation entries to see whether self-improvement goals have been met.

QUALITY ASSURANCE

Although QI is a comprehensive process to prevent problems, total abandonment of periodic inspection would be naïve. One method used to monitor health care is quality assurance (QA) programs, which ensure conformity to a standard. QA focuses on clinical aspects of the provider's care, often in response to an identified problem. Many QA activities focus on process standards (e.g., documentation, adherence to practice standards). The focus may be asking questions such as "Did the nurse document the response to the pain medication within the required time period?" instead of "Did the patient receive adequate pain relief postoperatively?" In

TABLE 2.3 Comparison of Traditional Quality Assurance and Quality Improvement Processes

	Quality Assurance (QA) Process	Quality Improvement (QI) Process
Goal	To improve quality	To improve quality
Focus	Discovery and correction of errors	Prevention of errors
Major tasks	Inspection of nursing activities Chart audits	Review of nursing activities Innovation Professional development
Quality team	QA personnel or department personnel	Interprofessional team
Outcomes	Set by QA team with input from staff	Set by QI team with input from staff and patients

contrast, QI may examine process, structure, and outcome standards. The similarities and differences between QA and QI are summarized in Table 2.3.

One of the methods most often used in QA is chart review or chart auditing. Chart audits may be conducted using the records of active or discharged patients. Charts are selected randomly and reviewed by qualified healthcare professionals. In an internal audit, staff members from the same hospital or agency that generated the records examine the data. External auditors are qualified professionals from outside the organization who conduct the review. An audit tool containing specific criteria based on standards of care is applied to each chart under review. For example, auditors might compare documentation related to use of restraints for medical-surgical purposes with the criterion "Licensed independent practitioner evaluates patient in person within 4 hours of application." Auditors note compliance or lack of compliance with each audit criterion and report a summary of these findings to the appropriate manager or committee for corrective action.

Because the focus of the chart audit is on detecting errors and determining the person responsible for

them, many staff members tend to view QA negatively. The nurse manager must reinforce that QA is not intended to be punitive but instead is an opportunity to improve patient care at the unit level. For example, to reinforce the importance of documentation, providing the standard of care for documentation and assisting the RN in reviewing several charts is an appropriate educational tool to reinforce policies and procedures or standards regarding documentation. The manager has the responsibility to communicate the importance of daily QA activities and how unit-based monitoring ties into the overall QI program. Moreover, many institutions incorporate both the participation in and the results of QA into annual performance appraisals or clinical ladders.

In collaboration with the Robert Wood Johnson Foundation (RWJF), the IHI's work, *Transforming Care at the Bedside (TCAB)*, created a framework for change on medical-surgical units built around improvements in four main categories: safe and reliable care, vitality and teamwork, patient-centered care, and value-added care processes. These small changes were designed to be tested quickly so that if failure occurred, not many resources or much time was wasted. The common core of most projects is patient safety. Further, the IHI's *Global Trigger Tool for Measuring Adverse Events* is one of the most widely used ways to determine overall level of harm to patients in a healthcare organization (more information at *www.ihi.org*).

Choosing Wisely is a multidisciplinary approach to helping both healthcare providers and patients make wise decisions related to various care conditions (learn more at *www.choosingwisely.org/*). The Choosing Wisely campaign is an initiative of the American Board of Internal Medicine (ABIM) Foundation to encourage conversations between patients and their healthcare professionals about what care is genuinely necessary. The American Academy of Nursing adopted this strategy as a major way to influence patients and their health, and to promote quality and safety.

EXERCISE 2.5 Review the Choosing Wisely website (www.choosingwisely.org) and review recommendations for graduated compression stockings in surgical patients for preventing venous thromboembolism (VTE) after surgery. Consider whether the suggestions found at Choosing Wisely reflect your local practices. If not, what are the differences? What ideas do you have about the reason for these differences?

RISK MANAGEMENT

Every year, The Joint Commission creates specific goals for specific settings. Introduced as safety goals for hospitals, these statements have expanded to other settings, such as critical access hospitals and to clinical specialties, such as behavioral health. These goals are based on an analysis of issues pertinent to the specific focus. Box 2.6 identifies examples of goals for hospitals for 2021.

QM and risk management are related concepts that emphasize the achievement of quality-outcome standards and the prevention of patient-care problems. Risk management also attempts to analyze problems and minimize losses after an adverse event occurs. These losses include incurring financial loss as a result of malpractice or absorbing the cost of an extended length of stay for the patient, negative public relations, and employee dissatisfaction. Moreover, the inclusion of safety standards in TJC guidelines further emphasizes the importance of risk management. Specific goals exist for hospitals, ambulatory, behavioral health, critical access hospital, and home care settings. For example, an additional goal of reducing the risk of patient harm resulting from falls applies to home care settings. The TJC website carries the most up-to-date patient safety goals for all patient care settings.

The risk management department has several functions, which include the following:
- Defining situations that place the system at some financial risk, such as medication errors or patient falls
- Determining the frequency of occurrence of those situations

> ## BOX 2.6 National Patient Safety Goals for Hospitals
>
> - Improve the accuracy of patient identification.
> - Improve the effectiveness of communication among caregivers.
> - Improve the safety of using medications.
> - Reduce patient harm associated with clinical alarm systems.
> - Reduce the risk of healthcare–associated infections
> - The hospital identifies safety risks inherent in its patient population.
> - Prevent wrong site, wrong procedure, and wrong person surgery.
>
> Copyright © The Joint Commission, 2021b. Reprinted with permission.

- Intervening and investigating identified events
- Identifying potential risks or opportunities to improve care

Each individual nurse is a risk manager who has the responsibility to identify and report unusual occurrences and potential risks. Active involvement in quality and risk management by direct caregivers, however, is a challenge complicated by staffing issues and increased demands on the nurse. Increased nursing staffing in hospitals is associated with better care outcomes. Consistent evidence shows that more favorable RN-to-patient ratios is associated with a reduction in hospital-related mortality, failure to rescue, and other nursing-sensitive outcomes, as well as reduced length of stay. Similarly, favorable patient care environments, including improved patient-to-nurse ratios and adequate nurse staffing, are associated with lower rates of serious complications or adverse events (Aiken & Sloane, 2020). Another barrier to improving patient safety is fear of punishment, which inhibits people from acknowledging, reporting, or discussing errors. One way to minimize errors is to monitor threats to patient safety continually and to recognize that individual errors often reflect organizational and system failures. For example, targeting nurse-to-patient load and work schedules, including 12-hour shifts and overtime, can reduce potential errors from human factors such as fatigue, stress, and distractions. Rotating shifts may have a negative effect on nurses' stress levels and job performance because of sleep disruption and intershift recovery, and working longer hours may have a negative effect on patient outcomes. Understaffing, emotional exhaustion, performing nonnursing care, and tension with patients, families, and members of the interprofessional team contribute to nurses' intent to leave the profession and create a negative practice environment (Sasso et al., 2019). Nurse managers must monitor nurse fatigue and facilitate scheduling decisions (e.g., limiting extra days and overtime) to give nurses an opportunity to recuperate and to sleep on their days off since fatigue jeopardizes patient safety.

Both risk management and QM deal with changing behavior, prevention, focus on the customer, and attention to outcomes. The following clinical examples illustrate how QM and risk management complement each other. First, the implementation of lift teams reduces employee injuries associated with lifting heavy or fully dependent patients and simultaneously, for the patient, decreases adverse events associated with difficult transfers. The implementation of lift teams reflects managing both quality and risk. Second, adherence to the universal safety verification known as "time out" before beginning a surgical procedure ensures perioperative safety within a TQM framework. A third example, the use of teach-back, ensures that quality teaching and health literacy learning has occurred and that risks are minimized by asking patients to explain in their own words what they need to know or do. Asking a question such as, "Please tell me, what will you do to take care of yourself when you get home?" provides the nurse with an opportunity to check understanding and reteach information if needed. Although nursing managers would prefer that all staff intrinsically embrace risk management practices aimed at patient and staff safety, accountability for safety can be one aspect of performance evaluations. Active involvement of staff in risk management activities is key to prevention of adverse events. Nurse managers should conduct safety rounds and praise employees for using safe practice as part of best practice standards. This philosophy reinforces that risk management not only benefits the patient but also works to keep individual employees safe in the workplace.

Adverse-event reduction is a key strategy for reducing healthcare mortality and morbidity because patients who suffer adverse events are at risk of death or permanent disability. Nurses have always played a pivotal role in the prevention of adverse events and can reduce negative outcomes with a focus on accurate assessment, early identification, and correction of potentially adverse situations. Also, adherence to best practice standards and ensuring quality standards for high-risk/high-volume practices (e.g., restraint use, medication reconciliation) can reduce adverse events. The NQF and CMS define never events as errors in medical care that are clearly identifiable, preventable, and serious in their consequences for patients and that indicate a real problem in the safety and credibility of a healthcare facility. Examples of never events (or events that should never happen) include surgery on the wrong body part, a foreign body left in a patient after surgery, mismatched blood transfusion, a major medication error, a severe pressure ulcer acquired in the hospital, and preventable postoperative deaths. Now that many third-party payers are following the CMS lead in withholding payment for preventable complications of care, no member of the healthcare team can fail to recognize the implications of quality care in their organization's overall success. In contrast to never events, always events should occur

100% of the time and include healthcare actions such as hand hygiene and accurate patient identification.

A comprehensive quality and risk program would proactively identify and reduce risks to patient safety through completion of a failure mode and effects analysis (FMEA) on select high-risk situations as advanced by TJC. FMEA is a systematic, proactive method for evaluating a process to identify where and how it might fail and to assess the relative impact of different failures to identify the parts of the process that are most in need of change. Nurses should be able to recognize near misses and sentinel events and participate with an interprofessional team in the root-cause analysis. A sentinel event is a serious, unexpected occurrence involving death or severe physical or psychological harm, such as inpatient suicide, infant abduction, or wrong-site surgery. Similarly, a near miss is an unplanned event that did not result in injury, illness, or damage but had the potential to do so. A near miss highlights an imminent problem that must be corrected and can provide useful lessons in terms of risk analysis and reduction. TJC calls for voluntary self-reporting of sentinel events by both inpatient institutions and home health agencies and announces sentinel events via news releases when the events apply to other organizations. See Box 2.7 for the most common sentinel events reported in healthcare. After a sentinel event is identified, a root-cause analysis is performed by a team that includes those directly involved in the event and those in leadership positions. This process is very similar to the QI process described in this chapter except that the root-cause analysis is a retrospective review of an incident to identify the sequence of events with the goal of identifying the root causes. The root-cause analysis leads to the development

---

BOX 2.7 Most Common Healthcare Sentinel Events (2020)

- Fall
- Unintended retention of a foreign object
- Suicide
- Wrong-site surgery
- Assault/rape/sexual assault
- Fire
- Clinical alarm response
  - Self-harm
  - Medication management

of specific risk reduction strategies; in certain situations, the plan must be reported to TJC.

Whereas reporting to TJC illustrates external reporting to regulatory or accrediting agencies, an internal method of communicating risks or adverse events is through electronic safety reporting systems or incident reporting. Incident reports are kept separate from the patient's medical record and should serve as a means of communicating an incident that caused or could have caused harm to patients, family members, visitors, or employees. Aggregated incident reports should be used to improve quality of care and decrease future risk. Trending data can illuminate systems issues that need to be modified to reduce risk and achieve quality patient care. Although an incident report may not be warranted for a unit-specific problem or an interdepartmental issue in which no adverse event occurred (e.g., delay in diagnosis or treatment), communication at the appropriate chain of command is essential to improve quality. Nurse managers are often responsible for investigating and remedying each identified hazard, which can result in safety being approached in a reactionary and overly narrow way. An effective approach to developing a high-reliability organization, a healthcare agency that employs best practices for quality care and patient safety, must use a systems perspective that allows the manager to look beyond the individual nurse and focus on the entire practice environment (Sherwood, 2019).

Evaluating Risks

In gathering data about unusual occurrences, the risk management team may involve perspectives from numerous disciplines to discover underlying problems that a single discipline might miss. Risk managers also use multiple data sources, data collection techniques, and perspectives to collect and interpret the data. Quantitative methods such as questionnaires or records of medication administration can be combined with qualitative methods such as open-ended question interviews. Actionable plans for reducing the incidence of common preventable adverse events such as medication administration errors (wrong patient, time, dose, drug, or mode of delivery) could result from assessment and analysis of both quantitative and qualitative data. Quality and risk strategies aimed at targeting high-volume and high-risk occurrences are essential. Moreover, accountability for quality efforts to third-party payers, including the federal government, on programs such as pay-for-performance, in which healthcare

systems receive additional payment incentives if specific quality targets are achieved, and public reporting, in which quality data are made available for comparison, has significant implications for nurses. Opportunities include participation on QI teams, data collection, and involvement in the implementation of quality initiatives.

However, recognizing errors does not always translate into reporting errors. The lack of agreement as to what constitutes error influences the willingness of healthcare professionals to report errors and subsequently affects whether they develop strategies that could reduce future risk. A lack of consensus exists regarding whether patients and families should be informed about healthcare errors. Building an organizational culture of quality and safety may have implicit or explicit pressure to achieve performance standards, particularly those that are publically reported or linked to payment (Bliss et al., 2020).

Approaches to patient safety and risk management require healthcare providers to challenge their attitudes that errors are an unfortunate but inevitable part of patient care. Diminished resources and challenges in the work environment have the potential to compromise communication among providers and to contribute to an environment in which unsafe practices are overlooked or excused. For example, communication errors between nurses and other healthcare providers may result from hurried exchanges in crowded hallways or in the midst of a busy nursing station. Breakdown in communication among healthcare professionals is the most common cause of serious injuries and death in healthcare settings. Not surprisingly, each of the National Patient Safety Goals is directly or indirectly related to communication. Use of common language when communicating critical information helps prevent misunderstandings and creates a culture of quality and safety. **SBAR** has become a best practice for standardizing communication between healthcare providers. SBAR stands for situation, background, assessment, and recommendation (IHI, 2022b). Because adverse patient outcomes commonly are a result of communication failures, The Joint Commission's National Patient Goals added standardization of hand-off communication, the verbal and written exchange of pertinent information during transitions of care. A team approach to quality and risk management is needed to promote optimal outcomes. Nurses have a responsibility to provide quality care. Thus, they must serve in leadership roles to ensure a culture of integrated quality, safety, and risk management.

EXERCISE 2.6 Describe an error that occurred in the organization where you practice that resulted in harm to the patient and one that did not. If you cannot access information about an error, use one of the sentinel events cited in Box 2.7 as an example to consider. What would you suggest to prevent a reoccurrence? Decide under what circumstances you would inform the patient and family and under what circumstances you would withhold the information.

IMPACT OF CULTURAL CONCEPTS AND PRINCIPLES ON QUALITY AND SAFETY

A diverse workforce brings a richness of perspectives to quality and safety. Cultural diversity is a term used to describe a vast range of cultural differences among individuals or groups, whereas cultural sensitivity describes the affective behaviors in individuals—the capacity to feel, convey, or react to ideas, habits, customs, or traditions unique to a group of people. Cultural awareness is the self-examination and in-depth exploration of one's own cultural background and subsequent attitudes and behaviors. It involves the recognition of one's biases, prejudices, and assumptions about individuals who are different. Cultural competency is mastery of the ability to understand, appreciate, and interact with people from cultures and belief systems different from one's own. See Box 2.8 for actions in the workplace for creating diversity, equity, and inclusion.

When assessing staff and patient diversity, nurse leaders or managers can ask these questions to guide their actions:
- What is the cultural representation of the workforce? Of the patient population?

BOX 2.8   **Key Actions for Creating Diversity, Equity, and Inclusion to Support Quality and Safety in the Workforce**

- Identify and challenge unconscious biases.
- Understand team differences.
- Create a respectful practice environment.
- Provide flexible scheduling to honor cultural practices.
- Support ongoing professional development.
- Create social support systems.
- Create effective communication systems.
- Empower staff through shared governance.

- What type of team-building activities are needed to create a cohesive workforce for effective healthcare delivery?
- What awareness training and educational offerings are needed to assure quality and safety?

The ANA has a commitment to eliminating discriminatory practices against nurses as well as patients. The ANA *Code of Ethics for Nurses with Interpretive Statements* (2015) helps the nurse recognize that effective healthcare must be provided to culturally diverse populations in the United States and throughout the world. Although nurses may be inclined to impose their own cultural values on patients and staff, avoiding this affirms the respect and sensitivity for the values and healthcare practices associated with different cultures. This is reinforced by the ANA revised position statement (2016), *The Nurse's Role in Ethics and Human Rights: Protecting and Promoting Individual Worth, Dignity, and Human Rights in Practice Settings.* The value of human rights is placed at the forefront for nurses whose specific actions are to promote and protect the human rights of every individual in all practice care environments. Similar statements are made with an international emphasis, including the *Code of Ethics for Nurses* (2012) from the International Council of Nurses (ICN), which places emphasis on providing care to vulnerable populations and on nurses' professional values, such as respectfulness, responsiveness, compassion, trustworthiness, and integrity.

Throughout history, the emphasis and support has been on recipients of care, such as patients, but the same attentiveness is needed in the workforce. Patients are aware of how they are treated, and they also see how staff interact with each other.

Impact of Health Disparities on Quality and Safety

Causes of disparities in healthcare include poor education, health behaviors of the minority group, inadequate financial resources, and environmental factors. Disparities in healthcare that relate to safety and quality of care include provider–patient relationships, access to care, treatment regimens that do not necessarily reflect current evidence, provider bias and discrimination, mistrust of the healthcare system, and refusal of treatment. Disparities in disease and in healthcare services might affect the healthcare providers in the workplace in relationship to their ethnic or racial group. Increasing healthcare providers' knowledge of such disparities is necessary to more effectively manage and treat diseases related to ethnic and racial minorities.

The healthcare system in the United States has consistently focused on individuals and their health problems. It has failed, however, to recognize the religious and cultural differences, beliefs, symbolisms, and interpretations of illness of some people as a group. As healthcare moves toward provision of care for populations, culture can have an even greater influence on approaches to care. *The Future of Nursing 2020–2030: Charting a Path to Achieve Health Equity* (NAM, 2021) emphasizes how nurses can reduce health disparities and promote health equity.

Leading and managing cultural diversity in an organization means managing personal thinking and helping others think in new ways. Nursing leaders need a workforce that can provide culturally competent care—in essence, not having this can lead to unsafe care. In addition, nursing's goal is to create a workforce that reflects the population it serves. This diversity can occur across roles, including advanced practice registered nurses, managers, and chief nurse executives.

Although the literature has addressed multicultural needs of patients, it is sparse in identifying effective methods for nurse managers to use when working with multicultural staff. Differences in education and culture can impede patient care, and jeopardize quality and safety. For example, staff members may be reluctant to admit language problems that hamper their written communication. They may also be reluctant to admit their lack of understanding when interpreting directions. Psychosocial skills may be problematic as well, because many non-Westernized countries encourage emotional restraint. Staff may have difficulty addressing issues that relate to private family matters. The lack of assertiveness and the subservient physician–nurse relationships of some cultures are other issues that provide challenges for nurse managers. Unit-oriented workshops arranged by the nurse manager to address effective assertive techniques and family involvement as it relates to cultural differences are two ways of assisting staff with cultural work situations. Respecting cultural diversity in the team fosters cooperation and supports sound decision-making, improving quality of care.

Nurse leaders and managers who ascribe to a positive view of culture and its characteristics effectively acknowledge cultural diversity among patients and staff. This includes providing culturally sensitive care to patients while simultaneously balancing a culturally diverse staff. For example, cultural diversity might mean being sensitive to or being able to embrace the emotions of a large multicultural group comprising staff and patients. Unless we understand the differences, we cannot come together and make decisions that are in the best interest of the patient. Culture must be construed more broadly to include differences in health beliefs and practices by race, color, ethnicity, national origin, economic status, sex, gender identity or expression, sexual orientation, age, religion, and disability or physical challenge. To understand and value diversity, nurse managers need to approach every staff person and every patient as an individual. Failure to address cultural diversity leads to negative effects on performance and staff interactions as well as on quality and safety.

DEALING EFFECTIVELY WITH CULTURAL DIVERSITY

The first individuals in most organizational structures who have to address cultural diversity are the leaders and managers. They have to give unwavering support to embracing diversity in the workplace rather than using a standard cookie-cutter approach. Creating a culturally sensitive work environment involves a long-term vision and financial and healthcare provider commitment. Leaders and managers need to make the strategic decision to design services and programs especially to meet the needs of diverse cultural, ethnic, and racial differences of staff and patients. Policies in healthcare organizations prohibit discrimination based on several aspects. Such policies, however, do not necessarily succeed at promoting a culturally aware environment. One benefit of creating a culturally aware environment is the opportunity to address the question of how people see workplace psychological safety. It is often influenced culturally and the opportunity to discuss safety from different perspectives enriches everyone's understanding of a broader societal context as well.

Nurse managers hold the key to making the best use of cultural diversity. Managers have positions of power to begin programs that enrich the diversity among staff. For example, capitalizing on the knowledge that all staff bring something unique to the patient promotes better quality care outcomes. One method that can be used is to allow staff to verbalize their feelings about particular cultures in relationship to personal beliefs. Another is to have two or three staff members of different ethnic origins present a patient-care conference, giving their views on how they would care for a specific patient's needs based on their own ethnic values. Even in organizations where no organizational strategy is evident, a nurse manager and committed team can be effective in improving their cultural competency. Addressing the potential for structural racism is another example of creating a diverse view of the workplace.

IMPLICATIONS IN THE WORKPLACE

Embracing cultural differences will also enhance the QSEN initiative. The overall goal of the QSEN initiative is to prepare nurses with the knowledge, skills, and attitudes (KSAs) needed to continuously deliver quality and safe patient care. With this initiative, we see the need to respect all patients and staff irrespective of their cultural differences to empower patient- and family-centered care, which is one of the QSEN initiative competencies. This component recognizes the patient or designee as the source of control and full partner in providing compassionate and coordinated care based on respect for a patient's preferences, values, and needs.

All nurses, regardless of their titles or positions, have a role in improving the workplace and patient care by attending to the implications of culture in healthcare. Because the culture of the workplace has been shown to be highly influential in people's perception of their work and their intent to stay, being sensitive to what else could be done to enhance the workplace, including inclusion, has potential for positive outcomes.

CONCLUSION

Nurses are key to creating a culture of quality and safety (IHI, 2022a). Every nurse must challenge any act that appears unsafe and stop actions that are not in the patient's best interest. Being proactive is insufficient in itself; examining practices and conditions that support errors is critical, as is sharing knowledge that can change practice. In this challenging context, nurses continue to provide care and the organizational foundation that supports patient care performed in a safe, effective, and efficient manner. Nurses who serve as leaders and managers have additional opportunities to create conditions in which ideas are heard, problems are solved, and the best evidence is used. Everyone in an organization must be invested in quality and safety; nurses play a crucial role in quality improvement, quality management, and quality assurance. As organizations addressed system errors, supporting organized quality and safety programs became even more important. Being able to address both clinical and system issues of risk contributes to improved quality. Frontline nurses must become aware of the work that happens at executive levels in their agencies and at the national and international level on behalf of patient safety. Creating a positive environment, ensuring appropriate staffing and equipment, intervening and supporting others in doing so in cases of incivility, and supporting the use of the best evidence in practice all create a safer patient environment. Inequities in healthcare access and delivery require emphasis on how culture impacts care; healthcare agencies must invest in inclusive environments to improve the quality and safety of healthcare for all.

THE SOLUTION

To decrease wait times, the triage process was modified. Here is what we did. After the patient enters the ED, the patient is sent to the triage area where the nurse and physician simultaneously evaluate and triage the patient. The team determines level of acuity and the provider then can place orders promptly. Laboratory work is complete in triage, and the patient is taken to imaging, if required, which decreases wait time and gets care to the patient promptly. If the patient is noncritical then the patient is sent to a new area of the department, the Vertical Transition Unit (VTU). While in the VTU area, the patient is further evaluated by a medical provider and further testing, small procedures, or imaging is completed. The patient is then sent back to the waiting room to await results. VTU is an important area of the department as it provides prompt care to noncritical patients and saves beds in the department for critical patients. The waiting room was also redesigned and covered outdoor seating was provided to account for times when the department is busy and patients are unable to be triaged promptly. The entire ED was involved in the process change and communication among all staff—nurses, physicians, and paramedics—was key to creating a smooth transition to the new system. The process change resulted in decreased wait times and quicker discharges, which ultimately allowed for more people to be seen and more beds available for sick patients.

Would this be a suitable approach for you? Why?

Emily Lezcano

REFLECTIONS

What issues related to safety and quality have you seen in a clinical setting? Were you comfortable with the actions taken to improve care? How will you use the material from this chapter to promote quality and reduce risk with the patients for whom you provide care? Write a one-paragraph summary with a specific example.

BEST PRACTICES

A growing body of literature exists that links the hospital practice environment with safety and quality of care. A strong correlation has been established between practice environments and nurse outcomes, including nurse job satisfaction, burnout, and intent to leave, as well as patient outcomes, including mortality and failure to rescue. Increased nurse staffing is associated with reduced patient mortality, reduced failure to rescue, and decreased length of stay. Nurses report more positive job experiences and fewer concerns about quality care, whereas patients had a significantly lower risk of death and failure to rescue in hospitals with better care environments, the best nurse staffing levels, and the most highly educated nurses. Similarly, missed cares that jeopardize quality and safety in nursing homes are associated with nurse burnout and decreased job satisfaction. A best practice would be to look at the data that a hospital might have related to these factors to determine whether it is a positive work environment for quality patient care.

Nurse specialty certification and baccalaureate education have consistently been associated with better patient outcomes. Staffing levels are an important predictor of nurse-assessed risks, including nursing-sensitive outcomes. Empowering nurses and adequately resourcing practice environments to support patient care enhances job satisfaction and nursing retention.

Nurse managers and leaders have several options for improving nurse retention and patient outcomes, including improving RN staffing, moving to a more educated nurse workforce, and facilitating a positive care environment. Hospitals with practice environments that include investment in development of staff, QM, and good nurse–physician relations (e.g., Magnet® designation) are associated with better nurse and patient outcomes. Nurse managers who promote an empowered workplace and facilitate teamwork support higher-quality care, less patient risk, and more satisfied nurses. Investment in practice settings that promote diversity, equity, and inclusion has great potential to improve quality, assure safety, and reduce risk. Again, these are factors to consider in evaluating places to work when concerned about quality of care.

TIPS FOR PROMOTING QUALITY AND SAFETY

- Use the NAM (formally IOM) recommendatons to frame your actions.
- Keep current with the evidence and best practices.
- Be prepared to intervene in unsafe situations.
- Embrace that anything measured and recorded can be improved.
- Concentrate QI energies on factors that are most important to patient quality and safety.
- Collaborating to prevent problems is more effective than fixing problems after they occur.
- Listen for differences and seek clarity.
- Value diversity, equity, and inclusion.
- Be proactive in creating a culturally competent workplace.

REFERENCES

Agency for Healthcare Research and Quality. (2018). *TeamSTEPPS 2.0. American Nurses Association.* Retrieved from https://www.ahrq.gov/teamstepps/instructor/index.html.

Agency for Healthcare Research and Quality. (n.d.). Quality indicators. https://qualityindicators.ahrq.gov/.

Aiken, L. H., & Sloane, D. M. (2020). Nurses matter: More evidence. *British Medical Journal Quality and Safety, 29,* 1–3.

American Nurses Association (ANA). (2015). *Code of ethics for nurses with interpretative statements.* MD: Silver Spring. nursesbooks.org.

American Nurses Association (ANA). (2016). *The nurse's role in ethics and human rights: Protecting and promoting individual worth, dignity, and human rights in practice settings.* MD: Silver Spring. nursesbooks.org.

Arnetz, B., Goetz, C., Arnetz, J., Sudan, S., vonSchagen, J., & Piersma, K. (2020). *Enhancing health care efficiency to achieve the Quadruple Aim: An exploratory study.* NCBI Resources. 13. Retrieved from https://www.ncbi.nlm.nih.gov/pmc/articles/PMC7393915/.

Bliss, K., Chambers, M., & Rabur, B. (2020). Building a culture of safety and quality: The paradox of measurement. *Nursing Economic$, 38*(4), 178–184.

Boylan, M. R., Suchman, K. I., Korolikova, H., Slover, J. D., & Bosco, J. A. (2019). Association of Magnet nursing status with hospital performance on nationwide quality metrics. *Journal of Healthcare Quality, 41*(4), 189–194.

Bragadóttir, H., Kalisch, B. J., & Bergthóra Tryggvadóttir, G. (2019). The extent to which adequacy of staffing predicts nursing teamwork in hospitals. *Journal of Clinical Nursing, 28*(23–24), 4298–4309.

Brooks Carthon, J. M., Hatfield, L., Plover, C., Dierkes, A., Davis, L., Hedgeland, T., Sanders, A. M., Visco, F., Holland, S., Ballinghoff, J., Del Guidice, M., & Aiken, L. H. (2019). Association of nurse engagement and nurse staffing on patient safety. *Journal of Nursing Care Quality, 34*(1), 40–46.

Bulechek, G. M., Butcher, H. K., Dochtermann, J. M., & Wagner, C. M. (2019). *Nursing interventions classification (NIC)* (7th ed.). St. Louis, MO: Elsevier.

Cengiz, A., & Yoder, L. H. (2020). Assessing nursing students' perceptions of the QSEN competencies: A systemic review of the literature with implications for academic programs. *Worldviews on Evidence-Based Nursing, 17*(4), 275–282.

Centers for Medicare & Medicaid Services (CMS). (2021). *Hospital compare.* Retrieved from https://www.cms.gov/Medicare/Quality-Initiatives-Patient-Assessment-Instruments/HospitalQualityInits/HospitalCompare.

Centers for Medicare & Medicaid Services (CMS). (2021b). *HCAHPS: Patients' Perspectives of Care Survey.* Retrieved from https://www.cms.gov/Medicare/Quality-Initiatives-Patient-Assessment-Instruments/HospitalQualityInits/HospitalHCAHPS.

DNV Healthcare. (2022). *Hospital accreditation.* Retrieved from https://www.dnvglhealthcare.com/accreditations/hospital-accreditation.

Drew, J., & Pandit, M. (2020). Why healthcare leadership should embrace quality improvement. *The British Medical Journal (Quality Improvement Supplement),* 49–51.

Djukic, M., Stimpfel, A. W., & Kovner, C. (2019). Bachelor's degree nurse graduates report better quality and safety educational preparedness than associate degree graduates. *The Joint Commission Journal on Quality and Patient Safety, 45*(3), 180–186.

GoLeanSixSigma. (n.d.). DMAIC — The 5 phases of Lean Six Sigma. Retrieved from https://goleansixsigma.com/dmaic-five-basic-phases-of-lean-six-sigma/.

Harrison, J. M., Aiken, L. H., Sloane, D. M., Brooks Carthon, J. M., Merchant, R. M., Berg, R. A., & McHugh, M. D. (2019). In hospitals with more nurses who have baccalaureate degrees, better outcomes for patients after cardiac arrest. *Health Affairs, 38*(7), 1087–1094.

Havaei, F., MacPhee, M., & Dahinten, V. S. (2019). Effect of nursing care delivery models on registered nurse outcomes. *Journal of Advanced Nursing, 75*(10), 2144–2155.

Herdman, T. H., Kamitsura, S., & Lopes, C. T. (2021). *NANDA International: Nursing diagnoses: Definitions and classifications 2021–2023* (12th ed.). New York: Thieme Medical Publishers.

Institute for Healthcare Improvement (IHI). (2022a). *Develop a culture of safety.* Retrieved from www.ihi.org/resources/Pages/Changes/DevelopaCultureofSafety.aspx.

Institute for Healthcare Improvement (IHI). (2022b). *SBAR tool: Situation-background-assessment-recommendation.* Retrieved from http://www.ihi.org/resources/Pages/Tools/SBARToolkit.aspx.

Institute for Healthcare Improvement (IHI). (2022c). *Transforming care at the bedside.* Retrieved from http://www.ihi.org/sites/search/pages/results.aspx?k=transforming+care+at+the+bedside.

Institute for Healthcare Improvement (IHI). (2022d). *Triple aim for populations.* http://www.ihi.org/Topics/TripleAim/Pages/default.aspx.

Institute of Medicine (IOM). (2000). *To err is human: Building a safer health system.* Washington, DC: National Academies Press.

Institute of Medicine (IOM). (2001). *Crossing the quality chasm: A new health system for the 21st century.* Washington, DC: National Academies Press.

Institute of Medicine (IOM). (2003). *Health professions education: A bridge to quality.* Washington, DC: National Academies Press.

Institute of Medicine (IOM). (2004). *Keeping patients safe: Transforming the work environment of nurses.* Washington, DC: National Academies Press.

Institute of Medicine (IOM). (2010). *The future of nursing: Leading change, advancing health.* Washington, DC: National Academies Press.

International Council of Nurses. (2012). *The ICN code of ethics for nurses.* Geneva, Switzerland: Author.

Moorhead, S., Johnson, M., Maas, M., & Swanson, E. (2018). *Nursing outcomes classification (NOC)* (6th ed.). St. Louis, MO: Elsevier.

Peimbert-García, R. E., Matis, T., & Cuevas-Ortuño, J. (2020). *Systematic review of literature on Lean and Six Sigma in healthcare and directions for future research. In Proceedings of the International Conference on Industrial Engineering and Operations Management.* Dubai: UAE.

McKenzie, L., Shaw, L., Jordan, J. E., Alexander, M., O'Brien, M., Singer, S. J., & Manias, E. (2019). Factors influencing the implementation of a hospital-wide intervention to promote professionalism and build a safety culture: A qualitative study. *Joint Commission Journal on Quality and Patient Safety, 45*(10), 694–705.

Mundy, S., Cooper, L. S., & Mate, K. S. (2022). The quintuple aim for health care improvement a new imperative to advance health equity. *JAMA, 327*(5), 521–522.

National Academy of Medicine (NAM). (2021). *The future of nursing 2020-2030: Charting a path to achieve health equity.* Retrieved from https://nam.edu/publications/the-future-of-nursing-2020-2030/.

Press Ganey. (2020). *National database of nursing quality indicators. Press Ganey.* Retrieved from https://www.healthlinks.me/web/ndnqi.html.

QSEN Institute. (2020). *Competencies.* Retrieved from http://qsen.org/competencies/pre-licensure-ksas/.

Rogers, E. M. (2003). *Diffusion of innovations* (5th ed.). New York, NY: Simon & Schuster.

Sherwood, G. (2019). A global call to action: Cultivating a safety mindset. *International Nursing Review, 66*(1), 1–3.

Sasso, L., Bagnasco, A., Catania, G., Zanini, M., Aleo, G., & Watson, R. (2019). Push and pull factors of nurses' intention to leave. *Journal of Nursing Management, 27*(5), 946–954.

The Joint Commission (TJC). (2021a). *Accountability measures.* Retrieved from https://www.jointcommission.org/measurement/measures/.

The Joint Commission (TJC). (2021b). *2021 Hospital national patient safety goals.* Retrieved from https://www.jointcommission.org/-/media/tjc/documents/standards/national-patient-safety-goals/2021/simplified-2021-hap-npsggoals-final-11420.pdf.

The Joint Commission (TJC). (2021c). *Sentinal events statistics released for 2020.* Retrieved from https://www.jointcommission.org/resources/news-and-multimedia/newsletters/newsletters/joint-commission-online/march-24-2021/sentinel-event-statistics-released-for-2020/.

White, E. M., Aiken, L. H., Sloane, D. M., & McHugh, M. D. (2020). Nursing home work environment, care quality, registered nurse burnout and job dissatisfaction. *Geriatric Nursing, 41*(2), 158–164.

Wynendaele, H., Willems, R., & Trybou, J. (2019). Systematic review: Association between the patient–nurse ratio and nurse outcomes in acute care hospitals. *Journal of Nursing Management, 27*(5), 896–917.

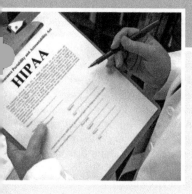

3

Ethical and Legal Issues in Nursing

Arica Brandford

ANTICIPATED LEARNING OUTCOMES

- Apply the principles included in state nurse practice acts, including scope of practice and unprofessional conduct.
- Apply various legal principles when acting in leading and managing roles in nursing practice settings.
- Evaluate informed-consent issues, including patients' rights in research and health literacy, from a nurse manager's perspective.
- Analyze how employment laws benefit professional nursing practice.
- Analyze ethical principles and codes and institutional policies that influence nursing practice.
- Apply best practices to assist staff in addressing legal and ethical situations, particularly when the law and ethics overlap.

KEY TERMS

apparent agency
autonomy
beneficence
code of ethics
bill of rights
breach of the duty
causation
confidentiality
corporate liability
damages
duty
employment laws
ethical considerations
failure to warn

fidelity
harm
health literacy
indemnification
independent contractor
informed consent
justice
law
liability
liable
licensure
medical
medical malpractice
moral distress

negligence
non-maleficence
nurse practice act
paternalism
personal liability
privacy
respect for others
respondeat superior
standard of care
statute
unprofessional conduct
veracity
vicarious liability
whistleblowing

THE CHALLENGE

In my role as a staff nurse in a busy Level 1 trauma emergency center, staff members are often confronted with questions about family presence during lifesaving techniques. Should the family or other loved ones be allowed to be present during cardiopulmonary resuscitation? Did the presence of family members hinder the ability of staff members to provide appropriate and competent care? Did their presence in some way benefit the patient? Was there a legal right for family members to be present during this time?

The issue of family presence was being addressed on a case-by-case basis. The primary healthcare professional has the final say in whether family (1) can be present,

(2) are given the option of being present, or (3) are tactfully escorted to another area of the unit. I continued to be ambivalent, especially when an 18-month-old girl was transported to the emergency center after falling from the family boat into a lake. Cardiopulmonary resuscitation was being given as the child was admitted; her mother was with her and her father was coming with other family members. The mother was escorted to the waiting area, crying, "I want to be with my baby!"

What would you do if you were this nurse?

Acacia Syring, BSN, RN
Staff Nurse Emergency Center, PeaceHealth Southwest Washington Medical Center, Vancouver, Washington

INTRODUCTION

The role of professional nursing continues to expand and incorporate increasingly higher levels of expertise, specialization, autonomy, and accountability from both legal and ethical perspectives. This evolving role continually creates new concerns for nurses, nurse managers, and nurse leaders and a heightened awareness of the interaction of legal and ethical principles. Areas of concern include professional nursing practice, legal issues, ethical principles, labor–management interactions, and employment. Each of these areas are addressed in this chapter. Although this chapter emphasizes the perspective of the nurse manager, all nurses benefit from understanding the legal and ethical aspects of managing, if only to understand the guidelines their managers are, or should be, following. Furthermore, all nurses have accountability for their practice and compliance with laws, professional standards, and ethical principles.

PROFESSIONAL NURSING PRACTICE: NURSE PRACTICE ACTS

The scope of nursing practice, those actions and duties that are allowable by the profession, is defined and guided by each state in the nurse practice act. The state nurse practice act, which is controlled through legislative action and approved (or vetoed) by the governor, is the most important piece of legislation for nursing because it affects all facets of nursing practice. Furthermore, the act is the law within a state or U.S. territory, and state boards of nursing cannot grant exceptions, waive the act's provisions, or expand practice outside the act's specific provisions.

Nurse practice acts define three categories of nurses: licensed practical or vocational nurses (LPNs and LVNs, respectively), licensed registered nurses (RNs), and advanced practice registered nurses (APRNs) including certified registered nurse anesthetists (CRNAs). The various state nurse practice acts set educational and examination requirements, provide for licensing of individuals who have met these requirements, and define the functions of each category of nurse, both in general and in more specific terminology. The nurse practice act must be read to ascertain what actions are allowable for the three categories of nurses. In the few states where separate acts for LPNs/LVNs, RNs, and APRNs exist, the acts must be reviewed at the same time to ensure that all allowable actions are included in one of the acts and that no overlap exists between the acts. In addition, nurse managers should understand that individual state nurse practice acts may vary among states in defining or delineating nursing practice, especially for advanced nursing roles.

Each practice act also establishes a state board of nursing. The main purpose of state boards of nursing is to ensure enforcement of the act to protect the public. The board enforces the act by regulating those practitioners who come under its provisions and preventing individuals not addressed within the act from practicing nursing. To protect the public, all those who present themselves as nurses must be licensed to practice within the state. The National Council of State Boards of Nursing (NCSBN) is a membership organization consisting of all U.S. state and territorial boards of nursing (except Puerto Rico). The NCSBN maintains a database (NURSYS) that enables states to enter and access current information regarding licensure and discipline of nurses throughout the country. The NCSBN's website features a public portion that allows individuals access to certain nonconfidential information that is valuable to the nurse manager and employer.

The various boards of nursing develop and implement rules and regulations regarding the discipline of nursing, which must be reviewed in conjunction with the nurse practice act. Often, any changes within the state's definition of nursing practice occur through modifications in the rules and regulations rather than in the act itself. This mandates that nurses and their nurse managers must periodically review both the state act and the board of nursing rules and regulations.

Because each state has its own nurse practice act and state courts have jurisdiction for the state, nurses are well advised to review and understand the provisions of the state's nurse practice act. This is especially true in the areas of diagnosis and treatment; states vary on whether nurses can diagnose and treat or merely assess and evaluate. Thus, an acceptable action in one state may be the practice of medicine in another state. This designation is particularly important when reviewing the scope of practice for licensed practical/vocational nurses and legislative limitations for advanced practice registered nurses.

The nurse practice act may state that unprofessional conduct is a violation of the statute. Deliberate definition of what constitutes unprofessional conduct is usually found in rules and regulations. Typical examples of unprofessional conduct include practicing outside of designated scope of practice, boundary issues; practicing while impaired; violating patient confidentiality; failing to supervise persons to whom nursing functions are delegated; inaccurate recording, falsifying, or altering a patient or healthcare provider record; sexual misconduct; and violating patient privacy rights via social media.

Licensure and Nursing Practice Acts

With the advent of the Nurse Licensure Compact (NLC), commonly referred to as "the Compact," the need to know and understand provisions of state nurse practice acts has become even more critical. Multistate licensure permits an RN or LPN/LVN licensed in one state to practice legally in states belonging to the NLC without obtaining additional state licenses (National Council of State Boards of Nursing, 2022). In addition to the NLC, in 2020 the NCSBN adopted the advanced practice registered nursing compact. The NCSBN developed the Model APRN Compact Legislation, which states must utilize to be eligible to join. Seven states must enact the APRN compact for it to be fully implemented. For the purposes of the law, the state nurse practice act that regulates the practice of the RN is from the state in which the client resides, not the state in which the nurse holds the license. Nurses residing in Compact states who have a Privilege to Practice may care for a patient in another Compact state. For example, a nurse in Compact state A may provide nursing care to a patient in Compact state B via a telephonic nursing advice or triage service program. Nurses practicing under provisions of the Compact work with patients in a variety of states through such electronic capabilities as telenursing, Internet applications, and telecommunications technology such as telephone triage and advice. Others work for agencies or clinics that serve patients across state borders. Many healthcare systems include facilities and practices in more than one jurisdiction. The enhanced Nurse Licensure Compact (eNLC) became effective in most U.S. jurisdictions in 2018 as requirements for a multistate practice privilege changed from the previous NLC in a concerted effort to enable all states to join. As of January 2022, thirty-nine (39) jurisdictions are a part of the eNLC (National Council of State Boards of Nursing, 2022).

All nurses must know applicable state law and use the nurse practice act for guidance and appropriate action. Nurse managers have this same basic responsibility to apply legal principles in their practice. However, they are also responsible for monitoring the practice of employees under their supervision and for ensuring that personnel maintain current and valid licensure. The NCSBN provides the employer the ability to subscribe to its E-Notify program to make nurse managers aware of nurses whose licenses are due for renewal. Subscription to E-Notify also alerts the nurse manager to any discipline the state board may have imposed on the nurse. Unless nurses and nurse managers remain current with the nurse practice act in their state or with nurse practice acts in all states in which nurse managers supervise employees, a potential for liability exists.

NEGLIGENCE AND MEDICAL MALPRACTICE

Nurse managers serve as coaches and practice experts for the nurses whom they supervise. Nurse managers must have a full appreciation for this area of the law. Negligence and malpractice continue to be the major causes of legal action brought against nurses. Managers cannot guide and counsel others unless the managers are fully knowledgeable of the components and key differences of these areas of law.

Negligence

Negligence, as defined by *Black's Law Dictionary* (2019), is the "failure to exercise the standard of care that a reasonably prudent person would have exercised in a similar situation; any conduct that falls below the legal standard established to protect others against unreasonable risk of harm, except for conduct that is intentionally, wantonly, or willfully disregardful of others' rights; the doing of what a reasonable and prudent person would not do under the particular circumstances, or the failure to do what such a person would do under the circumstances". To recover damages for negligence two standards must be met; First, the "existence of a duty on the part of the defendant to protect the plaintiff from the injury complained of, and second an injury to the plaintiff from the defendant's failure." (*Black's Law Dictionary*, 2019). Negligence applies to both the manager and the direct care nurse. Many experts equate negligence with carelessness, a deviation from the care that a reasonable person would deliver. If managers are careless in their responsibilities, they could be found negligent. The same applies to the direct care nurse. A scenario appears in Case Example Box 3.1.

Medical Malpractice

Medical Malpractice is a civil action for damages that generally arise from professional misconduct or unreasonable lack of skill. Malpractice concerns professional

CASE EXAMPLE BOX 3.1

Direct Care Nurse and Manager Scenario

The direct care nurse demonstrates behaviors consistent with substance use. The nurse's peers immediately report to the nursing manager a strong scent of alcohol coming from the nurse as well as slurred speech and movements. The nurse manager receives this information but fails to address the nurse and the suspected substance use. In the interim, after a dangerous accident occurs with a patient.

Rationale for Nursing Manager Negligence

In this scenario, the nursing manager is negligent. The nursing manager is held to the standard or reasonable care. What would a reasonably prudent nursing manager do in this situation? A reasonably prudent nurse manager in the same situation would have addressed this incident, removed, the nurse from the floor, and reported the possible impairment. It is important to remember not only does the direct care nurse has a duty/standard of care, but the nurse manager also has a duty/standard of care to protect the patient from harm due to the actions of the nurse given the information presented.

actions and is the failure of a person with professional education and skills to act in a reasonable and prudent manner. Issues of malpractice have become increasingly important to the nurse as the authority, accountability, and autonomy of nurses have increased. The same types of actions may be the basis for either negligence or malpractice, though some actions are often seen as malpractice because only the professional person would be performing the action. Specific examples include drawing blood for arterial blood gas analysis via a direct arterial puncture or initiating blood transfusions. Common allegations and/or causes of malpractice or negligence among nurses include the failure to follow standards of care, to use equipment responsibly, to document, to communicate, and to access and monitor patients (Reising, 2012; Brous, 2019; Brous, 2020).

Commonalities: Negligence and Medical Malpractice

Negligence and medical malpractice have two commonalities. Both negligence and malpractice concern actions that are a result of omission (the failure to do something that the reasonable, prudent person or nurse would have done) or commission (acting in a way that causes injury to the patient). They also concern nonintentional actions—though there is injury to a patient, the individual who caused the harm never intended to hurt the patient.

It is important to recognize that medical malpractice usually stems from a nurse's negligence to competently perform his or her job. However, not every negligent act of a nurse will constitute medical malpractice, but only when the acts or omissions complained of involve special skills not ordinarily possessed by lay persons.

Elements of Medical Malpractice

Four elements must be present in a successful medical malpractice suit. All these factors must be met before a court might find liability against the nurse and/or institution. These four elements are described in Table 3.1.

In a medical malpractice case based on negligence of a nurse, the plaintiff must establish the standard of care applicable to the nurse, a violation by the nurse of that standard of care, and a causal connection between the nurse's alleged negligence and the plaintiff's resultant injuries. *Mitter v. Touro Infirmary*, 874 So. 2d 265 (La. Ct. App. 4th Cir. 2004).

Duty/Standard of Care

The first element is duty owed to the patient, which involves (1) the existence of the duty and (2) the nature of the duty. The existence of the duty of care is generally established by showing the valid employment of

TABLE 3.1   Elements of Malpractice Examples

Elements	Examples
Duty/Standard of Care	Duty to the patient
Breach of Duty/Standard of Care	Provider breached that duty
Causation	Causal connection between the breach of duty/standard of care and actual harm/injury to the patient
Damages	Actual Harm/Injury must result in damages such as future medical needs and costs

the nurse within the institution. The nature of duty is the legal obligation nurses have to patients. These legal obligations are known as the duty of reasonable care. A nurse's conduct must be measured by that of other nurses in the same or similar locality and under similar circumstances. *Lattimore v. Dickey*, 239 Cal. App. 4th 959, 191 Cal. Rprt. 3d 766 (6th Dist. 2015). As the Literature Perspective shows, the concept of duty of care is complex, with implications. The more difficult part is to determine the nature of the duty, which involves the standard of care that represents the minimum requirements for acceptable practice or how one conducts oneself. Standards of care are

LITERATURE PERSPECTIVE

Resource: Dowie, I. (2017). Legal, ethical and professional aspects of duty of care for nurses. *Nursing Standard*, *32*(16-19), 47–52.

The author first points out that duty of care is not unique to professionals because we all have societal duties of care, such as ensuring safety when we drive or walk. Of course, because nurses, among other professionals, have specialized knowledge, they have a higher duty of care in terms of issues related to health. The author reminds us that our duty extends to the control of the environment, such as a spillage on the floor posing a hazard. When nurses leave a unit for a break and they have sought coverage for their patients by someone who was equally well qualified to provide care, they would not likely be found to have violated the principle of being fair, just, or reasonable. The author

cites how in England even not attending to such aspects as personal hygiene can be seen as a neglect of duty of care.

The distinction is made between the legal duty of care, which typically does not apply outside of the employment situation, and the ethical duty of care, which suggests we would respond in emergencies even if we were outside of our workplace and functioning primarily as a citizen.

Implications for Practice
Two key points can be derived from this article. The first is that the idea of duty of care is not a distinct consideration in the United States. The second, and perhaps more important in today's world, is that we are not legally bound to respond in emergency situations such as disasters; we are ethically expected to respond to the best of our ability.

established by reviewing the institution's policy and procedure manual, the individual's job description, and the practitioner's education and skills. Also reviewed are pertinent standards established by professional organizations, journal articles, and standing orders and protocols.

Several sources may be used to determine the applicable standard of care. The American Nurses Association (ANA), as well as a cadre of specialty nursing organizations, publishes standards for nursing practice. Accreditation standards, such as those published yearly by The Joint Commission (TJC), also assist in establishing the acceptable standard of care for healthcare facilities. In addition, many states have healthcare standards that affect individual institutions and their employees. Because these standards form the base for further controlling one's practice, nurses need to review these standards, question those that are impractical or no longer relevant in current practice and advocate for high quality, evidence-based standards that reflect safe patient care.

Nurse managers are directly responsible for ensuring that standards of care, as written in the hospital policy and procedure manuals, are current and that all nursing staff follow these standards of care. Should a standard of care be revised or changed, nurse managers must ensure that all staff members who are expected to implement this altered standard are apprised of the revised standard. If the new standard entails new skills, staff members must be educated about this revision and acquire the necessary skills before they implement the new standard. For example, if the institution alters a policy regarding a specific skill to be implemented, the nurse manager must first ensure that all nurses who will be performing this skill understand how to perform the skill safely, know possible complications that could occur and the most appropriate interventions to take should those complications occur. The nurse manager may work with others, such as clinical nurse educators, in attaining the desired outcomes.

Breach of the Duty/Standard of Care

The second element required in a medical malpractice case is breach of the duty of care owed the patient. Once the standard of care is established, the breach or falling below the standard of care is relatively easy to show. For instance, to determine the appropriate standard of care, expert witnesses give testimony in court on a case-by-case

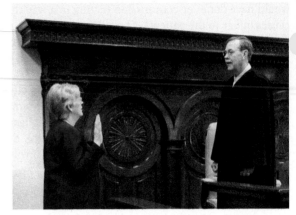

Fig. 3.1 Nurse serving as an expert witness.

basis, assisting the judge and jury in understanding nursing standards of care. In medical malpractice suits, nurses serve as expert witnesses. Their testimony helps the judge and jury understand the applicable standards of nursing care (Fig. 3.1).

Opinions of experts attesting to the standard of care may differ depending on whether the injured party is trying to establish the standard of care or whether the defendant nurse's attorney is establishing an acceptable standard of care for the given circumstances. The injured party will attempt to show that the acceptable standard of care is at a much higher level than that shown by the defendant, hospital, and staff. An example appears in Case Example Box 3.2.

Causation

The third element of a medical malpractice suit is causation. In this situation, the nurse's actions or lack of actions directly caused the patient's harm. A direct relationship must exist between the failure to meet the standard of care and the patient's injury. Merely breaching this standard of care is insufficient to show medical malpractice; a direct cause–effect factor must be present. For example, *O'Shea v. State of New York* (2007) concerned a patient who sustained an accident in which two fingers were severed while using a power saw. The patient permanently lost the two fingers when the nursing staff failed to follow the order for an immediate orthopedist consultation.

The resultant harm/injury must be physical, not merely psychological or transient. In other words, the patient must incur some physical harm before medical malpractice will be found against the healthcare provider.

CASE EXAMPLE BOX 3.2 An older case example, *Sabol v. Richmond Heights General Hospital* (1996), shows the importance of duty to the patient. A patient was admitted to a general acute care hospital for treatment after attempting to commit suicide by drug overdose. While in the acute care facility, the patient became increasingly paranoid and delusional. A nurse sat with the patient and tried to calm him. Restraints were not applied, because the staff feared this would compound the situation by raising the patient's level of paranoia and agitation. The patient jumped out of bed, knocked down the nurse who was in his room, fought his way past two nurses in the hallway, ran off the unit, and jumped from a third-story window, fracturing his arm and sustaining other relatively minor injuries.

Expert witnesses for the patient introduced standards of care pertinent to psychiatric patients, specifically those hospitalized in psychiatric facilities or in acute care hospitals with separate psychiatric units. The court ruled that the nurses in this general acute care situation were not professionally negligent in this patient's care. The court stated that the nurses' actions were consistent with basic professional standards of practice for medical-surgical nurses in an acute care hospital. They did not have, nor were they expected to have, specialized psychiatric nursing training and would not be judged as though they did.

Although some specific exceptions exist to the requirement that a physical injury must result, they are extremely limited and usually involve specific relationships, such as the parent–child relationship. Pain and suffering are allowed only when they accompany actual physical injuries.

Damages

The fourth and final element of a medical malpractice suit is damages. The injured party must be able to prove damages. Damages are vital, because medical malpractice is nonintentional. Thus, the patient must show financial harm before the courts will allow a finding of liability against the defendant nurse and/or hospital. Acceptable damages may be for immediate as well as future medical costs. Damages may include compensatory (economic), and noneconomic damages such as loss of enjoyment of life, pain, suffering, and loss of companionship.

A nurse manager must know the applicable standards of care and ensure that all employees of the institution meet or exceed them. The standards must be reviewed periodically to ensure that the staff members remain current and attuned to advances in technology and newer ways of performing skills. If standards of care appear outdated or absent, the appropriate committee within the institution should be notified so that timely revisions can be made. Finally, the nurse manager must ensure that all nursing employees meet the standards of care. This may be done by (1) performing or reviewing all performance evaluations for evidence that standards of care are met, (2) reviewing randomly selected patient records for standards of care documentation, and (3) inquiring of employees what constitutes standards of care and appropriate references for standards of care within the institution.

EXERCISE 3.2 You are the nurse manager for a skilled nursing facility that will now accept patients requiring long-term ventilator support. How should you begin to ensure that all of the staff in the facility are educated in the care of ventilator-dependent patients, know what complications to anticipate, and know how to respond should these complications arise? Should all staff members be educated in this skill?

Liability: Personal, Vicarious, and Corporate

Personal liability defines each person's responsibility and accountability for individual actions or omissions. Even if others can be shown to be liable for a patient injury, everyone retains personal accountability for one's actions. The law, though, sometimes allows other parties to be liable for certain causes of negligence. Known as vicarious liability, or substituted liability, the doctrine of respondeat superior (let the master answer) makes employers accountable for the negligence of their employees. The rationale underlying the doctrine is that the employee would not have been able to cause the wrongdoing unless hired by the employer, and the injured party would be allowed to suffer a double wrong if the employee was unable to pay damages for the wrongdoings. Nurse managers can best prevent these issues by ensuring that the staff they supervise know and follow hospital policies and procedures and continually deliver safe, competent nursing care or raise issues about policies and procedures through formal channels. This is where proactive followers shine—they raise critical questions, find loopholes, point out consistent workarounds and so forth in an effort to improve practice.

Nurses often believe that the doctrine of vicarious liability shields them from personal liability—they believe that the institution may be sued but not the individual nurse or nurses. However, patients injured because of substandard care have the right to sue both the institution and the nurse. This includes potentially suing the direct care nurse's manager if the manager knowingly allowed substandard and unsafe care to be given to a patient. In addition, the institution has the right under indemnification to countersue the nurse for damages paid to an injured patient. The principle of indemnification is applicable when the employer is held liable based solely on the actions of the staff member's negligence and the employer pays monetary damages because of the employee's negligent actions.

Corporate liability holds that the institution has the responsibility and accountability for maintaining an environment that ensures quality healthcare delivery for consumers. Corporate liability issues include negligent hiring and firing issues; failure to maintain safety in the physical environment; and lack of a qualified, competent, and adequate staff. In Wellstar Health System, Inc., v. Green (2002), a hospital was held liable to an injured patient for the negligent credentialing of a nurse practitioner. Nurse managers must be aware of trends in court cases and implications for persons in leadership positions because court outcomes follow precedents. In September 2015, the owner of a peanut butter manufacturing facility in Georgia was sentenced by a federal judge to 28 years in prison for the *Salmonella*-related deaths of nine persons (U.S. vs Parnell, Parnell, Lightest & Wilkerson, 2015.) The essence of the case was the knowledge of the person in a leadership position of the presence of *Salmonella* and his failure to take remedial action. Although this case didn't relate to a healthcare facility, it validated the idea that leaders have accountability for actions within organizations. The literature argues that hospital administration (which may include nurses in leadership positions) are not immune from criminal and civil liability, particularly in situations in which hospital-acquired infections (HAIs) cause harm. If defendants have knowledge of the danger and risk posed by HAIs in the facility but take no action to correct the situation, hospital administration may not be immune from civil and criminal prosecution for serious injury and death resulting from HAIs. They may also be held responsible for the failure to take remedial action once they had knowledge of the HAI (Ricciardi, 2015).

Nurse managers play a key role in assisting the institution to avoid corporate liability. For example, nurse managers ensure that staff members remain competent and qualified; that personnel within their supervision have current licensure; and that incompetent, illegal, or unethical practices are reported to the proper persons or agencies. Nurse managers also play a pivotal role in whether a nurse remains employed on the unit or is discharged or reassigned.

Perhaps the key to avoiding corporate liability is ensuring that all members of the healthcare team fully collaborate and work with other disciplines to ensure quality, competent healthcare regardless of the care setting. Such collaboration is a competency that must be mastered across disciplines.

Causes of Medical Malpractice for Nurse Managers

Nurse managers are charged with maintaining a standard of safe and competent nursing care within the institution. Several potential sources of liability for medical malpractice among nurse managers may be identified; thus, guidelines to prevent or avoid these pitfalls should be developed.

Assignment, Delegation, and Supervision

Assignment is the transfer of both the accountability and the responsibility from one person to another. This is typically what happens between professional staff members. The nurse manager assigns patient care responsibilities to other professional nurses working in the same unit of the institution or community healthcare setting. The level of accountability for the nurse manager who assigns as opposed to delegates is obvious, although some accountability can occur in both instances. The degree of knowledge concerning the skills and competencies of those one supervises is of paramount importance. The doctrine of respondent superior has been extended to include "knew or should have known" as a legal standard in both assigning and delegating tasks to individuals whom one supervises. If it can be shown that the nurse manager assigned or delegated tasks appropriately and had no reason to believe that the nurse to whom tasks were assigned or delegated was not competent to perform the task, the nurse manager potentially has no or minimal personal liability. The converse is also true: if it can be shown that the nurse manager was aware of incompetence in

EXERCISE 3.3 You are the nurse manager on a busy 38-bed surgical postoperative unit. A newly postoperative patient, Mrs. R., requires assistance with feeding, and you note that an unlicensed nursing personnel has been delegated to feed her. Reading Mrs. R.'s care plan, you also note that she is an older adult, has had periods of confusion, and has had difficulty swallowing since her surgery. Determine whether this is the right circumstance for such delegation. What are your next actions and why?

a given employee or that the assigned or delegated task was outside the employee's capabilities, the nurse manager becomes substantially liable for the subsequent injury to a patient.

Nurse managers have a duty to ensure that the staff members under their supervision are practicing in a safe and competent manner. The nurse manager must be aware of the staff members' knowledge, skills, and competencies and should know whether they are maintaining their competencies. Knowingly allowing a staff member to function below the acceptable standard of care subjects both the nurse manager and the institution to potential liability. This point is illustrated in Case Example Box 3.3.

As this case illustrates, delegation is both a process and a condition (Potter et al., 2010). It is a process of delegating appropriate tasks and activities to others while also being a condition because a mutual understanding must be held by both the delegator and the delegatee of

CASE EXAMPLE BOX 3.3 In *Estate of Travaglini v. Ingalls Health* (2009), an 84-year-old patient was admitted to the hospital with general complaints of "not feeling well." At the time of his admission, the physician told the admitting nurse that the patient had dysphagia and must be observed whenever he was eating or trying to swallow liquids. At 10:00 that evening, an aide came to the patient's room and left a sandwich for him to eat. Shortly afterward, the patient's roommate heard the patient choking and summoned help. At autopsy, it was confirmed that he had aspirated the turkey sandwich, and that this was the cause of the cardiopulmonary arrest that killed the patient. Though liability was found against the aide and her supervisor, the court also upheld a verdict of $500,000 against the hospital.

the specific results expected and the means of attaining those results.

Delegation, used in nursing practice throughout history, has evolved into a complex, work-enhancing strategy that has the potential for varying levels of legal liability. Before the early 1970s, nurses used delegation to direct the multiple tasks performed by the various levels of staff members in a team-nursing model. Subsequently, the concept of primary nursing and assignment became the desirable nursing model in acute care settings, with the focus on an all-professional staff requiring little delegation but considerable assignment of duties. By the mid-1990s, a nursing shortage had again shifted the nursing model to a multilevel staff, with the return of the need for delegation. Regardless of the nursing model used, nurse managers must fully understand and implement delegation principles effectively and properly.

Nurse managers need to know certain definitions regarding this area of the law. Delegation involves at least two people, a delegator and a delegatee, with the transfer of authority to perform some type of task or work. A working definition could be that delegation is the transfer of responsibility for the performance of an activity from one individual to another, with the delegator retaining accountability for the outcome. In other words, delegation involves the transfer of responsibility for the performance of tasks and skills without the transfer of accountability for the ultimate outcome. Examples include an RN who delegates patients' personal care tasks to certified nursing assistants who work in a long-term care setting. In delegating these tasks, the RN retains the ultimate accountability and responsibility for ensuring that the delegated tasks are completed in a safe and competent manner.

Typically, delegation involves tasks and procedures given to unlicensed nursing personnel, such as certified nursing aides, orderlies, assistants, attendants, and technicians. However, delegation can also occur with licensed staff members. For example, if one RN has the accountability for an outcome and asks another RN to perform a specific component of the overall function, that is delegation. This is typically the type of delegation that occurs between professional staff members when one member leaves the unit or work area for a meal break.

Delegation is complex because it involves the delegation relationship and communication. It also involves trusting others because both the delegator and the delegatee have shared accountability for certain tasks and duties. Interventions are needed to improve this relationship and communication effectiveness, which directly affects the quality of competent care delivery. Multiple players, usually with varying degrees of education and experience and different scopes of practice, are involved in the process. Understanding these variances and communicating effectively to the delegatee involve an understanding of competencies and the ability to communicate with all levels of staff personnel.

The field of nursing management involves supervision of various personnel who directly provide nursing care to patients. Supervision is defined as the active process of directing, guiding, and influencing the outcome of an individual's performance of an activity. The nurse manager retains personal liability for the reasonable exercise of assignment, delegation, and supervision activities. The failure to assign, delegate, and supervise within acceptable standards of professional nursing practice may constitute medical malpractice. In addition, failure to delegate and supervise within acceptable standards may extend to direct corporate liability for the institution.

Duty to Orient, Educate, and Evaluate

Most healthcare institutions have continuing education/professional development departments to orient nurses who are new to the institution and to supply in-service education addressing new equipment, procedures, and interventions to existing employees. Professional development may also provide ongoing learning opportunities for staff. Nurse managers also have a duty to orient, educate, and evaluate. Nurse managers and their representatives are responsible for the daily evaluation of whether nurses are performing safe and competent care. The key to meeting this requirement is reasonableness and is determined by courts on a case-by-case basis. Nurse managers should ensure that they promptly respond to all allegations, whether by patients or staff, of incompetent or questionable nursing care. Nurse managers should thoroughly investigate such allegations, recommend options for correcting the situation, and follow up on recommended options and suggestions.

For example, in *Marinock v. Manor at St. Luke's* (2010), the nursing facility had experienced multiple problems with patients falling or being dropped during

Hoyer lift transfers because some staff members were unaware of how to properly secure patients in the sling before beginning the transfer. These incidents apparently did not lead to additional training. Subsequently, an 82-year-old patient was dropped during a transfer from one bed to another bed, resulting in a femur fracture. The patient's lawsuit resulted in a $310,000 judgment against the facility for failure to properly orient and train its personnel.

EXERCISE 3.4   In a landmark study, the National Academy of Medicine (formerly the Institute of Medicine) (1999) outlined six characteristics for a safe healthcare system, noting that incorporating these six characteristics created a culture of safety. For example, culture focuses on effective systems and teamwork to accomplish the goal of safe, high-quality patient care. Review the National Academy of Medicine report and consider how nurse managers might begin to apply the characteristics of a culture of safety to the facts in the *Marinock v. Manor at St. Luke's* (2010) lawsuit. (https://www.ncbi.nlm.nih.gov/books/NBK2673/)

Failure to Warn

Another area of potential liability for nurse managers is failure to warn potential employers of staff incompetence or impairment. Information about suspected addictions, violent behavior, and incompetency is of vital importance to subsequent employers. If the institution has sufficient information and suspicion to warrant the discharge of an employee or force a resignation, subsequent employers should be advised of those issues. In addition, the state board of nursing or agency that oversees disciplinary actions of professional and unlicensed healthcare staff. Nursing staff should also be notified whenever a cause to dismiss an employee for incompetency or impairment exists unless the employee voluntarily enters a peer assistance program.

One means of supplying this information is using qualified privilege to certain communications. In general, qualified privilege concerns communications made in good faith between persons or entities with a need to know. Most states recognize this privilege and allow previous employers to give factual, objective information to subsequent employers. Note, however, that the previous employee must have listed the nurse manager or institution as a reference before this privilege arises.

Staffing Issues

Three issues arise under the general term *staffing*. These include (1) maintaining adequate numbers of staff members in a time of advancing patient acuity and limited resources, (2) floating staff from one unit to another, and (3) using temporary or "agency" staff to augment the healthcare facility's current staffing. Though each area is addressed separately, common to all three of these staffing issues is the requisite of collaboration among nurse managers in addressing the needs for the entire institution or healthcare agency.

Accreditation

Accreditation standards, such as those of TJC and the Community Health Accreditation Program (CHAP) as well as other state and federal standards, mandate that healthcare institutions provide adequate staffing with qualified personnel. This applies not only to the number of staff but also to the legal status of the staff. For instance, some areas of an institution—such as critical care areas, post anesthesia care areas, and emergency care centers—must have greater percentages of RNs than LPNs/LVNs. Other areas, such as the general nursing areas and some long-term care areas, may have equal or lower percentages of RNs to LPNs/LVNs or nursing assistants. Whether understaffing exists in each situation depends on the number of patients, care acuity scores, and number and classification of staff. Courts determine whether understaffing existed on an individual case basis.

California was the first state to adopt legislation that mandated fixed nurse-to-patient ratios, passing this historic legislation in 1999 (Cal. Health & Saf. Code. 1999. Sec. 1276.4). These types of ratios require set nurse-to-patient ratios based solely on numbers of patients within given nursing care areas and do not consider issues such as patient acuity, level of staff preparation, or environmental factors. Though a first step toward beginning to ensure adequate numbers of nurses, many states favor the concept of safe staffing rather than specific nurse-to-patient ratios. Generally, these safe staffing measures call for a committee to develop, oversee, and evaluate a plan for each specific nursing unit and shift based on patient care needs, appropriate skill mix of RNs and other nursing personnel, the physical layout of the unit, and national standards or recommendations regarding nursing staffing. Nurse managers must also know whether their states require public posting of the staffing plan (See Chapter 11 for more information on Staffing).

As early as 2011, federal legislation was introduced as the Registered Nurse Safe Staffing Act and included such provisions as a required public reporting of staffing information, a procedure for receiving and investigating complaints, and allowing the imposition of civil monetary penalties for each known violation (Registered Nurse Safe Staffing Act, 2011). The proposed legislation also included provision for nurse managers to work with direct care nurses to establish safe staffing based on variable factors. Because staffing has major implications for quality, legislation will be introduced and refined over several sessions. To date, there is no federal staffing legislation. (See Chapter 11 for more information on staffing legislation.)

Although the institution is ultimately responsible for staffing issues, nurse managers may also incur liability because they directly oversee numbers of personnel assigned to a given unit. Courts have looked to the constant exercise of professional judgment, rather than reliance on concrete nurse-to-patient ratios, in cases involving staffing issues. Thus, nurse managers should exercise sound judgment to ensure patient safety and quality care rather than rely on exact nurse-to-patient ratios. For liability to incur against the nurse manager, it must be shown that a resultant patient injury was directly caused by staffing issues and not by the incompetent or inappropriate actions of an individual staff member. To prevent nurse managers' liability, they must show that enough competent staff were available to meet nursing needs.

Guidelines for nurse managers in inadequate staffing issues include alerting hospital administrators and upper-level managers of concerns. First, however, nurse managers must do whatever is under their control to alleviate the circumstances, such as approving overtime for adequate coverage, reassigning personnel among those areas they supervise, and restricting new admissions to the area. Second, nurse managers have a legal duty to notify the chief nursing officer, either directly or indirectly, when understaffing endangers patient welfare. One way of notifying the chief nursing officer is through formal nursing channels, for example, by notifying the nurse manager's direct supervisor. Upper management must then decide how to alleviate the staffing issue, either on a short-term or long-term basis. Appropriate measures could be closing a unit or units, restricting elective surgeries, hiring new staff members, or temporarily reassigning personnel from other departments. Once nurse managers can show that they acted appropriately, used sound judgment given the circumstances, and alerted their supervisors of the serious nature of the situation, the institutions and not the nurse managers become potentially liable for staffing issues.

Mandatory Overtime

Several states prohibit the use of mandatory overtime by nurses. Generally, these laws state that the healthcare facility may not require an employee to work in excess of agreed to, predetermined, and regularly scheduled daily work shifts unless an unforeseeable declared national, state, or municipal emergency or catastrophic event occurs that is unpredicted or unavoidable and that substantially affects or increases the need for healthcare services. In addition, many of these laws define "normal work schedule" as 12 or fewer hours, protect employees from disciplinary action or retribution for refusing to work overtime, and establish monetary penalties for the employer's failure to adhere to the law. Some states also mandate that healthcare facilities are required to have a process for complaints related to patient safety. Note that nothing in these laws negates voluntary overtime. The pandemic experienced during 2020–2022 is an example of when normal work schedules were thrown into havoc.

Floating

Floating staff from unit to unit is the second issue that concerns overall staffing. Institutions have a duty to ensure that all areas of the institution are staffed adequately. Units temporarily overstaffed because of low patient census or a lower patient acuity ratio usually float staff to units that are understaffed. This means staff are temporarily assigned to another unit. Although floating nurses to areas with which they have less familiarity and expertise can increase potential liability for the nurse manager, leaving another area dangerously understaffed can also increase potential liability.

Before floating staff from one area to another, the nurse manager should consider staff expertise, patient-care delivery systems, and patient-care requirements. Nurses should be floated to units as comparable to their own unit as possible. This requires the nurse manager to match the nurse's home unit and float unit as much as possible or to consider negotiating with another nurse manager to cross-float a nurse. For example, a manager might float a critical care nurse to an intermediate care unit and float an intermediate care unit nurse to a general medical-surgical unit. Or the nurse manager might consider floating the general unit nurse to the postpartum unit and floating a postpartum nurse to labor and delivery. Open communications regarding staff limitations and concerns, as well as creative solutions for staffing, can alleviate some of the potential liability involved and create better morale among the floating nurses. A positive option is to cross-train nurses within the institution so that nurses are familiar with two or three areas and can competently float to areas in which they have been cross-trained. Nurses have the right—and obligation—to indicate their abilities in relation to the expected performance. Some organizations create dedicated float pools, meaning this is a regularly assigned area from which nurses are assigned throughout the organization. Some hospitals use this as an assignment area for new graduates to help them determine where they want to work and to develop multiple skills quickly.

Temporary Staff

The use of temporary or "agency" personnel has increased liability concerns among nurses and nurse managers. Previously, most jurisdictions held that such personnel were considered independent contractors and, thus, the institution was not liable for their actions, although their primary employment agency did retain potential liability. However, courts have begun to hold the institution liable under the principle of apparent agency. *Apparent authority* or *apparent agency* refers to the doctrine whereby principals become accountable for the actions of their agent. Apparent agency is created when a person (agent) holds oneself as acting on behalf of the principal; in the instance of the agency nurse, the patient cannot be sure whether the nurse works directly for the hospital (has a valid employment contract) or is working for a different employer. According to law, lack of actual authority is no defense. This principle applies when it can be shown that a reasonable patient believed that the healthcare worker was an employee of the institution. If it appears to the reasonable patient that this worker is an employee of the institution, the law will consider the worker an employee for the purposes of corporate and vicarious liability.

These trends in the law mean that nurse managers must consider the temporary worker's skills, competencies, and knowledge when delegating tasks and supervising the worker's actions. If a manager suspects that the temporary worker is incompetent, the manager must convey this fact to the agency. The nurse manager must also either send the temporary worker home or reassign the worker to other duties and areas. The same screening procedures should be performed with temporary workers as are used with new institutional employees. Those employed by the organization should treat temporary staff as if they were regular employees because that is how patients see them!

Additional areas that nurse managers should concentrate on when using agency or temporary personnel include ensuring that the temporary staff member is given a brief but thorough orientation to institution policies and procedures and is made aware of resource materials within the institution and documentation procedures. Also, nurse managers should assign a resource person to the temporary staff member. This resource person serves in the role of coach and advisor for the agency nurse and serves to prevent potential problems that could arise merely because the agency staff member does not know the institution routine or is unaware of where to turn for assistance. The resource person also assists with critical decision-making for the agency nurse.

Protective and Reporting Laws

Protective and reporting laws ensure the safety or rights of specific classes of individuals. Most states have reporting laws for suspected child and elder abuse and laws for reporting certain categories of diseases and injuries. Examples of reporting laws include reporting cases of sexually transmitted diseases, abuse of residents in nursing and convalescent homes, and suspected child abuse. Nurse managers are often the individuals who are responsible for ensuring that the correct information is reported to the correct agencies, thus avoiding potential liability against the institution.

Many states now also have mandatory reporting of incompetent practice, especially through nurse practice acts, medical practice acts, and the National Practitioner Data Bank. In addition, the NCSBN maintains an electronic license verification system (NURSYS) that monitors nurses' licensure status in all states and U.S. territories for discipline issues and licensure renewals. State boards submit data to NURSYS regarding disciplinary actions taken by the respective boards. Alerts are then sent to other U.S. jurisdictions in which the nurse is licensed. Special provisions may apply if nurses who struggle with substance abuse or misuse are enrolled in peer assistance programs.

Mandatory reporting of incompetent practitioners is a complex process, involving both legal and ethical concerns. Nurse managers must know what the law requires, when reporting is mandated, to whom the report must be sent, and what the individual institution expects of its nurse managers. When in doubt, seek clarification from the state board of nursing, hospital administration, or state professional nursing association. Some states hold the chief nursing officer (CNO) accountable for the nursing within the organization even if they do not all report through the CNO. Therefore, those in key leadership nursing positions need to know what the bigger picture involving nurses.

INFORMED CONSENT

Informed consent becomes an important concept for nurse managers in three different instances. First, direct care nurses may approach the nurse manager with questions about informed consent; thus, the nurse manager becomes a consultant for the direct care nurse. Second, the nurse manager is queried about patients' rights in research studies that are being conducted in the institution. Third, the issue of medical literacy has implications for the provision of valid informed consent by an ever-growing number of patients.

Informed consent is the authorization by the patient or the patient's legal representative to do something to the patient; it is based on legal capacity, voluntary action, and comprehension. Legal capacity is usually the first requirement and is determined by age and competency. All states have a legal age for adult status defined by statute; generally, this age is 18 years. Competency involves the ability to understand the consequences of actions or the ability to handle personal affairs. State statutes mandate who can serve as the representative for a minor or incompetent adult. The following types of minors may be able to give valid informed consent: emancipated minors, minors seeking treatment for substance abuse or communicable diseases, and pregnant minors.

Voluntary action, the second requirement, means that the patient was not coerced by fraud, duress, or deceit into allowing the procedure or treatment. Comprehension is the third requirement and the most difficult to ascertain. The law states that the patient must be given sufficient information in terms that the patient can reasonably be expected to comprehend to make an informed choice. Inherent in the doctrine of informed

BOX 3.1 Information Required for Informed Consent

- An explanation of the treatment or procedure to be performed and the expected results of the treatment or procedure
- Description of the risks involved
- Benefits that are likely to result because of the treatment or procedure
- Options to this course of action, including absence of treatment
- Name of the person(s) performing the treatment/procedure
- Statement that the patient may withdraw consent at any time

BOX 3.2 Elements of Informed Consent in Research Studies

- A statement that the study involves research, an explanation of the purposes of the research and the expected duration of the subject's participation, a description of the procedures to be followed, and identification of any procedures that are experimental
- A description of any reasonably foreseeable risks or discomforts to the subject
- A description of any benefits to the subjects or others that may reasonably be expected from the research
- A disclosure of appropriate alternative procedures or courses of treatment, if any, that may be advantageous to the subject
- A statement describing the extent, if any, to which confidentiality of records identifying the subject will be maintained
- For studies involving more than minimal research, an explanation as to any compensation and an explanation as to whether any medical treatments are available if injury occurs and, if so, what they consist of or where further information may be obtained
- An explanation of whom to contact for answers to pertinent questions about the research and research subjects' rights and whom to contact in the event of a research-related injury to the subject
- A statement that participation is voluntary, refusal to participate will involve no benefits to which the subject is otherwise entitled, and the subject may discontinue participation at any time without penalty or loss of benefits to which the subject is otherwise entitled

Source: *45 Code of Federal Regulations* (CFR), Sec. 46.116 (1991).

consent is the right of the patient to informed refusal. Patients must clearly understand the possible consequences of their refusal. In recent years, most states have enacted statutes to ensure that a competent adult has the right to refuse care and that the healthcare provider is protected should the adult validly refuse care. This refusal of care is most frequently seen in end-of-life decisions. Box 3.1 lists the information needed for obtaining informed consent.

Nurses often ask about issues concerning informed consent that involve the actual signing of the informed consent document, not the teaching and information that make up informed consent. Many nurses serve as witnesses to the signing of the informed consent document; in this capacity, they are attesting only to the voluntary nature of the patient's signature. No duty on the part of the nurse to insist that the patient repeat what has been said or what the patient remembers is present. If the patient asks questions that alert the nurse to the inadequacy of true comprehension on the patient's part or expresses uncertainty while signing the document, the nurse has an obligation to inform the primary healthcare provider and appropriate persons that informed consent has not been obtained.

A separate issue with informed consent concerns a patient who is part of a research study. Federal laws regulate this area because patients are generally considered to come under the heading of vulnerable populations. Whenever research is involved, such as a drug study or a new procedure, the investigators must disclose the research to the subject or the subject's representative and obtain informed consent. Federal guidelines have been developed that specify the procedures used to review research and the disclosures that must be made to ensure that valid informed consent is obtained.

The federal government mandates the basic elements of information that must be included to meet the standards of informed consent. Elements of informed consent are enumerated in Box 3.2.

The information given must be in a language that is understandable by the subject or the subject's legal representative. No exculpatory wording may be included, such as a statement that the researcher incurs no liability for the outcomes of the study or any injury to an individual subject. Subjects should be advised of the elements listed in Box 3.3.

BOX 3.3   Elements of Concern in Research Studies

- Any additional costs that they might incur because of the research
- Potential for any foreseeable risks
- Rights to withdraw at will, with no questions asked or additional incentives given
- Consequences, if any, of withdrawal before the study is completed
- A statement that any significant new findings will be disclosed
- The number of proposed subjects for the study

Source: *45 Code of Federal Regulations* (CFR), Sec. 46.101(b) (1991).

Excluded from these strict requirements are studies that use existing data, documents, records, or pathologic and diagnostic specimens if these sources are publicly available or the information is recorded so that the subjects cannot be identified. Other studies that involve only minimal risks to subjects, such as moderate exercise by healthy adults, may be expedited through the review process (Protection of Human Subjects, 1991, Section 46.110). Nurse managers must verify that staff members understand any research protocol with which their patients are involved.

The advent of the Health Insurance Portability and Accountability Act (HIPAA) of 1996 (Public Law [P.L.] 104-191) affected how health record information can be used in research studies. No separate permission need be secured from the patient to use medical record information if deidentified information is used. Deidentified information is health information that cannot be linked to an individual. Most of the 18 demographic items constituting the protected health information (PHI) must be removed before researchers are permitted to use patient records without obtaining the individual patient's permission to use/disclose PHI. The deidentified data set that is permissible for usage may contain the following demographic factors: gender and age of individuals and a three-digit ZIP code. Note that all individuals 90 years of age or older are listed as 90 years of age.

To prevent the onerous task of requiring patients who have been discharged from healthcare settings to sign such permission forms, researchers are allowed to submit a request for a waiver. The waiver is a request to forego the authorization requirements based on two conditions: (1) the use and/or disclosure of PHI involves minimal risk to the subject's privacy, and (2) the research cannot be done practically without this waiver. Additional information about HIPAA and confidentiality are covered later in this chapter.

Concerns over past abuses that have occurred in the area of research with children have led to the adoption of federal guidelines specifically designed to protect children when they are enrolled as research subjects. Before proceeding under these specific guidelines, state and local laws must be reviewed for laws regulating research on human subjects. In 1998, Subpart D: Additional Protections for Children Involved as Subjects in Research was added to the code (Protection of Human Subjects, 1998, 46.401 et seq.). These sections were added to give further protection to children when they are subjects of research studies and to encourage researchers to involve children, where appropriate, in research.

Health Literacy

A final issue with informed consent about which nurses and nurse managers should be cognizant concerns health literacy, or the degree to which individuals have the capacity to obtain, process, and understand basic health information, including services needed to make appropriate health decisions. Functional health literacy relates to the person's ability to act on the basic health information received. Comprehending medical jargon is difficult even for well-educated Americans; there are millions of Americans who do not have strong health literacy skills (Department of Health and Human Services, 2015). Comprehending medical instructions and terms may be impossible for individuals whose first language is not English, who cannot read at greater than a second-grade level, or who have vision or cognitive problems caused by aging or disabilities. These individuals have difficulty following instructions printed on medication labels (both prescription and over-the-counter), interpreting hospital consent forms, and even understanding diagnoses, treatment options, and discharge instructions.

Nurses play a significant role in addressing this growing problem. The first issue to address is awareness of the problem, because many patients and their family members hide the fact that they cannot read or do not understand what healthcare providers are attempting to convey. A second issue involves ensuring that the information and words nurses use to communicate with patients are at a level that the person can comprehend. One means to ensure that patients do understand patient discharge information and medication instructions is to give them a bottle of prescription medication and ask them to tell you how they would take the medication at home.

PRIVACY AND CONFIDENTIALITY

Privacy is the patient's right to protection against unreasonable and unwarranted interference with the patient's solitude. This right extends to protection of the person's reputation as well as protection of one's right to be left alone. Within a medical context, the law recognizes the patient's right to protection against (1) appropriation of the patient's name or picture for the institution's sole advantage, (2) intrusion by the institution on the patient's seclusion or affairs, (3) publication of facts that place the patient in a false light, and (4) public disclosure of private facts about the patient by the hospital or staff. Confidentiality is the right to privacy of the health record. Institutions can reduce potential liability in this area by allowing access to patient data, either written or oral, only to those with a "need to know." Persons with a need to know include physicians and nurses caring for the patient, technicians, unit clerks, therapists, social service workers, and patient advocates. This need to know usually extends to the house staff and consultants. Others wishing to access patient data must first ask the patient for permission to review a record. Administrative staff of the institution can access the patient record for statistical analysis, staffing, and quality-of-care review.

The nurse manager is cautioned to ensure that staff members both understand and abide by rules regarding patient privacy and confidentiality. "Interesting" patients should not be discussed with others, and all information concerning patients should be given only in private and secluded areas. All nurses may need to review the current means of giving reports to oncoming shifts and policies about telephone information. Many institutions have now added to the nursing care plan a place to list persons to whom the patient has allowed information to be given. If the caller self-identifies as one of those listed persons, the nurse can give patient information without violating the patient's

privacy rights. Patients are becoming more knowledgeable about their rights in these areas—some have been willing to take offending staff members to court over such issues. With the advent of social media, nurses must be cautious that their personal posts on Facebook, Twitter, Doxxing, or other platforms do not include pictures and/or information about their patients. This would constitute a violation of the patient's right to privacy and confidentiality. This would also be considered professional misconduct according to the nurse practice act.

The patient's right of access to one's own health record is another confidentiality issue. Although the patient has a right of access, individual states mandate when this right applies. Most states give the right of access only after the health record is completed; thus, the patient has the right to review the record after discharge. Some states give the right of access while the patient is hospitalized; therefore, individual state law governs individual nurses' actions. When supervising a patient's review of the patient's record, the nurse manager or representative should explain only the entries that the individual questions or about which the individual requests further clarification. The nurse makes a note in the record after the session indicating that the patient viewed the record and what questions were answered.

Patients also have a right to copies of the record at their expense. The health record belongs to the institution as a business record, and patients never have the right to retain the original record. This is also true in instances in which a subpoena is obtained to secure an individual's health record for court purposes. A hospital representative will verify that the copy is a "true and valid" copy of the original record.

An issue that is closely related to the health record is that of incident reports or unusual occurrence reports. These reports are mandated by TJC and serve to alert the institution to risk management and quality assurance issues within the setting. As such, incident reports are considered internal documents; thus, they are not discoverable (open for review) by the injured party or attorneys representing the injured party. In most jurisdictions where this question has arisen, however, the courts have held that the incident report was discoverable and, thus, open to review by both sides of the suit.

Therefore, prudent nurse managers complete and have staff members complete incident reports as though they will be open records, omitting any language of liability, such as, "The patient would not have fallen if Jane Jones, RN, had ensured the side rails were in their up and locked position." This document should contain only pertinent observations and care given the patient, such as x-rays that were obtained for a potential broken bone, medication that was given, and consultants who were called to examine the patient. Making any notation of the incident report in the official patient record is inadvisable because such a notation incorporates the incident report "by reference" and, thus, can be seen by the injured party or attorneys for the injured party.

PHI is at the crux of the confidentiality aspect of the law. The privacy standards limit how PHI may be used or shared, mandate safeguards for protecting the health information, and shift the control of health information from providers to the patient by giving patients significant rights. Healthcare facilities must provide patients with a documented Notice of Privacy Rights, explaining how PHI will be used or shared with other entities. This document also alerts patients to the process for complaints if they later determine that their information rights have been violated. Nurse managers have the responsibility to ensure that those they supervise uphold these patient rights as dictated by HIPAA and to take corrective actions should these rights not be upheld.

POLICIES AND PROCEDURES

Risk management is a process that identifies, analyzes, and treats potential hazards within a given setting; and it is everyone's job. The object of risk management is to identify potential hazards and eliminate them before anyone is harmed or disabled. Risk management activities include writing policies and procedures, which is a requirement of TJC. These documents set standards of care for the institution and direct practice. They must be clearly stated, well delineated, and based on current practice. Nurse managers should review the policies and procedures frequently for compliance and timeliness. If policies are absent or outdated, the nurse manager must request the appropriate person or committee to either initiate or update the policy.

> **EXERCISE 3.5** You are one of the Magnet champion direct care nurses on the Risk Management Committee. You work on a nursing unit where you have observed a recent incident fall report. In investigating incident reports filed by staff, you discover that this is the third incident this week in which a patient has fallen while attempting to get out of bed and sit in a chair. How would you begin to address this issue? Decide how you would start a more complete investigation of this issue. For example, is it a facility-wide issue or confined to one unit? Does it affect all shifts or only one? What safety issues are you going to discuss with your staff and how are you going to discuss these issues? Do these falls involve the same staff member?

EMPLOYMENT LAWS

The federal government and individual state governments enact laws that regulate employment. To be effective and legally compliant, nurse managers must be familiar with these laws and how the individual laws affect the institution and labor relations. Many nurse managers have come to fear the legal system because of personal experience or the experiences of colleagues, but much of this concern may be directly attributable to uncertainty with the law or partial knowledge of the law. By understanding and correctly following federal employment laws, nurse managers may decrease their potential liability by complying with both federal and state laws. As individual nurses have engaged in travel nursing, they would be wise to familiarize themselves with these laws because of the semi-independent nature of the and purpose of the legislation. Table 3.2 gives an overview of key federal employment laws.

Equal Employment Opportunity Laws

Federal laws have been enacted to expand equal employment opportunities by prohibiting discrimination based on gender, age, race, religion, handicap, pregnancy, and national origin. The Equal Employment Opportunity Commission (EEOC) enforces these laws. All states have also enacted statutes that address employment opportunities; the nurse manager should consider both when hiring and assigning nursing employees.

The most significant legislation affecting equal employment opportunities today is the amended Civil Rights Act of 1964. Section 703(a) of Title VII makes

TABLE 3.2 Selected Federal Labor Legislation

Year	Legislation	Primary Purpose of the Legislation
1935	Wagner Act; National Labor Act	Unions, National Labor Relations Board established; unionization rights established
1947	Taft-Hartley Act	Established a more equal balance of power between unions and management
1962	Executive Order 10988	Allowed public employees to join labor unions
1963	Equal Pay Act	Became illegal to pay lower wages based solely on gender
1964	Civil Rights Act	Protected against discrimination based on race, color, creed, national origin, etc.
1967	Age Discrimination in Employment Act	Protected against discrimination based on age
1970	Occupational Safety and Health Act	Established the development and enforcement of standards for occupational health and safety
1974	Wagner Amendments	Allowed nonprofit organizations to unionize and allowed collective bargaining in nursing
1990	Americans With Disabilities Act	Barred discrimination against workers with disabilities in the workplace
1991	Civil Rights Act	Addressed sexual harassment in the workplace
1993	Family and Medical Leave Act	Allowed work leaves based on family and medical needs
1996	Health Insurance Portability and Accountability Act	Provided for the phased introduction of a comprehensive system of mandated health insurance reforms
2010	Patient Protection and Accountability Act	Provided for the phased introduction of a comprehensive system of mandated health insurance reforms
2010	Health Care and Education Reconciliation Act	Amended the Patient Protection and Affordable Care Act to clarify budget resolutions

it illegal for an employer "to refuse to hire, discharge an individual, or otherwise to discriminate against an individual, with respect to his compensation, terms, conditions, or privileges of employment because of the individual's race, color, religion, sex, or national origin." The Equal Employment Opportunity Act of 1972 also amended Title VII so that it applies to private institutions with 15 or more employees, state and local governments, labor unions, and employment agencies.

The amended Civil Rights Act of 1991 further broadened the issue of sexual harassment in the workplace and supersedes many of the sections of Title VII. Sections of the new legislation define sexual harassment, its elements, and the employer's responsibilities regarding harassment in the workplace, especially prevention and corrective action. The Civil Rights Act of 1991 is enforced by the EEOC. The primary activity of the EEOC is processing complaints of employment discrimination. Three phases comprise processing complaints:

investigation, conciliation, and litigation. Investigation focuses on determining whether the employer has violated provisions of Title VII. If the EEOC finds "probable cause," an attempt is made to reach an agreement or conciliation between the EEOC, the complainant, and the employer. If conciliation fails, the EEOC may file suit against the employer in federal court or issue to the complainant the right to sue for discrimination under its auspices, including those relating to staffing practices and sexual harassment in the workplace.

The EEOC defines sexual harassment broadly, which has generally been upheld in the courts. Nurse managers must realize that it is the duty of employers (management) to prevent employees from sexually harassing other employees. The EEOC issues policies and practices for employers to implement, both to sensitize employees to this problem and to prevent its occurrence. Nurse managers should be aware of these policies and practices and seek guidance in implementing them if sexual harassment occurs in their units.

Employers may seek exceptions to Title VII on several premises. For example, employment decisions made based on national origin, religion, and gender (never race or color) are lawful if such decisions are necessary for the normal operation of the business, although the courts have viewed this exception very narrowly. Promotions and layoffs based on bona fide seniority or merit systems are permissible, as are exceptions based on business necessity.

Age Discrimination in Employment Act of 1967

The Age Discrimination in Employment Act of 1967 made discrimination against older men and women by employers, unions, and employment agencies illegal. A 1986 amendment to the law prohibits discrimination against persons older than 40 years. The practical outcome of this act has been that mandatory retirement is no longer allowed in the American workplace.

As with Title VII, some exceptions to this act exist. Reasonable factors other than age may be used when terminations become necessary. Reasonable factors may include a performance evaluation system or certain limited occupational qualifications, such as the tedious physical demands of a specific job.

Americans With Disabilities Act of 1990

The Americans with Disabilities Act (ADA) of 1990 provides protection to persons with disabilities and is the most significant civil rights legislation since the Civil Rights Act of 1964. The purpose of the ADA is to provide a clear and comprehensive national mandate for the elimination of discrimination against individuals with disabilities and to provide clear, strong, consistent, enforceable standards addressing discrimination in the workplace. The ADA is closely related to the Civil Rights Act of 1991 and incorporates the antidiscrimination principles established in Section 504 of the Rehabilitation Act of 1973.

The act has five titles; Table 3.3 depicts the pertinent issues of each title. The ADA has jurisdiction over employers, private and public; employment agencies; labor organizations; and joint labor–management committees. *Disability* is defined broadly. With respect to an individual, a disability is (1) a physical or mental impairment that substantially limits one or more of the major life activities of such individual, (2) a record of such impairment, or (3) an individual being regarded as having such impairment (ADA Amended Act, 2008). The effects of

TABLE 3.3   Americans With Disabilities Act of 1990

Title	Provisions
I	Employment: Defines the purpose of the act and who is qualified under the act as having a disability.
II	Public services: Concerns services, programs, and activities of public entities as well as public transportation.
III	Public accommodations and services operated by private entities: Prohibits discrimination against persons with disabilities in areas of public accommodations, commercial facilities, and public transportation services.
IV	Telecommunications: Intended to make telephone services accessible to individuals with hearing or speech impairments.
V	Miscellaneous provisions: Certain insurance matters; incorporation of this act with other federal and state laws.

Source: Americans with Disabilities Act of 1990, 42 U.S.C. § 12101 et seq. (1990).

this amended act were to allow the definition of disability to be as broad as possible and to disallow impairments that are transitory (6-month duration or less) and minor. It also allows the definition to include an impairment that is episodic or in remission if the disability substantially limits a major life event when not in remission.

The overall effect of the legislation is that persons with disabilities will not be excluded from job opportunities or adversely affected in any aspect of employment unless they are not qualified or are otherwise unable to perform the job. The ADA thus protects qualified individuals with disabilities regarding job application procedures, hiring, compensation, advancement, and all other employment matters.

The number of lawsuits filed under the ADA since its enactment is extensive. This is due in part to the fact that to prevent the act from being overly narrow, the determination of qualified individuals is done case by case, and the individual must show (1) evidence of having a physical or mental impairment, (2) that the impairment substantially limits one or more major life activities, and (3) that the individual is still able to perform the essential function of the employment position sought or in which the individual is currently employed.

CASE EXAMPLE BOX 3.4 The issue of reasonable accommodations was well illustrated by the court in *Zamudio v. Patia* (1997). The court stated that the employer would be required to inform Ms. Zamudio when a position became available for which the reasonable accommodation she required could be met. She would be allowed to apply, but "as a disabled employee seeking reasonable accommodation, she did not have to be given preference over other employees without disabilities who might have better qualifications or more seniority" (*Zamudio v. Patia, 1997*, at 808).

The ADA requires an employer or potential employer to make reasonable accommodations to employ persons with a disability. The law does not mandate that individuals with a disability be hired before fully qualified persons who do not have a disability; it does mandate that those with disabilities are not disqualified merely because of an easily accommodated disability. An example appears in Case Example Box 3.4.

Moreover, the court will not impose job restructuring on an employer if the person needing accommodation qualifies for other jobs not requiring such accommodation. In *Mauro v. Borgess Medical Center* (1995), the court refused to impose accommodation on the employer hospital merely because the affected employee desired to stay within a certain unit of the institution. In this case, an operating surgical technician who tested positive for HIV was offered an equivalent position by the hospital in an area where there would be no patient contact. He refused the transfer, desiring accommodation within the operating arena, and was denied such accommodation by the Michigan court.

The act also provides for essential job functions. These are defined by the ADA as those functions that the person must be able to perform to be qualified for employment positions. Courts have assisted in determining these essential job functions. For example, in *Moschke v. Memorial Medical Center of West Michigan* (2003), the court determined that the ability to take "on-call" work is an essential function of a surgical nurse's job. Such on-call work involves the ability of the surgical nurse to be available when emergency cases or scheduling problems require the staff to work beyond their assigned shifts. In *Laurin v. Providence Hospital and Massachusetts Nurses Association* (1998), the ability to work rotating shifts was held to be an essential job function.

The act specifically excludes the following from the definition of disability: homosexuality and bisexuality, sexual behavioral disorders, gambling addiction, kleptomania, pyromania, and current use of illegal drugs (ADA, 1990). Employers may hold persons with alcohol issues to the same job qualifications and job performance standards as other employees even if the unsatisfactory behavior or performance is related to alcoholism (ADA, 1990). As with other federal employment laws, nurse managers should have a thorough understanding of the law as it applies to the institution and their specific job description and should know whom to contact within the institution structure for clarification as needed.

Affirmative Action

The policy of affirmative action (AA) differs from the policy of equal employment opportunity (EEO). AA policy enhances employment opportunities of protected groups of people; EEO policy is concerned with implementing employment practices that do not discriminate against or impair the employment opportunities of protected groups. Thus, AA can be seen in conjunction with several federal employment laws. For example, in conjunction with the Vietnam Era Veterans' Readjustment Assistance Act of 1974, AA requires that employers with government contracts take steps to enhance the employment opportunities of veterans with disabilities who served during the Vietnam War era.

Equal Pay Act of 1963

The Equal Pay Act of 1963 makes it illegal to pay lower wages to employees of one gender when the jobs (1) require equal skill in experience, training, education, and ability; (2) require equal effort in mental or physical exertion; (3) are of equal responsibility and accountability; and (4) are performed under similar working conditions. Courts have held that unequal pay may be legal if it is based on seniority, merit, incentive systems, or a factor other than gender. The main cases filed under this law in the area of nursing have been by unlicensed staff.

Occupational Safety and Health Act

The Occupational Safety and Health Administration (OSHA) Act of 1970 was enacted to ensure that healthful and safe working conditions would exist in the workplace. Among other provisions, the law requires isolation procedures, placarding areas containing ionizing radiation, proper grounding of electrical equipment, protective storage of flammable and combustible liquids, and the gloving of all personnel when handling bodily fluids. The statute provides that if no federal standard has been established, state statutes prevail. Nurse managers should know the relevant OSHA laws for the institution and their specific area. Frequent review of new additions to the law also must be undertaken, especially in this era of acquired immunodeficiency syndrome (AIDS) and other infectious diseases.

Violence in the workplace is an issue that OSHA continues to address in its rules. Violence is perhaps the greatest hidden health and safety threat in the workplace today. Nurses, as the largest group of healthcare professionals, are most at risk of assault at work. In 1996, OSHA developed voluntary guidelines to protect healthcare workers and consumers. Relatively few states have laws that mandate employers to report incidents of workplace violence, although more states have enacted laws that strengthen or increase penalties for acts of workplace violence. Additionally, TJC created standards that address the incidence and prevention of workplace violence.

Another important workplace concern is the issue of safe patient handling, which refers to preventing injury to healthcare workers while ensuring that patients are protected as they are transferred or moved in healthcare settings. One of the common issues for nurses during transferring patients is the potential for, or actual harm of, back injury. Safe patient handling is a major concern and resource of the American Nurses Association (https://www.nursingworld.org/practice-policy/work-environment/health-safety/safe-patient-handling/). Additionally, some states have passed safe patient handling legislation to protect both patients and nurses.

In 2012, OSHA initiated its National Emphasis Program (NEP) for nursing and residential care facilities to focus on the workplace hazards that are the most common in the healthcare industry, including ergonomic stressors related to patient lifting. The desire is that this momentum will lead to federal laws that would require mechanical lifting equipment and friction-reducing devices for all healthcare workers, patients, and residents across all healthcare settings. Published in 2015, the "Inspection Guidance for Inpatient Healthcare Settings" memorandum further directs OSHA Regional Administrators and State Plans to focus inspections at these facilities to reduce five primary hazards: musculoskeletal disorders related to patient or resident handling, blood-borne pathogens, workplace violence, tuberculosis, and slips, trips, and falls.

Family and Medical Leave Act of 1993

The Family and Medical Leave Act (FMLA) of 1993 was passed because of the large numbers of single-parent and two-parent households in which the single parent or both parents are employed full-time, placing job security and parenting at odds. The law also supports the growing demands that aging parents are placing on their working children. The act was written to balance the demands of the workplace with the demands of the family, allowing employed individuals to take leaves for medical reasons, including the birth or adoption of children and the care of a spouse, child, or parent who has serious health problems. Essentially, the act provides job security for unpaid leave while the employee is caring for a new infant or other family healthcare needs. The act is gender neutral and allows both men and women the same leave provisions. Medical leave may be taken to care for a spouse, son, daughter, or parent of the employee when that person has a serious medical condition. Employees are also permitted to use medical leave for their own serious health condition.

To be eligible under the act, the employee must have worked for at least 12 months and worked at least 1250 hours during the preceding 12-month period. The employee may take up to 12 weeks of unpaid leave. The act allows the employer to require the employee to use all or part of any paid vacation, personal leave, or sick leave as part of the 12-week family leave. Employees must give the employer 30 days advance notice, or such notice as is practical in emergency cases, before using the medical leave.

On January 28, 2008, President George W. Bush signed the Family and Medical Leave Amended Act of 2008, which became effective January 16, 2009. The amendments permit a spouse, son, daughter, parent, or next of kin to take up to 26 work weeks of leave to care for a member of the U.S. Armed Forces, including a member of the National Guard or Reserves, who is undergoing medical treatment, recuperation, or therapy; is otherwise in outpatient status; or is otherwise on the temporary disability retired list for a serious injury or illness. In addition, the act permits an employee to take leave for any qualifying exigency arising out of the fact that the spouse or a son, daughter, or parent of the employee is on active duty (or has been notified of an impending call or order to active duty) in the Armed Forces in support of a contingency operation. In 2013, the FMLA was amended to address changes concerning calculating employee eligibility for FMLA leave, military caregiver leaves for veterans, qualifying exigency leave for parental care, tracking intermittent or reduced-schedule FMLA leave, and special leave provisions for flight crew employees.

Employment-at-Will and Wrongful Discharge

Historically, the employment relationship has been considered a "free will" relationship. Employees were free to take or not take a job at will and employers were free to hire, retain, or discharge employees for any reason. Many laws, some federal but predominantly state, have been slowly eroding this at-will employment relationship. Evolving case law provides at least three exceptions to the broad doctrine of employment-at-will.

The first exception is a public policy exception. This exception involves cases in which an employee is discharged in direct conflict with established public policy. Under this exception, an employer may not discharge an employee if it would violate the state's public policy doctrine or a state or federal statute. Some examples include discharging an employee for serving on a jury, reporting employers' illegal actions (better known as whistle-blowing, or the disclosure of information regarding misconduct within a workplace that either is illegal or endangers the welfare of others), and filing a workers' compensation claim. Most states and the District of Columbia recognize public policy as an exception to the at-will rule.

Several recent court cases attest to the number of terminations in healthcare settings that serve as retaliation for the employer. More commonly known as whistle-blowing cases, the healthcare provider in these cases is terminated for one of three distinct reasons: (1) speaking out against unsafe practices, (2) reporting violations of federal laws, or (3) filing lawsuits against employers. Essentially, whistleblower laws state that no employer can discharge, threaten, or discriminate against an employee regarding compensation, terms, conditions, location, or privileges of employment because the employee in good faith reported or caused to be reported, verbally or in writing, what the employee

had a reasonable cause to believe was a violation of a state or federal law, rule, or regulation. Most whistleblowers are internal; that is, they report misconduct to a fellow employee or supervisor within the agency. External whistleblowers are those who report misconduct to outside persons or entities. Examples appear in Case Example Boxes 3.5 and 3.6.

The second exception to wrongful discharge involves situations in which an implied contract exists. The courts have generally treated employee handbooks, company policies, and oral statements made at the time of employment as "framing the employment relationship" (*Watkins v. Unemployment Compensation Board of Review*, 1997). For example, in *Trombley v. Southwestern Vermont Medical Center* (1999), the court found that the employee handbook outlined the procedure for progressive discipline, mandating that such procedure be followed before a nurse could be terminated for incompetent nursing care.

The third exception to wrongful discharge is a "good faith and fair dealing" exception. The purpose of this exception is to prevent unfair or malicious terminations, and the courts use the exception sparingly. States also do not favor this exception—today, less than a quarter of the states recognize breach of such implied contracts.

CASE EXAMPLE BOX 3.5 *Martell v. Tarpon Springs Hospital* (2010) concerned a hospital surgical nursing supervisor with a spotless 14-year record who was fired 10 days after she voiced a complaint that the hospital administrator had falsified records. In these falsified records, the administrator had personally certified the number of hospital nurses' annual cardiopulmonary resuscitation retrainings, which neither he nor anyone else had done. During the trial, it was further disclosed that this same administrator had been fired from his previous employments for falsifying time records and for poor performance.

The jury in the case awarded the former nursing supervisor $425,000 as damages for compensation for emotional distress and the fact that her new employment paid less, had fewer benefits, and was less personally satisfying than her former position. The jury also noted that complaining about an illegal action by a superior was expressly protected by the state's whistleblower-protection law and that the hospital had no grounds on which to dismiss her.

CASE EXAMPLE BOX 3.6 Perhaps one of the best-known whistleblower cases involving nurses is what has become known as the Winkler County Nurses Lawsuit (Yoder-Wise, 2010). The case became nationally known after two registered nurses, Anne Mitchell and Vicki Galle, were terminated by the Winkler County Hospital in Kermit, Texas. The nurses first attempted to report a physician's behavior and negligent healthcare practices through designated hospital channels. When the hospital took no action, they reported the physician to the Texas Medical Board for serious misconduct, substandard care, and an inappropriate business partnership with the sheriff of Winkler County.

Although the usual procedure was for the medical board to investigate and keep the complainants' names confidential, the sheriff used the power of his position to learn that the reporting nurses had worked at the hospital for about 20 years and that each nurse was about 50 years old. That information allowed the sheriff to identify the two nurses; he then used his office to confiscate the nurses' computers, where he found the letter to the Texas Medical Board. The nurses were subsequently terminated and indicted on felony charges of misuse of official information, which could have resulted in their imprisonment for 10 years.

The criminal charges against Vicki Galle were dismissed the day before the trial was to occur, though the trial proceeded against Anne Mitchell. The trial lasted less than 4 days, with the jury returning a not guilty verdict. The nurses later filed successful civil lawsuits against the physician, Winkler County, the hospital and its administrator, the sheriff, and the district and county attorneys of Winkler County (*Mitchell & Galle v. Winkler County et al.*, 2010). Their cause of action included violations of their rights of free speech and due process, whistleblower retaliation, and interference with their business relationship, specifically their employment status.

Although this exception is rarely seen in nursing, it remains a valid exception to wrongful discharge of an employee.

Nurse managers are urged to know their respective state laws concerning this growing area of the law, particularly in conjunction with whistleblower laws. Managers should review institution documents, especially employee handbooks and recruiting brochures, for unwanted statements implying job security or other unintentional promises. Managers are also cautioned not to say anything during the preemployment negotiations and interviews that might be construed as implying job security or other unintentional promises to the potential employee. To prevent successful suits for retaliation by whistleblowers, nurse managers should carefully monitor the treatment of an employee after a complaint is filed and ensure that performance evaluations are conducted and placed in the appropriate files. The nurse manager should also take steps to correct the whistleblower's complaint or refer the complaint to upper management so that it can be addressed effectively. If the complaint is about the nurse manager and is made by a direct care nurse, for example when a 360-degree evaluation approach is used, the direct care nurse should retain details to document the statements made in the evaluation.

Collective Bargaining

Collective bargaining, also called *labor relations*, is the joining together of employees for the purpose of increasing their ability to influence the employer and improve working conditions. Collective bargaining is defined and protected by the National Labor Relations Act of 1935 and its amendments; the National Labor Relations Board (NLRB) oversees the act and those who come under its auspices. The NLRB ensures that employees can choose freely whether they want to be represented by a particular bargaining unit, and it serves to prevent or remedy any violation of the labor laws. Chapter 14 provides further detail regarding collective bargaining and collective action.

PROFESSIONAL NURSING PRACTICE: ETHICS

Ethics may be distinguished from the law because ethics is internal to an individual, looks to the ultimate "good" of an individual rather than society as a whole, and concerns the "why" of one's actions. The law, comprising rules and regulations pertinent to society, is external to oneself and concerns one's actions and conduct. Ethics concerns the individual within society, whereas law concerns society. Law can be enforced through the courts, statutes, and boards of nursing, whereas ethics is enforced via ethics committees and professional codes.

Today, ethics and legal issues often become entwined, and it may be difficult to separate ethics from legal concerns. Legal principles and doctrines assist the nurse manager in decision-making; ethical theories and principles are often involved in those decisions. Thus, the nurse manager must be cognizant of both laws and ethics in everyday management concerns, remembering that ethical principles form the essential base of knowledge from which to proceed, rather than giving easy, straightforward answers.

Ethics is the study of standards of conduct and moral judgment and is an area of professional practice in which nurse managers should have a solid foundation because it is increasingly an issue in clinical practice settings. However, it remains an area in which many nurses feel the most inadequate. This is partially because ethics is much more nebulous than are laws and regulations. In ethics, right and wrong answers are usually not possible, just better or worse answers, and nurses seek mentorship and counseling from nurse managers when they encounter difficult situations. Thus, nurse managers must have a deep understanding of ethical principles and their application. Applying theory and research-based knowledge from nursing, the arts, humanities, and other sciences, a competency

highlighted in the 2021 AACN New Essentials, is important to maintaining an ethical practice (https://www.aacnnursing.org/Portals/42/AcademicNursing/pdf/Essentials-2021.pdf).

Theoretical framework related to Ethical Decision-Making

Nurses and other health care providers have an ethical obligation to provide care that (1) benefits the patient, (2) avoids or minimizes harm, and (3) respects the values and preferences of the patient (Varkey, 2021) and knowledge of the theoretical frameworks used to make ethical decisions are helpful to achieve these goals. Several schools of thought exist related to ethical decision-making theory.

Table 3.4 outlines the most common approach.

Although these approaches contradict each other, each of them has its own advantages and disadvantages in health care. When a conflict exists between these two theories in healthcare, the resulting ethical dilemmas must be addressed to reach an appropriate solution for patients and others (Tseng & Wang, 2021).

TABLE 3.4   Application Examples of Theoretical Principles

Theory/Contributor	Key Ideas	Application to Practice
Deontological Ethics Name comes from the Greek word, "deon", or duty Mainly attributed to Immanuel Kant, a German philosopher and economist in the late 1700s.	Based on the idea that every person has inherent dignity. Because of this dignity, everyone has a range of rights and obligations. Thus, all humans have a duty to others. We should do our duty, because it is the right thing to do, regardless of the outcome. We cannot control outcomes, but we can control our actions.	From a health care perspective, deontological ethics can be considered "patient-centered". Healthcare Providers focus on providing the "best care possible". The ethical decisions occur when determining what the best care is. Is it what the physician believes is best or what the client (and/or what the family or significant others want?
Utilitarian Ethics Jeremy Bentham, and John Stuart Mill, both English philosophers, are associated with the development of Utilitarian ethical thought. The most famous type of Consequentialism ethics.	Based on the view that all humans have the obligation to take the course of action that achieves the most positive outcome. The ultimate good is happiness. Utilitarian theory expands this thinking by holding that we ought to maximize this good to bring about the greatest amount of good for the greatest number.	From a health care perspective, utilitarianism can be considered society centered. For example, Public health initiatives, such as wearing masks or vaccine, are designed for the public good. However, the conflict with individual rights results in an ethical dilemma.

The difficulty in decision-making in specific clinical situations using theories with different perspectives can be lessened using bioethical principles. The bioethical principles used in healthcare include *beneficence* (doing good), *non-maleficence* (doing no harm), *autonomy,* which involves having respect for another, and *justice* (fairness for all). Beneficence includes veracity or truth-telling (full disclosure) and confidentiality. In health care situations, ethical principles are often in conflict with one another, resulting in an ethical dilemma for caregivers. The ethical principles below define the bioethical principles commonly used in healthcare and provides examples of clinical situations in which each principle is used.

Ethical Principles

Ethical principles, used daily in patient care situations, are equally paramount to the nurse manager. Ethical principles that nurse managers should consider when making decisions include the nine items listed in Table 3.5. Each of the principles is applied daily in clinical practice, though some principles are used to a greater degree than others.

TABLE 3.5	**Examples of Applications of Ethical Principles**		
Ethical Principle	**Definition**	**Example**	**Application to Leadership/ Management Practice**
Autonomy	All persons have intrinsic and unconditional worth, and should have the power to make rational decisions and moral choices, including being allowed to exercise his or her capacity for self-determination	The nursing staff supports a patient's decision to terminate active treatment in the case of terminal illness.	The Nurse Manager in the OR reassigns a nurse who objects to participate in a surgical procedure in conflict with that nurses' religious beliefs.
Beneficence	An obligation to act for the benefit of the patient and to protect and defend the rights of others, prevent harm, remove conditions that will cause harm, help persons with disabilities, and rescue persons in danger.	The nurse provides patient instruction regarding medication management and evaluates the effectiveness of this instruction.	The Nurse Manager provides instruction and support to a new graduate who has a lack of confidence in certain psychomotor skills.
Confidentiality	Obligation to not disclose confidential information given by a patient to another party without the patient's authorization. An obvious exception (with implied patient authorization) is the sharing necessary of medical information for the care of the patient from the primary physician to consultants and other members of the health-care team. There are some exceptions to patient confidentiality, including legally required reporting of gunshot wounds and sexually transmitted diseases and exceptional situations that may cause major harm to another (e.g., epidemics of infectious diseases, partner notification in HIV disease, relative notification of certain genetic risks, threats of violence against another, etc.	A relative of a patient asked the nurse to provide information regarding the patient's prognosis. The nurse refuses to give this information, citing confidentiality.	If the relative is not satisfied with the nurse's response, the Nurse Manager may become involved and include someone who can explain confidentiality and legal requirements in greater depth.

Continued

TABLE 3.5	**Examples of Applications of Ethical Principles—cont'd**		
Ethical Principle	**Definition**	**Example**	**Application to Leadership/ Management Practice**
Fidelity	Fidelity means keeping one's promises or commitments.		Nurse Managers abide by this principle when they follow through on any promises they have previously made to employees, such as a promised leave, a certain shift to be worked, or a promotion to a preceptor position within the unit.
Justice	Fair, equitable, and appropriate treatment of persons.	The nurse advocates for sufficient staffing, so that all patients on the unit will have equal access to care.	The Nurse Manager supports this advocacy.
Non-maleficence	An obligation not to harm the patient. This includes do not kill, cause pain or suffering or offense, or deprive others of the goods of life. This ethical principle requires the provider to carefully weigh the benefits against the burdens of all interventions and treatments, avoiding those that are particularly problematic and choosing the best course of action for the patient.	The nurse creates a schedule and plan to ensure that an immobile patient is turned at least every two-hours and is frequently assessed for decubitus ulcers.	The Nurse Manager requests additional nursing staff because of the high patient care acuity of the unit, despite the negative impact on the unit's staffing budget.
Paternalism	The principle of paternalism allows one person to make partial decisions for another and is most frequently deemed to be a negative or undesirable principle. Paternalism, however, may be used to assist persons to make decisions when they do not have sufficient data or expertise. Paternalism becomes undesirable when the entire decision is taken from the employee.	Nurses use this principle in a positive manner by assisting employees in deciding major career moves and plans, helping the staff member more.	The Nurse Manager seeks input from the employee on career goals and aspirations. The nurse manager does not mandate decisions but provides opportunities in alignment with the nurse's wishes.
Respect	Many consider the principle of respect for others as the highest principle. Respect for others acknowledges the right of individuals to make decisions and to live by these decisions. Respect is the first principle enumerated in the American Nurses Association's Code of Ethics for Nurses.	Nurses use this principle to promote ethical behaviors including respect for self and others including peers and patients. Respect for others transcends cultural differences, gender issues, and racial concerns.	Nurse Managers positively reinforce this principle daily in their actions with employees, patients, and peers because they serve as leaders and models for staff members and others in the institution.

TABLE 3.5   Examples of Applications of Ethical Principles—cont'd

Ethical Principle	Definition	Example	Application to Leadership/ Management Practice
Veracity (Truth-telling)	An autonomous patient has not only the right to know about his/her diagnosis and prognosis, but also has the option to forgo this disclosure. However, the physician must know which of these two options the patient prefers.	A patient tells the nurse that he does not understand his diagnosis or prognosis. When the nurse informs the physician of the patient's concern, the physician indicates that the patient has, in fact, received this information. The nurse advocates for the patient and requests that the physician repeat the instructions.	If the physician in the situation refuses to provide additional information to the patient, the nurse reports this to the Nurse Manager who will request that the chief of medicine intervene in the situation.

Adapted from Varkey, B. (2021). Principles of clinical ethics and their application to practice. *Medical Principles and Practice, 30*(1), 17–28.

Codes of Ethics

Professional codes of ethics are formal statements that articulate values and beliefs of a given profession, serving as a standard of professional actions and reflecting the ethical principles shared by its members. Professional codes of ethics generally serve the following purposes:

- Inform the public of the minimum standards acceptable for conduct by members of the discipline and assist the public in understanding a discipline's professional responsibilities.
- Outline the major ethical considerations of the profession.
- Provide to its members guidelines for professional practice.
- Serve as a guide for the discipline's self-regulation.

The Code of Ethics for Nurses (ANA, 2015) should be the starting point for any nurse faced with an ethical issue. The first American nursing code was adopted in 1950, focusing on the character of the nurse and the virtues that were essential to the profession. In 1968, the code shifted to a duty-based ethical focus. In 2001, the ANA Code of Ethics for Nurses blended these duty-based ethics with a historical focus on character and virtue. In 2015, the revised provisions and interpretive statements were developed with an eye toward the future based on knowledge gained from the past. The code is regularly updated to reflect changes in health care structure, financing, and delivery. The Code of Ethics for Nurses (ANA, 2015) has nine points that guide nurses in understanding the extent of their commitment to the patient, themselves, other nurses, and the nursing profession. Further provisions in the code assist nurses in understanding that patients, whether as individuals or as members of families, groups, or communities, are their first obligation and that nurses must not only ensure quality care but also protect the safety of these patients. Nurses and their nurse managers should ensure that the provisions of the code are incorporated into nursing care delivery in all clinical settings. Along with establishing the ethical standard for the disciplines, the nursing code of ethics provides a basis for ethical analysis and decision-making in clinical situations.

Ethical Decision-Making Framework

Ethical decision-making involves reflection on many factors, such as intended outcomes, resources available, professional organizational directives, and likely and unintended consequences. When making decisions, nurses need to combine all these elements using an orderly, systematic, and objective method. Ethical decision-making models assist in accomplishing this goal.

For most nurses, ethical decision-making models are considered only when complex ethical dilemmas present in clinical settings. In truth, however, nurses use ethical decision-making models each time an ethical situation arises, although the decision-making model may not be acknowledged or fully appreciated (Hyatt, 2017). Ethical dilemmas involve situations in which a choice must be made between equally unacceptable options that nurses perceive they can accept and reasonably justify on a moral plane or in which there is not a more favorable or appropriate choice that dominates the situation (Hyatt, 2017).

Ethical decision-making is always a process. To facilitate this process, the nurse manager must use all available resources, including the institutional ethics committee, and communicate with and support all those involved in the process. Some decisions are easier to reach and support than others. Allowing sufficient time for the process contributes to a supportable option being reached.

Moral Distress

Nurses experience stress in clinical practice settings as they are confronted with situations involving ethical dilemmas. Moral distress most often occurs when one is faced with situations in which two ethical principles compete, such as when the nurse is balancing the patient's autonomy issues with attempting to do what the nurse knows is in the patient's best interest. Moral distress also may occur when the nurse manager is balancing a direct care nurse's autonomy with what the nurse manager perceives to be a better solution to an ethical dilemma. Though the dilemmas are stressful, nurses must make decisions and implement those decisions. The American Nurses Association developed the Exploring Moral Resilience Toward a Culture of Ethical Practice: A Call-to-Action Report (ANA, 2017) to identify potential individual and organizational strategies and interventions to approach ethical challenges and moral distress in nursing practice, as well as establish goals to strengthen moral resilience.

Seen as a major issue in nursing today, moral distress is experienced when nurses cannot provide what they perceive to be best for a given patient. Examples of moral distress include constraints caused by financial pressures, limited patient care resources, disagreements among family members regarding patient interventions, and/or limitations imposed by primary healthcare providers. Moral distress may also be experienced when actions nurses perform violate their personal beliefs.

The impact of moral distress can be quite serious. Moral distress compromises patient care and that moral distress may be manifested in such behaviors as avoiding or withdrawing from patient care situations. Additional behaviors include failure to act as a patient advocate, which often further contributes to patient discomfort and suffering.

Moral distress occurs when professionals cannot carry out what they believe to be ethically appropriate actions. A bibliometric analysis revealed that from 1984 to 2015, 239 articles on moral distress were published, with an increase after 2011. Most of them (71%) focused on nursing. Of the 239 articles, 17 empirical studies were systematically analyzed. Moral distress correlated with organizational environment (poor ethical climate and collaboration), professional attitudes (low work satisfaction and engagement), and psychological characteristics (low psychological empowerment and autonomy) (Lamiari et al., 2017).

Nurse managers can best assist nurses experiencing moral distress by remembering that such distress may be lessened through adequate levels of knowledge regarding nursing ethics and its application, acknowledging that such distress does occur, and serving as an advocate for nurses. In this latter role, the nurse manager advocates for improvement in conditions that may directly influence moral distress, such as additional staff during periods of high patient acuity, additional counselors to work with patients' family issues and disputes, and the implementation of in-service education and/or education concerning better communication among all levels of healthcare practitioners. These positive aspects of leadership may significantly reduce the level of moral distress encountered by direct care nurses and greatly increase their job satisfaction. Furthermore, nurses in leadership positions experience moral distress that direct care nurses do not. However, those sources of distress are the same types that direct care nurses experience—those issues simply are seen from a different perspective.

Moral Disengagement

Moral distress may result in negative emotions such as anxiety, fear, sadness, and anger. These feelings can escalate, resulting in a sense of moral disengagement in individuals, often leading to nursing behaviors that put patients at risk. A nurse who is disengaged in this way may act in an unethical manner for which they feel little

RESEARCH PERSPECTIVE

Resource: Zhao, H., & Xia, Q. (2019). Nurses' negative affective states, moral disengagement, and knowledge hiding: The moderating roles of ethical leadership. *Journal of Nursing* Management, *2019*, 357–370.

Zhao & Xia (2019) explored the impact of moral disengagement by nurses and the role nurse managers may play in reducing such disengagement and resulting potential harm to patients. Nurses who experience negative emotions, particularly in response to work-related pressures over time, may find that their actions tend to "narrow" to quick and decisive negative behaviors, such as escapism or attack. If actions are not taken to reduce these feelings, the nurse may respond by hiding certain important knowledge from other members of the team. Not sharing this information may result in potential to harm patients. For example, Zhao & Xia (2019) describe an example of such behavior when the nurse "believes it is alright to turn off patient call lights during night shifts in order to ensure a quiet night".

Zhao & Xia (2019) found that ethical leadership by nurse managers will reduce the impact of negative affective emotions, the staffs' knowledge-hiding behaviors, and moral disengagement.

Implications for Practice

The nurse manager plays a significant role in reducing negative effects of moral disengagement by nurses under their supervision. Initially, evaluating the potential of negative affective emotions in a candidate seeking employment is important. In addition, addressing environmental factors, such as inadequate staffing patterns or other problems affecting staff moral which may be influencing such negative emotions, is a key role of the nurse manager.

or no guilt. The Research Perspective of Zhao & Xia (2019) provides an understanding of this phenomenon.

Ethics Committees

With the increasing numbers of ethical dilemmas in patient situations and administrative decisions, healthcare providers are increasingly turning to hospital ethics committees for guidance. Such committees can provide both long-term and short-term assistance. Ethics committees provide structure and guidelines for potential problems, serve as open forums for discussion, and function as true patient advocates by placing the patient at the core of the committee discussions.

To form such a committee, the involved individuals should begin as a bioethical study group so that all potential members can explore ethical principles and theories. The composition of the committee should include nurses, physicians, clergy, clinical social workers, nutritional experts, pharmacists, administrative personnel, and legal experts. Once the committee has become active, individual patients or patients' families and additional representatives of members of the healthcare delivery team may be invited to committee deliberations.

Ethics committees traditionally follow one of three distinct structures, although some institutional committees blend the three structures. The autonomy model facilitates decision-making for competent patients. The patient-benefit model uses substituted judgment (what patients would want for themselves if capable of making their preferences known) and facilitates decision-making for the incompetent patient. The social justice model considers broad social issues and is accountable to the overall institution.

In most settings, the ethics committee already exists, because complex issues divide healthcare workers. In many centers, ethical rounds, conducted weekly or monthly, allow staff members who may later become involved in ethical decision-making to begin reviewing all of the issues and to become more comfortable with ethical issues and their resolution.

Blending Ethical and Legal Issues

Blending legal demands with ethics is a challenge for nursing. No case better portrays this type of difficult decision-making than does the case of Theresa (Terri) M. Schiavo. The Case Example Box 3.7 describes this situation. What feelings does this famous case bring up for you? What would you have done if you had been one of the nurses caring for this patient? What if you were the nurse manager?

Whichever side of the case one supported, the plight of Terri Schiavo created numerous ethical concerns for the nurses caring for her as well as for the nurse managers in the clinical setting. Issues that created these conflicts ranged from working with feuding family members, to multiple media personnel attempting to cover the story, to constant editorial and news stories invading the

CASE EXAMPLE BOX 3.7 Ms. Schiavo suffered a cardiac arrest in February 1990, sustaining a period of approximately 11 minutes during which she was anoxic. She was resuscitated and, at the insistence of her husband, was intubated, placed on a ventilator, and eventually received a tracheotomy. The cause of her cardiac arrest was determined to be a severe electrolyte imbalance that was directly caused by an eating disorder. In the 6 years preceding the cardiac event, Ms. Schiavo had lost approximately 140 pounds, going from 250 to 110 pounds.

During the first 2 months after her cardiac arrest, Ms. Schiavo was in a coma. She then regained some wakefulness and was eventually diagnosed as being in a persistent vegetative state (PVS). She was successfully weaned from the ventilator and was able to swallow her saliva, both reflexive behaviors. However, she was not able to eat food or drink liquids, which is characteristic of PVS. A permanent feeding tube was placed so that she could receive nutrition and hydration.

Throughout the early years of her PVS, no challenge was made to the diagnosis or to the appointment of her husband as her legal guardian. Four years after her cardiac arrest, a successful lawsuit was filed against a fertility physician who failed to detect her electrolyte imbalance. A judgment of $300,000 went to her husband for loss of companionship and $700,000 was placed in a court-managed trust fund to maintain and provide care for Ms. Schiavo.

Sometime after this successful lawsuit, the close family relationship that Ms. Schiavo's husband and her parents had began to erode, and the public first became aware of Ms. Schiavo's plight. As her court-appointed guardian noted (Wolfson, 2005): "Thereafter, what is for millions of Americans a profoundly private matter catapulted a close, loving family into an internationally watched blood feud. The result was a most public death for a very private individual. Theresa was by all accounts a very shy, fun loving, and sweet woman who loved her husband and her parents very much. The family breach and public circus would have been anathema to her" (p. 17).

The court battles regarding the removal or retention of her feeding tube were numerous. There was adequate medical and legal evidence to show that Ms. Schiavo had been correctly diagnosed and that she would not have wanted to be kept alive by artificial means. Laws in the state of Florida, where Ms. Schiavo was a patient, allowed the removal of tubal nutrition and hydration in patients with PVS. The feeding tube was removed and later reinstated after a court order.

In October 2003, there was a second removal of the feeding tube after a higher court overturned the lower court decision that had caused the feeding tube to be reinserted. With this second removal, the Florida legislature passed what has come to be known as Terri's Law. This law gave the Florida governor the right to demand that the feeding tube be reinserted and appoint a special guardian to review the entire case. The special guardian ad litem was appointed in October 2003. Terri's Law was later declared unconstitutional by the Florida Supreme Court, and the U.S. Supreme Court refused to overrule that decision.

In early 2005, during the last weeks of Ms. Schiavo's life, the U.S. Congress attempted to move the issue to the federal rather than Florida state court system. Finally, the Federal District Court in Florida and the 11th Circuit Court of Appeals ruled that there was insufficient evidence to create a new trial, and the U.S. Supreme Court refused to review the findings of these two lower courts (Wolfson, 2005). Ms. Schiavo died on March 31, 2005; she was 41 years old.

privacy of this individual, to masses of people lined at the borders of the hospice center insisting that she be fed, to individual emotions about the correctness of either keeping or removing the feeding tube. One issue remains clear: the nurse managers and nurses caring for this particular patient had a legal obligation to either remove or reinsert the feeding tube based on the prevailing court decision or legislative act. Their individual reflections about the correctness or justice of such court decrees were secondary to the prevailing court orders.

Nurse managers should ensure that nurses whose ethical values differ from court orders are given opportunities to voice their concerns and feelings, mechanisms for requesting reassignment, and time for quiet reflection. Although no deviance can occur from one's legal obligation, the nurse manager must ensure that the emotional and psychological well-being of those whom the nurse manager supervises are also recognized. Merely acknowledging that such discord can occur and allowing positive means to express this concern may be the best solution in handling these difficult legal and ethical patient situations.

Other Ethical Concerns for Nurses

Other issues of concern involve autonomy and independent practice among nurses, quality of care in home and community settings, and development of nurses as leaders in the healthcare delivery field. Issues that continue to permeate ethical concerns for nurses include the patient's right to refuse healthcare; issues surrounding death and

LITERATURE PERSPECTIVE

Resource: Muller, L. S. (2019). Legal and Regulatory Issues: Competency vs. Capacity. *Professional Case Management, 24(2)*, 95–98.

Nurse Leaders, managers, and followers must be able to apply legal and ethical principles to specific patient situations. This article discusses the legal and ethical concepts of patient autonomy, competency, and capacity, applying these concepts to the case management process. However, these concepts have meaning for nurses in any clinical setting. Below are definitions of these related concepts discussed, all of which should guide nursing practice.

Client/Patient Autonomy is an ethical standard that makes it clear that the role of healthcare professionals is not to dictate what they think is best for the patient, but rather to provide tools that help them make informed decisions. The American Hospital Association **Bill of Rights** states that, " except in emergencies when the patient lacks the ability to make decisions and the need for treatment is urgent, the patient is entitled to a chance to discuss and request information related to the specific procedures and treatments available, risk involved, possible length of recovery, and reasonable medical alternatives, along with accompanying risks and benefits, including financial consequences." (AHA Patient's Bill of Rights - APRA https://www.americanpatient.org/aha-patients-bill-of-rights/).

Two additional legal concepts are associated with the patient's ability to make decisions regarding care. The first, **Competency**, refers to the ability to reason and make decisions from a legal perspective. An individual's competency to contract or give permission for health care service is documented by signing a Consent for Treatment.

However, an individual's ability to make these decisions may be compromised, due to:
- Mental Illness
- Profoundly low intelligence

- Being younger than 18 years old or an adult with diminished mental acuity
- Under Anesthesia or other medications that reduces decision-making ability
- Alteration in consciousness for any reason

Such conditions may be temporary or permanent. Regardless, the presence of such a condition result in a patient not being able to "make a contract," which in healthcare, makes a patient's signature on a Consent for Treatment invalid.

If an individual is thought to be incompetent for any reason, determining who can make needed medical decisions is facilitated when he or she has a signed Advanced Directive for Healthcare. This legal instrument designates a representative to make healthcare decisions for the patient, which permits required care to continue. In some cases, courts may be involved in determining whether the patient has the potential to make a potential life-altering decision. Court action is typically required when no Advanced Directive is available and a complex treatment is proposed, the patient refuses treatment or demands to leave the hospital when medical professionals believe the action is unsafe.

Implications for Practice

Nurses have an obligation to advocate for the patient. As a result, nurses must use effective assessment skills, including good listening, when a Consent for Treatment is required. Being sensitive to patient behaviors and statements that may be clues to their lack of comprehension is critical. Should there be concern that a patient's decision-making is impaired, the nurse should try not to wait until faced with a time-sensitive or potentially dangerous decision must be made to consult with others regarding the patient's competence.

---

dying, including the issues of hydration and nutrition for patients in persistent vegetative states; nurses' ability to be patient advocates in today's healthcare structure; and the ability to perform competent, quality nursing care in healthcare delivery systems that often reward cost-saving measures rather than quality healthcare delivery. As with ethical dilemmas in patient care, the more expertise and time one has to resolve issues, usually, the better the outcome. In actual practice, legal and ethical principles are often intertwined, requiring nurses to consider both, and which may not always align. The Literature Perspective below describes ways in which both legal and ethical concepts of patient autonomy, competency, and capacity interact.

CONCLUSION

In addition to knowing and understanding legal terms and issues related to clinical concerns, formal leaders and managers need to know employment law, union laws, the nursing practice act, and numerous other legal findings. Though each state may have distinctive laws governing being a manager and working in a healthcare organization, the key decisions tested in court or laws that govern all healthcare operations within the United States are ones with which we must all be familiar. *In addition, ethical dilemmas often coincide with legal problems, requiring the nurse manager to deal with both.* Legal and ethical aspects present additional opportunities for nurses to exhibit leadership capabilities.

THE SOLUTION

Staff members and nursing leadership began by working together to understand the varied viewpoints of the healthcare team. We attempted to understand why some of the primary healthcare providers allowed family members to be present and other primary healthcare providers insisted that family members not be present during resuscitation efforts. When asked, primary healthcare providers often noted that the behaviors and attitudes of the family members were a factor in their decision. They noted that one could not know in advance whether the family members might be hostile or belligerent and thus distract or prevent the healthcare team from being able to provide necessary care. Additionally, no clear hospital policy existed. Many of these primary healthcare providers were more comfortable in not having the family members present, and the current practice was to assign a chaplain and social worker to provide supportive services as well as comfort and information to family members when such situations arose. Thus, the family members, though not present within the patient's room, were also not alone during this time and had the opportunity to ask questions.

We then looked at the issue from an ethical perspective. For many patients and family members, being present during this crucial time could have many positive effects, thus, beneficence and respect for others were the two ethical principles that most clearly seemed to support family presence. Seeing for themselves and understanding that everything possible was being done to save their loved one's life were the most positive outcomes to support family presence. Family members could later have an opportunity to more fully question why certain aspects were performed, and the nursing staff as well as the primary care provider could then explain in more detail answers to the family members' questions.

Viewing the literature about this topic was enlightening. We discovered that this topic has continually been studied, dating back to the early 1980s. These studies almost uniformly noted that family presence did not alter the effectiveness of the healthcare team's interventions, nor did family presence interfere with the duration of resuscitative efforts or selection of medications. Some of the more recent studies addressed the issue of interference by family members and noted that very few family members were aggressive or in conflict with the team's performance and that family members excluded from being present expressed regret at not having been present during resuscitation. Interestingly, some of the reviewed studies continued to question how to best determine which family members should be given the option of viewing resuscitation measures or whether all families should be given this option. At present, we continue to explore possible guidelines concerning family presence during resuscitation, recognizing that such a complex issue cannot be rapidly resolved.

Would this be a suitable approach for you? Why?

Acacia Syring

REFLECTIONS

Consider a situation you may have observed in the clinical area that made you wonder if the action taken was legal or ethical. What triggered that thought for you? What did you think you would have done differently? Did you consider reporting the concerns? Consider what you would do if you believed the client you were assigned to care for had not had the duty of reasonable care earlier in the care process. What would be your responsibility? What resources might you draw upon?

THE EVIDENCE

State boards of nursing have worked diligently to uphold high standards of accountability to the public. One example is the enhanced nurse licensure compact agreement. When nurses face ethical or legal concerns, they have resources available through their employment setting, the state board of nursing, and the state professional nursing association.

TIPS FOR INCORPORATING LEGAL AND ETHICAL ISSUES IN PRACTICE SETTINGS

- Read the state nurse practice act, ensuring compliance with the allowable scope of practice.
- Apply legal principles in all healthcare settings.
- Understand and follow state and federal employment laws.
- Follow the Code of Ethics for Nurses (ANA, 2015), and Nurses' Bill of Rights in all aspects of healthcare delivery.
- If available, use Ethics Committees to deal with ethical dilemmas.

- Remember that no right and wrong answers exist in ethical situations, merely better or worse solutions. Consider all aspects and consult with others before proceeding if there are unanswered questions.

- If legal and ethical issues are contradictory, legal aspects must be adhered to first.

CASE STUDY 3.1   NEXT-GENERATION NCLEX® CASE STUDY

Case Study

Next-Generation NCLEX® case studies are included in select chapters to familiarize you with these new testing items for the NGN exam.

Learning Outcome: Use the bioethical principle of autonomy to determine the most likely condition of the client, the actions of the Interprofessional team and the parameters the team is most likely to monitor.

Cognitive Skills: Recognize Cues, Analyze Cues, Prioritize Hypotheses, Generate Solution, Take Action, and Evaluate Outcomes.

A client is making a weekend home visit to an 88-year-old male recently admitted to a home health service.

History: The client had an ATK amputation of the L leg 2 years ago, resulting from poorly controlled diabetes. One month ago, the client was admitted to the hospital for a non-healing diabetic foot ulcer. The treatment included negative-pressure wound therapy. During this hospitalization, the ulcer became deeper and more extensive. The client's continued high blood glucose levels accelerated his peripheral arterial disease and complicated the treatment.

Social Hx: Client lives alone. Spouse of 60 years died last year. No other family.

Recommendation: Client refused amputation and was discharged home.

Physician Discharge Orders

1. Home Health RN and Home Health aide for personal care daily.
2. Dressing change on the R foot
3. AIC and point of care blood glucose test during visit

Nurse's Notes of Current Visit

Client lying in a hospital bed in the living room of his small home. The Home Health aide has been caring for client for 8 hrs/day. The client's church provides for an evening meal and members of an Out-Reach group in the church are taking turns spending the night with the client. Client states: "I only want to die. Since my spouse died, I have nothing to live for. I WILL NOT have that amputation!"

Hemoglobin A1C = 7.0 (5.7–6.5)

Blood glucose = 280 mg/dL (70–130)

Wound on the R foot covers the entire heel with yellow, foul-smelling discharge which saturates the dressing. Red streaks radiate two inches above the ankle.

Question

This case study presents an example of a bioethical dilemma, requiring the interprofessional team, collaborating with the client, to determine this client's plan of care. Assuming that the team is using **AUTONOMY** as the bioethical principle to guide the plan of care, complete the bow-tie question below by identifying the **condition** that the client will most likely experience, the two **actions** that the interprofessional team will most likely take, and the two parameters the team is most likely to monitor.

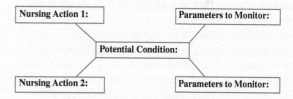

Nursing Action 1	Potential Condition	Parameters to Monitor
a. Physician will prescribe a mood elevator for patient.	a. Client remains in home with adequate support.	a. Assessment of client's emotional state.
b. Physician will make a referral to therapist to help client make a final decision.	b. Client elects to go to a long-term care facility.	b. Assessment of client's physical condition.
c. Social worker will make arrangements for admission to a long-term care facility.	c. Client remains at home with current level of support from the church.	c. Assessment of client's willingness to return to acute care facility for further treatment.
d. Social worker will collaborate with the client's church to seek additional assistance for evening/night care.	d. Client is readmitted to the acute care facility.	d. Assessment of client's willingness to transfer to a long-term care facility.

REFERENCES

American Association of Colleges of Nursing (AACN). (2021). *The Essentials: Core Competencies for Professional Nursing Education.* Retrieved from https://www.aacnnursing.org/Portals/42/AcademicNursing/pdf/Essentials-2021.pdf.

Age Discrimination in Employment Act of 1967, P.L. 90-202, 29 United States Code 621 (December 15, 1967).

American Nurses Association (ANA). (2015). *Code of ethics for nurses.* American Nurses Publishing.

American Nurses Association (ANA). (2017). *Exploring Moral Resilience Toward a Culture of Ethical Practice: A Call to Action Report.* Retrieved from https://www.nursingworld.org/~4907b6/globalassets/docs/ana/ana-call-to-action-exploring-moral-resilience-final.pdf.

Americans with Disabilities Act of 1990, Public Law 101-336, 104 Statutes 327 (July 26, 1990).

Americans with Disabilities Amended Act of 2008, Public Law 110-325 (September 25, 2008).

Black's law dictionary. (2019). (11th ed.). St. Paul, MN: West Publishing Company.

Brous, E. (2019). The Elements of a Nursing Malpractice Case, Part 1: Duty. *American Journal of Nursing, 119*(7), 64–67.

Brous, E. (2019). The Elements of a Nursing Malpractice Case, Part 2: Breach. *American Journal of Nursing, 119*(9), 42–46.

Brous, E. (2019). The Elements of a Nursing Malpractice Case, Part 3A: Causation. *American Journal of Nursing, 119*(11), 54–59.

Brous, E. (2020). The Elements of a Nursing Malpractice Case, Part 3B: Causation. *American Journal of Nursing, 120*(1), 63–66.

Brous, E. (2020). The Elements of a Nursing Malpractice Case, Part 4: Harm. *American Journal of Nursing, 120*(1), 63–66.

Civil Rights Act of 1964, P. L. 88-352, 78 Statutes 241, § 703 et seq. (July 2, 1964).

Civil Rights Act of 1991, P. L. 102-166 (November 21, 1991).

Department of Health and Human Services, Office of Disease Prevention and Health Promotion. (2015). Health Literacy Online: A guide to simplifying the user experience. Retrieved from https://health.gov/healthliteracyonline/.

Dowie, I. (2017). Legal, ethical and professional aspects of duty of care for nurses. *Nursing Standard, 32*(16-19), 47–52.

Equal Employment Opportunity Act of 1972, 78 Statutes 253; 42 U.S.C. 2000e (March 24, 1972).

Equal Pay Act of 1963, P. L. 88-38, 77 Statutes 56 (June 10, 1963).

Estate of Travaglini v Ingalls Health. (2009). WL 4432565 (Ill. App., November 24, 2009).

Family and Medical Leave Act of 1993, P. L. 103-3, 107 Statutes 6 (February 5, 1993).

Family and Medical Leave Amended Act of 2008, P. L. 110-181, 122 Statutes 128 (January 28, 2008).

Health Insurance Portability and Accountability Act of 1996, Public Law 104-191, 100 Statutes 2548 (August 21, 1996).

Hyatt, J. (2017). Recognizing moral disengagement and its impact on patient safety. *Journal of Nursing Regulation, 7*(4), 15–19.

Lamiari, G., Borghi, L., & Argentero, P. (2017). When healthcare professionals cannot do the right thing: A systematic review of moral distress and its correlates. *Journal of Health Psychology, 22*(1), 51–67. https://doi.org/10.1177/1359105315595120.

Laurin v. Providence Hospital and Massachusetts Nurses Association, 150F.3d 52 (1st Cir., 1998).

Lattimore v. Dickey, 239 Cal. App. 4th 959, 191 Cal. Rprt. 3d 766 (6th Dist. 2015).

Marinock v. Manor at St. Luke's, 2010 WL 3233125 (Ct. Com. Pl. Luzerne Co., Pennsylvania, January 29, 2010).

Mitchell & Galle v. Winkler County et al., CV 00037-RAJ, Document 42, Winkler County Trail Court, filed April 18, 2010.

Martell v. Tarpon Springs Hospital, 2010 WL 5485106 (Cir. Ct. Pinellas Co., Florida, September 29, 2010).

Mauro v. Borgess Medical Center, 4:94 CV 05 (Mich., 1995).

Mitter v. Touro Infirmary, 874 So. 2d 265 (La. Ct. App. 4th Cir. 2004).

Muller, L. S. (2019). Legal and Regulatory Issues: Competency vs. Capacity. *Professional Case Management, 24*(2), 95–98.

Moschke v. Memorial Medical Center of West Michigan, 2003 WL 462374 (Mich. App., February 21, 2003).

National Academy of Medicine (formerly Institute of Medicine). (1999). *To err is human: Building a safer health care system.* Washington, DC: The National Academies Press.

National Council of State Boards of Nursing (2022). *Licensure Compacts.* Retrieved from https://www.ncsbn.org/compacts.htm.

National Labor Relations Act, P. L. 74-198, 49 Statutes 449 (July 5, 1935).

Occupational Safety and Health Administration Act of 1970, P. L. 91-595, 84 Statutes 1590 (December 29, 1970).

O'Shea v. State of New York, WL 1516492 (N.Y. Ct. Cl., January 22, 2007).

Potter, P., Deshields, T., & Kuhrik, M. (2010). Delegation practices between registered nurses and nursing assistive personnel. *Journal of Nursing Management, 18,* 157–165.

Protection of Human Subjects, 45 Code of Federal Regulations, Sec. 46.111, 46.101(b), 46.110, 46.116 (1991).

Protection of Human Subjects, 45 Code of Federal Regulations, Sec. 46.401 et seq. (1998).

Registered Nurse Safe Staffing Act of 2011. United States House Bill 876/United States Senate Bill 58. Retrieved from http://legiscan.com/US/comments/HB876/2011; http://legiscan.com/US/bill/SB58/2011.

Reising, D. L. (2012). Make your nursing care malpractice proof. *American Nurse Today, 7*(1). Retrieved from https://www.myamericannurse.com/make-your-nursing-care-malpractice-proof/.

Ricciardi, C. L. (2015). Hospital administration not immune–criminal and civil liability: A risk for health care administrators. In *Becker's Hospital Review 2015* ASC Communications.

Sabol v. Richmond Heights General Hospital, 676N. E.2d 958 (Ohio App. 1996).

Trombley v. Southwestern Vermont Medical Center, 738 A.2d 103 (Vt., 1999).

Tseng, P. E., & Wang, Y. H. (2021). Deontological or utilitarian? An eternal ethical dilemma in Outbreak. *International Journal of Environmental Research and Public Health, 18*(16), 8565.

U.S. vs Parnell, Parnell, Lightsey & Wilkerson, U.S. District Court for Middle District of GA, 2015.

Varkey, B. (2021). Principles of clinical ethics and their application to practice. *Medical Principles and Practice, 30*(1), 17–28.

Vietnam Era Veterans' Readjustment Assistance Act of 1974, 38 United States Code § 4212 (1974).

Watkins v. Unemployment Compensation Board of Review, 689 A.2d 1019 (Pa. Commonwealth, 1997).

Wellstar Health System, Inc. v. Green, WL 31324127 (Ga. App., October 18, 2002).

Wolfson, J. (2005). Erring on the side of Theresa Schiavo: Reflections of the special guardian ad litem. *The Hastings Center Report, 35*(3), 16–19.

Yoder-Wise, P. (2010). More serendipity: The Winkler County trial. *The Journal of Continuing Education in Nursing, 41*(4), 147–148.

Zamudio v. Patia, 956F. Supp. 803 (N.D. Ill., 1997).

Zhao, H., & Xia, Q. (2019). Nurses' negative affective states, moral disengagement, and knowledge hiding: The moderating roles of ethical leadership. *Journal of Nursing Management, 2019*, 357–370.

4

Toward Justice

Karen A. Quintana and Susan Sportsman

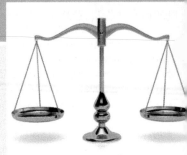

ANTICIPATED LEARNING OUTCOMES

- Evaluate the concepts of Diversity, Equity, Inclusion, and Belonging with cultural considerations in your staff and patients.
- Evaluate the use of concepts and principles of acculturation, culture, cultural diversity, and cultural sensitivity in leading and managing situations.
- Analyze inequities in healthcare (health disparities) and what nurses can do to minimize them.
- Evaluate individual and societal factors involved with cultural diversity.
- Value the contributions that a diverse workforce can make to the care of a diverse population of people.

KEY TERMS

acculturation	cultural sensitivity	healthy people
belonging	culture	implicit bias
cross culturism	diversity	inclusion
cultural competency	equity	justice
cultural diversity	ethnicity	social determinants of health
cultural humility	ethnocentrism	systemic racism
cultural imposition	global	transcultural nursing care
cultural marginality	health disparities	transculturalism

THE CHALLENGE

I work with a diverse group of men and women. They have various perspectives on how to approach their day and assignments. We additionally have a wide range of ages and experience levels which can lead to disagreements and frustrations. Our goal is a strong team. More novice nurses can often feel overwhelmed or intimidated. Our interaction is not only limited to diverse nursing staff, but also to diverse physicians, interdisciplinary teams, and various students (medicine, nursing, pharmacy, etc).

These differences can definitely lead to challenges within the team. My biggest challenge is allowing everyone to be themselves while respecting the differences of others, whether that be thoughts, plans, approaches to care, or reactions to stress.

Nancy Leal, MSN, RN, CPN, CNML
Nursing Department Director for Pediatrics and Pediatric Intensive Care Unit, University Medical Center, Lubbock, Texas

INTRODUCTION

This chapter is entitled "toward justice" to reflect the constant need to be sensitive to the needs of others and how we all can contribute to making society, healthcare, and the workplace more just places. The idea of diversity, equity, inclusion, and belonging (DEIB) applies to all of the "isms" in society—age, disability, ethnicity, gender, lifestyle, race, religion and others. While changes have occurred over the past several decades, to some people, these changes are minor and lack true meaning in achieving a sense of belonging in the workplace or in society. In other words, much work remains.

The focus of diversity, equity, inclusion, and belonging (DEIB) and cultural considerations apply both to patients and staff. DEIB does not address comprehensive details about any specific culture or group. It does, however, provide guidelines for actively incorporating diverse aspects into the roles of leading and managing in today's healthcare world. The goal is to embrace cultural differences while understanding disparities through recognition and action. This is expressed as one of the core competencies in *The Essentials: Core Competencies for Professional Nursing Education,* by the American Association of Colleges of Nursing (AACN, 2021), under Domain 9: "Professionalism, one must integrate diversity, equity, and inclusion [and belonging] as the core of one's professional identity. Nurses must also demonstrate respect for individuals with diverse differences, communities, and populations."

Justice in healthcare is a critical component of social justice, where everyone deserves equal rights and opportunities, including good health and fair work environments. We all want to feel as if we belong in our work environment and society. Similarly, people want to feel that they deserve the same healthcare everyone else is afforded. The American Public Health Association notes that inequities in healthcare, also known as health disparities, are avoidable, unnecessary, and unjust. These inequities result from an unequal distribution of money, power, and resources based on race, class, gender, place, and other factors (American Public Health Association, 2021).

> **EXERCISE 4.1** Think about a patient for whom you have provided care. Consider whether social determinants of health might have played a role in that patient's health condition (*Healthy People 2030, 2020*).

SOCIAL DETERMINANTS OF HEALTH (SDH)

Social determinants of health (SDH) are defined by *Healthy People 2030* as environmental conditions that affect health, functioning, and quality of life risks and outcomes. The environmental conditions include where someone was born; how they live, learn, work, play, and worship; and their age (*Healthy People 2030*, 2020). In the last decade, scholars and public health practitioners have focused on this unequal distribution of resources, recognizing that social determinants of health—such as income and social status, social support networks, education, employment/working conditions, social environments, physical environments, personal health practices and coping skills, healthy child development, gender, and culture—all significantly influence healthcare outcomes. *The Future of Nursing 2020–2030: Charting a Path to Achieve Health Equity* discusses the importance of nurses addressing the SDH in planning, implementing, and evaluating care (National Academy of Medicine, 2021).

SOCIAL POLICIES AIMED AT REDUCING HEALTH DISPARITIES

The concern over the impact of social determinants on health has resulted in numerous organizational recommendations to address social determinants as part of the nation's efforts to achieve health equity.

World Health Organization (WHO)

The World Health Organization (WHO) developed goals designed to improve health outcomes, as follows (WHO, 2021).
1. Improve the circumstances that determine people's daily lives.
2. Identify and address structural drivers such as the social and economic forces in people's lives (inequitable distribution of power, money, and resources surrounding vulnerable people).
3. Identify measures and frameworks to develop and expand scholarship around the SDH while raising awareness of the inequitable distribution of social and healthcare services.

Healthy People Goals

In 1979, the U.S. Surgeon General issued a landmark report titled *Healthy People: The Surgeon General's Report* on *Health Promotion and Disease Prevention*. Then, in 1980, the U.S. Office of Disease Prevention and Health Promotion (ODPHP) released *Healthy People 1990*, which was followed in later decades by new iterations of the Healthy People initiative, with each building on the prior report (ODPHP, 2021). The purpose of the Healthy People initiative is to help individuals, organizations, and communities improve the health and well-being of U.S. citizens through public health priorities. Since the founding of the Healthy People initiative, these priorities have been published every decade, with the most recent priorities published in August 2020 (*Healthy People 2030*). In addition to developing goals for improving the health of the U.S. population, the Healthy People initiative provides (1) data that illustrates national progress toward achieving objectives; (2) evidence-based resources to help with program and policy development; and (3) tools to inspire action, encourage collaboration, and empower individuals, organizations, and communities to use the initiative. Two of the foundational principles of *Healthy People 2030* address the ongoing concern regarding health disparities through emphasis on SDH:

- Achieving health and well-being requires eliminating health disparities, achieving health equity, and attaining health literacy.
- Healthy physical, social, and economic environments strengthen the potential to achieve health and well-being.

Centers for Disease Control and Prevention (CDC)

First in 2013 and again in 2014, the *Morbidity and Mortality Weekly Report* (*MMWR*) from the Centers for Disease Control and Prevention (CDC) highlighted disparities across a wide range of diseases, behavioral risk factors, environmental exposure, social determinants, and healthcare access. The goal of these reports was to use the *MMWR* to emphasize health disparities so that all Americans would live longer, healthier, and more productive lives. The reports looked at 29 topics related to health outcome disparities, such as health behaviors, exposures to health hazards, and access to healthcare. Since issuing these reports, the CDC has maintained a website devoted to health equity, health disparities, and strategies (CDC, 2013). In addition, in 2014 and 2016, the CDC's Center for Minority Health published reports of effective public health programs that help mitigate health disparities. These reports describe evidence-based programs regarding traditional foods, asthma, colorectal disease, reduction of violence, and skills for people with disabilities (CDC, 2016).

PROGRESS TOWARD ACHIEVING HEALTH EQUITY

Despite recognizing disparities for decades and the overall improvements in population health over time, nurses will find that many disparities have persisted and, in some cases, widened. For example, recent data reported by the Kaiser Family Foundation (KFF) found that before the COVID-19 pandemic, people of color fared worse compared with their White counterparts across a range of health measures, including infant mortality, pregnancy-related deaths, prevalence of chronic conditions, and overall physical and mental health status. As of 2018, life expectancy among Black people was four years lower than that of White people, with the lowest expectancy among Black men (KFF, 2021a). In addition, people with low incomes of all races reported worse health status than those with a higher income, and lesbian, gay, bisexual, transgender, and queer (LGBTQ+) individuals experience certain health challenges at increased rates (KFF, 2021b).

The Kaiser Family Foundation also reported that although the Affordable Care Act (ACA) health coverage expansions resulted in coverage across groups, people of color and individuals with low incomes reported being at increased risk of being uninsured, which presented barriers to access to care. Unfortunately, increased insurance coverage first became static and then began dropping beginning in 2017 because of a number of federal policies, including less funding for outreach and enrollment assistance and approval of state waivers of parts of the ACA. These losses continued during the COVID-19 pandemic, as people lost jobs (KFF, 2021a).

The COVID-19 pandemic escalated the rates of illness and death in American Indian and Alaskan Natives (AIAN), Blacks, and Hispanics. The pandemic also took a disproportionate toll on the financial security and mental health and well-being of people of color, low-income people, LGBTQ+ people, and other underserved groups. According to a KFF survey, 6 in 10 Hispanic adults (59%) and about half of Black adults (51%) said that their household lost a job or income due to the pandemic compared with about 4 in 10 White adults (39%) who said the same. Adults with a household income under $40,000 were three times as likely as those with a household income of $90,000 or more to say they had trouble paying for basic living expenses in the past three months. Finally, as of April 2021, Black and Hispanic people were less likely to get a COVID-19 vaccine. In addition, while vaccination rates through May of 2021 increased across all groups, the gaps in vaccination rates for Black and Hispanic people persisted, which reflect the ongoing inequities that create barriers to healthcare for people of color and other underserved groups (Singh, Palosky, 2021).

IMPLICIT BIAS

While many of us would like to believe we hold no prejudice about any one or any group, Eberhardt (2019) suggested that we are all biased and that this hidden prejudice shapes our lives. As she explains, we learn from our experiences what is important to us—and that is often the "familiar", in other words, people who look, act, sound and behave as we do. We tend to prefer faces that look more like ours, as an example, than those that don't look like ours. This is called the other race effect. We all experience this phenomenon and it applies to other aspects of life too, whether we think about race or religion or height, or almost any other characteristic. Our challenge is to be aware when we experience that "gut instinct" (the stereotypical response) to rethink what led us to a conclusion that what we experienced was positive or negative. What evidence presented itself to make us think one way or another about a person or a situation? How will we test the evidence to determine if it is true or false? One way to begin is found in Exercise 4.2.

> **EXERCISE 4.2**   Harvard University offers Project Implicit, which allows anyone to choose from among a variety of association tests (faces and words). Go to implicit.harvard.edu and choose a topic to investigate your own implicit bias on a topic. When you complete the assignment (about 10 minutes), consider what you learned and remember: every one of us is human and we are shaped by our experiences. Unless we had deliberate experiences to cause us to examine prejudice, we are likely to have responses that are the stereotypes of who we are. Consider what you learned from participating in whichever of the options that the implicit assessments allow you to explore.

Impact of Clinician Implicit Bias on Health Equity

Bias comes in the form of explicit bias and implicit bias. Implicit bias is always present and found everywhere in all situations. It exists in every individual to some capacity, no matter how strongly they feel impartial. Specifically, bias includes stereotypes that can unconsciously affect our actions, comprehension, and decisions. Implicit bias encompasses positive and negative connotations and can contradict each other often (Kirwan Institute for the Study of Race and Ethnicity, 2015). The goals of education programs for health care professionals are to remain culturally competent, free of judgement or bias, and provide fair and equal care. We also hope patients are provided with equitable care regardless of their race, sexual orientation, or other identity. This can become a challenge for healthcare providers as their behaviors do not always align with their beliefs.

Healthcare clinicians' biases (often implicit) may be a factor that influences care of people of color. Racial bias among clinicians may lead to poorer communication and lower quality of care. Implicit biases directly lead to health disparities by influencing how health professionals make decisions and communicate within their clinical practice (Sukhera, Watling, & Gonzales, 2020). The problem of implicit biases is that they innately influence health professionals without their knowledge and despite their best intentions.

When looking at healthcare professionals and students and implicit bias, the subjects of mental health and obesity is often explored. Research by Sandhu, Arora, Brasch, and Streiner (2019) analyzed explicit and implicit attitudes of medical students, undergraduate students, and psychiatrists. They found that psychiatrists had the lowest scores regarding implicit bias compared to the students, and that being diagnosed with a mental illness also significantly reduced someone's explicit stigma, but not necessarily implicit stigma. Research by Yılmaz and Ayhan (2019) examined implicit bias of registered nurses and nursing students. They found that when compared to current registered nurses, nursing students were found to have fewer negative attitudes towards obesity.

Hoffman et al. (2016) found 73% of White medical students had at least one false belief about the biological difference between races. For example, many (wrongly) believed that Black people have a higher pain tolerance than White people. Black children with painful health issues such as appendicitis or sickle cell disease were less likely to receive appropriate pain management than White children.

Black women may face higher risks during pregnancy. Howell (2018) reported that Black women were 3 to 4 times more likely to die from a pregnancy-related cause than White women in America. Such discriminations were not only between Black and White people. Chen et al. (2018) found that Asian-Americans with symptoms of addictions were less likely to be diagnosed with addiction when compared with White Americans with the same symptoms.

IMPACT OF HEALTH DISPARITIES ON HEALTHCARE WORKERS OF COLOR

Healthcare workers of color or who are part of groups who have struggled with health disparities may have similar experiences as patients. A study from Harvard Medical School based on data from more than 2 million COVID Symptom Study app users in the United States from March 24 through April 23, 2021 found that healthcare workers of color were more likely to care for patients with suspected or confirmed COVID-19, more likely to report using inadequate or reused protective gear, and nearly twice as likely as White colleagues to test positive for the coronavirus. Healthcare workers of color were also more likely to report inadequate or reused personal protective equipment (PPE), at a rate 50% higher than what White workers reported. The rate of reporting inadequate PPE for Latinos was double that of White workers. These risks rise for workers who were treating COVID patients. This study, which focused on the frontline roles and PPE, highlights the problem of structural racism (Menni et al., 2021).

CURRENT INITIATIVES TO REACH HEALTH EQUITY AMONG PATIENTS AND STAFF

Dealing with health disparities continues to be a high priority at the national level. The Office of Minority Health, in addition to the initiatives previously discussed, developed three overarching equity priorities for fiscal years 2020 and 2021. These priorities comprised (1) supporting states, territories, and tribes in identifying and sustaining health equity-promoting policies, programs, and practices; (2) expanding the utilization of community health workers to address health and social service needs within communities of color, and (3) perhaps most importantly from the perspective of nurse leaders, managers, and followers, strengthening cultural competency among healthcare providers throughout the country (Ndugga & Artiga, 2021).

The term, cultural competency, laid a foundation for the goal of health equity or equality as a whole. The seminal work of Cross, Barzon, Dennis, & Isaacs (1989) defined cultural competency as a set of congruent behaviors, attitudes, and policies that come together in a system, agency or among professionals and enable that system. They come together to work effectively in cross cultural situations (Cross et al, 1989). To become culturally competence, an agency or person must value diversity, have the capacity for cultural self-assessment, be conscious of the dynamics inherent when culture interacts, have institutionalized cultural knowledge, and develop adaptations related to cultural diversity (Cross et at, 1989).

Cultural Competencies as a Path to Healthcare Justice

Nurse leaders, managers, and followers play a significant role in reducing health disparities and addressing the social determinants of health, which present barriers to appropriate healthcare. A strategy to address these barriers is to increase the cultural competencies of nursing staff. What steps should nurses take to strengthen cultural competency among nurses and our healthcare colleagues? The first step is to learn all we can about the concept of culture—our own and those of our clients, as well as the theoretical underpinnings of culture.

> **EXERCISE 4.3** In a group, discuss the values and beliefs of justice and equality. As a nurse, you may have strong values and beliefs, but you may never have observed their application in healthcare. Consider language, skin color, dress, practices (health and others) and gestures of patients and staff from other cultures. Consider your own. How will you learn and value what differences exist?

CONCEPTS OF CULTURE

What is culture? Does it exhibit certain characteristics? What is cultural diversity, and what do we think of when we refer to cultural sensitivity? Are culture and ethnicity the same? Various authors have different views. Cultural background stems from one's ethnic background, socioeconomic status, and family rituals, to name three key factors. Ethnicity can be thought of as large groupings of people who are "classified" based on mutual factors that distinguish one group from another. Those groupings might relate to culture, language, nations, race, religion, or a variety of other factors. This description differs from what is commonly used to identify racial groups. This broader definition encourages people to think about the diversity of the populations in the United States.

Understanding the impact of culture can be facilitated by considering the following four factors:

1. Culture develops over time and is responsive to its members and their familial and social environments.
2. A culture's members learn it and share it. It is passed on from one generation to the next.
3. Culture is essential for survival and acceptance.
4. Culture changes with difficulty. This explains why we can create a new policy or issue a new statement and little changes in actual practice.

For the nurse leader or manager, the characteristics of ethnicity and culture are important to keep in mind, because the underlying thread is that culture and ethnicity of staff and patients have been with them their entire lives. All people view their cultural background as normal; the diversity challenge is for others to also view it as normal and to assimilate various cultures into the existing workforce to care effectively for diverse patient populations. No one needs to convert to a different culture; everyone needs to respect each person's culture and what it means to that person.

EXERCISE 4.4 List some of the beliefs associated with your own culture. In what way are these characteristics different from those of some of your colleagues? How might these differences influence your nursing practice?

Definitions of terms related to culture can help the nurse leader, manager, or follower to be sensitive to the impact of culture Cultural diversity is the term currently used to describe a vast range of cultural differences among individuals or groups. Cultural diversity may also be referred to as multiculturalism, which recognizes and respects the presence of diverse people in society (Horace Mann School, 2021). Cultural diversity also recognizes that people are different and, despite these differences, they can live in harmony.

Cultural sensitivity describes the affective behaviors in individuals—the capacity to feel, convey, or react to ideas, habits, customs, or traditions unique to a group of people. People with such sensitivity embrace diversity by accepting differences while not imposing their own beliefs on others (Sherman, 2019).

Ethnocentrism classically is defined as "the belief that one's own ways are the best, most superior, or preferred ways to act, believe, or behave" (Leininger, 2002, p. 50), whereas cultural imposition is defined as "the tendency of an individual or group to impose their values, beliefs, and practices on another culture for varied reasons" (Leininger, 2002, p. 51). Such practices constitute a major concern in nursing and "a largely unrecognized problem as a result of cultural ignorance, blindness, ethnocentric tendencies, biases, racism or other factors" (Leininger, 2002, p. 51).

Cultural acculturation is an important concept for nurses to integrate into their practice. Spector (2017) addressed three themes involved with acculturation. (1) *Socialization* refers to growing up or being raised within a culture and taking on the characteristics of that group. All of us are socialized to some culture and, sometimes, changing behavior resulting from our culture can be painful. (2) Acculturation refers to adapting to the dominant culture in the environment where you live or work. An example of this might be using the words a particular society calls a particular food or how healthcare organizations are changing to blame-free environments to encourage safety disclosures. The overall process of acculturation into a new society is extremely difficult and involuntary. "America" has a core culture and numerous subcultures. For example, think how differently people in rural American regions dress from those in urban centers or how a city looks on a Saturday night versus a Sunday morning. In other words, subcultures expand on how the core culture might be described. "Acculturation also refers to cultural or behavioral assimilation and may be defined as the changes of one's cultural pattern to those of the host society" (Spector, 2017, p. 25). (3) *Assimilation* refers to the change that occurs when people move from one country to another or from one part of a country to another. The person may become like the members of a dominant culture. They face different social and nursing practices, and individuals now define themselves as members of the dominant culture. An example of this might be when nurses no longer say they are from their country of origin. They say they are from where they currently live and practice.

Providing care for a person or people from a culture other than one's own is a dynamic and complex experience. The experience, according to the classic work of Spence (2001, 2004), might involve "prejudice, paradox and possibility" (Spence, 2004, p. 140). Spence used *prejudice* to describe conditions that enabled or constrained interpretation based on one's values, attitudes, and actions. By talking with people outside their "circle of familiarity," nurses can enhance their understanding of their own personally held prejudices.

Prejudices "enable us to make sense of the situations in which we find ourselves; yet they also constrain understanding and limit the capacity to come to new or different ways of understanding. It is this contradiction that makes prejudice paradoxical" (Spence, 2004, p. 163). *Paradox,* although it may seem incongruent with prejudice, describes the dynamic interplay of tensions between individuals or groups. We have the responsibility to acknowledge the "possibility of tension" as a potential for new and different understandings derived from our communication and interpretation. Therefore, *possibility* presumes a condition for openness with a person from another culture (Spence, 2004).

Multiculturism, also known as pluralism, reflects a positive interaction among different cultures. Successful multiculturism may build the bonds of community among various groups interacting in healthcare. Cross culturalism, on the other hand, refers to comparisons between two or more different cultures to develop ways to work together, a skill that is helpful for nurse leaders, managers, and followers.

Cultural humility helps us explore cultural competency as a process rather than an outcome. Hook et al. (2013) visualized cultural humility as the "ability to maintain an interpersonal stance that is other-oriented (or open to the other) in relation to aspects of cultural identity that are most important to the [person]" (p. 2).

When exploring cultural humility, we find three factors, first described by Tervalon and Murray-Garcia (1998), help shape our understanding of the process:

1. A lifelong commitment to self-evaluation and self-critique
2. A desire to fix power imbalances
3. An aspiration to develop partnerships with people and groups who advocate for others

The first factor, a lifelong commitment to self-valuation and self-critique, looks at our lives as never being finished with learning. The idea of lifelong learning is a hallmark of being a professional and, as with clinically based learning, we need to incorporate our newly acquired knowledge into our approach to others. We must remain humble to a point of being able to look at ourselves critically. We need to maintain the desire to learn more. Specifically, "We must continue learning about the cultures of others throughout our lives because we are ever-changing based on what is going on with us and our patients" (Stewart, 2019, p.1).

The second factor involves a desire to fix imbalances where none should exist. The work related to the social determinants of health is an example of this factor. This factor acknowledges that everyone brings value to our lives. Everyone holds important information in the big picture. An example is a pediatric nurse practitioner (PNP) obtaining a health history, review of systems, and physical assessment of the pediatric patient with the parents. The PNP interviewing the child and parent is not the expert in the child's life, symptoms, or strengths as compared with the child and parents. The PNP holds special knowledge that the child and parents do not, but the child and parents hold knowledge of self outside of that scope.

The PNP, who is the expert in pediatric scientific knowledge, and the child and parents, the experts in the personal history, must collaborate for successful outcomes. Similarly, the members of a team are each experts in their own lives. The leader's task is to facilitate the sharing of the "how I see it" perspective so that broad considerations are made rather than quick, often stereotyped, decisions. Although Stewart (2019, p. 1) is addressing the role of physician and patient relationships, the same holds true for nurse and patient relationships: "We must be humble about our level of knowledge regarding our patients' beliefs and values, aware of our own assumptions and prejudices, and active in redressing the imbalance of power inherent in the physician-patient relationship." Additionally, the same is true for our relationships with our professional teams.

The final factor in cultural humility is aspiring to develop partnerships with people and groups who advocate for others. Individuals can create positive change, but groups can have a more profound impact, and a more inclusive perspective, on communities and systems; and a diverse group can be exceptionally powerful. Change cannot occur on an individual level without the correction of power imbalances within a larger system. "We must recognize the importance of institutional accountability" (Stewart, 2019, p. 1). Practicing all three factors of cultural humility helps strengthen patient-centered care, as it gives us a greater understanding of people and their differences while providing the respect and responsiveness needed to foster openness to their differences. Such understanding also helps nurses and other healthcare workers from different cultures work well together.

Cultural marginality is defined as "the resulting sense of being between two cultures or more, living at the edges of each, but rarely at the center" (Bennett, 2014, p. 269). This "betweenness" is a time when managers might perceive disinterest in cultural considerations. This situation might reflect cognitive processing of information that is not yet reflected in effective behaviors. Marginalization was originally proposed as a nursing theory by J. M. Hall in 1994. This theoretical approach then evolved to incorporate a global perspective (Hall et al., 1994, 1999). The original theory looked at seven properties of marginalization: Intermediacy, Differentiation, Power, Secrecy, Reflectiveness, Voice, and Liminality. When the perspective changed into a global view, additional properties were presented: Exteriority, Constraint, Eurocentrism, Economics, Seduction, Testimonies, and Hope (Hall, 1999). "From the early 2000s to 2018, marginalization was applied to a broader range of patients by different research teams who used multiple variants of the definition proposed by Hall and colleagues" (Baah et al., 2019).

Marginalization and SDH are interconnected concepts that, when examined together, can "highlight the relationship between them and aid in developing interventions to address the effects of this reciprocal relationship and the inequity that exists in the distribution of health promoting services across social strata" (Baah et al., 2019).

When healthcare providers can identify the marginalized patients' challenges, they can also develop and offer supportive measures as prevention or targeted therapy.

LEININGER'S THEORY OF TRANSCULTURAL NURSING CARE

Theory is helpful in applying concepts important to practice in actual clinical situations. Madeleine Leininger (2002) recognized that recurrent behavioral patterns in children appeared to have a cultural basis and that the lack of understanding of their culture reduced the nurse's ability to support culturally appropriate health and wellness care. This observation was the beginning of Leininger's development of the Theory of Transcultural Nursing Care (see Theory Box). The central purpose of the theory is "to discover and explain diverse and universal culturally based care factors influencing the health, well-being, illness, or death of individuals or groups" (p. 190). Nurses can use Leininger's model to provide culturally congruent, safe, and meaningful care to patients or clients of diverse or similar cultures.

Providing quality and humane care is difficult to accomplish if the nurse does not have knowledge of the recipient's culture as it relates to care. Leininger believed that "culture reflects shared values, beliefs, ideas, and meanings that are learned and that guide human thoughts, decisions, and actions. Cultures have manifest (readily recognized) and implicit (covert and ideal) rules of behavior and expectations. Human cultures have material items or symbols such as artifacts, objects, dress, and actions that have special meaning in a culture" (Leininger, 2002, p. 48). Leininger (2002) stated that her views of cultural care are "a synthesized construct that is the foundational basis to understanding and helping people of different cultures in transcultural nursing

THEORY BOX

Cultural Care Theory

Theory/Contributor	Key Ideas	Application to Practice
Leininger (2002): transcultural nursing care.	The theory is explicitly focused on the close relationships of culture and care on well-being, health, illness, and death. It is holistic and multidimensional, generic (emic, folk) and professional (etic) care and has a specifically designed research method (ethnonursing).	Care is the essence of nursing, and culturally based care is essential for well-being, health, growth, and survival and for facing handicaps or death.

practices" (p. 48). Accordingly, "quality of life" must be addressed from an emic (insider) cultural viewpoint and compared with an etic (outsider) professional's perspective. By comparing these two viewpoints, more meaningful nursing practice interventions will evolve. The same is true for collegial relationships. This comparative analysis will require nurses to include global views in their cultural studies that consider the social and environmental context of different cultures.

Transculturalism sometimes has been considered in a narrow sense as a comparison of health beliefs and practices of people from different countries or geographic regions. However, culture can be construed more broadly to include differences in health beliefs and practices by age, disability or physical challenge, economic status, ethnicity, gender, race, or sexual preference. Thus, when concepts of transcultural care are discussed, we should consider differences in health beliefs and practices not only between and among countries but also between and among all of the other cultural factors. This requires us to consider multiple factors about all individuals.

IMPACT OF DIVERSITY IN HEALTHCARE

Sometimes we want to highlight the differences between and among cultures. For example, when a particular unit has excellent safety scores, we want to know more about what that culture does differently from other cultures. Other times, we want to create an emphasis on similarities. An example of this might be how people celebrate some holiday, even though they might do so in a variety of ways. Those celebrations often involve food, family (in the broadest sense) and rituals—such as decorations, clothing, practices and so forth. Sharing what each of us do so we understand how the differences have a common core.

Because of the ethnic, cultural, and lifestyle diversity of potential patients and healthcare staff, nurses must work to foster respect for this diversity. To do this, we need to accept three key principles discussed earlier: multiculturalism, cross-culturalism, and transculturalism. Each of those principles operates in the workplace. Sometimes, we want to maintain distinct cultures. For instance, we may advocate for equality if a particular unit has excellent safety scores. Anyone who wanted to make all cultures alike—and, thus, increase safety incidents—would be seen as foolish. Healthcare organizations have, as an example, provided various ways to celebrate holy days based on the cultural mix of staff and

patients. These practices are designed to acknowledge the individuals who comprise the organization.

Nurse leaders and managers who ascribe to a positive view of culture and its characteristics effectively acknowledge cultural diversity among patients, staff and each other. This includes providing culturally sensitive care to patients while simultaneously balancing a culturally diverse staff. For example, cultural diversity might mean being sensitive to or being able to embrace the emotions of a large multicultural group comprising staff and patients. Unless we understand the differences, we cannot come together and make decisions that are in the best interest of a patient. Nurse leaders and managers must not only apply the principles of cultural competency to the care of patients but must also use these concepts in their relationships with staff.

Although the literature has addressed multicultural needs of patients, few effective methods for nurse managers to use when working with multicultural staff are identified. Differences in education and culture can impede patient care, and uncomfortable situations may emerge from such differences. For example, education differences between physicians and nurses, or nurses with different level of education, may result in poor communication or conflict that negatively affect care. Staff members may be reluctant to admit language problems that hamper their verbal and written communication. They may also be reluctant to admit their lack of understanding when interpreting directions. They may also be biased against a team member of a different culture, a different profession, or a different work setting.

Assessment of psychosocial behaviors must also be framed from a cultural perspective because some non-Westernized countries encourage emotional restraint (Wang et al., 2020). Staff may have difficulty addressing issues that relate to private family matters. Non-Asian nurses may have difficulty accepting the intensified family involvement of Asian cultures. The lack of assertiveness and the subservient physician–nurse relationships of some cultures are other issues that provide challenges for nurse managers. Unit-oriented workshops arranged by the nurse manager to address effective assertive techniques and family involvement as it relates to cultural differences are two ways of assisting staff with cultural work situations. Respecting cultural diversity in the team fosters cooperation and supports sound decision-making.

From the perspective of the nurse leader or manager, the principle of multiculturalism is particularly important given the numerous cultures that exist not only within the patient population but also among the staff. Consider some of the following cultures that may be present in healthcare patients and staff.

Diversity in the RN Population

Since nurses make up the largest part of the U.S. healthcare system, a major strategy for nurses to contribute to improvement of health disparities is to increase the number and percentage of nurses who represent diversity in race, ethnicity, and gender. Among the numerous reports addressing issues in nursing, the Institute of Medicine (now the National Academy of Medicine), in conjunction with the Robert Wood Johnson Foundation (RWJF), convened a group of prominent nurses, physicians, and policy makers to consider the future of nursing. The result of their work, *The Future of Nursing: Leading Change, Advancing Health* (2010) addressed the need for diversity of nurses as one of the goals to be pursued and therefore required the creation of a new workforce to address the diverse population (Institute of Medicine, 2011).

EveryNurse.org describes seven steps a nurse can use to provide culturally sensitive patient care (see Literature Perspective).

In 2016, the National Academy of Medicine published *Assessing Progress on the Institute of Medicine Report, The Future of Nursing.* One of the findings of this report was the need to continue to make promoting diversity in the nursing workforce a priority (Committee for Assessing Progress, 2016).

The third National Academy of Medicine report, *Future of Nursing 2020–2030: Charting a Path to Achieve Health Equity,* as its name suggests, focuses its recommendations on achieving health equity. Major recommendations from this report include a substantial increase in the number, types, and distribution of members of the nursing workforce. In addition, all nurses must increase their knowledge of social determinants of health to better understand the people for whom we provide care (National Academy of Medicine, 2021).

What strides in increasing the diversity of the nursing workforce have been made in the first decade of the 21st century. A survey of the National Council of State Boards of Nursing (NCSBN) in 2021 also found a lack of diversity among nurses. This was echoed by the 2021 American Organization for Nursing Leadership (AONL) president, Mary Ann Fuchs, in the Voice of Nursing Leadership (2021). The AONL Board of Directors took a stand and focused on changing their bylaws, appointing diverse board members and developing educational material to support the need for inclusion with members who represented diverse populations. They also created a Diversity and Belonging Committee with the vision to drive a diverse nursing community. They developed this group in an effort to face racism head on as a public crisis.

LITERATURE PERSPECTIVE

Resource: EveryNurse Staff. (2022). Seven Steps to Become a More Culturally Sensitive Nurse. Retrieved from https://everynurse.org/7-steps-culturally-sensitive-nurse/.

Everynurse.com is a resource for nursing students and professional nurses. Their mission is to support the career aspirations of students and nurses by offering expert advice, volunteer opportunities, and financial aid support for career advancement. The authors explore the cultural growth in the US and estimations for future. They note that only 19% of the RN workforce is from a racial or ethnic minority background. They explore Transcultural Health Care: A Culturally Competent Approach by Dr. Larry D. Purnell, PhD, RN, FAAN. Through this approach, the authors note "cultural competence is learning about how cultural differences may impact healthcare decisions and being able to modify care to align with that patient's culture." The article continues with barriers such as language challenges, cultural traditions, health literacy, and cultural assumptions. The authors end the article with seven steps

a nurse can use to provide culturally sensitive care. They explain in detail the step, but also how you as the nurse can utilize them in a "What you can do" section. These steps are further explained and include: 1. Awareness, 2. Avoid making assumptions, 3. Learn about other cultures, 4. Build trust qand rapport, 5. Overcome language barriers, 6. Educate patients about medical practices, and 7. Practice active listening.

Implications for Practice

Each of these tips are valuable in strengthening culturally sensitive healthcare. A point the authors stress is the fact that being culturally sensitive is no longer a choice, but a necessity. They end with an excellent point, "The payoff is significant though—culturally sensitive care builds provider to patient trust and rapport, increases treatment acceptance and opens the door for continuing education about important health matters in cultural communities that need it."

Table 4.1 provides a snapshot drawn from *The Future of Nursing 2020–2030* of the diversity of the RN population in the United States by identifying that the percentage of minority RNs is slowly increasing over time. While this is encouraging, *The Future of Nursing 2020–2030* report recognizes that more must be done to better meet the needs of the diverse U.S. population. Currently, several nursing associations in America and globally serve different cultures and ethnicities. The bridging commonality among these organizations is they all support the nurse. Nurses remain at the forefront of change with regard to human conditions and humanity as a whole. Nurse leaders need to understand these varied differences within individual nurses to successfully support their teams and workplaces. Table 4.2 shows a sample of the many culturally specific nursing organizations. The missions of each are quite similar, with the overarching

TABLE 4.1   Trends in the Diversity of the RN Nursing Workforce from 2000 to 2018

Characteristic of Diversity	2000	2004	2008	2018
Men	7.9%	99.5%	9.0%	12.7%
Women	92.1%	90.1%	90.4%	87.3%
White	79.1%	78.1%	75.0%	68.0%
Black/African-American	8.8%	8.9%	10.6%	12.0%
Asian	6.4%	7.5%	8.3%	9.1%
Hispanic	3.7%	4.1%	4.6%	7.4%
Other	1.9%	1.3%	1.4%	2.5%

Source: National Academy of Medicine (formerly Institute of Medicine). (2021). *The future of nursing 2020–2030: Charting a path to achieve health equity.* Washington DC: The National Academies Press.

TABLE 4.2   Sample of Nursing Organizations' Missions Related to Diversity

Nursing Organization	Mission
American Association of Men in Nursing (AAMN)—https://www.aamn.org	"….is to provide a framework for nurses, as a group, to meet, to discuss and influence factors, which affect men as nurses. Our mission is to shape the practice, education, research, and leadership for men in nursing and advance men's health. Our vision is to be the association of choice representing men in nursing."
Asian American/Pacific Islander Nurses Association (AAPINA)—https://aapina.org/our-mission-philosophy-and-goals/	"…serves as the unified voice for Asian American Pacific Islander (AAPI) nurses around the world. AAPINA strives to positively affect the health and well-being of AAPIs and their communities by: supporting AAPI nurses and nursing students around the world through research, practice, and education; facilitating and promoting networking and collaborative partnerships; and influencing health policy through individual and community actions."
National Association of Hispanic Nurses (NAHN)—https://nahnnet.org/mission	"…to advance the health in Hispanic communities and to lead, promote and advocate the educational, professional, and leadership opportunities for Hispanic nurses."
National Black Nurses Association (NBNA)—https://www.nbna.org/who	"…to serve as the voice for Black nurses and diverse populations ensuring equal access to professional development, promoting educational opportunities and improving health."
National Coalition of Ethnic Minority Nurse Association (NCEMNA)—https://ncemna.org/mission-and-vision/	"….to be the unified body advocating for equity and justice in healthcare."
Philippine Nurses Association of America (PNAA)—https://aanhpihealth.org	"…to uphold and foster the positive image and welfare of Filipino-American nurses, promote professional excellence, and contribute to significant outcomes to healthcare and society through education, research, and clinical practice."
Transcultural Nursing Society (TCNS)—https://tcns.org	"…to enhance the quality of culturally congruent, competent, and equitable care that results in improved health and well-being for people worldwide."

goals of positivity, equity, professional excellence, improvement of health, fostering nursing standards, and supporting diversity.

Most of the literature about the broad issue of cultural considerations has historically derived primarily from the business literature. Business has looked at gender, as one example, over several years.

Gender roles and our assumptions about them have a particular impact upon the relationships among nursing staff. Cultural differences among groups should not be taken in the context that all members of a certain group or subgroup are indistinguishable. For example, regarding gender differences, women are perceived to have a more participative management style. However, this does not mean that all male managers use an authoritative management model. Likewise, female managers may use multiple sources of information to make decisions, and this does not mean that all male managers make decisions on limited data. The norm for gender recognition should be that women and men be hired, promoted, rewarded, and respected for how successfully they do the job, not for who they are, where they come from, whom they know, or the gender they represent.

One of the concerns from the return to work from the pandemic is known as the proximity bias, which refers to the idea that leaders might be more positively influence by workers they actually see versus those who may do equally good or better work but do so from a remote location such as the home. Although men also may have chosen to remain working from home, more commonly women have remained at home to provide care for family (children and parents). All of these types of factors are examples of what leaders must be alert to in order to remain objective and fair and avoid stereotypes of someone in the workplace based on common perceptions of gender.

In today's workplace, female-male collaboration should provide efficacious models for the future. Gender does not determine response in any given situation. However, men reportedly seem to be better at deciphering what needs to be done, whereas women are better at collaborating and getting others to collaborate in accomplishing a task. Men tend to take neutral, logical, and objective stands on problems, whereas women become involved in how the problems affect people. Women and men bring separate perspectives to resolving problems, which can help them function more effectively as a team on the nursing unit. Men and women must learn to work together and value the contributions

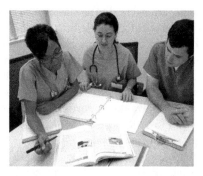

Fig. 4.1 Nurses have the opportunity to discuss diversity from various perspectives.

of the other and the differences they bring to any situation. Similar kinds of comparisons can be made related to other elements of diversity. Nurses have embraced information related to generational differences and have used religious and ethnic contexts as ways to begin dialogs about values and beliefs (Fig. 4.1).

LGBTQ + Populations

When promoting cultural competency within different lifestyles, nurses must also explore the nursing care of the LGBTQ+ (or the subsequent group recognitions) patients and staff. LGBT has been an acronym that is typically used to suggest homogeneity among these groups (Ard & Makadon, 2012; National LGBT Health Education Center, 2016). The acronym represents lesbian, gay, bisexual, and transgendered (and subsequent others) and has referred to the behavior, identity, and desire of each group. This acronym has grown to include various identities and now reflects lesbian, gay, bisexual, transgender, queer, and others (LGBTQ+). This broader group has long been addressed as a minority within a wide range of races, ethnicities, ages, and socioeconomic statuses. This group has often experienced discrimination, with healthcare needs not being addressed or discriminated in the workplace. People who identify themselves in this gender-diverse manner find challenges in accessing culturally competent health services. The *T*, representing *transgendered*, has long contained additional subcategories. This adds another layer of cultural understanding. For example, in healthcare settings, the term *Male to Female (MTF) transgendered* is used to describe a person born with male genitalia but who identifies as a female. *Female to Male (FTM) transgendered* is the reverse. Some people reject the nature of gender and see themselves as neither and commonly are referred to as *androgynous*. Consider how challenging it is for people in "traditional organizations" that might only recently have accepted women into leadership roles to now consider an employee who identifies as transgender. These challenges exist as readily in healthcare organizations as in other types of organizations and we have the opportunity to serve as role models for how to address policy and culture changes to create a new climate of acceptance.

More nurses and nurse managers must embrace the increasing diversity within this gender-identity community. This population has seen a history of bias, which has continued to challenge access to care despite increasing social acceptance. This bias was often found in healthcare and, until 1973, homosexuality was listed as a disorder in the *Diagnostic and Statistical Manual of Mental Disorders* (*DSM*) (National LGBT Health Education Center, 2016). This stigma and the related discrimination, combined with a lack of access to culturally competent and individualized healthcare, have resulted in health disparities for the gender-diverse community. Some of these health disparities include higher rates of smoking, depression, anxiety, substance use, and violence victimization. The Department of Health and Human Services' *Healthy People 2020* and the National Academy of Medicine. The Future of Nursing 2020-2030 Charting a Path to Achieve Health Equity, both acknowledge these disparities and have asked for steps to address them. A new report from The National Academies of Sciences, Engineering, and Medicine have also requested more data collected on the LGBTQ+ population in an effort to reduce gaps of care (2020). The report concludes with a recommendation to prioritize research into the health and well-being of sexual and gender diverse people, as well as research on development, implementation, and evaluation of services and programs that will directly benefit these populations.

One of the steps in addressing these disparities in the LGBTQ+ community starts with creating an inclusive environment for these patients. Something as simple as changing intake forms can provide a sense of belonging. "As of 2016, HRSA (Health Resources & Services Administration) requires health centers to report sexual orientation and gender identity data in the uniform data system" (The National LGBT Health Education Center, 2016). These forms of data, whether during the history-taking assessment, on paper forms, or electronically, should all pay attention to the sexual orientation and gender identity of the patient.

Providing such culturally competent care and understanding is not limited to patients in the healthcare setting. It also includes the staff within this community. Correct terminology and nonjudgmental support need to be provided to the nursing staff and other healthcare team members. Doing so will facilitate a positive and inclusive work setting. Taking steps to understand the varied cultures will also help clinicians ensure that their gender-diverse patients—indeed, all of their patients—receive the best level of healthcare possible.

When Hate and Anger Enter the Picture

The range of attitudes toward culturally diverse groups can be viewed along a continuum of intensity (Lenburg et al., 1995, p. 4) from hate to contempt to tolerance to respect and ending with celebration/affirmation. Managers need to be aware of this continuum so that they can apply strategies appropriately to the workforce—for example, contempt versus affirmation. Both responses are reflected in employee groups. The goal is to move from acknowledging differences to inclusion.

As nurses are on the forefront of cultural differences, they will encounter patients who have been affected by hate crimes or may personally be victims of hate crimes. Hate crimes are crimes in which the motivation for committing the crime is based on a bias, according to the United States Department of Justice (DOJ) (2020). The word "hate" truly reflects a bias against a group with a specific characteristic as defined by law, though not necessarily hate anger, rage, or a dislike for the group. According to the DOJ, most of these hate crimes are based on ethnicity, race, color, religion, sexual orientation, gender, gender identity, or disability. These crimes can include assault, murder, arson, vandalism, or threats, and can affect individuals, families, and communities.

A disparity exists between hate crimes that occur and those that are reported to law enforcement. This disparity is termed the Hate Crime Reporting Gap. This disparity only fuels further distress because when reports of such crimes are accurate, it shows support for the victims and tells others these crimes are not tolerated. It also helps law enforcement understand the breadth of the problem within the community. Resources can then be allocated to prevent and address future attacks. Nurses and healthcare providers, as well as institutions, have the responsibility to report these accurately. Health facilities need policies to instruct on how to report these incidents.

People with disabilities have expressed concerns about various aspects of living conditions that some of us might consider minor; and in the process we all benefitted when their voices were heard. Consider, for example, the presence of ramps on street corners. They were designed to allow people with motor movement disabilities to navigate from one corner to the other without having to step up on to or down off of a curb. As a result, we all benefited. Those of us who are slightly unsteady on our feet can cross more readily; we can pull luggage or personal grocery carts more easily; we can push wheel chairs easily from one side of the street to the other; and people who use walkers can simply keep on walking as opposed to trying to lift or lower their walkers. Even younger children on bicycles or tricycles are safer because they don't bounce up or down a curb or ride in the street until they get to a driveway or alley.

Culture in Organizations

Specific cultures may not only be found in gender, racial, and ethnic populations but also in other teams and organizations that focus on a specific mission or goal. An organizational culture is defined by the shared values, attitudes, and practices of the organization. Applying the principles of culture in teams and organization is important as nurses work in any system. As an example, healthcare has adopted a culture known as "Just Culture" from other complex, high-risk industries, such as the airline industry, to improve care in the institutions (Siewert, Brook, Swedeen, Eisenberg & Hochman, 2019).

Just Culture is built on two important values: justice and safety. Valuing justice can be seen by policies and actions that represent fairness to the workforce. Valuing safety is demonstrated by a commitment to reducing at-risk behaviors, design of safe methods of care, including establishing reporting of unsafe aspects of care, as well as a learning environment that uses potential or actual errors to improve systems of care. The Research Perspective provides more information about Just Culture from a nursing perspective.

Organizational culture can also mean "how we do things here." The mission and values may appear on a plaque on the wall. However, the real test of the culture is seeing how those words are enacted in care on the clinical units or in interactions among employees. On a micro level, the culture also dictates how we dress, how we address each other, how we tolerate gossip, and so forth.

RESEARCH PERSPECTIVE

Resource: Paradiso, L., & Sweeney, N. (2019). Just culture. Its more than policy. *Nursing Management, 50(6)*, 38–45. https://doi.org/10.1097/01.NUMA.0000558482.07815.ae.

This quantitative, correctional, cross-sectional study examined the relationship between trust, just culture, and error reporting in a large urban teaching hospital. The study used a convenience sample from 1,500 clinical nurses and 80 nurse leaders. The primary means of data collection was a self-administered, anonymous survey. The Just Culture Assessment Tool (JCAT) was used to measure just culture in a hospital setting. The Survey of Hospital Leaders was used to measure perceptions of an organization's culture. Six domains analyzed were feedback and communication, openness of communication, balance, quality of error reporting process, continuous improvement, and trust. Significant differences between perceptions of nurse leaders and clinical nurses were found. More than 90% of nurse leaders felt each employee is given a fair and objective follow up process regardless of his or her involvement in an event. Less than 65% of clinical nurses agreed with that statement. Most clinical nurses did not trust nurse leaders to do the right thing and often felt staff members were blamed when involved in an event. Positive correlations were found between both groups when exploring trust more. When just culture is ingrained in the organization and its analysis of safety events, it's expected that fair treatment generates a sense of trust among employees. This may influence speaking up to report errors. There was also a positive correlation between trust and voluntary reporting of errors.

Implications for Practice
This study revealed differences between perceptions of trust and just culture between staff nurses and nurse leaders in this organization. This can be challenging when the organization feels they are just, but when the perceptions are too varied, the just culture is fractured. The study reinforced the need for open communication as a foundation for just culture. Nurse leaders can strengthen a just culture by implementing visible and meaningful system improvements while supporting outcomes and communication toward clinical nurses. This helps validate and encourage error identification.

Working "toward justice" requires sensitivity of the needs of others and contributions toward society, healthcare, and the workplace. Professors Grover, V. Murthy, P., & Bedzow, I. (2020) developed culturally sensitive healthcare tips in an effort for all public health workers to reach the same goal of cultural sensitivity. To achieve this, we must be aware of our own biases. How are we are going to move past them to support others? We must also accept that in a cultural disagreement, our culture's values aren't automatically correct over another's. This is a challenge to accept and move forward. It is important to provide an environment where patients, family, and staff can ask questions if needed. When we open our environment with a comfortable atmosphere (our welcoming and non-judgmental self) then we allow others to lower their fearful walls and ask for help. The open communication become a huge ally. Invite questions! Learn to read our patients and staff. And be polite. Some may like a friendly and joke infused dialog, while others find that unprofessional. Work consistently toward developing and strengthening our own cultural competency. Always explore how we can embrace these differences and grow toward our justice.

Choosing an Employer That Values Diversity

Choosing an organization that is consistent with the nurse's own values is critical for a successful employment experience. One of the issues that has come to the forefront of many discussions in recent years is the acknowledgment that some organizations have supported systemic racism for some time. Banaji, Fiske, & Massey (2021) define systemic racism as occurring when racially unequal opportunities are intrinsic to the operation of a society's structures. It is a unified arrangement of racial differentiations and discrimination across different generations (2021). This term refers to an almost invisible presence of a cultural factor that often has existed for years that upholds different treatment of people based on one factor, in this case, race. It accounts for microaggressions; lack of promotions, especially above a certain level within an organization; a profiling of patients, even in our documentation; and numerous other ways of carrying forward past practices that were based on assumptions about people of color. To a lesser degree this same attribution has occurred related to other factors. Not one of us is likely to change the system; yet all of us being aware of such practices have the ability to identify them and call them into question and then terminate

them. Our ability and commitment to advocate for practices that help to eliminate such perspectives is an example of demonstrating our competency in employing a participatory approach to nursing care specifically as it relates to diversity (AACN, 2021). Although bringing about change in systemic racism is likely to be a slow process, the potential to revolutionize an organization is huge. Many organizations have multiple values—such as concern for patients and staff and emphasis on safety and patient-centered care—that the nurse seeking employment must consider. The extent to which the organization actualizes the need to attract a diverse nursing staff is also important. Asking questions of colleagues who work (or have worked) for the organization is an effective strategy for assessing the organization's commitment to diversity and inclusion. Equally important is asking pertinent questions during the interview process. Box 4.1 provides questions that are framed to solicit information regarding diversity and inclusion plans of the organization. When interviewing with an organization, the nurse should choose two or three of these questions and ask them of everyone involved in the interview process. A comparison of the responses will provide an understanding of the consistency with which the organization integrates values of diversity and inclusion into the organizational culture.

EXERCISE 4.5 Think back to an organization where you have worked or had clinical experiences. Do you believe that diversity and inclusion was a value of that organization? What is the evidence for your conclusion?

BOX 4.1   Selected Questions to Assess Employers' Commitment to Diversity and Inclusion

1. What are the core values of this organization?
2. How would you describe the organization's culture?
3. What does diversity and inclusion mean here?
4. Are there specific programs to increase diversity in the organization?
5. Does the organization have diversity and inclusion initiatives?

Adapted from Verduce, C. P. (n.d.). Questions students can ask in interviews to tell if a company really cares about diversity and inclusion. Indiana Tech Career Center.

CONCLUSION

Patient-centered care ensures that patients' individual values and needs will guide the best care for them. Healthcare providers must be culturally aware and culturally competent in order to secure the trust necessary for this care. When we are culturally competent, we are able to care for diverse populations and work in diverse settings with the common goal of equity for all through cultural proficiency. Trying to work with and care for different people can often lead to many challenges and opportunities. No matter how hard someone tries to remain fair, unbiased, and honorable toward differences, people make mistakes. Our goal is to minimize those mistakes in an effort to provide inclusion and equity for all. This must remain a goal in healthcare. We need to remember not to lose faith in humanity and the goodness within people—*all* people. When this becomes hard to remember, think about Mahatma Gandhi and his profound words, "You must not lose faith in humanity. Humanity is like an ocean; if a few drops of the ocean are dirty, the ocean does not become dirty." The takeaway is that we need to work as a team to help foster a diverse environment that benefits our patients as much as our colleagues. We will run into challenges, but those challenges will not ruin all of the hard work driving equity for all in healthcare and as a society. In fact, those challenges are likely to enrich us.

THE SOLUTION

As a nursing leader, understanding what each of your team needs from you is of the utmost importance. I do this by making sure I get to know each person as an individual first, then using that bond and connection to understand how they will work with their team. Each will respond differently according to their beliefs and culture, but with a greater understanding of what each person feels is most important, you can combine that energy to create a dynamic and productive team. Always keep an open mind, never trying to instill your beliefs on others.

As your teammates learn to appreciate you for that, they become more flexible and open with you about what they need from you as a leader to help them reach their full potential. You never want to create a work environment that does not let each person be who they are as that is where they find their value as an individual. Content and well cared for nurses, have content and well cared for patients.

Nancy Leal

REFLECTIONS

Find a quiet spot to reflect on the following questions. You may choose to record your answers to share with others or keep as goals for yourself.

- The purpose of asking yourself these questions is to consider how you are different from others—even someone who looks and talks like you do.
- Who are you and where are you from? Sharing personal things about yourself is coming from a place of connecting and not from a place of bragging.

If you are in a group, keep a list of descriptors as you interact with everyone and celebrate their unique differences and similarities.

- What would your organization look like if it were more diverse and inclusive?
- What would we gain (in healthcare) if we were more diverse and inclusive?
- What is one thing we can do to positively affect belonging?

TIPS FOR PRACTICE/BEST PRACTICES

To provide culturally sensitive care toward your team or patients, you must remember the following:

- Be aware of your own biases. How are you going to move past them to support others? You need to accept that in a cultural disagreement, one culture's

values aren't automatically correct over another's. This is a challenge to accept and move forward.

- Ask questions that are relevant to the current situation. Avoid those that aren't. Personal questions can make a person feel uncomfortable, but if necessary for treatment/care, then do so in a comforting and respectful manner.

- Keep your communication relevant to the situation. Avoid sharing your judgments or opinions that are not relevant and could make others feel uncomfortable.
- Allow time, whenever possible, for people to process choices or decisions. We tend to rush in healthcare as we have other people waiting for us to take care of them. Step aside and try to give people time to think about their treatment options or team suggestions. Time is so valuable but also critical for people to process information rather than jump to conclusions and make hasty decisions.
- Provide an environment in which patients, family, and staff can ask questions if needed. When you create a comfortable atmosphere, then you will inspire others to lower their fearful walls and ask for help. The open communication allow others to drop their inhibitions.
- Be polite. Learn to read your patients and staff. Some may like a friendly and joke-infused dialog while others could find that unprofessional. Learn to read cues and remain polite at all times.
- Listen! Listen to your patient or staff's concerns or questions. Listen to the tone of their words. How can you provide feedback that is personal and not defensive? This is challenging but critical to this relationship.
- Minimize generalizations about different groups. It is easy to think that everyone from a certain group or culture has the same attributes. However, differences within a group do exist and generalizing people in this manner can become a barrier to trust and communication.
- Work consistently toward developing and strengthening your own cultural competency. How can you embrace cultural differences? Our goals in healthcare are to provide the best care possible to our patients and colleagues. We need to understand differences to provide the best care possible.
- Bring kindness, respect, and honesty to your table—every day.

REFERENCES

American Association of Colleges of Nursing (AACN). (2021). *The Essentials: Core Competencies for Professional Nursing Education.* Author.

American Public Health Association (APHA). (2021). *Social justice and health.* Retrieved from https://apha.org/what-is-public-health/generation-public-health/our-work/social-justice.

Ard, K. L., & Makadon, H. G. (2012). *Improving the health care of lesbian, gay, bisexual and transgender (LGBT) people: Understanding and eliminating health disparities.* Boston: The National LGBT Health Education Center, The Fenway Institute, Brigham and Women's Hospital, and Harvard Medical School.

Baah, F. O., Teitelman, A. M., & Riegel, B. (2019). Marginalization: Conceptualizing patient vulnerabilities in the framework of social determinants of health—An Integrative review. *Nursing Inquiry, 26*(1), e12268.

Banaji, M.R., Fiske, S.T., & Massey, D.S. (2021). Systemic racism: individuals and interactions, institutions and society. *Cognitive Research, 6,* 82. https://doi.org/10.1186/s41235-021-00349-3.

Bennett, J. M. (2014). Cultural marginality: Identity issues in global leadership training. https://doi.org/10.1108/S1535-120320140000008020.

Centers for Disease Control and Prevention (CDC). (2016). *Strategies for reducing health disparities: Selected CDC-sponsored interventions, United States, 2016.* Retrieved from https://www.cdc.gov/minorityhealth/strategies2016/index.html.

Centers for Disease Control and Prevention (CDC). (2013). *Attaining Health Equity.* Retrieved from https://www.cdc.gov/nccdphp/dch/programs/healthycommunitiesprogram/overview/healthequity.htm.

Chen, A. W., Iwamoto, D. K., & McMullen, D. (2018). Model minority stereotypes and diagnosis of alcohol use disorders: Implications for practitioners working with Asian Americans. Journal of Ethnicity in Substance Abuse, 17(3), 255–272. https://doi.org/10.1080/15332640.2016.1175990.

Cross, T., Bazron, B., Dennis, K., & Isaacs, M. (1989). *Towards A Culturally Competent System of Care, Volume I.* Washington, DC: Georgetown University Child Development Center, CASSP Technical Assistance Center. **ERIC Number:** ED330171.

Eberhardt, J. L. (2019). Biased: *Uncovering the hidden prejudice that shapes what we see, think, and do.* Penguin Books.

EveryNurse Staff. (2022). Seven Steps to Become a More Culturally Sensitive Nurse. Retrieved from https://everynurse.org/7-steps-culturally-sensitive-nurse/.

Fuchs, M. A. (2021). American Organization for Nursing Leadership. Voice of the President, March 2021. https://www.aonl.org/news/voice/mar-2021/voice-of-the-president.

Grover, V., Murthy, P., & Bedzow, I. (2020). 11 Tips for Providing Culturally Sensitive Healthcare. *Medbridge*. https://www.medbridgeeducation.com/blog/2020/06/11-tips-for-providing-culturally-sensitive-healthcare/.

Hall, J. M., & Carlson, K. (2016). Marginalization: A revisitation with integration of scholarship on globalization, intersectionality, privilege, microaggressions, and implicit biases. *Advances in Nursing Science, 39*(3), 200–215. (PubMed: 27490876).

Hall, J. M. (1999). Marginalization revisited: Critical, postmodern, and liberation perspectives. *Advances in Nursing Science, 22*(2), 88–102. (PubMed: 10634190).

Hall, J. M., Stevens, P. E., & Meleis, A. I. (1994). Marginalization: A guiding concept for valuing diversity in nursing knowledge development. *Advances in Nursing Science, 16*(4), 23–41. (PubMed: 8092811).

Altman, S. H., Butler, A. S., & Shern, L. (Eds.). (2016). Committee for Assessing Progress on Implementing the Recommendations of the Institute of Medicine Report; Institute of Medicine; National Academies of Sciences, Engineering, and Medicine. In *Assessing Progress on the Institute of Medicine Report The Future of Nursing*. Washington, DC: National Academies Press.

Healthy People 2030. (2020). *Social determinants of health*. Retrieved from https://health.gov/healthypeople/objectives-and-data/social-determinants-health.

Hoffman, K. M., Trawalter, S., Axt, J. R., & Oliver, N. (2016). Racial bias in pain assessment and treatment recommendations, and false beliefs about biological differences between blacks and whites. *PNAS, 113*(16), 4296–4301.

Hook, J. N., Davis, D. E., Owen, J., Worthington Jr., E. L., & Utsey, S. O. (2013). Cultural humility: Measuring openness to culturally diverse clients. Journal of Counseling Psychology, 60(3), 353–366. https://doi.org/10.1037/a0032595.

Howell, E. A. (2018). Reducing disparities in severe maternal morbidity and mortality. *Clinical Obstetrics and Gynecology, 61*(2), 387–399. https://doi.org/10.1097/GRF.0000000000000349.

Kaiser Family Foundation (KFF). (2021a). *Disparities in health and health care: 5 key questions and answers*. Retrieved from https://www.kff.org/racial-equity-and-health-policy/issue-brief/disparities-in-health-and-health-care-5-key-question-and-answers/.

Kaiser Family Foundation (KFF). (2021b). *New analysis: In pursuit of a national vaccination benchmark, Hispanic and Black people's rates projected to lag behind*. Retrieved from www.kff.org/racial-equity-and-health-policy/press-release/new-analysis-in-pursuit-of-a-national-vaccination-benchmark-hispanic-and-black-peoples-rates-projected-to-lag-behind.

Kirwan Institute for the Study of Race and Ethnicity. (2015). Understanding Implicit Bias. Retrieved from http://kirwaninstitute.osu.edu/research/understanding-implicit-bias/.

Horace Mann School. (2021). *Why ICIE—Identity, Culture, and Institutional Equity*. Retrieved from https://www.horacemann.org/our-school/office-for-identity-culture-and-institutional-equity/why-icie-identity-culture-and-institutional-equity.

Institute of Medicine. (2011). *The future of nursing: Leading change, advancing health*. Washington, DC: The National Academies Press.

Leininger, M. (2002). Essential transcultural nursing care concepts, principles, examples, and policy statements. In M. Leininger, & M. R. McFarland (Eds.), *Transcultural nursing: Concepts, theories, research & practice* (3rd ed.). New York: McGraw-Hill Medical Publishing Division.

Lenburg, C. B., Lipson, J. G., Demi, A. S., Blaney, D. R., Stern, P. N., Schultz, P. R., et al. (1995). *Promoting cultural competence in and through nursing education: A critical review and comprehensive plan for action*. Washington, DC: American Academy of Nursing.

Menni, C., Klaser, K., May, A., Polidori, L., Capdevila, J., Panayiotis, L., et al. (2021). Vaccine side-effects and SARS-CoV-2 infection after vaccination in users of the COVID Symptom Study app in the UK: a prospective observational Study. *The Lancet*. Retrieved from https://www.thelancet.com/journals/laninf/article/PIIS1473-3099(21)00224-3/fulltext.

Merriam-Webster. (2021). *Ethnicity*. Retrieved from https://www.merriam-webster.com/dictionary/ethnicity.

Merriam-Webster. (2021). *Cross Culturalism*. Retrieved from https://www.merriam-webster.com/dictionary/cross-cultural.

National Academies of Sciences, Engineering, and Medicine. (2020). *New Report Calls for More Comprehensive Data on LGBTQI+ Well-Being*. Office of News and Public Information. https://www.nationalacademies.org/news/2020/10/new-report-calls-for-more-comprehensive-data-on-lgbtqi-well-being.

National Academy of Medicine (formerly Institute of Medicine). (2021). *The future of nursing 2020–2030: Charting a path to achieve health equity*. Washington DC: The National Academies Press.

National LGBT Health Education Center. (2016). *Understanding the health needs of LGBT people*. Retrieved from https://www.lgbtqiahealtheducation.org/wp-content/uploads/LGBTHealthDisparitiesMar2016.pdf.

Ndugga, N., & Artiga, S. (2021). *Disparities in health and health care: 5 Questions and answers*. Retrieved from: Kaiser Family Foundation. http://kff.org/racial-equity-and-health-policy/issue-brief/disparities-in-health-and-health-care-5-key-question-and-answers/.

Office of Disease Prevention and Health Promotion (ODPHP). (2021). *History of health people*. Retrieved from https://health.gov/our-work/national-health-initiatives/healthy-people/about-healthy-people/history-healthy-people.

Paradiso, L., & Sweeney, N. (2019). Just culture. Its more than policy. *Nursing Management, 50*(6), 38–45. https://doi.org/10.1097/01.NUMA.0000558482.07815.ae.

Sandhu, H. S., Arora, A., Brasch, J., & Streiner, D. L. (2019). Mental Health Stigma: Explicit and Implicit Attitudes of Canadian Undergraduate Students, Medical School Students, and Psychiatrists. *Canadian Journal of Psychiatry, 64*(3), 209–217. https://doi-org.ric.idm.oclc.org/10.1177/0706743718792193.

Siewert, B, Brook, O. R., Swedeen, S., Eisenberg, R. L., & Hochman, M. (2019). Overcoming human barriers to safety event reporting in radiology. *RadioGraphics, 39*(1), 251–263. https://doi.org/10.1148/rg.2019180135.

Singh, R., & Palosky, C. (2021). *New Analysis: In Pursuit of a National Vaccination Benchmark, Hispanic and Black People's Rates Projected to Lag Behind.* Retrieved from https://www.kff.org/racial-equity-and-health-policy/press-release/new-analysis-in-pursuit-of-a-national-vaccination-benchmark-hispanic-and-black-peoples-rates-projected-to-lag-behind/.

Sherman, F. (2019). Cultural sensitivity skills in the workplace. CHRON. Retrieved from https://smallbusiness.chron.com/cultural-sensitivity-skills-workplace-20375.html.

Spector, R. E. (2017). *Cultural diversity in health and illness* (9th ed.). Upper Saddle River, NJ: Pearson Prentice Hall.

Spence, D. (2001). Prejudice, paradox, and possibility: Nursing people from cultures other than one's own. *Journal of Transcultural Nursing, 12*(2), 100–106.

Spence, D. (2004). Prejudice, paradox and possibility: The experience of nursing people from cultures other than one's own. In K. H. Kavanaugh, & V. Knowlden (Eds.), *Many voices: Toward caring culture in healthcare and healing.* Madison, WI: The University of Wisconsin Press.

Stewart, A. (2019). *Cultural humility is critical to health equity.* American Academy of Family Physicians. Retrieved from https://www.aafp.org/news/blogs/leadervoices/entry/20190418lv-humility.html.

Sukhera, J., Watling, C., & Gonzalez, C. (2020). Implicit Bias in Health Professions: From Recognition to Transformation. *Academic Medicine, 95*(5), 717–723. https://doi.org/10.1097/ACM.0000000000003173.

Tervalon, M., & Murray-Garcia, J. (1998). Cultural humility versus cultural competence: A critical distinction in defining physician training outcomes in multicultural education. *Journal of Health Care for the Poor and Underserved, 9*(2), 117–125.

U.S. Department of Justice (DOJ). (2020). Hate Crime Statistics 2020. https://www.justice.gov/hatecrimes/hate-crime-statistics.

Verduce, C. P. (n.d.). Questions students can ask in interviews to tell if a company really cares about diversity and inclusion. Indiana Tech Career Center. Retrieved from https://wmich.edu/sites/default/files/attachments/u446/2021/Questions%20Students%20Can%20Ask%20in%20Interviews%20to%20Tell%20If%20a%20Company%20Really%20Cares%20About%20Diversity.pdf.

Wang, D., Gee, G. C., Bahiru, E., Yang, E. H., & Hsu, J. J. (2020). Asian-American and Pacific Islanders in COVID-19: Emerging disparities amid discrimination. Journal of General Internal Medicine, 35(12):3685–3688. https://doi.org/10.1007/s11606-020-06264-5.

World Health Organization (WHO). (2021). *Social determinants of health.* Retrieved from https://www.who.int/health-topics/social-determinants-of-health#tab=tab_1.

Yilmaz, H. O., & Ayhan, N. Y. (2019). Is there prejudice against obese persons among health professionals? A sample of student nurses and registered nurses. *Perspect Psychiatric Care, 55*(2), 262–268. https://doi.org/10.1111/ppc.12359.

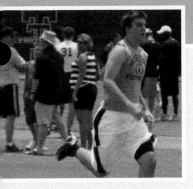

5

Healthy Workplaces, Healthy Workforce

Mary Ann T. Donohue-Ryan

ANTICIPATED LEARNING COMPETENCIES

- Define the concepts of healthy workplace and healthy workforce.
- Discuss the impact of unhealthy workplaces on nurses in the acute care, community, and ambulatory settings.
- Apply strategies that decrease the impact of work-related stress and burnout.

- Compare and contrast strategies employed by successful leaders, managers, and followers within teams, in organizations, and in systems that promote healthy personal and professional behaviors.
- Evaluate organizational and regulatory policies that promote safe and effective work environments at the local, state, national, and global levels.

KEY TERMS

burnout
delegation
depersonalization
documentation burden
employee assistance program
fatigue

general adaptation syndrome (GAS)
healthy work environment
healthy workforce
lateral workplace violence
overwork

role issues
perfectionism
self-limiting thoughts
time management
unhealthy work environment

THE CHALLENGE

My role is a new one: I am the first director of nursing (DON) in my hospital and in the entire system, with responsibility in administrative, clinical, and strategic operations. The DON is responsible for assisting the organization's CNO with human resource, regulatory, and nursing practice/excellence projects, along with strategic patient flow responsibilities. Many inpatient units, including Medicine, Geriatrics, Pulmonary, Behavioral Health, and the Palliative Care/Hospice Units and the administrative off-shift nurse managers report to me. I am actively involved in High Reliability Organization (HRO) activities, nursing quality/Joint Commission preparedness, Magnet®-related quality data and reporting, Department

of Health regulatory matters, and Master Facility Planning. I am the advisor for the system Nurse Practice Council, Co-Chair of the System-wide Hospital Acquired Infection (HAI) Device Reduction Committee, and several other ad hoc committees/council work as assigned.

When I first assumed the DON position, it became really hard for me to turn off my day. The role expectations resulted in so much more internal pressure than what I had been accustomed to as an ICU staff nurse and manager. I also have two children and a husband to go home to, yet I often found myself at the point of physical and emotional exhaustion at the end of the day. I would never turn off my phone, thinking that in order to prove to myself and others

(Continued)

INTRODUCTION

How would you know if a future or current workplace is healthy or not? Is it possible to assess the organizational landscape prior to accepting a position? Once you are on the job, will the unit/department/agency ever feel like the best fit, or even an "OK" fit for you? What can you do when a "great" workplace turns into "not so great" and becomes, instead, nearly intolerable and toxic in nature? Very importantly, what do you do when you find yourself trying to work within an unhealthy practice environment? People in the largest employment sector in many communities, such as healthcare workers in hospitals, ambulatory clinics, long-term care, and other health-related organizations, must achieve and exceed standards for their own personal health and well-being. Everyone wants to work in a positive, cohesive, and collaborative environment, no matter what the setting. A busy inpatient unit, ambulatory department, or telehealth initiative that serves the community all have the potential to be extremely stressful. Understanding your role-specific responsibilities in this stressful environment is your first priority. Then, leveraging your power as nurse leader, manager, and participant-follower creates healthier organizations no matter where you practice. Regardless of the setting or situation, everyone's talent can be "nourished to flourish" and, thus, contribute mightily to world-class patient, family, and community outcomes. Ultimately, in a healthy work environment, every member of the team is viewed as a true partner in a caring community and, thus, their physiologic and mental health is optimized now and into the future.

HEALTHY HEALTHCARE WORKPLACE

A healthy workplace is the cornerstone to successful patient safety initiatives, with better outcomes for patient satisfaction, the workforce, across organizations, and, according to the federal government, are known for their potential to produce thriving local communities. The *Healthy People*

2030 initiative, launched by the U.S. federal government in 1979, set defined goals as well as benchmarks, with the aim to improve the health and well-being of all communities of the United States by the year 2030 (Office of Disease Prevention and Health Promotion, n.d.). In 2008, the Triple Aim of healthcare improvement was first posited by Berwick et al. (2008), consisting of *care*, *health*, and *cost*. In their seminal 2014 article, Bodenheimer and Sinsky recommended the introduction of the Quadruple Aim, adding the fourth aim, *improving the work life of health care clinicians and staff*, which must be achieved before we can hope to realize the ultimate goal of true population health in this country (Bodenheimer & Sinsky, 2014). Similarly, the World Health Organization (WHO, 2020) issued a declaration about the importance of prioritizing health and safety concerns in order to ensure the existence of high functioning, supportive health systems across the globe. In 2022, the Quintuple Aim was proposed (Nundy, Cooper, & Mate, 2022) and became the expectation (Institute for Healthcare Improvement (IHI), 2022). The fifth aim adds to the other four elements by acknowledging the need for advancing health equity. Together these five elements are designed to improve health care, the reason we all engage in the work we do.

How is a healthy workplace defined? Similar to physiological definitions of health and wellness, a positive workplace is much more than the simple absence of dangerous, negative, or potentially harmful or pathological characteristics. According to the American Nurses Association (ANA, 2021a), a healthy work environment is safe, empowering, and satisfying. Contained within our profession's Nurses Bill of Rights, for example, are components that aim to "protect the dignity and autonomy of nurses in the workplace" (ANA, 2021b). Further, these rights are not optional—they are very essential, designed to emphasize basic human respect and safety within the healthcare environment in order to bring about safe and effective nursing care delivery and the best in professional practice. Specifically, a healthy work environment is associated with fostering nurses' well-being and advancing health-promoting lifestyles (Chung et al., 2020), a positive patient safety climate, and workforce satisfaction, leading to decreased turnover of staff (Bowles et al., 2019).

The term "magnet" in the context of the nursing work environment was first used to describe a nearly gravitational force that exists when hospitals create and sustain positive clinical and work cultures. A *magnet* nursing culture is so strong that nurses who choose such hospitals in which to work are less likely to leave their jobs (ANA, 2021c). Historically, it is the Magnet® Recognition Program of the American Nurses Credentialing Center (ANCC), based on the foundational American Academy of Nursing (AAN) landmark study by McClure and colleagues in 1983, that remains today a global phenomenon. Outcomes associated with the Magnet® designation positively influence nurse recruitment and retention, patient loyalty, physician engagement, and a number of superior clinical outcomes (Thew, 2020a). Magnet® hospitals are often where the best in nursing and patient care outcomes are possible (McClure et al., 1983). Therefore, when hospital leadership commits to the standards of excellence as defined within the Magnet® domains of Transformational Leadership, Structural Empowerment, Exemplary Professional Practice and New Knowledge, Innovations and Improvements (ANA, 2021d), a strong association is established between an excellent nursing practice environment and higher-quality performance for patients, the community, and its staff that positively impacts the entire organization. As is typical in Magnet®-designated organizations, nurses are regularly surveyed for their degree of satisfaction with their unit, department, and hospital. A robust professional practice model and a career progression track exists, along with a career progression track, a care delivery system that endorses a supportive novice-to-expert orientation, a deep commitment to a lifelong learning approach (continuing education), and, importantly, a shared governance philosophy that ensures a voice at the decision-making table for nurses at every level of the organization.

True to the original Magnet® research study findings, today's Magnet® hospitals outperform their peers in measures of nurse satisfaction, recruitment, and retention compared with those that are not (Press Ganey, 2020). Magnet® organizations foster a sustainable culture in which professionals are able to connect their personal caring values to an environment that consistently demonstrates a high degree of professional support, provides recognition in the form of compensation with other incentives, and fulfills an abiding commitment to the staff who comprise their workforce.

Other programs that align, define, and reward a positive work environment include the American Association of Critical Care Nurses Beacon Award for Excellence (AACN, 2021), the Emergency Nurses Association Lantern Award (ENA, 2021), the Academy of Medical-Surgical Nurses' PRISM Award (AMSN, 2021), and the DAISY Award (Daisy Foundation, 2021). Common criteria include excellence in leadership, staffing and staff engagement, communication, knowledge management and adult learning, access to the highest quality of evidence-based science to enrich the provision of patient care, patient and staff advocacy, nurses who participate in research activities and, ultimately, contribute to the achievement of superior performance improvement outcomes. Regardless of the specific award program, or even in the absence of any specific award designation itself, actual participation in the journey to excellence is what matters more than what any particular award represents. As in all journeys that involve setting measurable goals with increasing complexity and innovation, professional nurses and the outcomes of the care that they provide prosper when the work environment consistently surpasses industry standards for career growth opportunities (Pappas & Rushton, 2020). In 2022, the Quintuple Aim became the expectation (Nundy, Cooper, & Mate, 2022).

IMPACT OF UNHEALTHY HEALTHCARE WORKPLACES AND WORKFORCES

Conversely, both the day-to-day as well as the long-term impacts of an unhealthy work environment are entirely all too well known. As one example, nurses who work in areas where they are exposed to lateral violence suffer physiological and psychological consequences (Flannery, 2020), which is also associated with poor longitudinal health outcomes (Havaei et al., 2020). Without exception, the nature of nursing is that we are all highly engaged with patients and their families, who suffer with emotions of pain and grief usually associated with either acute (short-term) or chronic (long-term) physiologic, mental, or terminal illnesses. Consequently, without successful, intentional self-care interventions, nurses may develop emotional symptoms such as anxiety, depression, or anger; physical manifestations such as fatigue, headache, and insomnia; mental changes such as a decrease in sleep, concentration, and memory; and behavioral changes such as smoking, drinking, mood changes, crying, and outbursts for no outward apparent reason.

FACTORS THAT CONTRIBUTE TO UNHEALTHY WORK ENVIRONMENTS

Role Issues

Role issues are key fundamental stressors for nurses. Viewed as having interfacing components, role problems contain varying degrees of ambiguity, role conflict, and role overload (Orgambidez & Benitez, 2021) and may have a positive correlation to career burnout. Role problems are particularly acute, uncomfortable, and difficult for new graduates, whose lack of clinical experience and organizational skills, combined with the rapid bombardment of very new situations, expectations of multigenerational colleagues, and a steep learning curve about complex procedures, may all escalate feelings of overwhelming stress. Conflict between what was learned in the university classroom or limited clinical exposure in actual practice settings only serves to compound the situation and can make a hard situation even worse.

Personal "triggers" are events or situations that have a profound effect on specific individuals. A personal trigger might be a specific event, as in the death of a loved one, an automobile accident, losing a job, getting married, a new relationship, divorce, the birth of a child, or just about any major life event. These events are in addition to everyday personal stressors, such as balancing work/school/home, experiencing a bad day, not getting the chance to consistently eat a meal or take break time at work, and/or facing a long, hazardous daily commute. Negative self-talk, pessimistic thinking, self-criticism, and overanalyzing situations can also be significant ongoing stressors. During periods of high stress, particularly when we are fatigued with no immediate chance at rejuvenation, we may default to negative self-limiting thoughts when that is the only coping mechanism available in a less-than-ideal psychological toolkit. This results in a never-ending cycle and a no-win outlook on life. Usually stemming from unrealistic self-beliefs, such as harsh expectations, taking things personally, all-or-nothing thinking, exaggerating when things go in the wrong direction, or even your family of origin's "style" of coping, perfectionism is our own worst enemy and not unusual among nurses.

Compounding bleak thinking are poor and unhealthy lifestyle choices, such as the overuse of caffeine, lack of a routine exercise schedule, consuming a fat-ridden diet, patterns of inadequate sleep, insufficient leisure/paid time off, excessive alcohol intake/needing alcohol to relax or to fall asleep, the use of recreational/prescription drugs, and cigarette smoking. All of these have a direct effect on the person's perceived stress level. Unfortunately, a vicious lose-lose cycle may take center stage and rule out the potential of hope, a new, more positive direction in one's life, or any viable way to a different reality.

Gender Roles

Approximately 9.6% of the nation's approximately 4 million licensed registered nurses in the United States are men (Health Resources and Services Administration, 2018 [most recent source]). Most nurses are women who go home at the end of their shift to traditional responsibilities, including managing the household and caring for young children and aging parents at the same time, all the while balancing or ignoring their own health needs. When added to the already stressful workday of the nurse, these home responsibilities often contribute to a higher level of distress. Men may have those same experiences, because the "traditional" roles in society are changing to the extent that many men have those same stressors. Thanks to the entry of Generation Y (those born in the 1980s) and the Millennials (born between 1980 and 1996) into the workforce, the importance of work–life balance has become increasingly emphasized. Yet, this has not entirely translated into improvements in the American workplace. However, Millennials and Generation Z (born between the mid- to late-1990s to 2010s), also known as the Zoomers, are now making up more of the larger share of the nursing workforce, with positive work cultures, flexible scheduling, opportunity for career advancement typified by lateral (not always hierarchical) training programs, and colleague relationships scoring at the top of their priorities, according to a large survey (Advisory Board, 2020). In a 2020 Advisory Board survey, Zoomers were more than three times as likely to switch jobs within the past year. The level of engagement for these Zoomers is also among the lowest, making them prime for recruitment campaigns of shrewd organizations that promise gym memberships, innovative staffing models, sign-on bonuses, and attractive pay scales (Adkins, 2020).

Owing to the shifting economy, especially with the global financial markets hit hard by the impact of the recent COVID-19 pandemic, spouses, partners, and adult children may all be underemployed and/or experience sharply reduced work, resulting in reduced or nonexistent health benefits. Adult children, siblings, or even grand-children may have returned to live at home. Therefore, many nurses are shouldering the burden of a second full-time or weekend job and need to work significant over-time hours in order to contribute to strapped household budgets. Lack of financial security means that in times of severe economic hardships (such as in a national eco-nomic recession) or regional threats to the local economy (such as in a severe hurricane, a global pandemic, or a lo-cal industrial plant closing) living from paycheck to pay-check makes even the thought of going to the gym, much less pursuing career advancement activities or planning for retirement, totally out of reach. Financial insecurity may actually impair career opportunities in another way. Some nurses may be too afraid to seek a better position because of the real concerns of perhaps not succeeding or not liking the new job, leading to the possibility of need-ing to leave the position or potentially being laid off, thus, losing health and other employee benefits. All of these concerns are barriers to advancement and what could have been a much-needed change of pace.

Cultural Incompetence and Systemic Racial Inequity

Several tragic events have dramatically illustrated the great racial and cultural divide in the United States. Directly tied to the murders of Black men while in the hands of police officers, a national reckoning of historic proportions is taking place. Such thinking calls for the examination of racial justice that extends to the well-being of communities of color as well as the impact of social determinants of health. Moreover, a closer look into discourse related to social inequities reveals nu-merous and complex issues among healthcare workers. According to Dill et al. (2020), the healthcare industry is in itself racialized and gendered, perpetuating stereo-types and constraining long-term career growth, espe-cially for individuals in direct-care roles. Black nurses and, in fact, all staff of color, report unfortunate inci-dents of racism from patients who may refuse to accept care from non-White caregivers (Caldwell & Pirani, 2020). This is also experienced as originating from the very organizations that employ them because the orga-nization fails to address such racist complaints by reas-signing nurses and not fully addressing the problem of racism head on. Hiring biases compound the problem, significantly limiting career advancement before the in-dividual has the opportunity to begin employment at a health care facility (Scepura, 2020).

According to the ANA's 36th president, Dr. Ernest Grant, an all-White management team is a problem because the table of organization ought to reflect the reality of the communities it serves. Racism in healthcare, according to Grant, is evidenced by fewer opportunities for education, unconscious bias, and stereotypes that limit full and effec-tive social change (Thew, 2020b). Nurses of color frequently do not call out racism in the workplace because their coun-terparts often cannot acknowledge the pain they encounter at work and in their personal lives (Roberts, 2021). Nurses who are educated outside of the United States and come to this country to work also report episodes of discrimination in the workplace (Baptiste, 2020). Unhealthy work envi-ronments that are hostile to immigrant workers do, in fact, impact physical and psychological well-being and outcomes of care. As a powerful and unremitting stressor, discrimi-nation is corrosive to professional roles and careers, self-esteem, and self-awareness, impairing professionals' ability to perform critical role functions (Roberts & Mayo, 2019; Gray, 2021). Changing the system is not the obligation of people of color. That obligation belongs to those who are currently in charge (Botelho & Lima, 2020).

Cultural Incompetence and the LGBTQ+ Community

According to the ANA Position Statement entitled Nursing Advocacy for LGBTQ+ Populations (ANA, 2021e), nurses must deliver "culturally congruent care and advocate for lesbian, gay, bisexual, transgender, queer, or questioning (LGBTQ+) populations." Inasmuch that there is growing awareness and advocacy for social ac-ceptance of patients, there is much less known about the experiences of staff who identify as LGBTQ+ and how to provide for their needs in the clinical professional work-place. A study by the Williams Institute at the University of California Los Angeles School of Law (Sears et al., 2021) found that 46% of LGBTQ+ workers reported receiving unfair treatment at some point in their ca-reers, ranging from being denied a promotion or raise, harassed, excluded from receiving overtime hours, or even fired. Lim et al. (2019) notes that leaders now have the opportunity to usher in a new era of inclusivity for a population that has been stigmatized for far too long. Because there is a lack of research in this area, Younas (2019) recommends that studies related to workplace ex-periences, coupled with peer and organizational support systems and educational needs of LGBTQ+ nursing stu-dents, are all highly critical areas for new knowledge and represent a call to action for our profession.

Staffing Shortages

Unequal, ineffective, and inappropriate nurse–patient staffing has been well documented in the research literature since at least the 1990s (Aiken et al., 1994; Needleman et al., 2002; Aiken et al., 2008). A more recent systematic review of the staffing research literature (Halm, 2019) corroborated the earlier findings: Better staffing and supportive practice environments remain associated with improved patient outcomes, such as fewer falls, ability to rescue, and reduction in a host of patient complications, such as mortality. For nurses, improved staffing leads to higher quality of care and safety ratings, less job dissatisfaction, and decreased burnout. Conversely, in hospitals with higher nurses' workload, worsening rates of in-hospital mortality, hospital-acquired infection, and medication errors in addition to falls are commonly found. Other measures of the impact of poor staffing include an increase in nurses' intentions to leave the organization and so-called abandonment of treatment when, because they are working below the industry standard for safe staffing, they cannot fully act on the medical protocols that are ordered for the patient (Assaye et al., 2020).

Unfortunately, a climate of poor staffing practices was in existence across hospitals *before* the COVID-19 pandemic. Nurses in one study scored in the "high burnout range" due to unacceptable workloads and dissatisfaction with their jobs; they were not likely to definitely recommend their hospitals. Not surprisingly, one in five nurses in the study had previously planned to leave their hospitals within the year when the COVID-19 pandemic reversed those plans, at least temporarily (Lasater et al., 2021). Travel nursing, once the domain of a small segment of the profession, grew by 44% between 2018 and 2019 (before the pandemic) (SimpliFi, 2021). By mid-2021, travel agencies boomed and the high pay they promised, along with attractive bonuses, left many hospitals even more short staffed than they were before COVID-19. Moreover, demand has overburdened already stressed hospitals and shifted available funds away from needed investments in the workplace to travel and staffing agencies. This has led to poor morale when existing nurses work side-by-side with former teammates who now earn far more pay because they are taking advantage of the lucrative contracts that agency and travel nursing affords them (Devereaux, 2021).The post-pandemic reality is projected to impact nurse staffing far into the future, with waves of retiring nurses, nurses leaving the bedside, the closure or merging of health systems due to the financial impact on hospitals, a worsening nursing faculty shortage, and the shift to telemedicine and technology—all posing new and previously unforeseen challenges for the acute care, ambulatory, and community settings (Hudson, 2020) and exacerbating tenuous workforce stressors.

Workplace Violence

Plainly put, lateral workplace violence occurs when leaders demonstrate a lack of accountability for team behaviors. Manifestations include cultures that blame and are characterized by passivity, overt or covert aggression, hostility, and lack of professional trust in each other as well as in local and executive leadership. When toxic leaders utilize fear and distrust and undervalue their team, they may be able to achieve short-term goals. However, in the long run, they fail to engender a sense of security about everyone's place and contributions within the organization (Weberg & Fuller, 2019). A global issue, negative workplace behaviors in healthcare are usually aimed at member(s) of a workgroup and include bullying and harassment (Hawkins et al., 2021), also called *lateral violence*. Direct care nurses report an increase in mental health problems with long-term, cumulative exposure to workplace violence. In at least one study, these nurses were two to four times more likely to report high levels of post-traumatic stress disorder (PTSD), anxiety, depression, and burnout compared with their colleagues with no exposure (Havaei et al., 2020). The pervasiveness of horizontal violence leads many nurses to conclude that there is an unspoken level of acceptance for it even as long-term damage is calculated. With this comes the realization that the full benefits of true teamwork will never be experienced (Tedone, 2020).

Another pandemic in healthcare exists: on-the-job violence from patients and families. It ranges from threatening behavior to physical assault. In health care, this violence is on the increase. According to Watson, Jafari, and Seifi (2020), the majority of physicians and nurses can recall at least one incident of violence directed at them during their careers. Such violence holds negative consequences for the delivery, quality, and accessibility of health care. Common among such episodes are shouting, swearing, and grabbing (Morse, 2021). No matter where the violence originates, it is now considered the new "reality shock" for nurses in that nurses in otherwise healthier environments may not expect it.

Therefore, they may be at more risk for burnout than nurses who have somehow "normalized" unsafe work conditions and have learned to deal with it one way or another (Havaei et al., 2020). As is true of other situations in which rights exist, obligations need to be stated so that patients, families, and even visitors understand the expectations for appropriate behaviors.

Impact of Electronic Documentation Burdens

Nurses face stress as they attempt to learn and then integrate multiple computer systems that may lack sufficient interfaces. This often leads to frustration when we must toggle between multiple screens in order to complete critical patient documentation. When healthcare software is not designed to be intuitive to the end user, nurses wind up spending an increasing amount of time in front of a device instead of spending time with their patients. In truth, reports detailing failure to enter data within organizational parameters are now easily retrievable, attributable, and, as some nurses fear, subject to discipline, as these reports present data in terms of transgressions rather than in terms of time saved at the bedside. Nurses experience documentation burden because we are constantly feeding *data hungry systems* put into a production workflow to solve seemingly isolated, focused tasks—such as entering a patient's vital signs, blood pressure, or blood glucose levels—without regard to the overall effect on workflow (Moy et al., 2021). Nurses may also need to bridge a staggering number of gaps to safely communicate with their providers whose workplaces may be technologically different or several upgrades behind in expensive systems. Provider systems may also have separate and distinct rules about documentation, ordering tests, and receiving results. These challenges are as likely to exist when communicating within the same hospital or clinics in the outpatient/ambulatory settings as they are with organizations situated halfway around the globe.

EXERCISE 5.1 Think of the last time you were in the clinical area. How often did you record the same piece of data (e.g., a finding in your assessment of the patient)? Remember to include all steps, from jotting down notes on a piece of paper or entering data into the computer to the final report of the day. What information processing tools could decrease the number of steps? Has this issue been raised in your unit meetings?

Exposure to Needlestick and Sharps Injuries

That nurses still face harm and fear from contamination arising from needlestick and sharps injuries (NSIs) is perplexing, as the introduction of engineered safety features has not satisfactorily reduced the worldwide incidence (Dulon et al., 2020). Thomas (2019, 2020) observed that not only is the problem underreported, most NSIs occur because the users are not trained properly in the features' special components and that factors such as inadequate sleep further contribute to occurrences. Preventing full disclosure by both nursing students and practicing nurses was the fear of retaliation, embarrassment, and the rather unscientific belief that the patient did not seem to be overtly dangerous or infectious to the nurse (Thomas, 2020). Cumbersome incident reporting mechanisms, the need to schedule follow-up appointments, and an environment of blame toward the practitioner can all contribute to a lack of reporting. Studies have linked NSIs with unhealthy work environments: D'Ettore et al. (2020) and Wang et al. (2019) observed that job stress and certain organizational characteristics—such as overwork, embarrassment, fear of being labeled as ignorant of hospital policy, and even the caregivers' perception of a stressful environment—all greatly influence the incidence of NSIs in healthcare organizations, for which no immediate solution exists.

Exposure to Infectious Agents and Hazardous Chemicals

Not in any current healthcare practitioner's lifetime experience had the fear of widespread potential for infection and death been greater than during the COVID-19 outbreak, when the first case arrived in the United States. Throughout the pandemic, lack of personal protective equipment (PPE) in this country exposed caregivers to persons known or suspected to have been infected with COVID-19. Contracting the COVID-19 virus threatened significant harm to frontline healthcare workers, though individuals and family members within the community still posed the highest risk of all (Van Beusekom, 2020). The long-term and immediate effects of contracting and surviving COVID-19 are as yet not fully known. At the outbreak of the pandemic, the vulnerability of healthcare workers to the fatal outcomes of the virus was also unknown. It is now estimated that there were 2,900 deaths in the first full year (Jewett et al., 2020). At the height of the pandemic, confronting one's own risk for exposure to a potentially deadly virus while simultaneously caring for patients who were critically ill, contributed to significant exposure to psychological trauma (Donohue-Ryan & Schneider, 2020). Other exposures to infectious agents that also carry with it the threat of disability or death have been well known to us as nurses, which include hepatitis B virus, hepatitis C virus, and human immunodeficiency virus (HIV) (Mengistu et al., 2021). An increase in outbreaks among nurses on the job is also tied to an increase in time burdens for clinical nurses and infection preventionist workloads (Hessels et al., 2019). This detracts from other patient care needs, such as direct care, prevention, and control activities, thereby increasing stress.

Incidence of Musculoskeletal Harm

While pulling or moving patients or equipment, nurses are at risk for developing acute as well as chronic physiologic injuries. While many acute care environments have instituted a zero-lift environment and state authorities have mandated safe patient handling programs, such as investments in costly lift technology, nurses often do not use the devices or do not use them correctly, often citing constraints, such as not having the equipment readily available or the belief that they are too time-consuming to locate and use (Hawkins, 2021). Again, the pressure to perform tasks in a pressure-filled work setting can cause immediate and long-term damage. As Zare et al. (2021) described in a systematic review and meta-analysis, a relationship is established between upper limb musculoskeletal disorders and a host of factors, including poor staffing, job dissatisfaction, work-related stress, and lack of organizational support. Needless to say, even the best use of body mechanics is no match for a disproportionate ratio of body weight between patient and nurse. Since the U.S. Bureau of Labor Statistics (BLS, 2021) reports that sprains, strains, tears, soreness, pain bruises, and contusions are the majority of workplace occupational injuries for nurses (as measured by days away from work), our own bodies are at risk on a daily basis.

Upheaval in the Organization

Stress in organizations may result from unrealistic or conflicting expectations originating from oneself or others, the pace and magnitude of change, human behavior, individual personality characteristics, the characteristics of the position itself, or the entire culture of the organization. Stressors may be unique to certain environments, situations, and persons or groups. Hospitals care for increasingly critically ill patients, which requires advanced competencies and complex knowledge in order

to become ever more adept at accomplishing required functions. In the ambulatory setting, where most patients receive their care in the communities in which they reside, uneven volume distribution, care model uncertainty, insufficient data for personalizing the patient experience, and emerging threats to volumes and growth are among the many challenges (Singh, 2021). Add to the scenario the constant disruption caused by healthcare mergers, buy-outs and acquisitions and it becomes difficult to overlook a most unpredictable financial outlook in the ambulatory and home care marketplace.

At the top of any healthcare organizational chart is the C-suite executive, where long-term employment, once the hallmark in many hospitals, is simply no longer the case. Tenure has been less than ideal for the Chief Nursing Officer (CNO), whose responsibility it is to set the vision for the professional practice environment among staff, fellow administrators, and the boards of trustees. Persolja and fellow researchers (2020) determined that involuntary turnover of CNOs has been rising throughout the world, attributed to political turbulence, lack of support by management, and the introduction of new CEOs, who, in turn, may displace the most senior nurses or even ask them to reapply for their own jobs. This results in lack of stability among the nursing staff, as the inability to obtain enduring support for patient care initiatives, a lack of trust toward fellow senior colleagues, and failure to see strategic initiatives through to a successful endpoint all can have dire consequences for the nursing and overall corporate infrastructure. The CNO plays such a key role in promoting transformational leadership that the ANCC Magnet® program requires that the senior nurse possess equal authority to other executives within the organization and must have access to the top-most decision-making bodies (ANA, 2021d). Without organizational equality, it would be nearly impossible for such leaders to be perceived by frontline nurses as having similar authority and strategic importance as their senior peers because, it would follow, neither would nursing itself in such an environment.

RESPONSES TO UNHEALTHY WORK ENVIRONMENTS

Stress

Stress is a consequence of or response to an event or stimulus. Stress is not inherently bad. Rather, each individual's interpretation determines whether the event is viewed as positive or threatening. Stress can provide us with the determination to land a brand new position that is a step up on the career ladder. Stress gives us the "edge" we all need to help us think quickly and clearly and to express our thoughts in ways that will best represent our hard work and talent—most appropriate for the interview process! Self-reflection should lead us to acknowledge the significant effects of stress on our lives, which result in major physiologic changes—its indelible effects on sleep, eating, and social interactions (Bani-Issa et al., 2020). Once we are honest with ourselves, stress becomes easier to anticipate, identify, and manage more effectively over time. However, when looking at job-related stressors, we need to understand that stressors typically fall into one of two categories: external (working and living conditions) and internal (worker characteristics).

Most nurses can easily recognize the origins of stress and its symptoms. For example, a healthcare organization may make demands on the nursing staff, such as an excessive workload or floating outside one's specialty, that nurses regard as placing undue burdens on their capacity to perform well or in a healthy manner. When we are unable to resolve the problem through overwork, with more staff, or by trying to see the situation another way, nurses may experience decreased job satisfaction, become depressed, and have negative patient outcomes (Schlak et al., 2021). We may also experience headaches, fatigue, an inability to concentrate, or other physical symptoms that are associated with a low level of job performance. If the stress persists, such symptoms may escalate and manifest themselves in decreased job performance, medical errors, or musculoskeletal or NSIs. Nurses may attempt to cope by becoming completely apathetic, a sign of burnout. Box 5.1 gives physical, mental, and spiritual/emotional signs of overstress in individuals.

A relationship exists between stress and the human immune system and a body of literature that ties unrelenting stress to immune dysregulation. The immune systems of those who are older or already sick are more prone to stress-related immune system changes, such as inflammation, delayed wound healing, poor responses to vaccines, and increased susceptibility to infectious disease processes (Canas-Gonzalez et al., 2020). Physical illnesses linked to stress include visceral adiposity (increase in body fat), type 2 diabetes, cardiovascular disease (hypertension, heart attack, stroke), musculoskeletal disorders, psychological

BOX 5.1 Signs of Overstress in Individuals

Physical

Physical signs of ill health:
- Increase in flu, colds, accidents
- Change in sleeping habits
- Chronic fatigue

Chronic signs of decreased ability to manage stress:
- Headaches
- Hypertension
- Backaches
- Gastrointestinal problems

Unhealthy coping activities:
- Increased use of drugs and alcohol
- Increased or decreased weight
- Smoking
- Crying, yelling, blaming, mood swings

Mental
- Dread of going to work every day
- Rigid thinking and a desire to go by all the rules in all cases; inability to tolerate any changes
- Forgetfulness and anxiety about work to be done; more frequent errors and incidents
- Returning home exhausted and unable to participate in enjoyable activities
- Confusion about duties and roles
- Generalized anxiety
- Decrease in concentration
- Depression
- Anger, irritability, impatience
- Blaming, negotiating

Spiritual/Emotional
- Sense of being a failure; disappointed in work performance
- Anger and resentment toward patients, colleagues, and managers; overall irritable attitude
- Lack of positive feelings toward others
- Cynicism toward patients, blaming them for their problems
- Excessive worry, insecurity, lowered self-esteem
- Increased family and friend conflict
- Disconnection from family and friends and usual sources of support and love

disorders (anxiety, depression), workplace injury, neuromuscular disorders (multiple sclerosis), suicide, cancer, ulcers, asthma, and rheumatoid arthritis. Stress can even cause life-threatening sympathetic stimulation.

Dynamics of Stress

Initially, increased stress produces increased performance. However, when stress continues to escalate or remains intense and unrelenting, overall performance suffers. Hans Selye's (1956) mid–20th-century investigations to decode the nature of and reactions to stress have been very influential in our present-day understanding of this very human phenomenon. In his classic theory, Selye described the concept of stress, identified general adaptation syndrome (GAS), and detailed a predictable pattern of response (see the Theory Box and Fig. 5.1;

THEORY BOX

Theories Applicable to Self-Management

Key Contributors	Key Ideas	Application to Practice
Maslow's Hierarchy of Needs: Maslow (1943) identified five need levels of every human.	Although recent research shows that the five levels are not always present or in order, it is reasonable that unmet needs motivate most employees most of the time.	Nurse wages should be sufficient to provide shelter and food. Job security and a social environment that rewards and recognizes nurse performance are important.
General Adaptation Syndrome: Selye (1956) is credited with developing this theory.	The "stress response" is an adrenocortical reaction to stressors that is accompanied by psychological changes and physiologic alterations that follow a pattern of fight or flight. The general adaptation syndrome includes an alarm, resistance, and adaptation or exhaustion.	Change, lack of control, and excessive workload are common stressors that evoke psychological and physiologic distress among nurses.
Complex Adaptive Systems: Plsek and Greenhalgh (2001).	This theory of unpredictable interactions between interdependent people and activities emphasizes the importance of innovation and rapid information sharing to improve performance.	Nurse engagement in self-managed groups and teams empowers organizations to shape their environment through controlled "experimentation" using the rapid-cycle plan-do-study-act (PDSA) improvement method in a high reliability organization (HRO) mindset.
The Pareto Principle: Hafner (2001).	The "Pareto Principle" refers to a universal observation of "vital few, trivial many." Pareto (1848–1923) studied distribution of personal incomes in Italy and observed that 80% of the wealth was controlled by 20% of the population. This concept of disproportion was observed in many areas. Although the exact values of 20% and 80% are not significant, the considerable disproportion is important to remember.	The 80–20 rule can be applied to many aspects of healthcare today. For example, 80% of healthcare expenditures are attributed to 20% of the population, and 80% of personnel problems occur in 20% of the staff. In quality improvement, 80% of improvement can be expected by removing 20% of the causes of unacceptable quality or performance. A nurse can also expect that 80% of patient-care time will be spent working with 20% of one's patient assignment. This concept may help explain sources of stress when nurses attempt to provide all patients in their assignment "equal time" in the mistaken belief that all patients need the same type of nursing care.

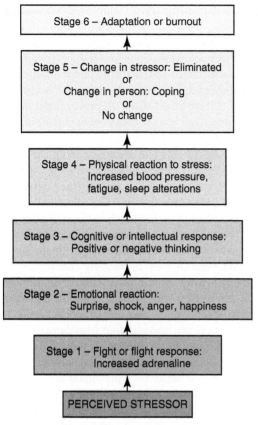

Stage 6 – Adaptation or burnout

Stage 5 – Change in stressor: Eliminated
or
Change in person: Coping
or
No change

Stage 4 – Physical reaction to stress:
Increased blood pressure,
fatigue, sleep alterations

Stage 3 – Cognitive or intellectual response:
Positive or negative thinking

Stage 2 – Emotional reaction:
Surprise, shock, anger, happiness

Stage 1 – Fight or flight response:
Increased adrenaline

PERCEIVED STRESSOR

Fig. 5.1 The stress diagram.

Lonsdale, 2020). The Theory Box also presents other key theories related to self-management. These are all particularly useful when presented with an unhealthy workplace.

More recent investigations of the relationship among the brain, immune system, and health (psychoneuroimmunology) have generated models that challenge Selye's thinking. Although Selye's position was that all people respond with a similar set of hormonal and immune responses to any stress, newer thinking posited that increased stress may actually connect humans to each other by increasing reward sensitivity for another person and prosocial behavior (Tomova et al., 2020). This is useful thinking when an entire work team seems to bond and form an alliance when there is bullying or any other unsupportive behavior on the part of someone else, who is either internal or external to the group.

Critical of stress research with predominately male subjects and, therefore, a male phenomenon, Taylor and fellow researchers (MacBride, 2020) proposed a model of the female stress response, the "tend and befriend," as opposed to the male's "fight or flight" model. The "tend and befriend" response is an estrogen and oxytocin–mediated stress response that is characterized by caring for offspring and befriending those around in times of stress to increase chances of survival. Here, an example would be when a work group, in the face of extreme stress, will continue to host birthday celebrations and plan recognition for graduates, retirements, and baby showers.

Unrelenting, Work-Related Stress

Burnout

Work-related stress can lead to poor physical and emotional health and injury on the job. Challenges (eustress) can be very positive when they motivate us to learn new skills, master our jobs, manage new situations, and help us mature and grow into knowledgeable, optimistic, caring professionals. For example, if you are involved in a job interview for an exciting new position, you will actually benefit from a certain amount of stress (eustress). This is a different phenomenon than *distress*, which can lead to unpleasant symptoms ranging from fatigue to exhaustion, feelings of inadequacy and failure, or even complete and total indifference, known as burnout. Sometimes, individuals cannot manage stress successfully through their own efforts and require targeted, short-term assistance. Examples of behavior related to stress that feels overwhelming are found in Box 5.1. Previous coping strategies that you have used in the past may furnish temporary relief or, perhaps, none at all. With a rising level of distress, one can feel overwhelmed or helpless and may become vulnerable to a mental or physical illness and feel burned out.

The classic view of burnout—a psychological term to describe the effects of prolonged emotional and physical exhaustion and diminished interest—is that it is caused by an unrelenting workload without relief (Celik et al., 2021). The source of the stressor(s) may exist in the environment, in the individual, or in the interaction between the individual and the environment. Some stressors, such as serious illness or death in the family, or the breakup of a relationship, occur in the personal world of the nurse. Usually, however, when we think of burnout, it is in the context of an unhealthy work environment. The Research Perspective emphasizes the importance of a health work environment, especially before nursing is expected to face another healthcare crisis. Burnout is not an objective phenomenon—it is not the accumulation of a certain number of stressors or limited to a certain type of stressor. Though highly individualized, the experience of burnout is that it has a significant impact, touches every area of our lives, and feels as though no help is available to get us out of it. How stressors are perceived, then, and how they are mediated as well as the individual's ability to adapt, are all crucial variables in determining their level of distress, particularly in a less-than-desirable workplace.

Nurses who are burned out feel as though their resources are depleted to the point that their entire well-being is at risk. A self-analysis usually uncovers the classic symptoms of burnout. First, a feeling of physical, mental, and emotional exhaustion is evident, obvious to oneself as well as to others within our social network. Frequently, it is our loved ones who are the first to point out that they are not seeing us at our best. Moss (2021) described that even prior to the recent COVID-19 pandemic, American workers were already stretched very thin, that emotional exhaustion was directly related to an unsustainable workload, and other factors persisted, contributing to an unhealthy workplace. For example, recent graduate nurses may value total, detailed care for individuals and may have little experience in caring for more than two or three patients simultaneously, let alone a full slate of patients to visit in a home healthcare agency. When confronted with the responsibility of caring for a group of six to eight acutely ill patients in a hospital, they may have difficulty adapting to the realities of the workplace. Coupled with fear of failure

and lack of peer/supervisor support, emotional exhaustion usually ensues. Emotional exhaustion, in turn, has a direct effect on levels of cynicism and somatization. A second characteristic of burnout is depersonalization, a state characterized by distancing oneself from the work itself and developing negative attitudes toward work in general (Elhadi et al., 2020). Depersonalization is commonly described as a feeling of being outside one's body, having the feeling of being a machine or robot, an "unreal" feeling of being in a dream, or being "on automatic pilot." Generally, subjective symptoms of unreality make the nurse uneasy and anxious. Others external to our situation may view this as callousness and rudeness. Nurses pushed to do too much in too little time, or who push themselves in some way, may distance themselves from patients as a means of dealing with emotional exhaustion. Also, nurses' personality characteristics may lean too heavily on the caregiving dimension, which often carries over into one's personal life. For example, caregiving individuals may be further challenged by life partners, families, and children who demand a disproportionate amount of time and energy. Thus, renewal and safe havens are unlikely to be available in such cases.

A decreased sense of professional accomplishment and competence is the third hallmark of burnout. Low professional efficacy has been found to be a function of higher levels of cynicism (Kajimu et al., 2021). *Efficacy* is the belief in one's capabilities to organize and execute goal-oriented activities. Nurses, like all humans, are more inclined to take on a task if they believe they can succeed. Lower levels of efficacy can lead nurses to believe that tasks are harder than they actually are. This can lead to a sense of failure, perceived helplessness, and, eventually, a full-blown crisis. At this point, one's coping skills are simply no longer as effective as they once were.

RESEARCH PERSPECTIVE

Resource: Whittington, K., Shaw, T., McKinnies, R. C., & Collins, S. K. (2021). Emotional exhaustion as a predictor for burnout among nurses. *Nursing Management, 52*(1), 22–28. https://doi.org/10.1097/01.NUMA.0000724928.71008.47

This is a quantitative study to explore and describe the experience of burnout among nurses in the United States, as measured by the Maslach Burnout Inventory and the Areas of Worklife Survey (AWS). Additionally, aspects of the nurses' work life were also studied. Seeking to build on the body of knowledge about the health and wellness of our nation's caregivers, the researchers sought to better understand the nature of burnout as the opposite of a joyful, highly productive workplace. Though nurse burnout often contributes to negative patient outcomes as well, there has been limited research linking the two phenomena. To study burnout, feelings of emotional exhaustion, depersonalization, and personal accomplishment were evaluated. Domains of workload, control, reward, community, fairness, and values were categories of the AWS that provided descriptive analysis among variables in addition to correlations between variables and linear regression modeling. Study participants were solicited via a national data distribution methodology; 93 nurses completed the survey. Of the participants, 89% were female, with an average age of 50.063 years. The majority, 62.4%, were employed in nursing for 16 years or longer. Most, 72%, were frontline staff. Of the participants, 40.9% were at their organization for 5 years of less, 13.6% for 6 to 10 years, 16.1% for 11 to 15 years, 11.2% for 16 to 20 years, and 10.1% for 21 + years. The remainder were retired or had left nursing altogether.

The concepts of workload, control, and community emerged as statistically significant, which reinforced the following key points about employers' obligations to provide a healthy workplace. (1) Positively impacting happiness/joy, improving patient satisfaction, and increasing nurse retention are all dependent on a wellness culture. (2) Nurses' perception of control in terms of how they manage their workload helps them manage stress. (3) Decision-making platforms empower nurses to create workflow arrangements that directly impact their practice.

(4) Mindfulness, break times. and group discussions must be supported. (5) A strong sense of community among nurses helps develop collaborative approaches to care delivery.

Implications for Practice

Burnout is a relentless experience that has the potential to undermine and derail careers. It also impacts patient care and has negative consequences for recruitment and retention. There is a relationship between workload, control over nursing practice, and a sense of community. These all have the capacity to either improve or detract from a healthy culture. It is critical that organizations refocus their workforce strategies. Nurses must be empowered to practice self-care measures so that they perceive that their employer supports them. The actual practice as well as the perception, is what has far reaching implications. In conclusion, building a strong culture is an imperative that must be addressed before the next global, regional, or local crisis presents itself. A healthy nurse and healthy workplace acts as an effective buffer against even the most formidable odds.

DEVELOPING A HEALTHY WORK ENVIRONMENT IN HEALTHCARE

A healthy work environment starts with healthy nurses. As nurses, we play the most significant role in promoting a healthy work lifestyle as long as we begin the journey with ourselves first. We know that healthcare is a stressful industry and that nursing is a stressful profession. It is also predicted that pressures upon nurses will increase in the future (Edmonson & Marshall, 2020). How we deal with challenges depends a lot on how we successfully recognize and practice the need for self-compassion in our lives so that we can develop a repository of coping skills. In order to do this, we as professionals must switch gears from a crisis intervention framework to long-term prevention for ourselves and others (Melnyk, 2020). Our eventual goal is to enhance nurses' ability to deal with stress by nurturing resilience, known as *psychological hardiness*. Successful stress management, such as developing hardiness, even in an unhealthy environment or during constant exposure to negative factors in the workplace, does not necessarily lead to stress reduction or its outright elimination. Kobasa, Maddi, and Kahn (1982) characterized successful stress management as the control of emotions and behaviors, perseverance, and a heightened sense of purpose, along with handling the continuous challenge

that is present in the face of stressful events. According to seminal researchers Lambert, Lambert, and Yamase (2003), how humans develop psychological hardiness is a blend of commitment, control, and challenge. These form a constellation that (1) dampens the effects of stress by challenging the perception of the situation and (2) decreases the negative impact of a situation by moderating both cognitive appraisal and coping. Nursing resilience is a cultivated characteristic that occurs when individuals strategically use education, coaching, peer review, self-reflection, spirituality, emotional intelligence, and other resources in bad to extremely bad situations and, despite overwhelming odds, continue to learn and grow (Cooper et al., 2021).

Workplace Stress Prevention

Nurses need to fully appreciate and recognize their unique stressors at home and on the job. Everyone experiences stress—the exhilaration of a joyous event as well as the negative feelings and unpleasant physical symptoms associated with a life situation that challenges us. Anticipation of an event such as meeting the parents of a new romantic partner or taking an exam in a really tough subject area precipitates stress. Learning what stress is, its dynamics, and how we individually experience it and determine effective strategies to manage it are all part of personal and professional growth. Because nurses tend to work in areas and situations that are extremely stressful, stress management skills have to be continuously adapted to new situations and strengthened over time through a commitment to lifelong learning and an attitude of being open to new ideas. Not everyone we encounter in life and in nursing is so open. Yet, resistance to change is a fundamental and normal consequence whenever a threat to the status quo is present (DuBose & Mayo, 2020). Even when an alternative way of dealing with a situation is presented to us, our first response should not be "no, I'm fine" when what we are really feeling is very far from "fine." Another common source of stress is our own unrealistic, unhealthy expectations, as well as the impact of leadership behaviors upon nurse burnout (Wei, Jiang, & Lake, 2020).

Emotional Intelligence

Daniel Goleman (1995; see also danielgoleman.info) is considered by many to be the undisputed, seminal author on emotional intelligence (EI). He observed that those who are the most successful in organizations are not necessarily more intelligent. Rising stars are distinguished from their peers because they have learned how to master their own emotions as well as their relationships. Such individuals, with average IQs, clearly outpaced those with even the highest IQs when principles are learned and refined over time. Managing EI, managing stress (or at least our response to it), and managing time, when possible, are three key strategies for healthy self-management.

EI is a critical leadership competency involving four skills: self-awareness, self-management, social awareness, and relationship management (Goleman, 2020). Briefly, *self-awareness* relates to how well we perceive our own emotions at the time we are experiencing them. This element is important because our emotions tell us how we are reacting to events and information. If you have an uncomfortable "gut" feeling and do not know what caused that sensation, you may want to practice deliberately thinking about it—and, importantly, your reactions—so that you gain a better understanding of yourself. Self-management is your response to being self-aware. You either act or do not act. We all know people who blurt out something they would rather not have said pubicly, as when a driver cuts them off on the road. That is an example of an immediate, although not very productive, act, especially if you are in the midst of a work-related phone call. Being a more self-aware "driver" may allow us as individuals to move from viscerally making a negative

response to instead focusing on "putting on the brakes," as it were, thinking of a calm response, and so forth. *Social awareness* relates to "reading" people. Are they happy, angry, distressed, hurt? The purpose of being socially aware is to gain critical information. Thus, listening and observing are two critical life skills to cultivate. The final element is *relationship management.* As you might suspect, it relies heavily on your abilities in the first three areas. It combines your awareness of self and others in an effort to execute clear communication. Through solid relationship management, even with people we may not like very much, we can be more effective in reducing personal and sometimes even organizational stress. In times of crisis, no matter what the origin is, clear communication is critical to being an effective communicator and in resolving the issue.

Personal competence includes the skills of self-awareness and self-management, particularly with respect to your own values and how well they line up to the behaviors observed in the workplace (Tye, 2020). Social competence involves the skills of social awareness and relationship management. The good news is that EI can be learned and is worth the investment. Emotionally intelligent managers possess greater insight into their staff and manage better because they provide support and guidance, serve as role models, and, one might infer, raise optimism and cohesiveness, with a natural give-and-take that results in growth (Preugschat, 2020). With the philosophy of "every nurse a leader," it follows that nurses' goals include growth and self-knowledge, learning to balance new as well as formerly held personal and professional objectives, and reorganizing time and activities to reach these goals. The so-called stress hardiness of nurses and leaders has long been thought to be essential to the survival of the nurse, giving rise to a professional alter-ego—the "supernurse culture" (Groves et al., 2020). In the past, seasoned nurses would pride themselves on being able to "take it," meaning silently work in, and even take on, negative behaviors that contribute to unhealthy work environments without ever openly challenging negative aspects of the workplace however unacceptable they might be. Nurses who spoke up or found themselves unable or unwilling to tolerate difficult conditions in the practice setting were labeled as "weak," "bad nurses," or often criticized behind closed doors as being "not a good fit" for the organization. However, we currently define hardiness as exemplified by control, commitment, and challenge.

These are important tools to refine throughout a career that contribute to positive outcomes for nurses and their patients (Desai, 2020).

In fact, organizations that make a significant investment in leadership development actually make it their strategic priority to connect and strengthen positive social support networks. Even the *perception* of transformational leadership mitigates against the toxic effects of burnout (Lai et al., 2020). Leaders in progressive and innovative thinking, called "thought leaders," suggest that the cultivation of stress hardiness produces nurse managers with a leadership style and resilience that improves overall working conditions. Fortunately, stress management can be taught and personal hardiness can be acquired when interventions at all organizational levels exist to mitigate against caregiver burnout and stress (Miller, 2016). In fact, during the COVID-19 pandemic, Liu (2020) observed that training for stress reduction was up by 4,000% in 2020. To further develop stress hardiness and resilience, we must actively improve our skills related to stress management, adaptive coping, healthy communication, and problem solving. The three key strategies—EI, time management, and stress management—are important ways to support one's talents, energies, and creativity and are the fundamental building blocks to healthy nurse behaviors.

Management of Stress

Individuals respond to stress by eliciting coping strategies that are a means of dealing with stress to maintain or achieve an improved sense of well-being or perceived work–life balance. Certain strategies may be ineffective because of reliance on excessive alcohol or prescription drug and substance use. Other methods—such as a dedicated physical exercise program, meditation, or professional counseling—are quite effective in helping restore a greater sense of well-being and overall health improvement. One effective way to deal with stress is to determine and manage its source. Discovering the origin of stress in patient care may be difficult because some environments have changed so rapidly that the nursing staff is overwhelmed trying to balance bureaucratic rules and limited resources with the demands of vulnerable human beings for whom they are caring.

An editorial in *Business News Daily* (Vasconcellos, 2020), observed that workplace politics, while seemingly inevitable, cause tension, prevent employees from performing at their full capacity, and detract from team and employee morale. Therefore, when in distress, nurses may need to step back and look at the moments that connect them more fully to their purpose and job enjoyment, such as deliberately disengaging from the politics of the workplace. Gossip, though often a source of intense discussion and speculation, does not do us very much good in the long run. However, identifying daily stressors and developing better management of the stress is often a watershed moment for new managers, on the way toward becoming a transformational leader. Such leaders actively create a plan to eliminate the stressor if possible, modify the stressor, and/or change the perception of the stressor (e.g., viewing mistakes as opportunities for new learning) and gaining practice over time with the *reframing* technique. *Reframing* is changing the way you look at things to make you feel better about them or to obtain a different perspective. For example, an individual who is difficult to deal with may be viewed instead as someone who lacks understanding about how to create an assignment and is in need of a peer coaching session or perhaps needs to have a totally different experience that might, in the end, contribute to improvements in patient care.

A situation can be seen in multiple ways. It is less stressful to take the view that there is always an aspect of our lives (including the rapidly changing healthcare environment) that is bound to be unpredictable and remain a mystery at times and not something for which we always have to take responsibility, thereby increasing stress. In their seminal article, Plsek and Greenhalgh (2001) observed that according to Complex Adaptive Systems (see the Theory Box), all systems are nested within other systems and all are in a state of constant interaction. Therefore, it would seem that taking one aspect of a situation out of proportion and fretting about it does little to achieve one's overall understanding of the so-called "big picture."

Of course, such on-the-job stressors are often counterbalanced by the rewards of patient appreciation, the joy of seeing a healthy baby born, or seeing firsthand the relief brought by a nursing intervention such as appropriate pain medication or repositioning of an uncomfortable limb. Given the nature of nursing practice, nurses must be alert to our own individual signs of stress and be able to develop self-awareness about our goal to achieve some measure of work–life balance. Each of us has to understand how many hours in a day, how many shifts in a row, and, conversely, how many hours or days between shifts for refueling purposes "works" for us as human beings. We may be challenged to figure out what is reasonable for us in light of family, organizational, personal, and social expectations. As we know from our experience with a global pandemic, how we conserve our personal resources matters a great deal. We know that cultivating healthy lifestyle habits helps reduce stress in that getting adequate sleep, a balanced diet, regular exercise, and frequent social interactions with friends and colleagues are all excellent stress-buffering habits and, as such, that must be prioritized in our own lives.

According to Fernandez (2021), nearly one-quarter of all workers view their jobs as the top stressor in their lives. Fernandez looks to the scientific findings of neuroscience and behavioral and organizational research for the following survival tips: (1) exercise mindfulness, (2) compartmentalize your workload, (3) take detachment breaks, (4) develop mental agility, and (5) cultivate compassion. Practicing these skills can be challenging and may feel uncomfortable at first, yet the return on investment is essential to our overall well-being and, coupled with a solid return on investment for our organizations, makes self-care a win/win.

EXERCISE 5.2 Identify what stress you experience and how you usually manage it. Create and complete the following log at the end of every day for 1 week or locate and use a common app for your phone or other portable device. Review the log and note what situations (e.g., people, technology, values conflict) were the most common. Also, identify how you most often react to stress: physically, mentally, or emotionally and spiritually. Keeping this diary for a week is helpful to determine what stress triggers you encounter and, importantly, to learn more about your reactions. Enter a date and describe a situation and your response. Ask yourself whether the stress was good stress (eustress) or bad stress (distress). Then, with a trusted colleague, conduct a peer review about what more positive strategies could be used to deal with similar situations.

Date_____
Situation_____
Your response_____
Good stress or bad_____
Action (how you dealt with your response)

_____
Evaluation_____

Symptom Awareness and Management

Multiple stress-buffering behaviors can be used to reduce the detrimental effects of stress. Stressor-induced changes in the hormonal and immune systems can be modulated by an individual's behavioral coping responses. These coping responses help to buffer what Cross et al. (2020) refer to as "micro stresses" that frequently occur during a usual workday. These may include spending time developing a particular interest, such as getting in shape to finally run that 5K, playing a once-favorite instrument, engaging in leisure activities with friends and family, cultivating a strong faith/belief system, enjoying a sense of humor, developing realistic expectations, reframing challenging events, frequently fitting in aerobic exercise that raises cardiac output, taking the time to reap the benefits of meditation, and considering the practice of yoga or meditation techniques for self-care and stress reduction.

Everyone needs to balance work and leisure in one's life. Leisure time and stress are inversely proportional. If you find that time for work is more than 60% of awake time or if self-care is less than 10% of awake time and you find that stress levels increase accordingly, consider your own work/self-time ratio. Changes should be made to relieve stress, such as decreasing the number of work hours or finding some time for leisure activities. Caffeine is a strong stimulant and, in itself, a stressor. Slowly reducing caffeine and alcohol intake should result in better sleep and more energy. Positive social support can offer validation, encouragement, or advice. By discussing situations with others, one can reduce stress. A great deal of stress comes from our own self-talk, which causes stress in two ways. First, behaviors result from them, such as placing work before rest or pleasure. Second, out-of-touch beliefs may also conflict with those of other people, as may happen with colleagues and patients from different cultures. Articulating one's thoughts and finding common ground will help reduce anger and stress. Humor is a great stress reducer and laughter a great tension reducer. Other activities may include self-reflection in the form of guided imagery, journaling, or debriefing with a valued mentor or trusted peer. One could invest in the services of a life coach, a professional who teaches new skills such as learning to communicate well embedded within cultural, systemic, and contextual awareness (Rindone, 2021). Life coaches also recommend strategies to fix gaps in the leader's knowledge, such as reading a recommended article, attending a particular networking meeting, or even making a professional introduction that may launch a new career direction. Another valuable approach to self-care is taking the time to reconnect with lifelong career mentors, very important when we consider that we, as well as the teams we lead, are well worth it.

EXERCISE 5.3 According to Healthdirect, an Australian governmental health website, relaxation is a state that promotes well-being and, with it, the ability to manage one's own life in the best way possible (Healthdirect, 2021). While relaxation might be a difficult goal to achieve, its many benefits make it a desirable activity to learn how to do. For example, the following systematic relaxation technique can be used in the middle of a working day, the last thing at night, or at any time you feel tense or anxious. Review the information and strategies at the Atlantic Health System website, originally created to help the community during the COVID-19 pandemic. It has broad implications for sustaining mental health: *https://www.atlantichealth.org/about-us/ stay-connected/news/content-central/2020/covid-19- coronavirus/reduce-covid-19-anxiety.html*

Social Support

Social support in the form of positive work relationships, as well as nurturing family and friends, is an important way to buffer the negative effects of a stressful work environment. Although friendships may be formed with colleagues, the workload and shifting of staff from one unit to another sometimes make it difficult to establish and maintain close relationships with peers. For many people at work, the time spent with their managers and coworkers represents one of the strongest sources of community in their lives. The Gallup Organization created the Q-12 survey question: *I have a best friend at work.* Therefore, strong friendships with coworkers who will help people get through rough spots positively correlates with employee retention, customer metrics, productivity, and profitability (Abel HR, 2020). Leaders can provide regular recognition feedback through personal notes that are mailed to their team members' homes; annual Nurses' Week celebrations; or participation in the DAISY Foundation, a not-for-profit organization that formally recognizes the extraordinary contributions

of nurses (*http://daisyfoundation.org*). All of these approaches shape the organization's culture in a positive way that patients, families, and nurses value.

Early career nurses in their first positions, those who find themselves in an unfamiliar geographic area, or nurses who switch employers after a long tenure at another setting will want to be part of a collegial work group that furnishes emotional support and a sense of belonging to an endeavor that is greater than themselves. Too often, nurses overlook the benefits of active membership in their professional or specialty associations. Connections established at the beginning of one's career will offer the nurse an unending lifelong source of enthusiastic colleagues who are as passionate about their individual professional careers as they are about serving their profession. Opportunities to become active members help nurses discover and refine brand-new leadership skills in a warm, comfortable setting. Ongoing mentorship by seasoned nursing leaders from academia, private practice, and the ambulatory sectors is often free for the taking and adds dimension and a valuable perspective to nurses at every level. Such ongoing mentoring and coaching efforts may help nurses cope with workplace demands that seem to exceed their capabilities.

Resolution of stress in its early stages can be accomplished through a variety of techniques. Nurses must be able to reach a balance of caring for others and caring for self. Box 5.2 summarizes physical, mental, and emotional and spiritual strategies. When stress rises to unacceptable or even dangerous levels, colleagues can be supportive and perhaps even point out the stress level or recommend appropriate help (Fig. 5.2).

EXERCISE 5.4 Using the items in Box 5.2, identify what strategies you most commonly use. Then, find at least one strategy you never or rarely use and consider what prevents you from using that strategy more effectively.

Peers and followers can be supportive and help reduce stress by assisting with problem solving and presenting different perspectives. This is not "venting," which is pointless gossip, complaining or "trashing" one's job, work colleagues, or supervisor. Instead, being with supportive family and friends can provide an affirming, loving perspective and a much-needed respite

BOX 5.2   Stress-Management Strategies

Physical
- Accept physical limitations.
- Modify nutrition: moderate carbohydrate, moderate protein, high in fruits and vegetables, low caffeine, low sugar.
- Exercise: participate in an enjoyable activity five times a week for 30 minutes per session.
- Make your physical health a priority.
- Nurture yourself by taking time for breaks and lunch.
- Sleep: get enough in quantity and quality.

Mental
- Learn to say "no!"
- Use cognitive restructuring and self-talk.
- Use imagery.
- Develop hobbies or activities.
- Plan vacations and take them!
- Learn about the system and how problems are handled.
- Learn communication, conflict resolution, and time-management skills.
- Take continuing education courses.

Emotional/Spiritual
- Relax: use meditation, massage, yoga, or biofeedback.
- Seek solace in prayer.
- Seek professional counseling.
- Participate in support groups.
- Participate in networking.
- Communicate feelings.
- Identify and acquire a mentor.
- Ask for feedback and clarification.

Best Practices
- Remember the principle of placing oxygen on yourself first, always!
- Prioritize and regularly practice the art of self-compassion.
- Learn how to become an advocate for workplace safety and for a healthy work environment for you and for your colleagues.

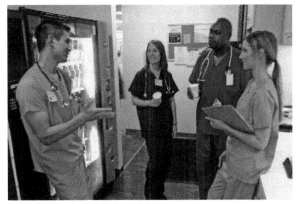

Fig. 5.2 Peers and followers can be supportive and help reduce stress.

from stress in the form of regular touchpoints, such as phone calls, emails, and texts as well as celebrations around birthdays, graduations, and seasonal holidays. We know that social isolation increases stress. When nurses find themselves in a never-ending cycle of work, sleep, school, and conflicting calendars with escalating pressures at home, relief must be actively sought. True social support allows us to relax, be playful, have fun, laugh, give a relief valve to emotions, and promote the enjoyment of life to the fullest.

Counseling

Persistent unpleasant feelings, problem behavior, helplessness, and withdrawal during prolonged stress may suggest the need for assistance from a mental health professional. Examples of problem behaviors include tearfulness or angry outbursts over seemingly minor incidents, traffic violations, major or subtle changes in eating and/or sleeping patterns, frequent unwillingness or a lack of desire to go to work, chronic complaining and negativity, passive-aggressive behaviors, and, unfortunately, reliance on alcohol and other substances that may veer into abuse territory. In such cases, the aforementioned coping strategies afford only temporary relief. Nurses with this level of distress often feel so overwhelmed or paralyzed that they believe that they simply cannot go on living this way. In these stressful situations, individuals may feel helpless and not see any way out. At this point, we may require professional assistance from an advanced practice psychiatric nurse, clinical psychologist, psychiatrist, licensed clinical social worker, spiritual director/counselor, clergy, or another mental health professional. Assistant nurse managers, nurse managers, and nursing supervisors often have the task of addressing and referring nurses to seek help for themselves before the stress escalates to a state of personal, family, or organizational crisis.

In some organizations, leaders may refer their peers, staff, or themselves to Employee Assistance Programs (EAPs). EAPs are a source of free, voluntary, confidential, short-term professional counseling and provide other services for employees via in-house staff or through a contract with an external mental health agency. This type of counseling can be effective because the counselors are usually already well aware of organizational issues and stressors in the workplace. Some nurses may put off getting help because of confidentiality concerns related to employer-recommended or employer-provided counseling services. However, mental health professionals are bound by their professional standards of confidentiality.

Those who seek counseling outside of the workplace may be guided in their selection of mental health professionals by a personal provider (physician or nurse practitioner), a knowledgeable colleague in the human resources department, or the most recent edition of their health insurance referral website. A phone call to the state nurses' association and an inquiry for lists of advanced practice registered nurses in adult psychiatric–mental health practice in your region will often yield significant results. When the problem underlying the distress is ethical or moral, a trained pastoral counselor or spiritual director may be very helpful. Some clergy and mental health professionals are certified in pastoral care or have earned a degree in another discipline such as psychology or spiritual direction counseling. Referrals can be obtained from hospital pastoral care departments or places of worship that affiliate with regional centers where certified counselors are available. When private counseling is being arranged, the health insurance contract should be checked to determine mental health benefits and the payment limitations and types of providers eligible for reimbursement.

Responsibilities of Leaders

These are uncertain times, an era marked by uncommon workplace pressures, fears about the future viability of the nation's healthcare infrastructure, and extreme political turbulence. Even at a time when the hospital industry is facing historic volatility, as non-profits and large for-profit chains struggle to maintain profitability and, in many cases, viability, nurse leaders must navigate and promote a healthy workplace. Especially in times that are less than optimal, the leader's singularly important role is to create vision and lead with clarity (Weston,

2020). Though it is not necessarily a new responsibility for leaders, high-focus coordination, deft orchestration with human resources, alignment with administrative colleagues, and support from the boards of trustees are all dependent on relationships that have not yet been fully engaged in the healthcare industry (Edmonson & Marshall, 2021). In order to achieve even baseline goals in staffing metrics, for example, or to address practice environment improvements, such as when unit budgets include enough time for staff to attend council meetings and seek out off-unit educational programs or even to obtain the consulting services of an external organizational expert, the support of fellow executive leadership is crucial. Candidates for advertised positions in organizations where a recent upheaval has occurred or when a previously award-winning facility is suddenly turning over numerous senior staff members or in danger of losing significant recognition, such as when Magnet© status is jeopardized or eroding Leapfrog Hospital Safety Results, or when there is a distinct lack of visibility of the top-most corporate executives in the ambulatory, outpatient, or inpatient areas, conducting a thorough assessment amid such alarming and unfruitful trends would be wise. This is a prime opportunity to network with your professional association colleagues in order to gather reputational information before accepting a job offer in settings that ought to set off alarm bells to prospective candidates.

The work of creating and sustaining a healthy work environment is everyone's responsibility (Dimino et al., 2020). However, leaders are in a distinct position to set the tone for the organization and serve as gatekeepers because they set the stage and provide crucial coaching through the implementation phase of change (Nursing CE, 2021). Nurse leaders who are well prepared for their roles and are highly supportive to staff promote autonomy, control of practice, organizational support, collegial interaction, affiliation, conflict management, and a sense of belonging that are all so very important (Reinhardt et al., 2020). Chief nursing officers, along with their senior teams, strategize and foster innovations in the hospital, ambulatory care, and home health settings that advance a healthy work environment to the next level of success. As Raso et al. (2020) observed, if leaders are the anchor for a healthy work environment, it follows that authentic nurse leadership behaviors serve as its cornerstone.

On the other hand, leaders who fail to do their part to strengthen the professional work environment—and are either unempowered, unsupported, or otherwise uninvolved in taking their team on a quality wellness journey—miss prime opportunities for advancement of health and well-being in themselves and others. Instead of writing off such leaders, Pinekenstein and Pawlak (2020) prescribe a new model, CALM©, a customized advanced leader model for enhancing career and well-being based on professional organizational recommendations for strategic development. Contained within the CALM© model are strategies to help the leader to engage in a comprehensive self-assessment; envision future roles; evaluate the education and experience necessary to achieve one's career goals; set up strategic networking, mentoring and coaching, with defined leadership opportunities; institute foundational elements of self-care; and, finally, construct a solid gap analysis and customized plan. Key to the CALM© model is knowledge of yourself, without which an upward career trajectory is either not sustainable or not possible.

We know that transformational leaders positively influence healthy workplace behaviors by focusing in on the key concepts that are linked to nurse retention, such as affiliation, a sense of belonging, and authentic support of staff (Reinhardt et al., 2020), all the while being tuned in to threats to a positive environment. This may include the fear of harm while working in an unsafe work area, when leaders may unrealistically expect their staff to continue to be productive and care for patients' needs. Especially as it concerns horizontal violence, leaders must strongly support policies, education, and zero tolerance to ensure that the culture of safety in a high reliability environment embraces nurses as equally as it includes patients and their families (Flannery, 2020). Leaders who are attuned to the importance of budget and finance likewise evaluate innovative staffing models for their ability to promote a healthy work environment by anticipating rather than reacting to workforce needs (Kester et al., 2019). Openness to new ways of solving the problems of new-nurse retention, where simulation learning and gaming may create innovative methods to achieve practice readiness and improve patient outcomes, is a distinctive leadership trait (Sitterding et al., 2019).

Responsibilities of Managers

Despite the best intentions of even the most diligent nurse manager, one significant potential minefield in leadership behaviors is the nurse manager's inability to astutely assess the work environment. Cassidy (2020) found that a gap exists between how nurse managers rate their work environment and what the frontline clinical staff believe about what constitutes a healthy work environment. In order to bridge the two, it is recommended that nurse managers communicate and educate about issues as they arise, team up with their direct staff to devise solutions, and, most importantly, empower everyone in their unit, work area, or department to collaborate and innovate for a more positive future. As a manager, you need to establish a work culture, with the help of trusted mentorship, that invites dialogue about the culture for which everyone is ultimately responsible. In addition, managers should examine their own behavior as a source of their staffs' stress via peer review, coaching, and regularly scheduled leadership rounds. Nurse managers and supervisors can and must continue to articulate clinical and workplace issues as they work to control existing environmental stressors on their own units. Above all, their job is to mitigate stress so that frontline staff can deliver the highest-quality care. Imagine if an airplane pilot had to incorporate and manage the personal stress of every passenger on her plane that day? Delivering first-rate, high-quality care in a complex environment, even as the world recovers from COVID-19 and prepares itself for future global pandemics, places unprecedented stress upon nurses—more than any other professional group (Mitchell et al., 2020). Nurse leaders have the opportunity to develop their competencies in how they access and appraise the best available scientific evidence in management decision-making, especially in light of an uncertain future (Majers & Warshawsky, 2020).

Since social support and counseling can alter how stressors are perceived, a growing body of research is demonstrating how online mental health programs are effective in improving managers' confidence and strengthening workplace practices around mental health (Gayed et al., 2019). Wellness champions, a role recently initiated to improve colleagues' health and well-being, is only one strategy toward defining healthy workplaces, yet their introduction is a valuable asset (Mitchell et al., 2020). Such coaches may bring in awareness of another key component that has been frequently overlooked, such as sleep and its relationship to a healthy workforce. Employer-sponsored efforts to improve sleep hygiene and promote healthier habits have been connected to self-reported improvements in sleep duration and quality and fewer self-reported sleepiness complaints (Redeker et al., 2019). Due to the relationship between satisfactory sleep and subjective reports of stress among female healthcare professionals, evaluating cortisol levels and regularly examining shift work patterns may be needed to promote health, productivity, and workplace safety (Bani-Issa et al., 2020).

Effective leadership that is shared and time management that supports involvement at the level of direct care nurse in the unit can modify or even remove stressors altogether. Historically, nurses have had limited formal authority as individuals in most hierarchical organizations. In a survey of millennial nurses, a study by Faller and Gogek (2019) found that there is a higher emphasis than ever before on the quality of leadership. Shared governance, defined by Tim Porter-O'Grady when he first described the pioneer efforts of Vanderbilt University Medical Center in the 1980s, is a professional practice model founded on the cornerstone principles of partnership, equity, accountability, and ownership (Porter-O'Grady, 2019). Shared governance is highly dependent on effective leaders who work collaboratively with active and vocal participation by staff. Chief nursing executives and the managerial and administrative groups in which they participate must continually advocate for nursing resources and influence policy and resource allocation. Yet, a strong connection between nursing leadership and the voices of the frontline clinical teams must exist to bring needed resources and support and to link all efforts directly to the point of care, to the nurses themselves, and ultimately to patients and their families embedded within the communities we serve.

In some cases, a controlling or autocratic style of management is appropriate, such as in emergency or disaster situations and when working with a large percentage of new and inexperienced team members. For the most part, however, professional nurses need, want, and deserve the latitude to direct their activities within their sphere of competence. "Letting go" of autocratic power and learning more about the power in delegating important functions to team members means that the nurse leader trusts the personal integrity and professional competence of the entire team. It does not mean abdicating accountability for achieving accepted standards of patient care and agreed-upon outcomes. Such an attitude offers ample opportunity to provide invaluable coaching that has the potential to teach, motivate, and guide others toward reaching their full potential.

Assistance with problem solving is another way to reduce environmental stressors. Nurse leaders may provide technical advice, refer staff to appropriate resources, or mediate conflicts. Often, nurse leaders enable staff to meet the demands of their work more independently by providing time for continuing education and preparation for national board certification. Such nurse leaders make it possible for frontline staff to attend internal and external professional meetings to enhance their clinical competence and learn new ways to exert control over their own workplace.

A major way in which nurse leaders can reduce stress is to be supportive of staff. Support is not equated with being a friend or buddy; rather, it is helping one's peers accomplish good care, develop professionally, and feel valued personally. Leaders can ensure that the expected workload is in line with the nurses' capabilities and resources. They can work to ensure meaningfulness, stimulation, and opportunities for nurses to use their skills.

Nurses' roles and responsibilities need to be clearly and publicly defined. Work schedules should be posted as far in advance as possible and should be compatible with what is known about patient safety and respect for their team members' private lives and educational schedules. Encouraging innovation and experimentation, as in self-scheduling, for example, can motivate staff and give them a sense of greater control over their environment. Affirming a good idea, finding resources for further study, or implementing a promising new procedure or proposal by a direct care nurse are all characteristic of supportive leadership. Being supportive even when things are not necessarily going well is also possible. For example, when staff members struggle with their methods of coping with overwork and other stressors, supportive leadership behaviors include helping staff members recognize the need to avoid passive coping strategies that fuel helplessness and lower the standards of care through active, engaged coaching.

Nurse leaders must be sensitive to the distress of the nursing staff and acknowledge it without themselves becoming therapists or counselors, which would present a role conflict. Support may involve raising the staff's knowledge of counseling resources and truly getting to know each and every staff member. The Literature Perspective addresses an example of the point during the pandemic.

Nurse managers also must be careful to avoid diagnostic labels and to maintain strict confidentiality. This is difficult to do, for example, when a nurse's practice is impaired by alcohol or drug use. Sometimes, the staff on the entire unit and even staff on other units may already be aware of the impairment. When distress relates to the personal life of staff, managers should focus on the effect of such situations on workplace performance and ask for outside assistance, if necessary, to help team members work through the events. The individual who has produced the stress can then hopefully be welcomed back to the job after recovery in a goal-directed program designed to aid the person in appropriate coping approaches.

In addition, leaders can enhance the workplace by recognizing and dealing effectively with their own stressors. Maintaining a sense of perspective as well as a sense of humor is important. Some stressors, in fact, can be minimized by posing three questions:

1. Is this event or situation important? Stressors are not all equally significant. Do not waste energy on minor stressors.
2. Does this stressor affect me or my unit? Although some situations that produce distress are institution-wide and need group action, others target specific units or activities. Do not borrow stressors from another unit. Individuals can "cross-pollinate" stressors by spreading gossip about the misfortunes or negative perceptions of other units' team members.
3. Can I change this situation? If not, then find a way to cope with it or, if the situation is intolerable, make plans to change positions or employers. This decision may require continuing the journey to lifelong knowledge, such as gaining additional skills that may produce long-term career benefits.

Keeping stressful situations in perspective can enable nurses to conserve their energies to cope with those stressful situations that are truly important, that are within their domain, or that can be changed or modified.

Goal Setting

The first steps in stress management are goal setting and developing a plan to reach the goals. Set goals that are reasonable and achievable. Do not expect to reach long-term goals overnight—*long-term* means just that. Give yourself time to meet the goals. Determine many short-term goals to reach the long-term goal, giving yourself a frequent sense of goal achievement.

LITERATURE PERSPECTIVE

Resource: Dimino, K., Learmonth, A. E., & Fajardo, C.C. (2021). Nurse managers leading the way: Reenvisioning stress to maintain healthy work environments. *Critical Care Nurse, 41*(5), 52–58.

The authors note that even without considering the extraordinary burden placed on nurses throughout the world by the COVID-19 pandemic, numerous challenges within the "normal" workplace are ever present—such as unrelenting stress, understaffing, incivility, and perceived lack of support. Now that COVID-19 has brought with it additional issues—such as shrinking staff levels, fear of contagion, burnout, and more—nurse managers must expand their own skills and abilities to care for their staff and learn to embody the AACN Standards for Establishing and Sustaining Healthy Work Environments. Because COVID-19 has been such a severe crisis, it is more than appropriate that nurses must be recognized as having performed disaster nursing during a major public health emergency. Nurse managers and nurses themselves need finely tuned tools, therefore, to be able to assess and respond to the extreme challenges of the workplace by learning more about their own stress responses during this unprecedented time in our collective consciousness. Elements of emotional intelligence such as self-awareness, self-regulation, motivation, empathy, and social skills, when maximized to their full potential, are aligned with key actions that truly make a difference to staff. Finally, leaders are encouraged to consistently provide messaging to staff that they are valued, that the leaders are there for them, and that what is important to staff are the same things that matter to their leaders—also moving forward in a strong, decisive, and stable manner.

Implications for Practice

Nurse managers have the responsibility and the opportunity to help their staff heal and thrive from the stressors of work in everyday professional nursing as well as during the COVID-19 pandemic and beyond. Utilizing resources and reimagining them so that they are incorporated into burnout mitigation strategies are critical keys to staff and manager wellness.

Give yourself flexibility. If the path you chose last year is no longer appropriate, change it. Write your goals, date the entry, keep it handy, and refer to it often to give yourself a progress report. Very often, goals are an important discussion point of the annual performance evaluation process. The time for reviewing goals ought not to be the period immediately preceding this year's discussion. Unfortunately, too often this is the case. Successful people will prefer to mutually set goals frequently throughout the year and address, encourage, and recognize progress toward achievement during monthly meetings and at specific hallmark times

---

EXERCISE 5.5 Create a goal statement related to some competency you wish to achieve or improve in this quarter. Using a Gantt chart approach, designate timelines and activities to meet this goal. Print the chart and enter it in your phone to track your progress.

Managing Information and Clutter

The first step in managing information is to assess the source. Once you have identified the sources of your particular stressors, such as clutter, you will have a better idea of how to deal with the information. Track incoming information for a few days. Patterns will begin to emerge and will give clues as to how to deal with it. You can generally predict that, using the Pareto principle, 80% of your incoming data comes from approximately 20% of your sources, and that 80% of useful information comes from 20% of information received (Audate, 2021) (see the Theory Box on p. 10). By developing information-receiving skills, you can quickly interpret the data and convert them to useful information, discarding unneeded data. Initially, you should delete that which is useless, and next, eliminate redundancies wherever possible. Label files and folders to which e-mail messages can be directed. Frequently delete emails or encourage administrative leaders to endorse systems that automatically archive older messages. Next, monitor the information flow and decide what to do with incoming data. Find and focus on the most important pieces, and then quickly narrow down the specific details you need. Identify resources that are most helpful and have them

readily available. Be able to build the big picture from the masses of data you receive. Finally, recognize when you have enough information to act.

Once you have mastered the receiving end of information, concentrate on your own information-sending skills. Remember, your information is simply another person's data! Try to keep your outflow short; make it a synthesis of the information. If your email message is more than a few sentences in length, your message may warrant a phone call or meeting instead. Finally, select the most appropriate mode of communication for your message from the technology available. You may be sending your information in written (memo or report) or verbal (face-to-face or presentation) form or via telephone, webinar or Zoom, voice mail, email, text, Twitter, or sanctioned forums such as Workplace from Facebook. Remember, the most important skill is to know when you have said enough.

Delegating

Delegation is a critical component of self-management for all frontline staff, nurse managers, and care managers. Appropriate delegation not only increases time efficiency but also serves as a means of reducing stress, as it promotes and prioritizes self-care. Delegation is discussed in depth in Chapter 14; and it is also appropriate to discuss briefly as a time-management strategy and as a healthy work behavior. Delegation works only when the delegator trusts the delegatee to accomplish the task and to report findings back to the delegator. The delegator wastes time when checking and redoing everything someone else has done. Delegation requires empowerment of the delegatee to accomplish the task. If the nurse does not delegate appropriately, with clear expectations that the task is an opportunity for growth, the delegatee will constantly be asking for assistance or direction. If the nurse does not understand delegation and does not use it appropriately, it can be a major source of stress as the nurse assumes accountability and responsibility for care administered by others.

Management of Time

A very close relationship exists between stress management, a healthy work environment, and time management. Time management is one method of stress prevention and reduction. Stress can decrease productivity and lead to poor use of time. Time management can be considered a preventive action to help reduce the elements of stress in a nurse's life.

Everyone has two choices when managing time: organize or "go with the flow." Everyone has only 24 hours in every day, and it is clear that some people make better use of time than others do. *How* people use time makes some people more successful than others. The effective use of time-management skills thus becomes an even more important tool to achieve personal and professional goals. Time management is the appropriate use of tools, techniques, and principles to control time spent on low-priority needs and to ensure that time is invested in activities leading toward achieving high-priority goals.

As the nurse's role in care management becomes more complex, the need for organizational tools increases. Tracking the care of groups of patients, either as a member of a care team or in a leadership capacity, can be overwhelming. Each nurse must devise a method for tracking care and organizing time as well as delegating and monitoring care provided by others. Although some nurses still depend on a physical paper shift flowsheet, many more now have the benefit of electronic tracking systems. Handheld smartphones or other devices provided by your organization and bar-code scanners for medication administration are great methods to track information plus increase patient safety and efficiency. The issue of patient confidentiality and organizational privacy cannot be overemphasized when entering data into any device. Check with your organization's privacy officer and policies to verify that you are on the right side of managing paper and electronic information. The unifying theme is that each activity undertaken should lead to goal attainment and that goal should be the number one priority at that time.

In terms of time management as an act of self-compassion, setting goals and actively working to reduce time stealers means you will have the extra time to accomplish them. Table 5.1 presents a classification scheme for time-management techniques. Table 5.2 provides ways to apply time-management strategies to practice.

TABLE 5.1 Classification of Time-Management Techniques

Technique	Purpose	Actions
Organization	Promotes efficiency and productivity	Organize and systematize things, tasks, and people. Use basic time-management skills.
Keep focused on goals	Focuses on goal achievement	Assemble a prioritized "to do" list daily, based on goals.
Tool usage	Uses the right tool for planning and preparation	Use tools such as a smartphone.
Time-management plan	Helps refocus, gain control, and use information	Develop a personal time-management plan appropriately.

TABLE 5.2 Time-Management Applications to Practice

Key Idea	Definition	Application to Practice
Losing track of time	Absorption in one aspect of a task, or distractions that prevent focus on a task, preventing successful resolution in a time-effective manner	Concentrate on results. Identify common "time stealers" and guard against them. Do not get caught up with technology, such as answering emails or responding to instant message alerts. Minimize distractions. Use an alarm or stopwatch feature on your smartphone or other device. Take a class on time management.

TABLE 5.2   Time-Management Applications to Practice—cont'd

Key Idea	Definition	Application to Practice
Doing too much	Competing priorities that vie for attention	Reduce the number of important projects that are due at the same time. Be realistic and limit major commitments. Give each major activity your undivided attention. Avoid multitasking whenever possible! Make a daily "to do" list and tick the items off as each is accomplished. Engage with a supervisor or mentor for advice/guidance on which project needs the most attention.
Learning to say "no" or "not now, please"	Politely declining requests for an additional project or assignment	Agreeing to tasks that are not in alignment with your individual personal/professional priorities may translate into frustration and resentment. Consider whether this task may be easily delegated to another individual. Discuss the request in detail so you may better understand its nature: Is it in alignment with the organization's overall goals or your family's primary needs at this time? Or is it someone else's "emergency" who needs a favor?
Procrastination	Putting off important tasks because they may not be enjoyable or involve a level of difficulty	Identify the reason for procrastination. Develop a PERT (Program Evaluation and Review Technique) chart or a Gantt chart (see Table 5.3) to help parse out complex assignments. Make that specific task your number one priority for the next opportunity. Select either the least attractive component or the easiest; tackle that part first. Reward yourself after you complete the task.
Complaining/ whining	Expressing dissatisfaction or annoyance	Stop and ask yourself, "What would the ideal resolution be?" and then take the risk to act on it. Discuss the scenario with a trusted friend/coworker/mentor or supervisor. Bring potential solutions so that you can move beyond complaining to effective problem solving. Spend time speaking with the parties involved or those with the power to improve the overall situation. Write yourself a letter describing the situation as well as options for correction. Look for solutions that are very simple or "outside the box" for you.
Perfectionism	The tendency to never completely finish a project or assignment because it is not yet acceptable	Continue to do your best. Find and share feedback with others who have similar assignments or projects or are in situations like yours. Once you receive feedback on your project, move quickly to incorporate it into your final submission and move on to the next assignment.
Interruptions	Avoidable or unavoidable occurrences that distract from one's ability to complete a prioritized task	Set workplace rules to limit lengthy emails and other distractions (see Box 5.3). Mentally, dive right back into the immediate task at hand.
Information overload	Proliferation of data that occurs too quickly to be able to interpret the information in an effective manner	Form or join study groups or other forms of knowledge communities. Learn to appreciate podcasts, email capsules of weekly healthcare news, or other professional organizations' and specialty associations' online news summaries.

TABLE 5.3   Sample Gantt Chart

Task	Accountability	Jan	Feb	Mar	Apr	May	June
1. Conduct literature search	Unit clinical nurse specialist	———————→					
2. Hold nursing practice committee meeting to review material	Chair, nursing practice committee		X				
3. Create report for the medical staff	Chair, nursing practice committee			————————————————→			
4. Disseminate findings to nursing and medical staff	Chair, nursing practice committee					——————————————————→	

BOX 5.3   Tips to Prevent Interruptions and Work More Effectively

- Ask people to put their comments in writing in an email—do not let them catch you "on the run." On this line of thinking, do not use others as you would a Post-it® note!
- Let the office or unit secretary know what information you need immediately.
- Conduct some private time in a separate room to keep from being interrupted.
- Be comfortable saying "no" and "not yet."
- When involved in a long procedure or home visit, ask someone else to cover your other responsibilities to increase your focus.
- Break projects into small, manageable pieces.
- Get yourself organized.
- Minimize interruptions—for example, allow voicemail to pick up the phone, shut the door.
- Keep your work surface clear. Have available only those documents needed for the task at hand.
- Plan where things should go on your desk or desktop, laptop, and smartphone.
- Create a "to do" folder or notebook.
- Use a "to be filed" folder for any papers—these should all be phased out in favor of an electronic storage system.
- Schedule time to work your way through the folders.
- Keep your manager informed of your goals and ask for input for additional insight.
- Plan to accomplish high-priority or difficult tasks early in the day.
- Develop a plan for the day and stick to it. Remember to schedule in some time for interruptions.
- Schedule time to meet regularly throughout the shift with staff members for whom you are responsible. Likewise, make sure you meet with the leader to whom you report.
- Make an effort to round with the night and weekend teams. Conduct early morning breakfasts so that night staff can meet with you away from the unit if possible.
- Recognize that crises and interruptions are part of the position.
- Be cognizant of your personal time-wasting habits and try to avoid them.

Setting Priorities as a Step in Time Management

Once goals are known, priorities are set. However, they may shift throughout a given period in terms of goal attainment. For example, working on a budget may take precedence at certain times of the year, whereas new staff orientation to a brand-new electronic medical record system is a higher priority at other times. Knowing what your goals and priorities are helps shape the "to do" list. On a nursing unit or as you work in a community setting, you must know your personal goals and current priorities. How you organize work may depend on geographic considerations, patient acuity, or some other schema.

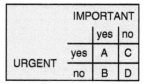

Fig. 5.3 Classification of priorities.

A particular strategy to assist in prioritization suggests that people generally focus on those things that are important and urgent. Clarity is enhanced about priorities by placing the elements of importance and urgency in a grid (Fig. 5.3) or by using the Covey Matrix (Mueller, 2015).

Typically, we tend to focus on those items in cell A because they are both important and urgent and, therefore, command our attention. Making shift assignments is an A task: it is both important to the work to be accomplished and commonly urgent because a time frame is specified during which data about patients and qualifications of staff can be matched. Conversely, if something is neither important nor urgent (cell D), it may be considered a waste of time, at least in terms of personal goals. An example of a D activity might be reading "junk" email or attention-grabbing department store or vacation advertisements. Even if something is urgent but not important (cell C), it contributes minimally to productivity and goal achievement. An example of a C activity might be responding to a memo that has a specific timeline but is not important to goal attainment. The real key to setting priorities is to attend to the B tasks, those that are important but not urgent. Examples of B activities are reviewing the organization's strategic plan or participating on organizational committees.

Organization

A number of simple routines for organization can save many minutes over a day and enhance your efficiency. Keeping a workspace neat or arranging things in an orderly fashion may be a powerful time-management tool and contribute to a healthy workplace. Rather than a system of "pile management," use "file management." Make yourself an organizational list. Although the traditional method of making lists is on physical paper, if you don't have a physical desk at work, you can use something else—a designated space, a tablet, a clipboard, or your phone. Consider how to translate this list into a non-desk format.

Determine your priority goals for the next day and have the materials ready to work on when you arrive. If you are fortunate to have the resources of a secretary or administrative assistant, even for very limited periods of the day, be sure to discuss with this individual how scheduling has the power to either maximize your day or sap your energy and strength.

Policies—Local, State, and National

The *Healthy Nurse, Healthy Nation*™ Grand Challenge (HNHN) campaign of the American Nurses Association, (ANA, 2021e; see *healthynursehealthynation.org*) is perhaps the best example of a strategic initiative designed to improve the health and well-being of nurses everywhere. A social movement, HNHN has as its goal to *transform the health of the nation by improving the health of the nation's 4 million registered nurses.* Five domains comprise the success of the model: activity, sleep, nutrition, quality of life, and safety. These domains are embedded in a web platform featuring resources and competitive walking and running events offering social connection to other nurses. You may go to your mobile platform's store and download the app for HNHN to keep motivated and achieve your own healthy targets for nutrition and exercise and contribute to a more positive workplace.

The leading nursing and healthcare organizations have also prioritized healthy work environments in position statements and policies. These include the American Association of Critical Care Nurses, the American Association of Colleges of Nursing, the International Council of Nurses, the American Hospital Association, and many others. Each has set definitions for what constitutes a healthy work environment and has created targets for realization of the associated goals. Of note, The *Healthy People 2030* initiative, launched by the U.S. federal government in 1979, has defined goals as well as benchmarks that aim to improve health and well-being in all communities of the United States (health.gov/healthypeople). Included within its program objectives are health conditions, health behaviors, populations, settings and systems, and social determinants of health. A review of the content in the *Workplace* section of the website prioritizes the importance of health promotion initiatives to address exposure to unhealthy toxins and other stressful immediate and long-term trauma associated with the COVID-19 pandemic, as well as on-the-job injuries, conflict, and violence suffered while at work.

Recent significant collaboration among key organizations includes a national commission to address racism in nursing (see https://www.nursingworld.org/practice-policy/workforce/clinical-practice-material/national-commission-to-address-racism-in-nursing/). Other examples, designed to raise awareness and create coalitions among nursing organizations, include the Organization of Nurse Executives of NJ and the Association of Women's Health, Obstetric and Neonatal Nurses. Membership in specialty and professional organizations has never been more urgent; your dues go directly to advocacy for health in our nation's nurses, our workplaces, and the communities in which we work and live.

Several state nurses associations have proactively created position papers and reports, especially when legislative efforts have been unsuccessful, to address challenging issues. Some of those issues relate to staffing, reporting unsafe conditions, reporting acts of incivility, and ways to document acuity levels of patients.

Massachusetts is one example of how a state hospital association's leaders created a program to increase hospital-to-hospital sharing of best practices and other safety improvement initiatives that may be used as a guidebook for other organizations and systems at the state and local level (Noga et al., 2021). Legislative examples include safe patient handling (Association of Occupational Health Professionals in Healthcare, 2020), where programs are mandated in acute, long-term, and ambulatory healthcare settings in states across the country. Another example is the national effort by the American Association of periOperative Nursing (AORN) to prevent staff exposure to surgical smoke in their Go Clear Award Program (see https://www.aorn.org/goclear). A well-orchestrated grassroots approach by the AORN, through partnership with state nurses' associations of the ANA, has led to numerous states enacting legislation that is designed to promote staff safety through the use of evacuation devices (Liu et al., 2019; AORN, 2021). Other examples include whistleblower protection and sexual harassment laws, plus protection from violence in the workplace. As policy varies from state to state, you need to become familiar with your own region and what you can do to promote a climate of advocacy for nurses' right to a safe and healthy environment.

CONCLUSION

A healthy workplace and healthy workforce are important concepts that drive the health and safety of an organization with outreach into the surrounding communities and society at large. To achieve a balance in life, minimize stressors, and achieve the best life, nurses must learn to create a lifestyle of self-compassion and contribute to a safe environment. Stressors and coping strategies need to be learned, prioritized, and used. By continuously developing innovative techniques, nurses can gain a sense of control to become far better nurses, and leaders, in the process.

THE SOLUTION

I've been in my role for four years now and I felt that it took me three years to truly feel in control and to be able to "project manage" all my responsibilities. At this point, I'm now able to build my own team, I hired a new psych manager, created an almost entirely new off-shift team—over 50% of that group had turned over due to advanced leadership opportunities for them. So, I'm happy that's been so successful because I've built a bond and established a great rapport with them, leaving me with more confidence that responsibilities—that I used to do entirely myself—are now in the hands of competent individuals.

As for me, there was a definite turning point. At a meeting of a committee I chair, the CLABSI and CAUTI reduction initiative groups, I asked for volunteers to take on components of our workplan. There was complete silence; nobody spoke up. In the silence of the room that day, I found myself announcing to the group that my new resolution was to become better at delegating—and this is what needed to happen. Immediately, everyone stepped up to ask why I hadn't asked them before. I used the opportunity to meet afterwards as a group in order to completely validate everyone's assessment of their strengths, interests, and schedules to take on additional responsibilities. The entire meeting, I can definitely say, was huge—I feel that the discussion actually fostered their professional growth as much as my own.

I've had access to graduate education and great leadership training right here at Atlantic Health System. Yet, it was my own personal discovery when I realized that I had amazing resources right here, yet I had never accessed them before. I knew I had to throw up a white flag. They were definitely there the whole time. From that experience, I learned how to intentionally prioritize. I know as nurses we are all so guilty of not prioritizing, and then the days overpower us. I constantly tell myself and others, "stop being the helper/do-er," and take accountability for planning for the day. Another thing is that I share an office with a "Millennial" and she writes in my calendar to schedule private time for myself. As it turns out, this actually helps me a lot—it helps to prioritize and focus so I'm more organized and less stressed out.

In the beginning, I along with my peers, treated emergencies such as COVID-19 exactly like a war. It demands high energy along with equally high exhaustion at an incredible pace, without a day off or even a break. I realized that nobody, not even me, can live that type of life for very long. As I am maturing more as a leader, I now realize I absolutely have to strategically plan my day to be effective—leaving room for focus time as well as the gym, time with family, or taking on something new altogether.

Would this be a suitable approach for you? Why?

Brandee Fetherman

REFLECTIONS

When you think about healthy behaviors in your personal life, how would you describe them? What impact does it have on your professional goals? How can you be more personally effective at becoming a healthier nurse? How can you help to make your own workplace healthier and more supportive of its team members?

BEST PRACTICE

Several studies referenced in this chapter identify unhealthy personal and work-related stressors we can all experience and how they affect us. Similarly, opportunities to understand the characteristics of poor work environments and their effect on our overall health are offered because they have shown effectiveness in raising awareness and promoting positive change. Nurses must stop all of these unhealthy practices and take on the role of being in charge of our own well-being and advocate that it has the same importance as patient well-being.

TIPS FOR SELF-MANAGEMENT

- Make your own health and that of your colleagues a priority and use strategies that keep yourself feeling cared for and in control.
- Think about and resolve to do at least one different healthy thing for yourself today and tomorrow.
- Make and keep personal physical and mental health appointments.
- Engage in online or in-person fitness or gym programs.
- Know your personal response to stress and self-evaluate (pulse check) frequently.
- Know what your high-priority goals are and use them to filter decisions.
- Refocus on your priorities whenever you begin to feel overwhelmed and stressed.
- Use organizational systems to declutter that meet your needs—the simpler, the better.
- Invoke a support structure in order to assess, manage, or remove unhealthy work characteristics.

REFERENCES

Abel, H. R. (2020). *In the news: friendships are an important component of workplace happiness, retention*. Retrieved from https://www.abelhr.com/in-the-news-friendships-are-an-important-component-of-workplace-happiness-retention.

Academy of Medical-Surgical Nurses (AMSN). (2021). *Unit Award—AMSN PRISM Award*. Retrieved from https://www.amsn.org/career-development/awards/unit-award-amsn-prism-awardr.

Adkins, A. (2020). *Millennials: The job-hopping generation*. Gallup Workplace: *Business Journal* https://www.gallup.com/workplace/231587/millennials-job-hopping-generation.aspx.

Advisory Board. (2020). *What's driving millennial and Gen Z nurses, according to a 1,250-nurse survey*. Daily Briefing. February 11, 2020. Retrieved from https://www.advisory.com/daily-briefing/2020/02/11/nurse-survey.

Aiken, L. H., Smith, H. L., & Lake, E. T. (1994). Lower Medicare mortality among a set of hospitals known for good nursing care. *Medical Care, 32*(8), 771–787. https://doi.org/10.1097/00005650-19940800-0002.

Aiken, L. H., Clarke, S. P., Sloane, D. M., Lake, E. T., & Cheney, T. (2008). Effects of hospital care environment on patient mortality and nurse outcomes. *Journal of Nursing Administration, 38*(5), 223–229.

American Association of Critical-Care Nurses. (2021). *Be a beacon of excellence for your community, hospital and patients*. Retrieved from https://www.aacn.org/nursing-excellence/beacon-awards.

American Nurses Association (ANA). (2021a). *Healthy work environment*. Retrieved from https://www.nursingworld.org/practice-policy/work-environment/.

American Nurses Association (ANA). (2021b). *The Nurses Bill of Rights FAQs*. https://www.nursingworld.org/practice-policy/work-environment/health-safety/bill-of-rights-faqs/.

American Nurses Association (ANA). (2021c). *Magnet® Recognition Program: About Magnet, Why Become Magnet?* Retrieved from https://www.nursingworld.org/organizational-programs/magnet/about-magnet/why-become-magnet/benefits/.

American Nurses Association (ANA). (2021d). *Magnet model—Creating a Magnet culture.* https://www.nursingworld.org/organizational-programs/magnet/magnet-model/.

American Nurses Association (ANA). (2021e). ANA Position Statement: Nursing Advocacy for LGBTQ+ Populations. https://www.nursingworld.org/practice-policy/nursing-excellence/official-position-statements/id/nursing-advocacy-for-lgbtq-populations/#:~:text=Statement%20of%20ANA%20Position,and%20acceptance%20of%20LGBTQ%2B%20populations.

American Nurses Association (ANA). (2021f). *What is the Healthy Nurse, Healthy Nation^TM Grand Challenge?* Retrieved from http://www.healthynursehealthynation.org.

Association of Occupational Health Professionals in Healthcare. (2020). Resource Guide/Beyond Getting Started. https://aohp.org/aohp/WORKTOOLS/PublicationsforYourPractice/BeyondGettingStarted.aspx.

American Association of periOperative Nursing. (2021). *Protect your team and patients from surgical smoke.* Retrieved from https://www.aorn.org/goclear.

Assaye, A. M., Wiechula, R., Schultz, T. J., & Feo, R. (2020). The impact of nurse staffing on patient and nurse workforce outcomes in acute care settings in low- and middle-income countries: A quantitative systematic review. *Joanna Briggs Institute Evidence Synthesis, 18*(0), 1–43. https://doi.org/10.1111/ijn.12812.

Audate, A. (2021). How the 80/20 rule can save your sanity in business. *Forbes.* https://www.forbes.com/sites/forbescoachescouncil/2021/11/22/how-the-8020-rule-can-save-your-sanity-in-business/?sh=46c2e7bc1e2f.

Baptiste, M. M. (2020). Workplace discrimination: An additional stressor for internationally educated nurses. *The Online Journal of Issues in Nursing.* Retrieved from http://ojin.nursingworld.org/MainMenuCategories/ANAMarketplace/ANAPeriodicals/OJIN/TableofContents/Vol-20-2015/No3-Sept-2015/Articles-Previous-Topics/Workplace-Discrimination-for-Internationally-Educated-Nurses.html?css=print.

Bani-Issa, W., Radwan, H., Al Marzooq, F., Al Awar, S., Al-Shujairi, A. M., Samsudin, A. R., Khasawneh, W., & Albluwi, N. (2020). Salivary cortisol, subjective stress and quality of sleep among female healthcare professionals. *Journal of Multidisciplinary Healthcare, 2020*(13), 125–140.

Berwick, D. M., Nolan, T. W., & Whittington, J. (2008). The Triple Aim: Care, health, and cost. *Health Affairs, 27*(3), 759–769.

Bodenheimer, T., & Sinsky, C. (2014). From Triple to Quadruple Aim: Care of the patient requires care of the provider. *Annals of Family Medicine, 12*(6), 573–575.

Botelho, M. J., & Lima, C. A. (2020). From cultural competence to cultural respect: A critical review of six models. *Journal of Nursing Education, 59*(6), 311–318. https://doi.org/10.3928/01484834-20200520-03.

Bowles, J. R., Batcheller, J., Adams, J. M., Zimmerman, D., & Pappas, S. (2019). Nursing's leadership role in advancing professional practice-work environments as part of the Quadruple Aim. *Nursing Administrative Quarterly, 43*(2), 157–163.

Bureau of Labor Statistics (BLS), U.S. Department of Labor. (2021). *Occupation snapshot, registered nurses, 2015–2019.* January, 2021. Retrieved from https://www.bls.gov/iif/oshwc/case/osn-registered-nurses-2015-19.htm.

Canas-Gonzalez, B., Fernandez-Nistal, A., Ramierez, J. M., & Martinez-Fernandez, V. (2020). Influence of stress and depression on the immune system in patients evaluated in an anti-aging unit. *Frontiers in Psychology, 2020*(11), 1844. https://doi.org/10.3389/fpsyg.2020.01844.

Caldwell, M., & Pirani, F. (2020). Racism against Black nurses is a historic problem that still exists today. In *Pulse: Digital Magazine for Nurses in the Southeast.* Retrieved from https://www.ajc.com/news/racism-against-black-nurses-historic-problem-that-still-exists-today/WXgpiNAYHIuIKnoZRdZnxI/.

Cassidy, L. (2020). To have a healthy work environment, mind the gap. In *ICU Management & Practice.* January 13, 2020. Retrieved from https://healthmanagement.org/c/icu/post/to-have-a-healthy-work-environment-mind-the-gap?fbclid=IwAR1UZR-WgLHgJSWx7VRigGuklM-xxo-dT0T7j3s4vhDQs8-zsajTU9qn51z4.

Celik, S. U., Aslan, A., Coskun, E., Coban, B., Haner, Z., Kart, S., Skaik, M. N. I., Kocer, M. D., Ozkan, B. B., & Akyol, C. (2021). Prevalence and associated factors for burnout among attending general surgeons: A national cross-sectional survey. *British Medical Journal, 21.* https://doi.org/10.1186/s12913-020-06024-5. 39 (21).

Chung, H. C., Chen, Y. C., Chang, S. C., Hsu, W. L. O., & Hsieh, T. C. (2020). Nurses' well-being, health-promoting lifestyle and work environment satisfaction correlation: A psychometric study for development of nursing health and job satisfaction model and scale. *International Journal of Environmental Research in Public Health, 17,* 3582. https://www.mdpi.com/1660-4601/17/10/3582.

Cooper, A. L., Brown, J. A., & Leslie, G. D. (2021). Nurse resilience for clinical practice: An integrative review. *Journal of Advanced Nursing.* February 9, 2021. Epub ahead of print https://www.mdpi.com/1660-4601/17/10/3582.

Cross, R., Singer, J., & Dillon, K. (2020). Don't let the microstresses burn you out. In *Harvard Business Review.* Retrieved from https://hbr.org/2020/07/dont-let-micro-stresses-burn-you-out.

Daisy Foundation. (2021). *About us.* Retrieved from https://www.daisyfoundation.org/about.

Desai, N. (2020). *The 3Cs of psychological hardiness.* The Emotional Wellness Platform. Retrieved from https://weqip.com/the-3cs-of-psychological-hardiness.

D'Ettore, G., Pellicani, V., & Greco, M. (2020). Job stress and needlestick injuries in nurses: A retrospective observational study. *ACTA Biomed for Health Professions*, *91*(S.2), 45–49. https://doi.org/10.23750/abm.v91i2-SA8824.

Devereaux, M. (2021). Travel nurses 'a double-edged sword' for desperate hospitals. In *Modern Healthcare*. Retrieved from https://www.modernhealthcare.com/labor/travel-nurses-double-edged-sword-desperate-hospitals.

Dill, J., Akosionu, O., Karbeah, J., & Henning-Smith, C. (2020). Addressing systemic racial inequity in the health-care workforce. Health Affairs Blog. In *Health Affairs*. Retrieved from https://www.healthaffairs.org/do/10.1377/forefront.20200908.133196.

Dimino, K., Brown, J., & Fernandes, B. (2020). Creating a healthy work environment is every nurse's responsibility. In *My American Nurse*. Retrieved from https://www.myamericannurse.com/creating-a-healthy-working-environment-is-every-nurses-responsibility/.

Dimino, K., Learmonth, A. E., & Fajardo, C. C. (2021). Nurse managers leading the way: Reenvisioning stress to maintain healthy work environments. *Critical Care Nurse*, *41*(5), 52–58. https://doi.org/10.4037/ccn2021463.

Donohue-Ryan, M. A., & Schneider, M. A. (2020). Supporting staff during the COVID-19 pandemic: A case report. In *My American Nurse*. Retrieved from https://www.myamericannurse.com/supporting-staff-during-the-covid-19-pandemic-a-case-report/amp/.

Dubose, B. M., & Mayo, A. M. (2020). Resistance to change: A concept analysis. In *School of Nursing and Health Science Faculty Scholarship* (p. 29). https://digital.sandiego.edu/nursing_facpub/29.

Dulon, M., Strangziner, J., Wendeler, D., & Nienhaus, A. (2020). Causes of needlestick and sharps injuries when using devices with and without safety features. *International Journal of Environmental Research and Public Health*, *17*(23), 8721. https://doi.org/10.3390/ijerph17238721.

Edmonson, C., & Marshall, J. (2020). Keeping the human in health care human capital: Challenges and solutions for RNs in the next decade. *Nurse Leader*, *18*(2), 130–134.

Edmonson, C., & Marshall, J. (2021). Creating a healthier workplace environment in an era of rising workforce pressures. *Nursing Administrative Quarterly*, *45*(1), 52–57.

Elhadi, M., Mxherghi, A., Elgzairi, M., Alhashimi, A., Bouhuwaish, A., Biala, M., Abuelmeda, S., Khel, S., Khaled, A., Alsoufi, A., Elmabrouk, A., Alshiteewi, F. B., Hamed, T. B., Alhadi, B., Alhaddad, S., Elhadi, A., & Zaid, A. (2020). Burnout syndrome among hospital healthcare workers during the COVID-19 pandemic and civil war: A cross-sectional study. *Frontiers in Psychiatry*, *11*, Article 579563. https://doi.org/10.3389/fpsyt.2020.57963.

Emergency Nurses Association (ENA). (2021). *ENA Lantern Award*. Retrieved from https://www.ena.org/about/awards-recognition/lantern.

Faller, M., & Gogek, J. (2019). Break from the past: survey suggests modern leadership styles needed for millennial nurses. *Nurse Leader*, *17*(2), 135–140.

Fernandez, R. (2021). *5 ways to boost your resilience at work*. Strategic Leaders. Retrieved from http://strategicleaders.com/5-ways-boost-resilience-work/.

Flannery, J. (2020). *Perceptions of nurses' ability to provide safe care in unhealthy work environments*. Walden Dissertations and Doctoral Studies. 8608 https://scholarworks.waldenu.edu/dissertations/8608.

Ford, S. (2019). Exclusive: High level of racial discrimination faced by nurses revealed. In *Nursing Times*. October 2, 2019. https://www.nursingtimes.net/news/workforce/exclusive-high-level-of-racial-discrimination-faced-by-nurses-revealed-02-10-2019/.

Gayed, A., Bryan, B. T., LaMontagne, A. D., Milner, A., Deady, M., Calvo, R., Mackinnon, A., Christensen, H., Mykletun, A., Glozier, N., & Harvey, S. (2019). A cluster randomized controlled trial to evaluate HeadCoach: An online mental health training program for workplace managers. *Journal of Occupational and Environmental Medicine*, *61*(7), 545–551.

Goleman, D. (1995). *Emotional intelligence*. New York: Bantam Books.

Goleman, D. (2020). What people (still) get wrong about emotional intelligence. *Harvard Business Review*. Retrieved from https://hbr.org/2020/12/what-people-still-get-wrong-about-emotional-intelligence.

Gray, K. (2021). *The effect discrimination, microaggressions can have on people of color*. National Association of Colleges and Employers. January 11, 2021. Retrieved from https://www.naceweb.org/diversity-equity-and-inclusion/best-practices/the-effect-discrimination-microaggressions-can-have-on-people-of-color/.

Groves, P. S., Farag, A., & Bunch, J. (2020). Strategies for and barriers to fatigue management among acute care nurses. *Journal of Nursing Regulation*, *11*(2), 36–43.

Halm, M. (2019). The influence of appropriate staffing and healthy work environments on patient and nurse outcomes. *American Journal of Critical Care*, *28*(2), 152–156. https://doi.org/10.4037/ajcc2019938.

Havaei, F., Astivia, O. L. O., & MacPhee, M. (2020). The impact of workplace violence on medical-surgical nurses' health outcome: A moderated mediation model of work environment conditions and burnout using secondary data. *International Journal of Nursing Studies*, *109*(2020), 103666.

Hawkins, N., Jeong, S., & Smith, T. (2021). Creating respectful workplaces for nurses in regional acute care settings: Protocol for a sequential explanatory mixed methods study. *JMIR Research Protocols*, *10*(1), e18643. https://doi.org/10.2196/18678.

Hawkins, R. (2021). Ceiling lifts and safe patient handling and mobility programs. *My American Nurse*. February 17, 2021. Retrieved from https://www.myamericannurse.com/ceiling-lifts-and-safe-patient-handling-and-mobility-programs/.

Healthdirect. (2021). *Relaxation and mental health*. Retrieved from https://www.healthdirect.gov.au/relaxation.

Health Resources and Services Administration. (2018). *The US nursing workforce: Trends in supply and education*. Retrieved from https://www.ruralhealthinfo.org/assets/1206-4974/nursing-workforce-nchwa-report-april-2013.pdf.

Hessels, A., Kelly, A. M., Chen, L., Cohen, B., Zachariah, P., & Larson, E. (2019). Impact of infectious exposures and outbreaks on nurse and infection preventionist workload. *American Journal of Infection Control, 47*(6), 623–627.

Hudson, B. (2020). Navigating nurse staffing post-pandemic. In *Staffing Industry Analysts*. http://www.thestaffingstream.com/2020/07/21/navigating-nurse-staffing-post-pandemic/.

Institute for Healthcare Improvement (IHI). (2022). Triple Aim for populations. http://www.ihi.org/Topics/TripleAim.

Jewett, C., Lewis, R., & Bailey, M. (2020). More than 2,900 health care workers died this year – and the government barely kept track. In *Kaiser Health News*. Retrieved from https://www.pbs.org/newshour/health/more-than-2900-health-care-workers-died-this-year-and-the-government-barely-kept-track.

Kajjimu, J., Kaggwa, M. M., & Bongomin, F. (2021). Burnout and associated factors among medical students in a public university in Uganda: A cross-sectional study. *Advances in Medical Education and Practice, 12*, 63–75. https://doi.org/10.2147/AMEP.S287928.

Kobasa, S. C., Maddi, S., & Kahn, S. (1982). Hardiness and health: A prospective study. *Journal of Personality and Social Psychology, 42*(1), 168–177. https://doi.org/10.1037/0022-3514.42.1.168.

Kester, K. M., Lindsay, M., & Granger, B. (2019). Development and evaluation of a prospective staffing model to improve retention. *Journal of Nursing Management, 28*(2), 425–432.

Lai, F. Y., Tang, H. C., Lu, S. C., Lee, Y. C., & Lin, C. C. (2020). Transformational leadership and job performance: The mediating role of work engagement. *Organizational Research Methods, 10*(1). https://doi.org/10.1177/2158244019899085.

Lambert, V., Lambert, C., & Yamase, H. (2003). Psychological hardiness, workplace stress and related stress reduction strategies. *Nursing and Health Sciences, 5*, 181–184.

Lasater, K. B., Aiken, L. H., Sloane, S. M., French, R., Martin, B., Reneau, K., Alexander, M., & McHugh, M. D. (2021). Chronic hospital nurse understaffing meets COVID-19: An observational study. *British Medical Journal Quality & Safety, 30*, 639–647. https://qualitysafety.bmj.com/content/30/8/639.

Lim, F., Jones, P. A., & Paguirigan, M. (2019). A guide to fostering an LGBTQ+ inclusive workplace. *Nursing Management, 50*(6), 46–53.

Liu, J. (2020). *Training for this workplace skill is up nearly 4,000% in 2020*. CNBC.com. Retrieved from https://www. cnbc.com/2020/11/27/training-for-this-workplace-skill-is-up-nearly-4000percent-in-2020.html.

Liu, Y., Song, Y., Hu, X., Yan, L., & Zhu, X. (2019). Awareness of surgical smoke hazards and enhancement of surgical smoke prevention among the gynecologists. *Journal of Cancer, 10*(12), 2788–2799.

Lonsdale, D. (2020). Corona virus and the general adaptation syndrome. *Scholarly Journal of Emergency Medicine and Critical Care, 4*(1). https://doi.org/10.36959/592/385.

MacBride, E. (2020). Tend and befriend: How women may respond differently to the stress of the pandemic. *Forbes*. Retrieved from https://forbes.com/sites/elizabethmacbride/2020/04/29/tend-and-befriend-how-women-may-responding-differently-to-the-stress-of-the-pandemic/?sh=3cc9badd5955.

Majers, J. S., & Warshawsky, N. (2020). Evidence-based decision-making for nurse leaders. *Nurse Leader, 18*(5), 471–475.

Maslow, A. H. (1943). A theory of human motivation. *Psychological Review, 50*, 370–396.

McClure, M. L., Poulin, M. A., Sovie, M. D., & Wandelt, M. (1983). American Academy of Nursing, Task Force on Nursing Practice in Hospitals. In *Magnet Hospitals: Attraction and Retention of Professional Nurses*. Kansas City, MO: American Nurses Association.

Melnyk, B. M., Hsieh, A. P., Davison, J., Carpenter, H., Chofiet, A., Heath, J., Hess, M. E., Lee, P., Link, T., Marcus, J., Pabico, C., Poindexter, K., & Stand, L. (2020). Promoting nurse mental health. *American Nurse Journal., 16*(1), 20–59.

Mengistu, D. A., Tolera, S. T., & Demmu, Y. M. (2021). Worldwide prevalence of occupational exposure to needle stick injury among healthcare workers: A systematic review and meta-analysis. *Canadian Journal of Infectious Diseases and Medical Microbiology, 2021*. Article ID 9019534. https://doi.org/10.1155/2021/9019534.

Miller, E. T. (2016). Preventing burnout. *Rehabilitation Nursing, 41*, 65–66.

Mitchell, G. (2020). Danger of nurses quitting after COVID-19' if mental health overlooked. April 24, 2020. *Nursing Times*. Retrieved from https://www.nursingtimes.net/news/mental-health/danger-of-nurses-quitting-after-covid-19-if-mental-health-overlooked-24-04-2020/.

Mitchell, L., Amaya, M., Battista, L., Melnyk, B., Andridge, R., & Kaye, G. (2020). Manager support for wellness champions: A case study for consideration and practice implications. *Workplace Health & Safety*. https://doi.org/10.1177/2165079920952759.

Morse, S. (2021). Workplace violence in hospitals is preventable, says head of National Nurses United: Proposed bill would create OSHA standards in an effort to protect employees. *Healthcare Finance*. Retrieved from https://www.healthcarefinancenews.com/news/workplace-violence-hospitals-preventable-says-head-national-nurses-united#:~:text=Workplace%20violence%20 in%20healthcare%20is,were%20facing%20increased%20 workplace%20violence.

Moss, J. (2021). Beyond burnout out. *Harvard Business Review*. February 20, 2021. Retrieved from https://hbr.org/2021/02/ beyond-burned-out.

Moy, A. J., Schwartz, J. M., Chen, R. J., Sadri, S., Lucas, E., Cato, K. D., & Rossetti, S. C. (2021). Measurement of clinical documentation burden among physicians and nurses using electronic health records: A scoping review. *Journal of the American Medical Informatics Association*, 28(5), 998–1008. https://doi.org/10.1093/jamia/ocaa325.

Mueller, S. (2015). *Stephen Covey's time management matrix explained*. http://www.planetofsuccess.com/blog/2015/stephen-coveys-time-management-matrix-explained/.

Needleman, J., Buerhaus, P., Mattke, S., Stewart, M., & Zelevinsky, K. (2002). Nurse-staffing levels and the quality of care in hospitals. *New England Journal of Medicine*, 326(22), 1715–1722.

Noga, P. M., Dermenchyan, A., Grant, S., & Dowdell, E. B. (2021). Developing statewide violence prevention in health care: an exemplar from Massachusetts. *Policy, Politics & Nursing Practice.*, 22(2), 156–164. https://doi.org/10.1177/1527154420987180.

Nundy, S., Cooper, L., Mate, K. (2022). The Quintuple Aim for healthcare improvement: A new imperative to advance health equity. *Journal of the American Medical Association*, 327(6), 521–522.

Nursing CE. (2021). Civility Matters! Strategies to Inspire Healthy, Productive Work Environments. *Nursing CE*. Retrieved from https://www.cmelist.com/nursingce-civility-matters-strategies-to-inspire-healthy-productive-work-environments-free-course/.

Office of Disease Prevention and Health Promotion. (n.d.) Social determinants of health. *Healthy People 2030*. U.S. Department of Health and Human Services. Retrieved from https://health.gov/healthypeople/objectives-and-data/ social-determinants-health.

Orgambidez, A., & Benitez, M. (2021). Understanding the link between work engagement and affective organizational commitment: The moderating effect of role stress. January 19, 2021. *International Journal of Psychology*, 56(5), 791–800. https://doi.org/10.1002/ijop.12741.

Pappas, S., & Rushton, C. (2020). Leading the way to professional well-being. *My American Nurse*. Retrieved from https://myamericannurse.com/leading-the-way-to-professional-well-being/amp/.

Persolja, M., Marin, M., Caporale, L., Odasmini, B., Scarsini, S., Fiorella, V., DeLucia, P., & Palese, A. (2020). Chief nurse executives' involuntary turnover in times of health care reforms: Findings from an interpretive phenomenology study. *Health Services Management Research*, 33(24), 172–185. https://doi.org/10.1177/0951484820923923.

Pinekenstein, B., & Pawlak, R. (2020). Calm©: A customized advanced leader model for enhancing career and well-being. *Nurse Leader*, 18(1), 455–460.

Plsek, P. E., & Greenhalgh, T. (2001). The challenge of complexity in health care. *British Medical Journal*, 323(7313), 625–628.

Porter-O'Grady, T. (2021). *Shared governance*. Retrieved from http://www.tpogassociates.com/implementing-shared-governance/.

Porter-O'Grady, T. (2019). Principles for sustaining shared governance. *Nursing Management*, 50(1), 36–41. https:// doi.org/10.1097/01.NUMA.0000550448.17375.28.

Press Ganey. (2020). *Press Ganey Nursing Special Report: The Far-Reaching Impact of Nursing Excellence*. February 20, 2020. Retrieved from http://images.healthcare.pressganey. com/Web/PressGaneyAssociatesInc/%7B980c39eb-7cf2-4e71-8be4-694149ee8768%7D_2020_PG_Nursing_ Special_Report.pdf.

Preugschat, J. (2020). The benefits of emotional intelligence in the workplace. *Thrive Global*. Retrieved from https:// thriveglobal.com/stories/the-benefits-of-emotional-intel-ligence-in-the-workplace/.

Raso, R., Fitzpatrick, J. J., & Masick, K. (2020). Clinical nurses' perceptions of authentic nurse leadership and healthy work environment. *Journal of Nursing Administration*, 50(9), 489–494.

Rindone, A. (2021). Leaders need professional coaching now more than ever. *Harvard Business Review*. March 2, 2021. Retrieved from https://hbr.org/sponsored/2021/03/lead-ers-need-professional-coaching-now-more-than-ever.

Redeker, N. S., Caruso, C. C., Hashmi, S. D., Mullington, J. M., Grandner, M., & Morgenthaler, T. I. (2019). Workplace interventions to promote sleep health and an alert, healthy workforce. *Journal of Clinical Sleep Medicine*, 15(4), 649–657.

Reinhardt, A. C., Leon, T. G., & Amatya, A. (2020). Why nurses stay: Analysis of the registered nurse workforce and the relationship to work environments. *Applied Nursing Research*, 55(2020), 151316. https://doi.org/10.1016/j.apnr.2020.151316.

Roberts, D. C. (2021). The elephant in the room. *Nursing 2021*, 50(12), 42–46.

Roberts, L. M., & Mayo, A. J. (2019). Toward a racially just workplace. *Harvard Business Review*. Retrieved from https://hbr.org/2019/11/toward-a-racially-just-workplace.

Scepura, R. C. (2020). The challenges with pre-employment testing and potential hiring bias. *Nurse Leader*, 18(2), 151–156.

Schlak, A. E., Aiken, L. H., Chittams, J., Poghosyan, L., & McHugh, M. (2021). Leveraging the work environment to minimize the negative impact of nurse burnout on patient outcomes. *International Journal of Environmental Research and Public Health*, 18(2), 610.

Sears, B., Mallory, C., Flores, A. R., & Conron, K. J. (2021). *LGBT people's experiences of workplace discrimination and harassment.* Los Angeles School of Law, Williams Institute: University of California. Retrieved from https://williamsinstitute.law.ucla.edu/publications/lgbt-workplace-discrimination/.

Selye, H. (1956). *The stress of life.* McGraw Hill Book Company.

Simplifi. (2021). *Travel nurse job industry trends, 2018–2019.* Retrieved from https://www.simplifimsp.com/healthcare/travel-nurse-job-industry-trends-2018-2019.

Singh, S., Brand, R., & Davis, E. (2021). Ambulatory care: current landscape and challenges. *Avia Insights.* January 7, 2021. Retrieved from https://aviahealth.com/insights/ambulatory-care-current-challenges/.

Sitterding, M. C., Raab, D. L., Saupe, J. L., & Israel, K. J. (2019). Using artificial intelligence and gaming to improve new nurse transition. *Nurse Leader, 17*(2), 125–130.

Tedone, D. A. (2020). Eliminating workplace violence from the workplace. *Nursing 2020, 50*(8), 57–60. https://doi.org/10.1097/01NURSE.0000668440.64732.39.

Thew, J. (2020a). The impact of nursing excellence on 'pretty much everything in healthcare, *HealthLeaders. February, 28,* 2020. Retrieved from https://www.healthleadersmedia.com/nursing/impact-nursing-excellence-pretty-much-everything-healthcare.

Thew, J. (2020b). Nurses must fight against racism: ANA's president shares how. June 12, 2020. *HealthLeaders.* Retrieved from https://www.healthleadersmedia.com/nursing/nurses-must-fight-against-racism-anas-president-shares-how.

Thomas, L. M. (2020). Nursing faculty experiences with students' needlestick injuries. *Nurse Educator, 45*(6), 307–311.

Thomas, L. M. (2019). Underreporting of bloodborne pathogen exposures in nursing students. *Nurse Educator, 45*(2), 78–82. https://doi.org/10.1097/NNE.0000000000000696.

Tomova, L., Saxe, R., Klobl, M., Lanzenberger, R., & Lamm, C. (2020). Acute stress alters neural patterns of value representation for others. *NeuroImage, 209*(2020), 116497.

Tye, J. (2020). Living your values. *Nurse Leader,* 67–72. https://www.nurseleader.com/article/S1541-4612(22)00032-5/fulltext.

Van Beusekom, M. (2020). *High-risk COVID contact puts health workers, patients, families at risk.* Center for Infectious Disease Research and Policy. Retrieved from https://www.cidrap.umn.edu/news-perspective/2020/10/high-risk-covid-contact-puts-health-workers-patients-families-risk.

Vasconcellos, E. (2020). 6 types of office 'politicians' and how to handle them. *Business News Daily.* February 6, 2020. Retrieved from https://www.businessnewsdaily.com/3048-coping-office-politics.html.

Wang, C., Huang, L., Li, J., & Dai, J. (2019). Relationship between psychosocial working conditions, stress perception, and needlestick injury among healthcare workers in Shanghai. *BMC Public Health, 19,* 874. https://doi.org/10.1186/s12889-019-7181-7.

Watson, A., Jafari, M., & Seifi, A. (2020). The persistent pandemic of violence against health care workers. *The American Journal of Managed Care, 26*(12), e377–e379.

Wei, H., Jiang, Y., & Lake, D. M. (2020). The impact of nurse leadership styles on nurse burnout: A systematic literature review. *Nurse Leader, 18*(5), 439–450.

Weberg, D. R., Fuller, R. M. (2019). Toxic leadership: Three lessons from complexity science to identify and stop toxic teams. *Nurse Leader, 17*(1), 22–26.

Weston, M. J. (2020). Strategic planning in an age of uncertainty: Creating clarity in uncertain times. *Nurse Leader, 18*(1), 54–58.

Whittington, K., Shaw, T., McKinnies, R. C., & Collins, S. K. (2021). Emotional exhaustion as a predictor for burnout among nurses. *Nursing Management, 52*(1), 22–28. https://doi.org/10.1097/01.NUMA.0000724928.71008.47.

World Health Organization. (2020). *Keep health workers safe to keep patients safe: WHO.* Retrieved from https://www.who.int/news/item/17-09-2020-keep-health-workers-safe-to-keep-patients-safe-who.

Younas, A. (2019). Lesbian-, gay-, bisexual- and transgender-related inequalities within nursing: A neglected research area. *Journal of Advanced Nursing, 75*(7), 1374–1376.

Zare, A., Choobineh, A., Hassanipour, S., & Malakoutikah, M. (2021). Investigation of psychosocial factors on upper limb musculoskeletal disorders and the prevalence of its musculoskeletal disorders among nurses: a systematic review and meta-analysis. *International Archives of Occupational and Environmental Health, 94*(5), 1113–1136. https://doi.org/10.1007/s0040-021-01654-6.

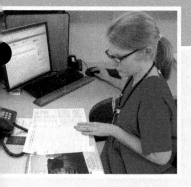

6

Translating Research Into Practice

Margarete Lieb Zalon

ANTICIPATED LEARNING OUTCOMES

- Value the nurse's obligation to use research evidence in practice.
- Analyze differences among research, evidence-based practice, practice-based evidence, comparative effectiveness research, outcomes research, and quality improvement.
- Formulate a clinical question that can be searched in the literature.

- Identify resources for critically appraising evidence.
- Describe the potential of "big data" in a connected healthcare system.
- Assess organizational barriers and facilitators for the translation of research into practice.
- Identify organizational strategies for translating research into practice.

KEY TERMS

big data
bundles
clinical guidelines
comparative effectiveness
    research (CER)
effectiveness
efficacy
evidence-based practice (EBP)
external validity
GRADE system
implementation science

internal validity
journal club
meta-analysis
outcomes
participatory action research
    (PAR)
patient-centered outcomes
    research
practice-based evidence (PBE)
practice-based research networks
    (PBRNs)

randomized controlled trial
    (RCT)
reliability
research
systematic review
system science
translating research into practice
    (TRIP)
translation science
validity

THE CHALLENGE

Surgical site infection (SSI) rates had increased significantly at our hospital. Literature reviews found that several evidence-based interventions existed that we could implement to help decrease these rates. We also identified specific interventions for patients undergoing hysterectomies and colon surgery. We believed, along with the staff, that we were using these interventions, but clearly we had more work to do to reduce our infection rates. Nurses who graduated in more recent years seemed to have an easier time in grasping the concept of

(Continued)

137

translating research evidence into practice. When I asked them if it is hard to put this information into practice, they would give me a look of confusion and say, "Isn't this what we are supposed to do?" Incorporating these practices seemed to be a harder challenge for those nurses who went to school years ago, not having had evidence-based practice included in their education. Nursing leadership met and decided that an intraprofessional approach would

be best, with the focus on basic techniques, especially asepsis. We decided that the best way to monitor this would be through observational audits but were concerned about the staff's reaction to the audits.

What would you do if you were this nurse?

Megan Lamoreux, BSN, RN, CNOR
Clinical Nurse Educator, Geisinger Wyoming Valley Medical Center,
Wilkes-Barre, PA

INTRODUCTION

When people or their loved ones require nursing care, they want that care to be based on the best research evidence available. For example, if someone needs to be on a ventilator, the family would want to be sure that the nurses providing the care were using best practices to prevent ventilator-associated pneumonia and were assessing for delirium, a common complication with serious life-altering consequences. The family would want to know that there is good communication among nurses and physicians on the clinical unit where the family member has been placed because research demonstrates that teamwork and collaboration lead to lower mortality and fewer errors. If their loved one also had a central venous catheter, the family would want to be sure that the nurse who removes that catheter is using an established procedure that minimizes the risk for introducing an air embolism into the circulation. And, when that person is discharged, the family would want to know that the nurses are using well-tested strategies to help transition the person safely to home, recover from the illness, and manage that illness. As a follower, leader, and manager, one should be concerned about incorporating research evidence not only into clinical practices but also into the management of systems of care. The challenge is how to (1) find the best research evidence; (2) incorporate the best evidence into practice in a meaningful manner; and (3) motivate nurses, nursing leadership, and organizational leadership to care about using evidence in practice amid all the other challenges faced in delivering high-quality nursing care.

Research is an integral part of professional practice and its hallmark is the creation of new knowledge. Research is a "systematic approach that relies on disciplined methods to answer questions or solve problems" (Polit & Beck, 2021, p. 2). Nurses, as professionals, have

an obligation to society that involves rights and responsibilities as well as a mechanism for accountability. These obligations are outlined in *Nursing's Social Policy Statement: The Essence of the Profession*, which outlines the profession's contract with society (American Nurses Association [ANA], 2010): "To refine and expand nursing's knowledge base, nurses use theories that fit with professional nursing's values of health and health care that are relevant to professional nursing practice. Nurses apply research findings and implement the best evidence into their practice ..." (p. 13). Using research is the responsibility of all nurses.

The *Code of Ethics for Nurses* (ANA, 2015, p. 27) directs that the "nurse, in all roles and settings, advances the profession through research and scholarly inquiry, professional standards development, and the generation of both nursing and health policy." Globally, the International Council of Nurses (ICN) *Code of Ethics for Nurses* indicates that the nurse is "active in expanding research-based current professional knowledge that supports evidence-informed practice" (ICN, 2021). The American Association of Colleges of Nursing (AACN, 2021) in its *Essentials: Core Competencies for Professional Nursing Education* identifies Scholarship for the Nursing Discipline as a domain with the expectation that nurses integrate best evidence into nursing practice. This includes generating questions for practice improvement, evaluating evidence, using best evidence, participating in efforts to improve nursing care, and evaluating practice outcomes.

Nursing research is designed to refine and expand the scientific foundation for nursing. On the national level, the National Institute of Nursing Research (NINR, n.d.), part of the National Institutes of Health, focuses on funding research that has the potential for the greatest impact on the health of the most people, advanced equity, diversity, and inclusion, addresses challenges to health, stimulates discovery, and finds solutions to enhance health.

Evidence-based practice (EBP) is derived from the widely used classic definition of evidence-based medicine: the integration of the best research evidence with clinical expertise and the patient's unique values and circumstances in making decisions about the care of individual patients (Straus et al., 2011). Use of the word "practice" denotes the use of evidence by all healthcare practitioners, including nurses. In EBP, clinicians drive the search for solutions to clinical problems based on the best available evidence, which is then translated into practice. EBP is a broader, more encompassing view of using research in practice. It is focused on searching for, appraising, and synthesizing the best evidence to address a clinical practice problem. EBP is more involved than reading a research study and identifying its practice implications. It involves systematically searching for the best evidence and making judgments about its application to patient care while considering patient preferences.

MAKING PRACTICE IMPROVEMENTS

Once decisions have been made about the best evidence that addresses a clinical problem, the next step is to make changes to improve clinical practice. The translation of evidence into practice involves all healthcare disciplines, and the integration of research with practice in a timely fashion is essential for quality healthcare. Tremendous variation exists in the lag time between the publication of research findings and integration of the results into practice. This lag time from research discovery to implementation is often cited as taking 17 years (Hanney et al., 2020), a time frame that seems intolerable in today's world. Even if the lag from publication to the use of findings were dramatically reduced, the gap is still measured in years, not months. We might believe that once a research study is published in a journal, clinicians read it immediately and then clinicians and/or policy makers use it to improve practice. For example, for more than 20 years, the National Institute of Child Health and Human Development implemented a public health campaign to prevent sudden infant death syndrome (SIDS) by educating the public about the importance of placing infants on their back to sleep. Now named "Safe to Sleep," the program includes recommendations for infants to sleep in their own space. Despite extensive campaigning that included both physicians and nurses,

50% of new mothers received no advice on infants' sleep location and 20% did not receive recommendations on breastfeeding or placing infants to sleep on their backs (Eisenberg et al., 2015). Subsequently, Specker et al. (2020) found that only 7.7% of new mothers received information about all eight American Academy of Pediatric recommendations for infant sleep. In consideration of the number of nurses who may have contact with a mother before her discharge with a new baby and shortly thereafter, this research indicates that additional efforts are needed to provide new mothers with information about evidence-based practices. EBP has the dual purpose of promoting the use of effective strategies to improve health outcomes and helping healthcare providers stop recommending ineffective, unsafe, or harmful strategies. When we think of the rapid development and deployment of a vaccine to address COVID-19 (coronavirus disease 2019), we have to be impressed with the numbers of people who were vaccinated worldwide in such a short time. That is not to say we should be satisfied with the numbers, though.

Research provides the foundation for nursing practice improvement. Examples include preoperative teaching, pain management, child development assessment, falls prevention, pressure-injury risk detection, incontinence care, transitional care, and family-centered care in critical care units. Research needs to be systematically evaluated to determine which interventions should be implemented to improve care outcomes. Practice changes may have greater likelihood of success when aligned with the organization's mission and goals. Practices that were once considered the standard of care may quickly become outdated. Some practices may have been carried out for many years without their scientific basis or effectiveness ever being examined or questioned. Adverse events precipitated by an outdated practice may prompt an organization to act more quickly to incorporate EBP. The latest research findings need to be incorporated into procedures using an evidence-based model when they are being updated by an organization.

> **EXERCISE 6.1** Identify a common activity that is part of your nursing practice and determine how the practice aligns with the organization's mission/vision, and whether any research supports the intervention or nursing care activity.

THE RELATIONSHIP BETWEEN RESEARCH AND EVIDENCE

Nursing research designs can be categorized in several ways, such as basic versus applied, qualitative versus quantitative, cross-sectional versus longitudinal, experimental versus descriptive, and retrospective versus prospective. Regardless of the design, some research is ready for implementation and some research may not warrant a change in practice. Readiness for implementation may be influenced by the strength of the research, which is determined by study design, sample size, ease of implementation, and the beliefs and values of clinicians.

The quality of care and the quality of the outcomes of care can be dramatically improved with the implementation of practices derived from a systematic evaluation of research evidence. Patients entrusted to our care are deserving of practices that are based on the best available evidence. Examining the evidence for a specific practice generally needs to go beyond examining the results of a single study. At times, a single well-designed study might be adequate for recommending and implementing a practice change. However, developing an EBP requires the development of a clearly written clinical question and a more thorough search of the literature, the review of single studies, meta-analyses, metasyntheses, critically appraised topics, systematic reviews, and clinical guidelines.

Research evidence must be appraised and placed in the context of patient, family, and community values. Nurse managers and leaders may not necessarily be the ones conducting research, evaluating research evidence, or developing evidence-based guidelines, but they will be facilitating the application of research findings in practice. The end results of care are known as the *outcomes* of care. These are important to a public that wants to know what is best and what was improved. Outcomes of care may include whether a new mother received the correct advice about safe sleep practices, whether a person with diabetes is able to maintain a hemoglobin A1c value that is less than 6.5, or whether a critically ill patient develops a central line–associated bloodstream infection (CLABSI). Improving the outcomes of care involves different approaches, such as identifying EBPs, comparative effectiveness research, participatory action research, practice-based evidence, and quality improvement. It also requires

understanding how innovations are incorporated into practice, identifying appropriate strategies for translating research into practice, and sustaining the practice improvement within the context of the organization's culture and policies. Frontline nurses and nurse leaders face many decisions along the way to effectively implement evidence derived from research into daily care practices.

FROM USING RESEARCH TO EVIDENCE-BASED PRACTICE

Individual nurses may apply research findings to their own practice. However, nurses' broader responsibility to society includes activating the change process in translating research into practice. Research use can be in a variety of forms: enlightenment, implementation of a research-based protocol, or the widespread adoption of standards based on research findings. Ultimately, multiple factors influence how a research finding is adopted, translated into practice, and sustained.

The movement to use research in practice paralleled the development of original nursing research. In the 1970s, three major projects facilitated research utilization: The Western Institute of Commission on Higher Education in Nursing (WICHEN), Conduct and Utilization of Research in Nursing (CURN), and the Nursing Child Assessment Satellite Training (NCAST). These projects used research findings to improve practice, which spawned the growth of demonstration projects to use research as well as research studies identifying factors that facilitated or created barriers to research utilization. The NCAST programs developed by Kathryn Barnard, PhD, RN, FAAN, a nurse researcher at the University of Washington, used assessments of mother–infant feeding behaviors to promote positive parent–child interactions and enhance the development of cognitive and language abilities. This has grown today to a suite of programs for professionals designed to provide nurturing environments for children (Parent-Child, 2020).

Subsequently, nurse researchers developed models to guide nurses in the steps of the research utilization process. Researchers also identified barriers to nursing research utilization: those within the nurse, the nature of the research, administrators, and the healthcare organization. Research, even when ready for implementation, was not necessarily readily embraced. At times, a new practice is not implemented until the costs of the practice are factored in and the research has been demonstrated to have an impact on the finances of a healthcare organization.

THE EVIDENCE-BASED PRACTICE MOVEMENT

The EBP movement is derived from the work of Archie Cochrane, who described the lack of knowledge about healthcare treatment effects and advocated for using proven treatments. Subsequently, the Cochrane Collaboration was established at Oxford University in 1993. About that time, Gordon Guyatt and his colleagues at McMaster University authored a series of articles in the *Journal of the American Medical Association* (*JAMA*) known as the *Users' Guides to the Medical Literature*, providing detailed steps for the analysis of different types of research studies.

In the 1990s, the focus changed to finding a research-based solution to clinical problems, not only in nursing but also in medicine and other disciplines. Healthcare organizations began to be more systematic in using research and evaluating patient outcomes. Federal government agencies provide support for EBP and research. See Table 6.1 for EBP resources under the auspices of federal agencies and other organizations. Global initiatives for EBP have been established around the world, some of which include centers for evidence-based nursing. Resources for learning EBP as well as repositories for EBP reviews and/or guidelines are included in Table 6.2.

The EBP movement has grown exponentially with scientific publications, establishment of collaboration centers, resources on the Internet, and grants focused specifically on translating research into practice, including resources devoted to nursing. The JBI (formerly known as the Joanna Briggs Institute), based in Australia, has a network of nursing collaborating centers and evidence-based synthesis and utilization groups around the world. These centers have teams of researchers critically appraising evidence and disseminating evidence-based protocols. The JBI also provides training programs in conducting systematic reviews, many of which are available from its collaborating centers. Nurses associations have developed evidence-based standards of practice, clinical guidelines, and EBP toolkits, many of which are publicly available on their websites (Table 6.3). Nurses are also members of interdisciplinary groups involved in guideline development. Many of these guidelines are available through some of the resources listed in Table 6.2.

Researchers and clinicians collaborate to address specific practice problems and advance healthcare. Health maintenance organizations are monitoring provider practices for patients' adherence to screening guidelines. Voluntary organizations providing support services for individuals not covered by health insurance are expecting that the agencies they fund provide evidence for the outcomes of their projects to more effectively meet community needs. Societal factors—such as the rising cost of healthcare, quality improvement initiatives, and the pressures to avoid errors—have resulted in an increased emphasis on research as a basis for practice decisions.

Healthcare professionals are expected to use evidence in practice. The National Academy of Medicine (formerly Institute of Medicine [IOM]) (Greiner & Knebel, 2003) in its landmark report on health professions education indicates that all healthcare professionals should be able to do the following:

- Know where and how to find the best possible sources of evidence.
- Formulate clear clinical questions.
- Search for relevant answers to those questions from the best possible sources, including those that evaluate or appraise evidence for its usefulness with respect to a particular patient or population.
- Determine when and how to integrate those findings into practice.

EBP is included in the Quality, Safety, and Education for Nurses (QSEN) competencies, which identify the knowledge, skills, and attitudes needed by nurses to improve the quality and safety of healthcare systems (QSEN Institute, 2020). Research-based competencies for EBP are being integrated into healthcare systems by including EBP in strategic plans and providing support through changes in organizational infrastructure, validation of staff competencies in EBP, and systematic oversight (Ost et al., 2020). Frontline nurses and nurse leaders need to participate in an organization's EBP initiatives. The critical importance of nurses having EBP competencies is illustrated in the results of a survey conducted by Melnyk and her colleagues (2020) in the Research Perspective.

TABLE 6.1   Selected Programs and Resources Supporting Evidence-Based Practice

Agency or Organization	Program or Resource	Description	Website
Agency for Healthcare Research and Quality (AHRQ)	Evidence-Based Practice Center (EPC)	Awards contracts for evidence reports and technology assessments for common, expensive, and/or significant for Medicare/Medicaid populations.	https://www.ahrq.gov/research/findings/evidence-based-reports/overview/index.html
	Effective Healthcare Program	Partners with researchers, healthcare organizations, and other stakeholders to conduct research, synthesize evidence, and support evidence translation, dissemination, and implementation. Includes comparative effectiveness reviews, effectiveness reviews, and technical briefs on patient-centered outcomes.	https://effectivehealthcare.ahrq.gov
	Practice-Based Research Networks (PBRNs)	Supports AHRQ in providing support to primary care PBRNs doing clinical and health services research	https://pbrn.ahrq.gov
Centers for Disease Control and Prevention (CDC)	Advisory Committee on Immunization Practices (ACIP)	Medical and public health experts who develop recommendations on the safe use of vaccines and related biological products in the U.S. civilian population.	https://www.cdc.gov/vaccines/acip/
	Guidelines and Recommendations	Repository for guidelines and recommendations developed by the CDC.	https://stacks.cdc.gov/
Patient-Centered Outcomes Research Institute (PCORI)	Clinical Effectiveness and Decision Science (CEDS)	Funds and manages CEDS research to compare effectiveness of different clinical options specifically for (1) assessment of prevention, diagnosis, and treatment options; (2) communication and dissemination research; and (3) accelerating patient-centered outcomes research and methodological research.	https://www.pcori.org/about-us/our-programs/clinical-effectiveness-and-decision-science
	Healthcare Delivery and Disparities Research	Compares patient-centered approaches to improve the equitability, effectiveness, and efficiency of care by improving healthcare systems and addressing disparities.	https://www.pcori.org/about-us/our-programs/healthcare-delivery-and-disparities-research/
U.S. Preventive Services Task Force (USPSTF)	Independent, volunteer national expert panel in prevention and evidence-based medicine	Makes evidence-based recommendations about clinical preventive services.	https://uspreventiveservicestaskforce.org

TABLE 6.2 Resources for Evidence-Based Health Care

Organization	Website
The Centre for Evidence-Based Medicine (CEBM)	cebm.net
Centre for Reviews and Dissemination (CRD)	https://www.york.ac.uk/crd/
The Cochrane Collaboration	https://www.cochrane.org/
ECRI Guidelines Trust®	https://www.ecri.org/solutions/ecri-guidelines-trust/
Guidelines International Network	https://g-i-n.net
The Helene Fuld Health Trust National Institute for Evidence-Based Practice in Nursing and Healthcare	https://fuld.nursing.osu.edu/
JBI (formerly known as the Joanna Briggs Institute)	https://joannabriggs.org/about-jbi
The Johns Hopkins Nursing Center for Evidence-Based Practice	https://www.hopkinsmedicine.org/evidence-based-practice
Improvement Science Research Network	http://isrn.net/
Knowledge Translation Canada (KT Canada)	https://ktcanada.org/
National Institute for Health and Care Excellence (NICE)	https://www.nice.org.uk/
National Health and Medical Research Council (NHMRC)	https://www.nhmrc.gov.au/
Sarah Cole Hirsch Institute at the Frances Payne Bolton School of Nursing, Case Western Reserve University	https://case.edu/nursing/research/centers-excellence/sarah-cole-hirsh-institute
Scottish Intercollegiate Guidelines Network (SIGN)	https://www.sign.ac.uk/

TABLE 6.3 Nurses Association Resources for Evidence-Based Practice

Association	Website
American Association of Critical-Care Nurses (AACN)	www.aacn.org
American Association of Neuroscience Nurses (AANN)	www.aann.org
American College of Nurse Midwives (ACNM)	www.midwife.org
American Nephrology Nurses Association (ANNA)	www.annanurse.org
Association for Radiologic and Imaging Nursing (ARIN)	www.arin.org
American Society of PeriAnesthesia Nurses (ASPAN)	www.aspan.org
Association of PeriOperative Registered Nurses (AORN)	www.aorn.org
Association of Rehabilitation Nurses (ARN)	www.rehabnurse.org
Association of Women's Health, Obstetric and Neonatal Nursing (AWOHNN)	www.awhonn.org
Emergency Nurses Association (ENA)	www.ena.org
Infusion Nurses Society (INS)	www.ins1.org
National Association of School Nurses (NASN)	www.nasn.org
Oncology Nursing Society (ONS)	www.ons.org
Registered Nurses Association of Ontario (RNAO)	www.rnao.ca
Wound and Ostomy Continence Nurses Society™ (WOCN Society)	www.wocn.org

RESEARCH PERSPECTIVE

Resource: Melnyk, B. M., Zellefrow, C., Tan, A., & Hsieh, A. P. (2020). Differences between Magnet and non-Magnet-designated hospitals in nurses' evidence-based practice knowledge, competencies, mentoring, and culture. *Worldviews on Evidence-Based Nursing, 17*(5), 337–347.

Melnyk et al. conducted a secondary analysis of data obtained from a survey of 2,344 nurses from 19 U.S. healthcare systems comparing the results of nurses in Magnet and non-Magnet facilities regarding EBP in four domains: knowledge, competencies, mentorship, and perceived organizational culture and readiness. The American Nurses Credentialing Center Magnet® Recognition Program uses a research framework to recognize healthcare organizations that retain excellent registered nurses. Much of the work in Magnet facilities focuses on the implementation and evaluation of EBPs to improve patient care, but numerous barriers remain. The researchers found that nurses in Magnet-designated facilities (n = 1,622) had higher scores in EBP knowledge, mentoring, and organizational culture than nurses in non-Magnet facilities (n = 638). However, no differences in self-rated EBP competencies were found. The mean scores for each of the 24 competencies were below average for both groups of RNs. In only one competency did the nurses in Magnet facilities have a significantly higher

score than non-Magnet facilities, that of formulating PICO(T) questions: *P*opulation, *I*ntervention, *C*omparison or *C*ontrol, *O*utcome (*T*ime Period). However, the group differences were very small.

Implications for Practice

While nurses in Magnet facilities have a stronger background for EBP—greater knowledge, more mentoring, and a more supportive organizational culture—that finding did not translate into higher levels of self-reported competencies. However, the nurses in Magnet facilities might have a slightly stronger foundation in EBP because they are more confident about developing clinical questions in the PICO(T) format. That did not translate into the competencies that would be necessary to complete an EBP project. Therefore, healthcare organizations, regardless of Magnet designation, need to focus on developing the EBP competencies of their staff. These competencies range from analysis of published studies to the implementation of an EBP workplace to sustaining a culture of EBP. Since the quality of care and the outcomes of care can be dramatically improved with the implementation of evidence-based nursing practices, nurses need to be supported in developing the EBP competencies to meet organizational goals.

EXERCISE 6.2 Select a practice guideline topic appropriate for implementation in your clinical setting. Select two guidelines on the same topic and determine which one might be more useful in your practice setting. Identify as many strategies as possible for disseminating the guideline's key points to direct care nurses at a clinical agency. Compare your list of strategies with that of a colleague. (Hint: Search the ECRI Institute for guideline topics, guidelines.ecri.org.)

COMPARATIVE EFFECTIVENESS RESEARCH

Although clinicians are concerned with identifying the best evidence for a practice, very often the benefits of a practice are unclear (Fig. 6.1). Comparing intervention effectiveness as well as the feasibility of implementation can aid in determining which intervention is the best one to use for a patient population. Comparative effectiveness research (CER) examines the evidence for the effectiveness, benefits, and harms of treatment options to improve the delivery of care and help with making

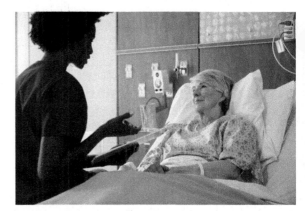

Fig. 6.1 The purpose of gathering and analyzing evidence is to improve patient care. (Copyright © monkeybusinessimages/iStock/Thinkstock.)

informed decisions to improve health and individual and population levels (Institute of Medicine, 2009). To understand CER, one needs to understand the difference between efficacy and effectiveness. Efficacy is when an intervention or treatment is tested in a rigorously designed research study such as a traditional randomized controlled trial (RCT). Careful attention is paid to internal validity, with carefully selecting the sample and consistency in delivering the intervention or treatment to determine whether it works. Once efficacy has been established, the next step is to test effectiveness—that is, determining what happens when the intervention is delivered in the real world of practice with variations in the setting and delivery of the intervention. CER, although it compares similar interventions, may also be considered part of research dissemination and implementation science. Many RCTs are considered CER studies because different interventions or doses of the intervention (e.g., number of treatments or length of treatment) are compared. An example of CER is an RCT study comparing a program, Mouth Care without a Battle, and standard care on the incidence of pneumonia in nursing home residents (Zimmerman et al., 2020). This study was a "pragmatic" trial conducted in seven intervention and seven nonintervention nursing homes in North Carolina over a two-year period. Significantly fewer cases of pneumonia occurred in the intervention group after the first year; the rate of pneumonia was higher, but not significantly so in the intervention group after the second year. This indicates that ongoing support may be needed for the sustainability of the mouth care intervention, which included instruction on the use of individualized techniques and products for mouth care. Although RCTs are commonly used in CER studies, many other designs can be used. These include large-scale observational studies, quasi-experimental (no randomization or double-blinding) studies and meta-analyses, and studies that mine data in electronic health records (EHRs).

PRACTICE-BASED EVIDENCE

With the growth of large databases, the use of EHRs, and sophisticated statistical techniques, examining practices in real-world situations and comparing the effectiveness of interventions is enhanced. Clinicians face challenges in achieving comparable outcomes to RCTs when trying to translate research into practice. Clinicians may also be faced with situations in which there are gaps in the literature resulting in the lack of definitive information about a course of action. Systematic reviews that include only RCTs may not always provide clear answers to a clinical question. Therefore, using evidence from a broader range of sources can provide direction for practice. For example, it would be unethical to conduct a clinical trial on the impact of e-cigarettes, yet we are learning about their harmful effects from population-based studies. Practice-based evidence (PBE) can help inform practice decisions by examining outcomes in the real world, which helps to close gaps in data in the absence of traditional RCTs. In clinical practice, patients may not be similar and the application of an intervention may have multiple variations. In PBE, the focus is on external validity, which answers the question of whether similar outcomes can be achieved in broader populations, in different settings, with different clinicians, and, most likely, limited resources (Vaidya et al., 2017). Quite often, PBE studies use observational designs comparing interventions on multiple outcomes in very large samples with study participants whose characteristics and care settings are diverse, mirroring real-world practice. Promising sources of evidence for PBE include participatory action research (PAR) and practice-based research networks, systematic reviews, and system science (Green & Allegrante, 2020). System science includes an examination of complex systems and how evidence-based strategies for improving health can be implemented within them. PBE designs need to be inclusive of stakeholders and a participatory approach that includes stakeholders in designing the research questions. As an example, this methodology was used in developing a protocol for the prevention of CLABSI in a pediatric oncology unit where the children are typically excluded from RCTs because of their higher risk for CLABSIs (Linder et al., 2017). A comprehensive analysis of research reports, their own data, and current practice standards led to the development of structured protocols, which when implemented led to a significant reduction in CLABSI rates.

Big data analytics can be used in PBE designs. It involves using technology to analyze large data sets to examine patterns and identify new relationships that, in turn, can be used to make improvements in healthcare. Big data involves four "v's"—volume, variety, velocity, and veracity—as illustrated in Box 6.1. Big data can be

---

BOX 6.1   Big Data's Four V's

Volume: Large quantities of data
Variety: Great variation in the data
Velocity: Data processing needs to occur close to the time of data acquisition
Veracity: Figuring out what are the true data and eliminating noise or artifact

descriptive (what happened), predictive (what might happen, or who is at risk), and prescriptive (action to impact outcomes). Nurse researchers are using big data science, drawing on multiple data sources in a variety of settings for research and to provide evidence-based care. For example, Park et al. (2020) used several machine learning methods that used EHRs and nurse staffing data to examine the relationships among factors associated with hospital-acquired catheter-associated urinary tract infections (HA-CAUTIs). The use of these methods can provide new insights that guide nursing practice. Nurses, when documenting their practice, generate large quantities of data that can be harnessed for making predictions about who might respond best to a certain intervention and for identifying the most promising interventions to be used for a patient with certain characteristics.

Big data analytics will be coupled with Connected Health (or C-health), which involves people using electronic devices, sensors, activity monitors, and other devices for remote patient monitoring. This generates vast amounts of data to be merged with data from more traditional healthcare sources. Nurses will need to understand how to use these data to provide individualized care for patients. Even though evidence-based practice centers have been established around the world that provide busy clinicians with high-quality evaluations of evidence, Zhu et al. (2019) make the case for the establishment of big data centers for nursing science in the Literature Perspective.

The promise of big data analytics linking personal and population data to make continuous improvement in the delivery of healthcare is the basis for what is known as a continuously learning healthcare system. The complexity and amount of data have increased exponentially, as has computing power. Learning healthcare systems use information from every interaction to continuously develop knowledge, provide feedback to patients and clinicians, and apply the best evidence to improve care (IOM, 2015). Learning healthcare systems use data and evidence to facilitate decision-making by patients and their healthcare providers by way of integration of healthcare improvement efforts with the science of implementation practice (Melder et al., 2020). They provide real-time access to knowledge, digital capture of the care experience, engaged and empowered patients, incentives for continuous improvement, transparency (making information available), strong leadership, and a supportive learning environment (IOM, 2013, p. 159). For example, in a learning healthcare system, potential errors in medication administration or handoffs could be identified so that system improvements can be made more quickly. Key stakeholders—including patients, frontline nurses, and nurse leaders—all have an integral role to play in the development of learning health systems. Nurses, in turn, will be able to practice more effectively because they are in a care environment that values the use of evidence in the delivery of care.

LITERATURE PERSPECTIVE

Resource: Zhu, R., Han, S., Su, Y., Zhang, C., Yu, Q., & Duan, Z. (2019). The application of big data and the development of nursing science: A discussion paper. *International Journal of Nursing Sciences, 6*(2), 229–234.

The authors make the case for big data in preventing the spread of disease, preventing waste of medical resources, and avoiding the high cost of health. They propose that the advancement of nursing science would be enhanced by big data centers that would have centralized processing, storage, transmission, exchange, and management. Such a center would integrate nursing science, informatics, analysis, and nursing research. A challenge in using big data is that different methods in each of these steps could result in different outcomes. A big data center for nursing science would help ensure the systematic uses of processes to interpret the data. Zhu et al. also point out challenges in using big data in that it describes relationships and not causality, may be incomplete, data sharing is incomplete, standardized terminology in nursing needs additional work, software limitations for nursing data, and insufficient numbers of nurses prepared in informatics.

Implications for Practice
Big data analytics has tremendous potential for the use of evidence in practice. For example, big data can be used to provide trend analysis to support decision-making and demonstrate nursing's value. The use of big data analytics in nursing is growing. Direct care nurses and nurse leaders need to understand the nature of big data so that they can advocate for its use to improve patient outcomes.

PARTICIPATORY ACTION RESEARCH

Participatory action research (PAR), sometimes also called community-based participatory research (CBAR), involves members from the community being studied, usually as part of an advisory board for a research project, to identify and refine (1) research questions, (2) strategies for engaging community members, and (3) potential challenges in carrying out the research project. The Patient-Centered Outcomes Research Institute (PCORI) recognizes the vital contributions of community stakeholders (patients, caregivers, clinicians, insurers, and more) by their inclusion as partners in every step of the research process so that the research is relevant to the community of interest (PCORI, 2018). The use of PAR is common in public health and community settings, but it is increasingly being expanded to other healthcare settings. For example, a rights-based PAR approach was used to create an innovative sexual health promotion intervention for young men in prisons, an often marginalized group that is at high risk for sexually transmitted infections, including HIV and viral hepatitis (Templeton et al., 2019). This involved listening to these young men and viewing them as the holders of rights, helping them to empower themselves. Nurses in the prison were considered to be duty bearers, that is, having a responsibility to provide appropriate sexual health education and treatment. The final outcome was a co-produced video tailored to the needs of these young men.[1] The PAR process included ongoing engagement of key stakeholders (young men in prisons and the nurses responsible for their care). Guiding principles for the collaboration included developing an active partnership, fostering co-ownership of the project, and building system change on local knowledge.

QUALITY IMPROVEMENT

Quality improvement uses an organization's data to improve both processes (how things are done) and outcomes, whereas evidence-based practice uses the best available evidence along with patient preferences to make clinical decisions, and research focuses on developing new knowledge. Quite often, these activities may overlap. For example, it is important to use validated tools to collect data for a quality improvement activity. Or, when beginning a new project, it may be critical to collect data beforehand so that you will know whether the results had an impact. The National Database of Nursing Quality Indicators (NDNQI), established by the ANA and now owned by Press Ganey, is used to collect data on nursing structures, processes, and outcomes, providing a comprehensive assessment of an organization's nursing care quality. The NDNQI includes data on nurse-sensitive outcomes such as falls, nosocomial infections, and pressure injuries. Nurse-sensitive outcomes are directly related to the quality of nursing care, in contrast to those outcomes that are more dependent on a multidisciplinary team effort. These measures also include nurse satisfaction and staffing. Hospitals receive unit-level data as well as benchmark comparisons with similar hospitals. This enables the staff to design practice improvement projects with standardized outcome measures. As might be expected, the NDNQI scores dropped during 2020 due to the severe staffing shortages as a result of the patient acuity from COVID-19.

Quality improvement projects often use EBP as a foundation for their activities. For example, a large medical center had established performance improvement (PI) teams for nurse-sensitive indicators (e.g., wound and skin care, CLABSIs, catheter-associated urinary tract infections). The teams had considerable experience in using evidence for quality improvement initiatives. The teams were mobilized for guidance in addressing quality issues related to altered care processes for patients with COVID-19 when they noticed an increase in healthcare associated infections in this population (Stifter et al., 2021). These experienced teams (frontline nurses, clinical nurse specialists, specialty nurses, leadership, and PI staff) examined their data, conducted intense case reviews, and then designed innovative strategies to maintain quality in the face of new circumstances and increased volume of patients. The experience of this facility necessitated by changes in caring for patients with COVID-19 demonstrated that a robust quality structure can facilitate the ongoing work that is needed to maintain quality. Physician specialty and other healthcare disciplinary organizations also collect quality indicators for specific procedures such as coronary artery bypass graft surgery and joint

---

[1] Available at https://www.youtube.com/watch?v=eXAWctsAKys& feature=youtu.behttps%3A%2F%2Fwww.youtube.com% 2Fwatch%3Fv%3DeXAWctsAKys&feature=youtu.be (short web address, https://tinyurl.com/yyar2hfs).

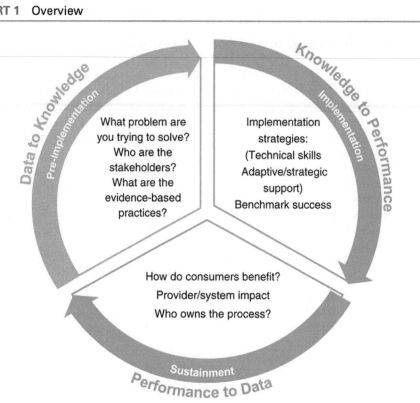

Fig. 6.2 Quality Enhancement Research Initiative Implementation Roadmap. (From Kilbourne, A. M., Goodrich, D. E., Miake-Lye, I., Braganza, M. Z., & Bowersox, N. W. [2019]. Quality Enhancement Research Initiative Implementation Roadmap: Toward sustainability of evidence-based practices in a learning health system. *Medical Care, 57* (10, Suppl 3), S286–S293. https://www.ncbi.nlm.nih.gov/pmc/articles/PMC6750196/figure/F1/.)

replacement to provide their members with benchmark data. The Quality Enhancement Research Initiative (QUERI) of the U.S. Department of Veterans Affairs is designed to use research evidence to improve practice. The complex process of implementing an EBP is illustrated by the QUERI roadmap (Fig. 6.2), which identifies strategies for pre-implementation, implementation, and sustainability to make practice improvements to enhance patient care (Kilbourne et al., 2019).

EVALUATING EVIDENCE

Frontline nurses and nurse leaders are called upon to take an active role in evaluating evidence, and integrating evidence into practice is an expected competency of professional practice. Evidence is best evaluated using a systematic process. EBP steps are illustrated in Box 6.2. The first steps are creating a spirit of inquiry and identifying the problem so that the relevant information can be obtained Melnyk and Fineout-Overholt (2019). Clinical questions should be put into the widely used PICOT

BOX 6.2 Steps of Evidence-Based Inquiry

0. Cultivate a spirit of inquiry.
1. Ask the burning clinical question in PICOT (**p**atient, **i**ntervention, **c**omparison, **o**utcome, and **t**ime frame) format.
2. Search for and collect the most relevant best evidence.
3. Appraise the evidence (i.e., rapid critical appraisal, evaluation, and synthesis).
4. Integrate the best evidence with one's clinical expertise and patient/family preferences and values in making a practice decision or change.
5. Evaluate outcomes of the practice design or change based on evidence.
6. Disseminate the outcomes of the EBP (evidence-based practice) decision or change.

From Melnyk, B. M., & Fineout-Overholt, E. [2019]. Making the case for evidence-based practice and cultivating a spirit of inquiry. In B. M. Melnyk & E. Fineout-Overholt [Eds.], *Evidence-based practice in nursing and healthcare: A guide to best practice* [4th ed.]. Philadelphia, PA: Wolters Kluwer.

TABLE 6.4   Asking the Right Question: The PICOT-D Format

Patient population	What is the patient population or the setting?
	This could be adults, children, or neonates with a certain health problem; or home, hospital, primary care, schools.
Intervention/ Interest Area	What is the intervention?
	This can be an intervention or a specific area of interest (e.g., electronic monitoring of self-care or postoperative complications).
Comparison	What is a comparison intervention?
	This might be a treatment or the absence of a risk factor (e.g., using social networks or group classes for diabetes self-management).
Outcome	What are the results?
	Measuring results can be accomplished with different methods. Sometimes, several methods are used to measure a single outcome. Examples may include complication rates, satisfaction, a nursing diagnosis, a nursing quality indicator, or completion of a rehabilitation program.
Time	What is the time frame for this intervention? Is time a relevant factor for this evaluation? For example, 1 week after discharge from a hospital, or 3 months later.
Digital	What data will be used? Where are the data located? What is the format for data extraction? Who are the data stewards from whom permission to use the data is needed? Examples of these might be readmission and chief nursing informatics officer.

From Elias, B. L., Polancich, S., Jones, C., & Conroy, S. (2015). Evolving the PICOT method for the digital age: The PICOT-D. *Journal of Nursing Education, 54*(10), 594–599.

format of *p*atient, *i*ntervention, *c*omparison intervention or group, *o*utcome, and *time* to facilitate searching for the appropriate evidence. Questions to be asked in developing a PICOT question are provided in Table 6.4. Identifying the question is often the most challenging step. Different strategies can be used to identify practice problems. One might conduct a survey of staff members or use a focus group methodology. The data from surveys or focus groups, or even informal interviews with staff, can be examined along with patient outcome data to address relevant practice problems. Collaboration between nurses and members of pertinent disciplines will enhance the success of an evidence-based project by early involvement in the project design and conception. When designing the PICOT question, additional consideration should be given to adding a digital component, making it into a PICOT-D question (Elias et al., 2015). This would include determining what data are to be used, the location of the data, data stewards (for permission to use the data), and format for extracting the data. If data are not easily obtained, then completing the project becomes labor-intensive, decreasing the likelihood of its completion. Once the clinical question has been identified, writing it down will help in moving on to the next step

of gathering evidence. Examples of questions to be asked using the PICOT-D format are provided in Table 6.4.

> **EXERCISE 6.3** Develop a clinical question using the PICOT (*p*atient, *i*ntervention [*i*nterest], *c*omparison, *o*utcome, and *t*ime) format. Do a search in PubMed or CINAHL with the key PICOT terms. Identify two potential sources of data that could be used to answer the clinical question.

Searching for Evidence

Searching for evidence is accomplished with effective database use. Some databases contain preprocessed evidence that has been synthesized and/or summarized, such as systematic reviews of evidence in addition to original single studies. Commonly used databases are listed in Table 6.5. Obtaining a librarian's assistance to navigate the databases is critical because identifying the correct search terms and taking advantage of new database features facilitates successful searching. Tracking search terms used provides consistency when using multiple databases. Preprocessed evidence can be found in the evidence-based resources listed in Tables 6.2 and 6.3.

TABLE 6.5   **Commonly Used Databases**

Database	Description
APA PsycINFO®	Abstract database of psychology and the behavioral and social science research literature from the 1800s to the present.
CINAHL: Cumulative Index to Nursing and Allied Health Literature	A comprehensive nursing and allied health abstract database that includes some full-text material such as state nurses association publications, nurse practice acts, research instruments, government publications, and patient education material from 1982 to the present.
Clinical Trials (clinicaltrials.gov)	Registry of publicly and privately supported clinical trials with human participants from around the world.
Cochrane Library (www.cochranelibary.org) Cochrane Database of Systematic Reviews (CDSR) Cochrane Central Register of Controlled Trials (CENTRAL) Database of Reviews of Effects (DARE) Cochrane Methodology Register (CMR) Health Technology Assessment Database (HTA) NHS Economic Evaluation Database	Six databases with different types of evidence and a seventh about Cochrane workgroups
EMBASE (https://www.embase.com)	Database for biomedical and pharmaceutical studies.
Google Scholar (https://scholar.google.com)	Contains scholarly literature, including articles, theses, books, court opinions, and online repositories.
MEDLINE (http://www.nlm.nih.gov/databases)	The largest component within PubMed, indexing over 5600 journals according to Medical Subject Headings (MeSH).
PubMed (https://pubmed.ncbi.nlm.nih.gov/)	The abstract database of the National Library of Medicine, providing access to over 26 million citations from the 1950s to the present. Includes ahead-of-print citations for articles.
PubMed Central (https://www.ncbi.nlm.nih.gov/pmc/)	Repository of full-text articles by participating publishers and authors complying with the NIH Public Access Policy. Linked with PubMed.
UpToDate (www.uptodate.com/)	Clinical decision resource for evidence-based practice.
Web of Science (https://clarivate.com/webofsciencegroup/solutions/open-access/	Publisher-independent global database with metadata links. Includes open access content.

An exhaustive and systematic review of multiple databases is necessary to obtain the latest and best evidence.

Evidence for a practice problem can come from a single research study, integrative literature review, meta-analysis, metasynthesis, clinically appraised topic, clinical guideline, or systematic review. Traditionally, evidence hierarchies (Fig. 6.3) have been used to guide evaluation, with evidence ranging from opinion at the lowest level to systematic reviews at the peak. Keep in mind that the hierarchy is fluid. With increased capacity to use large data sets for PBE and data analytics for real-time data analysis, observational data may provide powerful evidence for practice recommendations. No single established method of rating evidence is best for all situations. An evidence hierarchy can be used to compare the strength of the evidence when deciding which intervention might be the best. Researchers examining evidence and developing guidelines use a variety of different rating systems that include a hierarchy and key quality domains.

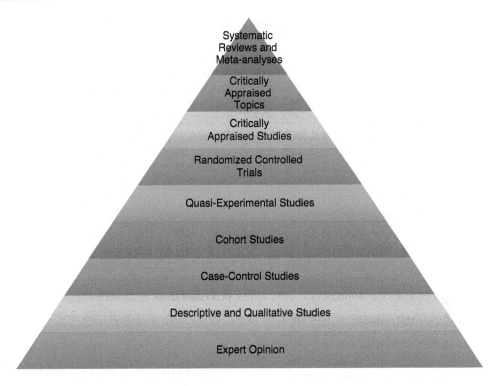

Systematic Reviews and Meta-analyses

Critically Appraised Topics

Critically Appraised Studies

Randomized Controlled Trials

Quasi-Experimental Studies

Cohort Studies

Case-Control Studies

Descriptive and Qualitative Studies

Expert Opinion

Systematic Review: Appraises evidence thoroughly in accordance with established standards and criteria

Meta-analysis: Synthesizes evidence using quantitative methods

Critically Appraised Topic: Evidence syntheses or clinical guidelines

Critically Appraised Study: Systematic appraisal of a single study

Randomized Controlled Trials: Experimental studies that include randomization and double-blinding

Quasi-Experimental Studies: Well-designed studies without randomization and/or blinding

Cohort Studies: Prospectively examine a population for a disease, outcome, or risk factor

Case-Control Studies: Compare people with a condition (cases) and those who do not have the condition (controls)

Descriptive Studies: Examine patterns occurring in a population

Qualitative Studies: Gain understanding of a phenomenon; develop theory

Expert Opinion: Opinions of authorities or experts in the field

Fig. 6.3 Hierarchy of evidence.

Appraising Evidence

Ultimately, when appraising multiple sources of evidence, nurses need to make decisions about the strength of the evidence and its application to a patient population. This is a critical step in focusing on the most valuable, relevant data for use in practice. Once the evidence is located, an appropriate and systematic method for rating or appraising the evidence is used along with analysis of its applicability to a clinical situation. Appraisal tools exist for evaluating different types of evidence from a single qualitative study, qualitative metasyntheses,

descriptive studies, randomized clinical trials, and clinical guidelines to systematic reviews. These tools generally include a series of steps for evaluating the quality of the research that is specific to the study design, type of review or guideline, and a strategy for determining the applicability of the evidence to one's practice.

Consistent with well-established hierarchies, much of the EBP literature has been devoted to evaluating randomized controlled trials (RCTs). These research studies include at least two groups and random assignment of participants to one group or another, either by a coin toss or by some other strategy, to test a treatment's efficacy. Preferably, such studies are double-blinded, with participants and those who are evaluating outcomes not knowing who has received the treatment. Although this design is generally considered the gold standard in terms of ranking individual studies, study quality is considered rather than merely the design. The number of RCTs conducted in nursing has been limited. In certain clinical trials, blinding recipients to interventions may be difficult to accomplish, as when delivering an intervention involving interaction with study participants. RCTs are not always an appropriate design for answering a research question and implementing them may not be possible for all of the research questions that need to be answered—for example, when evaluating the long-term consequences of vaping. Hence, appraisal methods need to include examining rigor and research quality in accordance with standards for that type of study.

Tools for Evaluating Vvidence

Consensus on checklists or guides for evaluating different types of research reports have been established by professional societies and interdisciplinary groups. See Box 6.3 for selected checklist resources for types of studies and guidelines that can assist in evaluating evidence

for nursing practice. Using these guides ensures that components critical to evaluation of rigor in study design is included in the appraisal process.

Checklists are usually designed so that a critical component's presence or absence is noted. It is also necessary to make a judgment about the strength of the evidence. The Grading of Recommendations Assessment, Development and Evaluation (GRADE) system, developed by consensus, is a widely used and well-established system to evaluate evidence (Neumann et al., 2016). The GRADE system evaluates evidence on a scale of high, moderate, low, and very low to indicate degree of certainty about evidence supporting a recommendation. Professional groups use grading systems for evidence when formulating practice recommendations for use in clinical guidelines. Grading the evidence is useful in making practice recommendations and in examining processes used to grade evidence, especially when two organizations have seemingly contradictory recommendations for clinical practice.

ASSESSING FOR APPLICABILITY TO PRACTICE

First, all research evidence needs to be examined, regardless of the studies included in the analysis, the types of study designs, their results, and appraisal systems used to evaluate them. Then, questions need to be answered about validity, reliability, and applicability of the findings. Validity answers the question of whether the results are true, that the study measured what it was supposed to measure because it was well designed (internal validity). Reliability answers the question of whether the similar results would be obtained if the study were repeated, such as if reliable instruments were used to measure the outcomes. Finally, if validity and reliability questions are answered, then it is possible to answer applicability questions: whether the study results can be applied to a patient population. Are the patients sufficiently like those in most of the studies examined? Is it feasible to make a practice change in a particular setting? What are the consequences of not making such a change?

Once evidence is appraised, new practice recommendations need to be integrated with clinical expertise and the preferences and values of patients, families, and communities in making the change. For example, in evaluating a research-based protocol for teaching

---

BOX 6.3   Selected Online Resources for Appraisal Checklists and Guides

Checklist Compilations
- CASP, Critical Appraisal Skills Programme Checklists: http://www.casp-uk.net/casp-tools-checklists
- EQUATOR Network, Enhancing the QUAlity and Transparency Of health Research: http://www.equator-network.org/

Internet Resources for Appraisal of Specific Research Designs
- AGREE, Advancing the Science of Practice Guidelines: https://www.agreetrust.org
- CONSORT, Consolidated Standards of Reporting Trials: http://www.consort-statement.org/
- PRISMA, Preferred Reporting Items for Systematic Reviews and Meta-Analyses: http://www.prisma-statement.org/
- SQUIRE, Standards for Quality Improvement Reporting Excellence: http://www.squire-statement.org/
- STROBE, Strengthening the Reporting of Observational Studies in Epidemiology: strobe-statement.org

oncology patients about preparing for a bone marrow transplant, the amount and type of information that would be desired by the patient need to be considered. In this instance, a qualitative research study might provide guidance for decision-making. For certain types of interventions, inclusion of patient preferences might not be appropriate, as in the example of implementing a protocol to reduce ventilator-associated pneumonia. However, frontline nurses need to be involved in planning the details. Determining patient preferences depends on the intervention's characteristics or change that is proposed.

The sheer quantity and complexity of information available illustrates the importance of frontline nurses and nurse leaders collaborating with nurse researchers. See Box 6.4 for an example of an academic–service partnership to promote the use of evidence in practice.

Frontline nurses and nurse leaders bring their clinical expertise, their assessment of clinically relevant questions, and their understanding of the patient population. Nurse researchers bring their capacity to appraise evidence to facilitate its application to the clinical setting. Together, practitioners and researchers can forge a partnership to develop an evidence-based solution to a clinical practice problem, which can then be systematically evaluated and disseminated to the wider community.

> **EXERCISE 6.4** Use the PubMed or CINAHL databases to search for a research study that has implications for your practice. Retrieve the full text of an original article to learn more about the patient population, details of the study design, outcome measures, results, and implications for practice.

BOX 6.4 Collaboration in Developing an Evidence-Based Protocol for Kangaroo Care

Clinician Perspective

We discovered there was interest in, but not common practice of, kangaroo care for premature babies. Many of the staff members in our facilities have a wealth of clinical experience. However, they really did not have the chance to learn about evidence-based practice in school. The students came to us to talk about our needs. When they finished their work, they presented their findings about the evidence for kangaroo care and thermoregulation at our regional perinatal center nursing leadership retreat. Initially, they were intimidated about presenting to a group of such experienced nurses. However, it was rewarding to see them become more confident about their work.

Since the student presentation, we have had an upsurge of interest in providing kangaroo care. It has helped us in overcoming resistance to its use. We are now working on how to most effectively implement kangaroo care because it takes concerted work and staff time to teach and prepare the parents. One of our hospitals is using the poster developed by the students as a training tool. I enjoyed working with the students in a way that produced a tangible outcome for everyone involved. Learning how to conduct research for evidence-based practice gave the students a skill that they will have as new nurses and can offer as a complement to their more experienced nursing colleagues as they begin their professional careers.

Sally Girvin, MPH, BS, RN, NP
Coordinator, New York Presbyterian Regional Perinatal Centers,
New York

Student Perspective

The eight of us who worked on this project were in the middle of our accelerated nursing program when it was assigned to us. We had to come up with an answerable clinical question, but because of our lack of clinical experience, we had only a vague idea of what to ask. We were able to develop our question after we talked with Sally and listened to her needs. We had spent some time in the neonatal intensive care unit and realized how hard it would be for the already busy nurses to take on this project. As students, we had the time.

When we went to the retreat to present our project, we thought no one would be interested in what we had done, that it might not be applicable, or that we had discovered something they already knew. The response was incredible. Our presentation created open debate. Some hospitals had kangaroo-care policies, some did not, some had them and did not follow them, and some people were unsure what they had in place. It really prompted people to look at their practices. It was a great experience to work with Sally and her colleagues and to see that what we did had an influence on policy. It was an experience that we can take with us wherever we go.

Elizabeth K. Kelly, BS, RN
Student at Columbia University School of Nursing, New York,
when this project was developed

TRANSLATION SCIENCE

Translation research and implementation science is known as translation science, the science of translating research into practice (TRIP). Translation science is a research area focused on testing interventions that are designed to facilitate using evidence to improve patient outcomes and population health and to determine what strategies work in a setting and why (Titler, 2014). *Translation science* is a term that is often used interchangeably with implementation science, which focuses on studying methods to facilitate the integration of research findings and evidence into healthcare policy and practice (Fogarty International Center, 2022). Numerous other terms are used, including *knowledge translation, knowledge uptake, knowledge exchange*, and *research utilization*, depending on the context and region of the world. Research is translated into practice on a continuum of diffusion-dissemination-implementation. Diffusion is an unfocused and passive adoption of new practices, dissemination is actively spreading new practices with specific strategies, and implementation is integrating practices into the care delivery processes of a clinical setting (Nilson, 2015).

> **EXERCISE 6.5** Review the Challenge at the beginning of the chapter and identify practices that would promote the translation of research findings into practice. Compare your strategies with those described in the Solution at the end of this chapter. What strategies do you think would be the most effective in sustaining the improvement over time?

Translating research into practice so that it becomes embedded in care processes involves careful planning and understanding of organizational dynamics and a commitment to seeing through all the intermediate steps. Frontline nurses and nurse leaders not only need to pay careful attention to the development of a clinical protocol or an evidence-based guideline but also must address the implementation process. When planning to translate a research finding into practice, considering what types of strategies have been most successful in implementing a practice in one's organization is important. For example, although results of a study protocol used in an RCT to decrease ventilator-associated events may have significantly improved patient outcomes, those same results may not be as dramatic when the protocol is implemented at institutions with varying resources and degrees of commitment to implementation. Even when evidence for a practice change is substantial, it might not be implemented in all settings. For example, details about the dorsogluteal intramuscular injection site have largely disappeared from fundamentals textbooks. Nurses in practice for many years might be unaware of the change, as dorsogluteal site instructions persist on the Internet. Some pharmaceutical companies still include the site as a recommended location in product literature for medications administered intramuscularly, and some healthcare agencies may still include the site in their procedure manuals. Therefore, it is important to not only embed the use of evidence into a practice setting but also to disseminate information about the EBP.

Strategies for TRIP can include using opinion leaders, educational programs, observations of behavior, auditing records, reminder systems, and incentives. It is necessary to determine how often and for how long a strategy should be used within an organizational context. For example, a neonatal fall/drop event is somewhat rare but has the potential to be devastating. A comprehensive newborn fall/drop event strategy was addressed with the creation of a newborn fall safety bundle by a multidisciplinary task force to be used in a healthcare system with a tertiary hospital, three community hospitals and four critical-access hospitals (Miner, 2019). Key to the strategy for implementation was treating all newborns as high risk for a fall/drop event and debriefing after such an event. Subsequently, fall/drop events were reduced from 6.66 to 4.06 events per 10,000 live births, with no events at the site for the pilot during the same time frame.

Choosing Wisely® is a program of the ABIM Foundation (a charitable arm of the American Board of Internal Medicine) designed to reduce unnecessary medical tests, treatments, and procedures. Professional societies representing different professional groups have identified questionable interventions and practices. Two examples of nursing practices identified as questionable include waking hospitalized patients at night when not clinically indicated and using restraints on hospitalized older adult patients (Choosing Wisely, 2021).

ORGANIZATIONAL STRATEGIES TO EMBED EVIDENCE-BASED PRACTICE INTO ORGANIZATIONS

Embedding EBPs into organizational systems and processes is challenging. Frontline nurses and nurse leaders need to work as partners in implementing EBPs. Frontline nurses bring knowledge of current clinical issues and nurse leaders bring knowledge of the organization in identifying how EBPs can be embedded into the organization. A strong shared governance program can facilitate these processes. The partnership between frontline nurses and nurse leaders needs to be extended to the executive level, interdisciplinary groups, and to the organization's stakeholders. For example, implementing a fall risk reduction program will not be successful without physician involvement, because physicians will need to be involved in reducing modifiable fall risk factors related to patient medications. Physical therapists are invaluable team members for a patient mobility program. Partnering with researchers can accelerate the implementation process and facilitate presenting evidence in a convincing manner. Providing key organizational decision makers with evidence regarding the safety of practices is critical for decision-making. Nurses can be highly effective in creating systematic approaches for decision-making processes related to EBP processes and for evaluating the system effectiveness.

Using a Framework

Integrating best evidence into practice can be facilitated by using a theoretical approach, model, or framework to understand complex interactions between clinicians and organizational leaders within the context of an organization's environment. These are important in helping nurses to understand barriers and facilitators of change within the context of their practice settings, which can then help in reducing the considerable evidence-to-practice time lag. Theories, models, and frameworks can guide specific strategies designed to enhance the implementation of an EBP. A scoping review conducted by Strifler et al. (2018) found nearly 600 studies that used 159 knowledge translation theories, models, or frameworks among them for change at the level of the individual, organization, community, and/or system. The Theory Box contains the key elements of the *integrated Promoting Action on Research Implementation in Health Services* (i-PARIHS) framework.

The complex factors that need to be considered by facilitators and activities that they carry out using the i-PARIHS framework (Harvey & Kitson, 2015) is illustrated in Fig. 6.4. Initially, facilitators focus on the nature of the innovation itself and then move the focus outward to the individuals who will be involved in implementing the innovation, the local context, and then the organizational context. Finally, the facilitator focuses on the external environment, examining regulatory and policy issues and interorganizational relationships and networks. The I-PARIHS framework can be used to understand what is most successful in implementing a practice change. Using the i-PARIHS framework, some of the questions that can be asked by nurses tasked with implementing an EBP include the following:

- How complex is the practice change? Does it require many steps to implement?
- How extensive is the education and preparation that nurses and members of other disciplines need for implementation?
- What type of support is provided by formal and informal nurse leaders?
- Are frontline nurses routinely included in planning proposed changes?
- What other resources are needed: staffing, financial, information technology?
- How will you know when you are successful? How will outcomes be measured?

THEORY BOX

Theory/ Contributor	Key Ideas	Application to Practice
i-PARIHS (Kitson & Harvey, 2016)	The framework focuses on the role of individuals in facilitating the innovation process. • Leadership role of facilitator to guide implementation • Variety of knowledge sources: research, clinical experience, patient preferences, local information • Recognition that some settings are more conducive to success • Using negotiation, shared understandings, and team approach	Success depends on quality and type of evidence (innovation), characteristics of the setting (context), and how evidence is introduced (impact on the individual)

Facilitator focus and activity

What the facilitator looks at
What the facilitator does

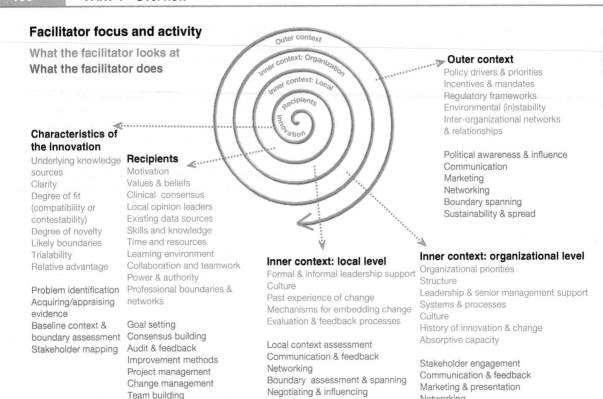

Outer context
Policy drivers & priorities
Incentives & mandates
Regulatory frameworks
Environmental (in)stability
Inter-organizational networks
& relationships

Political awareness & influence
Communication
Marketing
Networking
Boundary spanning
Sustainability & spread

Characteristics of the innovation
Underlying knowledge sources
Clarity
Degree of fit (compatibility or contestability)
Degree of novelty
Likely boundaries
Trialability
Relative advantage

Problem identification
Acquiring/appraising evidence
Baseline context & boundary assessment
Stakeholder mapping

Recipients
Motivation
Values & beliefs
Clinical consensus
Local opinion leaders
Existing data sources
Skills and knowledge
Time and resources
Learning environment
Collaboration and teamwork
Power & authority
Professional boundaries & networks

Goal setting
Consensus building
Audit & feedback
Improvement methods
Project management
Change management
Team building
Conflict management & resolution
Barriers/boundary assessment
Boundary spanning

Inner context: local level
Formal & informal leadership support
Culture
Past experience of change
Mechanisms for embedding change
Evaluation & feedback processes

Local context assessment
Communication & feedback
Networking
Boundary assessment & spanning
Negotiating & influencing
Policies & procedures
Structuring learning

Inner context: organizational level
Organizational priorities
Structure
Leadership & senior management support
Systems & processes
Culture
History of innovation & change
Absorptive capacity

Stakeholder engagement
Communication & feedback
Marketing & presentation
Networking
Boundary spanning
Negotiating & influencing
Policies & procedures

Fig. 6.4 The Promoting Action on Research Implementation in Health Services integrated framework (i-PARIHS framework): facilitation as the activity ingredient. (From *Implementing evidence-based practice in healthcare: A facilitation guide*, G. Harvey & A. Kitson. Copyright [© 2015] and Routledge. Reproduced by permission of Taylor & Francis Books, United Kingdom.)

- Can outcomes be measured without adding to nurses' workload?
- How will the project results be disseminated to key decision makers and stakeholders?
- Does the change have implications beyond the immediate practice setting?
- Will it be necessary to change policies, standards, or regulations?

Sustaining EBP in an organization requires leadership support, organizational capacity for EBP, and the capacity to implement specific practices. An important organizational impetus for EBP is The Joint Commission (TJC) with its annual publication of National Patient Safety Goals, which provide guidelines and bundles for their achievement. Bundles generally consist of 3 to 5 EBPs that have been shown to be grouped together and improve outcomes (Institute for Health Improvement, 2021). The challenge, however, is the extent to which nurses implement all of the bundle's elements. Connor (2018) found that pediatric nurses did not consistently implement all of the bundle elements for preventing CLABSIs and SSIs, with no differences between nurses in Magnet and non-Magnet facilities. The question raised is whether all of the bundle elements are necessary for achieving the outcomes and the extent to which fidelity to the elements impacts the outcomes. Successful implementation of EBP also includes integrating expectations for participation in EBP into job descriptions and recognition for EBP successes. Hospitals with Magnet Recognition® seek to provide an organizational environment that facilitates the implementation of EBP to improve quality.

EXERCISE 6.6 Using the information in Fig. 6.4 and the sample questions that should be asked using the I-PARIHS framework noted in the Theory Box, assess the capacity of your agency to implement an EBP. Identify one strategy to address a specific barrier to implementation.

BOX 6.5 Steps in Implementing an Evidence-Based Practice Change and Translating Research into Practice

1. Create an EBP team to develop and refine the PICOT question, evaluate the evidence, determine the change in practice, and develop a preliminary plan.
2. Identify stakeholders at the unit and organizational level.
3. Complete an environmental assessment of barriers and facilitators.
4. Develop a plan for minimizing barriers and enhancing facilitators.
5. Identify resources needed for implementation (e.g., staffing, information technology, data, publicity).
6. Refine the implementation plan.
7. Obtain necessary approvals (administrative, institutional review board).
8. Educate key stakeholders about the plan.
9. Implement the project.
10. Evaluate the outcomes.
11. Disseminate the results of the project to key stakeholders.

The consistent adoption of EBPs ultimately depends on a complex interaction of individual and organizational factors. Steps to implement an EBP change and TRIP are listed in Box 6.5. Nurse leaders are increasingly called upon to support individual nurses, implement strategies to enhance frontline nurses' use of evidence, and create an organizational infrastructure that promotes EBP.

ISSUES FOR NURSE LEADERS AND MANAGERS

Issues faced by nurse leaders and managers include lack of resources, limited staff expertise with respect to EBP, lack of knowledge about nursing research, and limited time for planning. Not all organizations can hire a full-time nurse scientist. Some organizations may not employ clinical nurse specialists (CNSs). This is shortsighted in view of the potential benefits CNSs provide related to improved patient outcomes and cost savings resulting from a reduction in adverse outcomes. However, this resource limitation is a reality faced in many organizations. Therefore, partnering with nurse researchers at a university could be invaluable. New graduates can partner with experienced nurses, who can demonstrate leadership skills and strengthen mentorship bonds. Faculty can partner with staff in a facility to provide consultation for a specific patient care problem, and agencies can partner together to address a specific practice problem.

COLLABORATION

Collaboration is critical to ensuring the success of implementation efforts. Collaboration can occur not only within an organization but also through practice-based research networks (PBRN) and data warehousing. Originally formed to address primary care research issues, PBRNs are being used in large healthcare organizations because they can integrate systems across multiple practice sites. Primary care PBRNs can register with the AHRQ. PBRNs have also been established to serve the needs of advanced practice registered nurses, school nurses, dentists, long-term care facilities, federally qualified health centers, and rural healthcare centers. The PBRNs share data to analyze common problems and make improvements in quality. Six large health systems, the Geisinger, GroupHealth Cooperative, Intermountain Healthcare, Kaiser Permanente, Mayo, and OCHIN are part of the Care Connectivity Consortium, which shares information across systems from their data warehouses. These warehouses have the capability of aggregating large quantities of data to facilitate analysis, reporting, and answering complex research questions. Frontline nurses and nurse leaders working in these settings can take advantage of these resources to obtain evidence that has immediate relevance for practice.

PREPARATION FOR EVIDENCE-BASED PRACTICE

Nurses' preparation for EBP is an organizational issue. Many nurses might not have had research or statistics courses in their basic nursing education or they had those courses many years ago. Even if nurses had research or EBP courses, they might not have had practice with the steps for developing EBP and implementing such practices into their daily workflow. New frontline nurses prepared with a bachelor's or higher degree have had research courses and more recent experience with EBP. Therefore, they are ideally suited to partner with more experienced nurses. A new nurse could assist in developing capacity for evaluating evidence by starting a monthly journal club. This involves reading a relevant research article and discussing how it might be applied to practice. Although nursing has general and specialty nursing research journals, *Evidence-Based Nursing*, *Worldviews on Evidence-Based Nursing*, and the *JBI Database of Systematic Reviews and Implementation Reports* are specifically devoted to EBP. *Implementation Science* is a journal devoted specifically to strategies for TRIP. Journal club discussions can be used to identify clinical practice problems. Healthcare system and university librarians can assist with gathering information and identifying articles.

The outcomes of EBP and TRIP initiatives need to be evaluated. Collecting outcome data before protocol implementation for a quality improvement activity is critically important in providing a subsequent basis for comparison. When implementing a protocol on one unit, consideration should also be given to the impact of staff casually talking with the staff working on other units. This might create competition, making it difficult to interpret the impact of the protocol. An important consideration is whether the implementation of an EBP project might be considered a research project. Considerable variation exists among institutions in the interpretation of what projects fall under the purview of the Institutional Review Board (IRB) and what is considered quality improvement (Carter, 2021). Therefore, consulting with the organization's IRB and/or quality improvement oversight committee early in the planning phase is critical. This ensures that ethical considerations have been addressed before implementation.

Nurses, other healthcare professionals, and the public might not be familiar with EBP. Publicizing positive outcomes of EBP efforts helps stimulate interest. When EBP is publicized in media or news alerts to colleagues in nursing and other disciplines, key organizational decision makers and stakeholders need to be notified.

Joining a professional association and signing up for alerts from key agencies provide nurses with access to the latest news, research, and standards impacting EBP. Specialty certification helps nurses to stay abreast of current practices and standards. Research evidence has a much better chance of being implemented if key stakeholders can understand its relevance. Sometimes, introducing important concepts in small increments can be effective. For example, a first step might be incorporating research into the revision of procedures and agency guidelines as they are reviewed. Subsequently, nurses and key stakeholders can be asked to identify clinical practice problems that create challenges in providing care to develop an EBP. Multiple strategies are needed for TRIP. They are also needed to change a culture to one that is driven by research and evidence-based standards for practice. Finally, if one should have the opportunity to implement an EBP, as much consideration needs to be given to planning for implementation using the change process as protocol development (see Chapter 15). Planning should include a thorough and frank discussion of how to minimize the barriers and maximize the facilitators of TRIP. Strategies to sustain the adoption of the practice over time need to be considered. Although the implementation of EBP is a very complex process, the increased emphasis on the use of sound evidence creates an exciting opportunity for frontline nurses and nurse leaders to demonstrate the value of nursing in improving patient care and healthcare outcomes.

CONCLUSION

Nurses are accountable to their patients to provide the best care possible. This means that nurses must translate research into practice. Numerous approaches to do so are possible. The challenge lies in more rapidly incorporating solid evidence into practice so that patients may benefit from that translation sooner than the current translation time of 17 years.

THE SOLUTION

The main challenge, as always, is getting buy-in from all parties, including staff, physicians, and others. We had to make sure everyone understood that this would not lead to anything punitive, nor were we just giving them extra work, but rather giving them the tools they needed for the best patient outcomes. We took the idea of the audits and the proposed process for them to our Unit Council for feedback about the proposed changes.

Observational audits were conducted over a period of two years and included four main parts. First was aseptic technique, which included those who scrubbed following policy, watching for possible contamination of the sterile field, appropriate surgical skin prep, and any excessive movement during the procedure. Second, counts were observed at the end of a case and during handoffs to ensure they were performed per policy. The third part concerned preparation for the case and included staff having all supplies and instruments, positioning devices, and anticipating the needs of the entire team. Lastly, we observed the universal protocol to ensure the timeout and all the components, including infection control practices, were being performed correctly and that staff were comfortable stopping the line when necessary. At first, staff thought we would be punitive if we found them doing something that was not best practice. But after we started, staff would come to us suggesting specific things that we should examine, such as skin preparation on multiple surgical sites or recommending surgical team members for further coaching. We encouraged staff to bring any issues, good or bad, or recommended changes back to the Unit Council.

Two other intraprofessional groups were also formed for specific specialty areas that had significantly higher infection rates. Both implemented several interventions found in literature reviews along with direct observation of those procedures to see if there were any breaks in sterile technique.

Since implementing these interventions, we have successfully and significantly decreased our SSI rates across the board, with zero infections for three types of surgeries. This was achieved by using a multifaceted approach and engaging all of those on the surgical team. Presently, we are overhauling these audits to continue the success we have shown so far. With continued observation, we hope to see even more consistently below national average SSI rates, but rates as close to zero as possible.

Would this be a suitable approach for you? Why?

Megan Lamoreux

REFLECTIONS

Think of a clinical practice problem on your unit where there is considerable variation in the nursing care provided, resulting in different outcomes among patients. To help you identify such a practice problem, think about when you have asked yourself, "Why are we doing this?" or "Why are we doing it this way?" Practices to consider are those that have (1) high volume, (2) important clinical outcomes, (3) significant adverse effects or safety implications, (4) reporting requirements for quality improvement or regulatory agencies, (5) serious financial implications, and (6) promote patient engagement through person-centeredness. What strategies might you use to bring this clinical practice problem to the attention of your colleagues and/or organizational leaders? Does the problem include other disciplines? If so, what can you do to facilitate collaboration and engage your colleagues in seeking solutions? What resources are available to you to determine the best EBP? What specific organizations might have standards to help guide your efforts?

BEST PRACTICES

Nurses' readiness for implementing EBP is important to the success of such programs. Numerous studies have been conducted across the globe to assess nurses' EBP competencies and their willingness to adopt EBPs. However, willingness to adopt EBP needs to be coupled with organizational support. Therefore, organizations embarking upon a formal EBP program need to conduct an assessment of their readiness for EBP. This will help to identify what is needed to prepare the nursing workforce for using EBP as well as well as organizational strengths that can be used to support a new program. Such an organizational assessment can also provide an assessment of opportunities for improvement in order to create a sustainable culture of inquiry (Pittman et al., 2019).

TIPS FOR DEVELOPING SKILL IN USING EVIDENCE AND TRANSLATING RESEARCH INTO PRACTICE

- Make a personal commitment to read articles reporting on research, EBP, and TRIP projects.
- Complete an online tutorial in EBP.
- Use your clinical experiences to develop relevant clinical questions.
- Obtain assistance from librarians, researchers, advanced practice registered nurses, and nurse leaders.
- Use the Patient, Intervention, Comparison, Outcome, and Time (PICOT) format to search for evidence on a clinical practice problem.
- Learn about your organization's sources of data that may be used to measure outcomes of care.

- Use a journal club to encourage your colleagues to join you in learning about EBP and evaluating research evidence.
- Examine EBP resources on a professional association's website.
- Volunteer to take part in a project that is focused on translating research into practice.
- Identify facilitators and barriers to translating research into practice in your setting and strategies to mitigate them.
- Volunteer for membership in an organization's shared governance council and/or quality improvement committees.

REFERENCES

American Association of Colleges of Nursing (AACN). (2021). *The essentials: Core competencies for professional nursing education.* https://www.aacnnursing.org/AACN-Essentials.

American Nurses Association (ANA). (2010). *Nursing's social policy statement: The essence of the profession.* Silver Spring, MD: Nursesbooks.org.

American Nurses Association (ANA). (2015). *Code of ethics for nurses with interpretive statements.* Silver Spring, MD: Nursesbooks.org.

Carter, E., Usseglio, J., Pahlevan-Ibrekic, C., Vose, C., Rivera, R. R., & Larson, E. (2021). Differentiating research and quality improvement activities: A scoping review and implications for clinical scholarship. *Journal of Clinical Nursing.* Retrieved from https://doi.org/10.1111/jocn.15668.

Choosing Wisely®. (2021). *Clinician lists.* Retrieved from http://www.choosingwisely.org/clinician-lists/.

Connor, L. (2018). Pediatric nurses' knowledge, values, and implementation of evidence-based practice and use of two patient safety goals. *Journal of Pediatric Nursing,* 41, 123–130. https://doi.org/10.1016/j.pedn.2018.04.003.

Eisenberg, S. R., Bair-Merritt, M. H., Colson, E. R., Heeren, T. C., Geller, N. L., & Corwin, M. J. (2015). Maternal report of advice received for infant care. *Pediatrics,* 136(2), e315–e322. https://doi.org/10.1542/peds.2015-0551.

Elias, B. L., Polancich, S., Jones, C., & Conroy, S. (2015). Evolving the PICOT method for the digital age: The PICOT-D. *Journal of Nursing Education,* 54(10), 594–599. https://doi.org/10.3928/01484834-20150916-09.

Fogarty International Center. (2022). *Implementation science news, resources and funding for global health researchers.* https://www.fic.nih.gov/researchtopics/pages/implementationscience.aspx.

Green, L. W., & Allegrante, J. P. (2020). Practice-based evidence and the need for more diverse methods and sources in epidemiology, public health and health promotion. *American Journal of Health Promotion: AJHP,* 34(8), 946–948. https://doi.org/10.1177/0890117120960580b.

Greiner, A. C., & Knebel, E. (Eds.). (2003). *Board on Health Care Services, Committee on the Health Professions Summit, Institute of Medicine. In Health professions education: A bridge to quality.* Washington, DC: National Academies Press.

Hanney, S. R., Wooding, S., Sussex, J., & Grant, J. (2020). From COVID-19 research to vaccine application: Why might it take 17 months not 17 years and what are the wider lessons? *Health Research Policy and Systems,* 18(1), 61. https://doi.org/10.1186/s12961-020-00571-3.

Harvey, G. & Kitson, A. (2015). Implementing evidence-based practice in health care: A facilitation guide. New York: Routledge.

Institute for Health Improvement (IHI). (2021). *Evidence-based care bundles.* http://www.ihi.org/Topics/Bundles/.

Institute of Medicine. (2009). *Initial national priorities for comparative effectiveness research.* The National Academies Press. https://doi.org/10.17226/12648.

Institute of Medicine (IOM). (2013). *Best care at lower cost: The path to continuously learning health care in America.* Washington, DC: National Academies Press.

Institute of Medicine (IOM). (2015). *Integrating research and practice: Health system leaders working toward high-value care: Workshop summary.* Washington, DC: National Academies Press.

International Council of Nurses (ICN). (2021). *The ICN code of ethics for nurses.* Revised 2021. Retrieved from https://www.icn.ch/system/files/2021-10/ICN_Code-of-Ethics_EN_Web_0.pdf.

Kilbourne, A. M., Goodrich, D. E., Miake-Lye, I., Braganza, M. Z., & Bowersox, N. W. (2019). Quality Enhancement Research Initiative Implementation Roadmap: Toward sustainability of evidence-based practices in a learning health system. *Medical Care, 57*(10, Suppl 3), S286–S293. https://doi.org/10.1097/MLR.0000000000001144.

Kitson, A. L., & Harvey, G. (2016). Methods to succeed in effective knowledge translation. *Journal of Nursing Scholarship, 48*(3), 294–302. https://doi.org/10.1111/jnu.12206.

Linder, L. A., Gerdy, C., Abouzelof, R., & Wilson, A. (2017). Using practice-based evidence to improve supportive care practices to reduce central line-associated bloodstream infections in a pediatric oncology unit. *Journal of Pediatric Oncology Nursing, 34*(3), 185–195. https://doi.org/10.1177/1043454216676838.

Melder, A., Robinson, T., McLoughlin, I., Iedema, R., & Teede, H. (2020). An overview of healthcare improvement: Unpacking the complexity for clinicians and managers in a learning health system. *Internal Medicine Journal, 50*(10), 1174–1184. https://doi.org/10.1111/imj.14876.

Melnyk, B. M., & Fineout-Overholt, E. (2019). Making the case for evidence-based practice and cultivating a spirit of inquiry. In B. M. Melnyk, & E. Fineout-Overholt (Eds.), *Evidence-based practice in nursing and healthcare: A guide to best practice* (4th ed., p. 17). Philadelphia, PA: Wolters Kluwer.

Melnyk, B. M., Zellefrow, C., Tan, A., & Hsieh, A. P. (2020). Differences between Magnet and non-Magnet-designated hospitals in nurses' evidence-based practice knowledge, competencies, mentoring, and culture. *Worldviews on Evidence-Based Nursing, 17*(5), 337–347. https://doi.org/10.1111/wvn.12467.

Miner, J. (2019). Implementation of a comprehensive safety bundle to support newborn fall/drop event prevention and response. *Nursing for Women's Health, 23*(4), 327–339. https://doi.org/10.1016/j.nwh.2019.06.002.

National Institute of Nursing Research (NINR). (n.d.). *Strategic plan.* Retrieved from https://www.ninr.nih.gov/aboutninr/ninr-mission-and-strategic-plan.

Neumann, I., Santesso, N., Aki, E. A., Rind, D. M., Vandvik, P. O., Alonso-Coello, P., et al. (2016). A guide for health professionals to interpret and use recommendations in guidelines developed with the GRADE approach. *Journal of Clinical Epidemiology, 72*, 45–55. https://doi.org/10.1016/j.jclinepi.2015.11.017.

Nilson, P. (2015, April 21). Making sense of implementation theories, models and frameworks. *Implementation Science, 10*(53). https://doi.org/10.1186/s13012-015-0242-0.

Ost, K., Blalock, C., Fagan, M., Sweeney, K. M., & Miller-Hoover, S. R. (2020). Aligning organizational culture and infrastructure to support evidence-based practice. *Critical Care Nurse, 40*(3), 59–63. https://doi.org/10.4037/ccn2020963.

Park, J. I., Bliss, D. Z., Chi, C. L., Delaney, C. W., & Westra, B. L. (2020). Knowledge discovery with machine learning for hospital-acquired catheter-associated urinary tract infections. *Computers, Informatics, Nursing: CIN, 38*(1), 28–35. https://doi.org/10.1097/CIN.0000000000000562.

Patient-Centered Outcomes Research Institute (PCORI). (2018). *The value of engagement.* Retrieved from https://www.pcori.org/engagement/value-engagement.

Parent-Child Relationship Programs at the Barnard Center. (2020). *About us.* Retrieved from https://www.pcrprograms.org/about/.

Pittman, J., Cohee, A., Storey, S., LaMothe, J., Gilbert, J., Bakoyannis, G., Ofner, S., & Newhouse, R. (2019). A multisite health system survey to assess organizational context to support evidence-based practice. *Worldviews on Evidence-based Nursing, 16*(4), 271–280. https://doi.org/10.1111/wvn.12375.

Polit, D. F., & Beck, C. T. (2021). *Nursing research: Generating and assessing evidence for nursing practice.* Philadelphia, PA: Wolters Kluwer.

QSEN Institute. (2020). *QSEN competencies.* Retrieved from https://qsen.org/competencies/pre-licensure-ksas/.

Specker, B. L., Minett, M., Beare, T., Poppinga, N., Carpenter, M., Munger, J., Strasser, K., & Ahrendt, L. (2020). Safe sleep behaviors among South Dakota mothers and the role of the healthcare provider. *South Dakota Medicine, 73*(4), 152–162. https://www.sdsma.org/SDSMA/Publications/South_Dakota_Medicine.aspx.

Stifter, J., Sermersheim, E., Ellsworth, M., Dowding, E., Day, E., Silvestri, K., Margwarth, J., Korkmaz, K., Walkowiak, N., Boudreau, L., Hernandez, L., Harbert, B., Ambutas, S., Abraham, A., & Shaw, P. (2021). COVID-19 and nurse-sensitive indicators: Using performance improvement teams to address quality indicators during a pandemic. *Journal of Nursing Care Quality, 36*(1), 1–6. https://doi.org/10.1097/NCQ.0000000000000523.

Straus, S. E., Richardson, W. S., Glasziou, P., & Haynes, R. B. (2011). *Evidence-based medicine: How to practice and teach EBM* (4th ed.). Edinburgh: Churchill Livingstone.

Strifler, L., Cardoso, R., McGowan, J., Cogo, E., Nincic, V., Khan, P. A., Scott, A., Ghassemi, M., MacDonald, H., Lai, Y., Treister, V., Tricco, A. C., & Straus, S. E. (2018). Scoping review identifies significant number of knowledge translation theories, models, and frameworks with limited use. *Journal of Clinical Epidemiology, 100*, 92–102. https://doi.org/10.1016/j.jclinepi.2018.04.008.

Templeton, M., Kelly, C., & Lohan, M. (2019). Developing a sexual health intervention with young men in prisons: A rights-based participatory approach. *JMIR Research Protocols, 8*(4), e11829. https://doi.org/10.2196/11829.

Titler, M. G. (2014). Overview of evidence-based practice and implementation science. *Nursing Clinics of North America*, *49*(3), 269–274. https://doi.org/10.1016/j.cnur.2014.05.001.

Vaidya, N., Thota, A. B., Proia, K. K., Jamieson, S., Mercer, S. L., Elder, R. W., et al. (2017). Practice-based evidence in community guide systematic reviews. *American Journal of Public Health*, *107*(3), 413–420. https://doi.org/10.2105/AJPH.2016.303583.

Zhu, R., Han, S., Su, Y., Zhang, C., Yu, Q., & Duan, Z. (2019). The application of big data and the development of nursing science: A discussion paper. *International Journal of Nursing Sciences*, *6*(2), 229–234. https://doi.org/10.1016/j.ijnss.2019.03.001.

Zimmerman, S., Sloane, P. D., Ward, K., Wretman, C. J., Stearns, S. C., Poole, P., & Preisser, J. S. (2020). Effectiveness of a mouth care program provided by nursing home staff vs standard care on reducing pneumonia incidence: A cluster randomized trial. *JAMA Network Open*, *3*(6), e204321. https://doi.org/10.1001/jamanetworkopen.2020.4321.

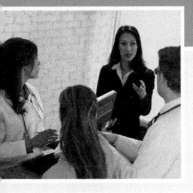

Gaining Personal Insight: Being an Effective Follower and Leader

Amy Boothe and Jeffery Watson

ANTICIPATED LEARNING OUTCOMES

- Value the need to gain insight into one's self to develop leadership capacity.
- Determine how insight into personal talents and abilities can help nurses be effective/resilient in their role of nurse and leader.

- Envision the goals of the Quintuple Aim.
- Differentiate between Leader, Effective Follower, and Ineffective Follower.
- Examine the characteristics and roles of Leader and Effective Follower within a healthcare team.

KEY TERMS

authentic leadership
effective follower
emotional intelligence
formal leadership
ineffective follower

informal leader
journaling
leader–follower relationship
moral courage
personal leadership

Quintuple Aim
reflection
value

THE CHALLENGE

Several months into my nursing career, I encountered a situation that would make me question current practices. As a newborn nursery nurse, I frequently had infants who struggled with low blood sugars after delivery. It can take several days for a newborn to acclimate to life outside the womb and so it is crucial to frequently assess infants for signs of distress. In an effort to address blood glucose issues, our unit had a hypoglycemia protocol that served as an algorithm for nurses to follow in the event that an infant's blood sugar started to drop. One sign we constantly assessed for was low temperature. In most instances, we would take temperatures twice a shift with a thermometer that could be purchased in any local pharmacy. This would allow new parents to become comfortable with using this tool and we could educate them on how to take an infant's temperature. If a newborn was in the nursery being assessed, we would frequently use a hospital-grade thermometer.

We had changed thermometer models and I began to notice that many of my babies began to be put on frequent blood sugar checks due to low temperatures. There had been conversations about this trend among nurses, but

(Continued)

nothing had really been done to address this issue. The general thought was that we were just experiencing a larger group of infants who had difficulties maintaining their glucose levels. The increase in blood sugar checks on infants had a negative effect on patient satisfaction. Parents were distressed that infants were having to have blood drawn frequently to ensure that blood sugars were stable.

During my assessments, I began to carry the hospital-grade thermometer with me to see if there was a difference in readings between the two types. What I began

to discover was that, at times, the generic thermometer would read 0.5 to 1 degree lower than the hospital-grade thermometer. This slight variation made a huge difference in whether or not an infant was placed on a hypoglycemic protocol.

What would you do if you were this nurse?

Amy McCarthy, MSN, RNC-MNN, NE-BC
Director of Nursing, Women and Infants Specialty Services,
Parkland Health and Hospital System

INTRODUCTION

Approximately 4 million people in the United States are registered nurses. That number seems enormous when we think of the numbers in other healthcare disciplines. Because we are so large in numbers, we have additional obligations in healthcare. One of those obligations is to capitalize on the role of leading and following in any position so that quality care is rendered.

Leadership is a journey. It is an iterative process, one that may take twists and turns and always contributes to our learning if we exhibit intentionality in our approach to learning. It begins with being an effective follower, and it never ends. Our task is to continue to develop personally and professionally so that our talents match the tasks we need to address, which evolve over our careers.

All members of the healthcare team have worked in a follower role at one point or another within their careers. However, being in a follower role does not place people into a passive or submissive role in which their thoughts and ideas are not valued. Being an effective follower means that you courageously challenge or champion leaders based on complex situations that arise within the healthcare environment (Chaleff, 2017). The relationship between leaders and followers is extremely important in the effectiveness of the entire team. Effective followers develop into effective and authentic leaders and managers with the experiential knowledge of how to create a constructive and trusting environment.

Being proactive about learning is a key strategy to developing effective followership that may evolve into effective leadership. We have to be mindful of our actions and the motivations behind those actions. The follower can either advance the leader's goals or divert and limit

progress. As an example, some people think about leadership in terms of power, "being in charge," and fame and glory. When someone exerts leadership from that perspective, the individual may have followers, but they commonly are not really engaged with the mission of the work they are doing. They may even behave very differently depending on the physical presence of the leader. An opposite example is when leadership derives from the desire to help others be their best. When leadership is exerted from that perspective, followers are engaged in the mission of their work and they behave consistently—with or without the formal leader being present.

Our task in leadership is to promote a focus on person-centered or population-centered care to provide the most accessible, inclusive, least costly, and highest-quality outcomes. To achieve that, we need the vision of each of us contributing something critical to the work at hand. In this view, leadership is shared. This means that one person may hold a title that conveys a position of ultimate authority, yet each person has the potential to step forward and lead when that person is the one most capable of supervising a particular element of work. Diversity in leadership can fuel healthcare organizations into caring for diverse populations within each community. This chapter explores established tools and strategies that will help you develop into an effective follower and leader.

DIFFERENCES BETWEEN LEADING AND FOLLOWING

Leading and following can be visualized within any organization, especially within healthcare organizations.

If we look into the behaviors of leaders and followers, we can dive into how they are used within nursing practice. We can see some differences and similarities in the characteristics of each one.

Leaders

When people think of leadership, they typically think of position. Those types of positions have official-sounding titles: president, chief executive, director, and the like. That type of leadership is positional and, therefore, formal. The assumption is that people in formal leadership roles exert influence over others and that they are "in charge." Within healthcare organizations and nursing practice, the word *leader* describes a person who does so much more. A leader within this context guides and gives direction to those who are perceived to be subordinate or reliant on them. The nursing leader performs the courageous act of releasing control to create an active learning and engaging environment. This release of control allows leaders to share the accountability of decision-making with other people within their supervision (Alegbeleye & Kaufman, 2020). Sharing accountability fosters a partnership of trust between leaders and team members or followers. Leaders supervise by inspiring team members to speak up and voice their opinions and concerns. The leader can handle and adapt to the unknown. Different leadership styles emerge during different crises and everyday situations.

Followers

Within nursing, followers are often the direct care or frontline nurses who are trusted to think critically, ask probing questions about care, and advocate for the patient. When we think about leadership, we often think only of one element of the equation—the leader. Yet without the follower role, leadership does not actually exist.

Another term for follower is informal leader. Informal leaders are those individuals who influence others because they are engaged with those who listen to and follow the informal leaders. These individuals are often the "behind the scenes" and "go-to" people who motivate others to act (Heard, 2018). They are more accessible to their coworkers and provide critical thinking, innovation, and ideas that support their organizational goals (Heard, 2018). Wise formal leaders acknowledge that they do not have all the answers and, thus, look to their informal leaders or followers, whose talents may differ from their own.

> **EXERCISE 7.1** Name five characteristics of a great leader. Think about a nursing leader you have observed. Does that person match those characteristics? Now, name five characteristics of a great follower. Have you seen a follower exhibit those characteristics? How are the two sets of characteristics similar? How are they different?

Effective Followers

The phrase effective followers identifies engaged and participating team members who think for themselves. Effective followers identify the practical aspects of nursing, provide input when needed, and ask questions to clarify. They have positive attitudes and support the leaders within their organization. Effective followers need leaders who foster professional growth. In return, effective followers can also influence the leader by using intelligent and experience-driven suggestions to solutions about patient care (Falls & Allen, 2020). Effective followers are loyal to the organization, fostering partnerships and supporting leadership in every area of nursing. Followers have the ability to self-manage; have commitment to their organizations; and have competence, focus, and courage (Watters et al., 2019). The effective follower has the potential to not only influence the leadership but also influence coworkers within the healthcare organization. Positive attitudes can be contagious and increase the morale of the entire unit and team. Fostering this type of atmosphere will most likely increase productivity and patient outcomes.

Ira Chaleff describes the courage it takes to become an effective follower within an organization. In these circumstances, followers use their own self-awareness when they courageously question or challenge leaders. Chaleff developed a self-assessment for followers to explain these behaviors. The intent of the self-assessment is to identify behaviors among followers that encourage reflection. Chaleff (2017) stated that this is a way to develop followers and help them identify the style of follower they are in order to move into an effective follower role (see the Literature Perspective).

LITERATURE PERSPECTIVE

Resource: Chaleff, I. (2017). In praise of followership style assessments. *Journal of Leadership Studies, 10*(3), 45–48.

The roles of the leader and follower are not always static. Most team members will occupy both roles interchangeably or simultaneously within the organizational setting. Chaleff describes the ability to move fluidly into and out of these roles as an area in which self-assessment of behaviors should occur. These assessments can be oriented toward the individual, group, or culture. The result will help identify what is needed to know about followers and how they react within their environment.

Implications for Practice

To be effective in any teamwork, all members of the team must be effective at what they do. Additionally, because leadership is shared and fluid, a leader must be equally capable of transitioning into the role of follower as the follower is in transitioning into the role of leader.

Ineffective Followers

The term ineffective followers describes static team members who rely solely on leadership for all direction and guidance (Malak, 2016). They do not challenge or champion leadership and have a hard time voicing their opinions or concerns because of the traditional hierarchy. The way that ineffective followers communicate is through complaining and pointing fingers—they hardly ever offer solutions. Ineffective followers are not flexible, and their main concern is putting in only their required number of hours. Ineffective followers who have gained influence can alter the workplace culture, placing different demands on the team and leader (Watters et al., 2019).

EXERCISE 7.2 Think of a time when you were involved in a great work relationship. What made the relationship great? Was it hierarchical, in which one person was always the leader and the other was always the follower? Or was it "give and take" depending on the situation? What kind of trust was present? Were you afraid to voice your opinion? Did the other person value your opinion?

LEADER–FOLLOWER RELATIONSHIP

Great leadership requires great followership. For a long time within healthcare organizations, the hierarchy of leaders and followers did not permit the development of the leader–follower relationship. The leaders were the source of knowledge and power, and the followers were submissive. This was more like a dictatorship than a true working relationship. Fortunately, a shift in thinking occurred away from hierarchies because, within a successful healthcare team, all members are active and contribute to the leadership processes and behaviors. In modern healthcare today, the relationship between leaders and followers is a true partnership built on trust and accountability. Communication opens up the engagement, increases the trust, and increases the influence to and from both leaders and followers within this relationship (Varpio & Teunissen, 2021).

"All team members are leaders and followers; together collaborators create the relationships that enable (or inhibit) success" (Varpio & Teunissen, 2021, p. 5). Simplifying this statement, leaders can become followers and followers can become leaders depending on the situation and expertise and experience of the nurse. With this knowledge, the emphasis on understanding the leader–follower relationship is more important to create a cohesive and productive team. Trusting and cohesive partnerships between leaders and followers are necessary in creating a safe, team-based work environment. This understanding helps new graduates to develop the capacity for leadership as required by the 2021 American Association of Colleges of Nursing (AACN) baccalaureate essentials.

A cohesive relationship between leaders and followers can reduce skill-based errors because followers are not afraid to challenge leaders by asking questions and speaking up about possible mistakes or missed steps. When the formal leader and the follower(s), or informal leader(s), are in concordance, great outcomes can be produced. When these relationships do not exist, a lot of energy is expended on working around the other person(s) and creating an appearance of productivity rather than actually being productive. The path to authentic leadership starts with being an effective follower. Most of the strategies seen in authentic leaders are mirrored in the characteristics and strategies of an effective follower. Box 7.1 lists the characteristics of both authentic leaders (Rosler, 2018) and effective followers (Chaleff, 2017; Falls & Allen, 2020). From the information in Box 7.1, we can see how the characteristics among authentic leaders and effective followers complement each other within the workplace. We will learn more about becoming an authentic leader later in this chapter.

BOX 7.1   Comparing Authentic Leader Characteristics and Effective Follower Characteristics

Leader	Effective Follower
Knows what they stand for	Understands values and principles
Understands strengths and weaknesses	Understands strengths and weaknesses
Leads by example	Leads by example
Is open and honest in communications	Engages in open and honest communication
Is true to individual values	Speaks up when ethical concerns arise
Admits when they do not know something	Asks thought-provoking questions
Considers input from all viewpoints before making a decision	Makes decisions based on the right thing to do
Is objective	Faces the fear of rejection and ridicule to speak up for the right thing
Knows the right thing to do, then does it	Knows the right thing to do, then does it

From Rosler, G. [2018]. Your journey to authentic leadership. *American Nurse Today, 13*(2), 40–41. https://www.myamericannurse.com/journey-authentic-leadership/; Chaleff, I. (2017). In praise of followership style assessments. *Journal f Leadership Studies, 10*(3), 45–48. https://doi.org/10.1002/jls.21490; Falls, A., & Allen, S. (2020). Leader-to-follower transitions: Flexibility and awareness. *Journal of Leadership Studies, 14*(2), 24–37. https://doi.org/10.1002/jls.21696.

THE CORE OF BEING A LEADER

Personal leadership is an integration of you, your ideas, and your personhood into the path you set for your life. It is the ability to lead from your core values and beliefs. Leadership is not a part that you play to fulfill a role responsibility; rather, it is a role responsibility that comes to life because of who you are. Incorporating your unique qualities into the role of leader is a function of both living and learning. Fig. 7.1 suggests that being a nurse is integral to who we are as individuals and that being a leader overlaps both nurse and person because we can exert leadership in our personal and professional lives. We are the sum of our life experiences, bringing the fullness of our personhood to the other roles we fulfill. In this case, we are referring to the role of nurse and leader.

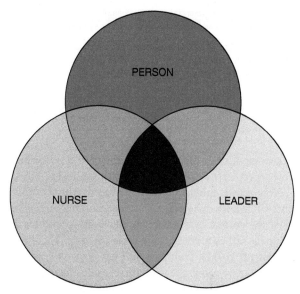

Fig. 7.1 Leadership integration.

Sometimes, all three elements intersect, indicating that all of the roles we assume in life are influenced by all others.

Kouzes and Posner (2017) developed one of the most widely used models for considering leadership (see the Theory Box). Although this model is used widely in other fields, the key for us is that it is used widely in nursing and healthcare. The five elements of their model begin with *modeling the way*. This means that if we want others to be civil, we must be civil to others. *Inspire a shared vision* is an expectation of a formal leader, yet effective followers contribute to this by taking such actions as translating a big-picture vision to the practicalities faced by team members. Members of the team, any of whom may exhibit leadership, have the obligation to *challenge the process*. We can all do this by asking questions or posing scenarios to help clarify how something is possible across a wide range of situations. *Enable others to act* refers to how we help others find the conditions that allow them to do their best. Finally, *encourage the heart* is about creating a positive work environment and self-renewal. Think for a moment about the feedback you receive. We expect feedback from those "above" us, such as team leader, manager, or clinical director. The question is: Do you provide that same type of feedback to your leader? People in leadership positions are in "the middle" between those they are accountable for and those they are accountable to. They receive feedback from those to whom they report. An opportunity to exert leadership is to provide feedback to those individuals who seldom

THEORY BOX

Theory/Contributor	Key Ideas	Application to Practice
Kouzes and Posner: The Leadership Challenge (2017)	Model the way. Inspire a shared vision. Challenge the process. Enable others to act. Encourage the heart.	This approach to leadership provides a view of how to lead and develop others and how to remain personally relevant in leadership.

receive input from those to whom they are accountable. How powerful you can be if you take this model to heart!

How do we enhance our current leadership competency? The answer begins with understanding one's self.

At the core of both effective followership and leadership is self-awareness. In his classic text, *The Four Agreements* (1997), Don Miguel Ruiz presents a set of agreements we can make with ourselves to enhance personal growth and awareness. These agreements focus on how we present ourselves to self and others and how we act in and interact with the world around us. They also can serve as the core of who we are as leaders (Table 7.1).

Be impeccable with your word means to always speak with integrity about yourself and others. As leaders, we must use language that reinforces integrity of practice and honors humanity. We demonstrate leadership when we speak in truth and follow through on our words. One of the most difficult agreements to master is *don't take anything personally*. What others say is reflective of their reality, not yours. You will encounter numerous opinions about you, your work, your ideas, your philosophies, and so forth. Deliberately destructive communications can be found in toxic environments where incivility is tolerated. Although personally based, these communications actually say more about the originator than the target.

In conversations, having the willingness to ask clarifying questions leads to success in the third agreement, *don't make assumptions.* Assumptions are created by your imagination when clear communication fails. Asking clear follow-up questions and listening with a desire to understand fills in the gaps where assumptions take hold. The fourth and final agreement is to *always do your best.* Numerous factors influence how you feel from day to day and even hour to hour. Yet you can commit to doing your best in each circumstance. You are able to release any looming self-judgment because you have put forth your best effort. In other words, you have good days, bad days, and in-between days. On each of those days and, indeed, in varying moments throughout the day, your best will vary. Yet, at the end of the day, you want to be able to say, "I did my best." Does that mean we would tolerate "I'm doing my best" (and having a bad day) as rationale for subpar performance? Of course not! The intent of this agreement is to strive to do our best every day.

TABLE 7.1	**Application of Ruiz Four Agreements**
Ruiz Four Agreements (1997)	**Effective Follower and Leader Implications**
Be impeccable with your word.	• Listening and engaging in discussion are vital trust-building activities. • Being honest with yourself and others is foundational to developing trust and reliability as an effective follower and leader.
Don't take anything personally.	• Personalizing every comment or action others make disrupts critical thinking. • Realizing opinions are not about you but are rather a reflection of the person voicing those views frees you from self-imposed judgment.
Don't make assumptions.	• Overcoming assumptions requires asking deeper questions to get the needed clarity. • Avoiding misunderstandings in healthcare is vital because of the risk to the health and safety of human life.
Always do your best.	• Committing to always doing your best acknowledges your humanness. • Doing your best enhances group performance by acknowledging where we are in our performance.

GAINING INSIGHT INTO SELF

Many organizations and educational programs address the task of developing leaders. Although we encourage you to explore and select those that meet your personal needs, our attempt here is to use broad concepts plus readily available, and least costly, strategies to help develop your insight into self. You may choose to use any of these strategies that fit your needs. The key point is that resources exist to help you understand who you are; capitalizing on the information those resources provide can enrich your talents as a leader.

Reflection and Reflective Practice

Developing leadership comes from knowing and understanding your authentic self (Kouzes & Posner, 2017). Learning from experience is a critical skill in developing your potential for leadership. Reflection, exploring the thoughts you have about your experiences, actions, and reactions, is an active process you can use to strengthen your ongoing professional growth. In his foundational work, Schön (1983) described reflection from two different perspectives: *thinking-in-action* and *thinking-on-action*. Thinking-in-action occurs when an individual employs existing knowledge to guide behaviors as a situation develops. Thinking-on-action is a recounting of the situation, inviting self-evaluation (Schön, 1983). We often think-in-action as we provide nursing care. We are not as diligent about thinking-on-action afterward (debrief or reflection). Adding this strategy can create new insights and lead to more effective performance.

Consider a cardiac arrest event in an acute care setting. The decision-making occurring in the midst of cardiopulmonary resuscitation (CPR) is an example of thinking-in-action. A post-CPR debriefing, reviewing all aspects of the event after the fact, is thinking-on-action—giving thoughtful consideration to individual and group performance as well as to any technical issues influencing the outcome. The same type of thinking occurs when you are in a situation in which you think harm may occur and you intervene immediately. How you decided to act and what you decided to do are thinking-in-action. After the fact, you consider the many factors leading up to the situation, what else you might have done (or done differently), and what you will do the next time such an event occurs. That is an example of thinking-on-action.

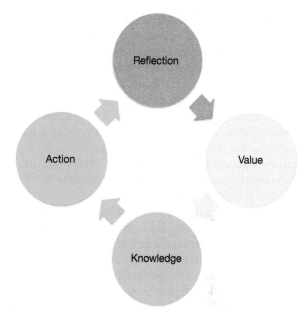

Fig. 7.2 The impact of reflection.

Reflection helps you assess the effect your choices have on both yourself and on those around you. Numerous models have been developed to guide reflection and reflective practice. Fig. 7.2 identifies four basic stages that are common to most reflective practice models: reflection, value, knowledge, and action.

The thinking-on-action type of reflection starts when you begin to think about the activities of the day. You may choose to take a broad view or focus on a single specific event. The list of questions in Exercise 7.3 is not exhaustive. However, you will notice that each experience you have invites other deeply personal questions as you explore the core of who you are as a leader.

> **EXERCISE 7.3** Think of what you did yesterday. You may have been in a clinical setting, at a religious service, out to dinner with friends, or at a meeting. As you do so, consider asking questions of yourself to guide the reflection: What happened? Why did I respond the way I did? What precipitated my behavior? Were my values in conflict with others? Did I honor the view of others?

In contemplating and grappling with probing questions, you release yourself to value specific aspects of each experience. Understanding develops about why you felt the way you did in the moment. You have the freedom to study the sources of input that influenced your behavior. You can contemplate different choices that might yield other outcomes. Over time, awareness is raised of your own conduct and you begin to distinguish more effective patterns for interaction.

Awareness is essential; however, successful leaders go well beyond being aware. Building on self-awareness, leaders cultivate personal insight and new knowledge. A key question at this stage of reflection is: What have I learned about myself and how can I take this knowledge into the future? Leaders embrace new knowledge, making sense of the events of the past and present to develop a plan of action for the future. For example, if you accept that learners learn in different ways, you do not simply tell your team something collectively. You find ways to provide something from the key senses to engage each member in gaining the knowledge you are sharing. You may use a graph to show progress of a new intervention. You may talk with your team about the importance of this work. You might even ask them to manipulate equipment to develop the sensation of a psychomotor skill.

The ultimate goal of reflection is to bolster your leadership acumen. The final stage of the process is action—putting what you have learned into practice. The action stage of reflection is where you test the new knowledge you have gained about yourself. You may discover only incremental improvement toward the desired outcome. If this is the case, you need not worry. With each cycle of reflection, you increase your understanding of the leader within. Reflection as part of leadership development is a lifelong iterative process. After you act, you recycle through the process again to learn more about what your values are, what knowledge you gained, and what action modifications or replacements you will test next.

A common outcome of reflection in your early stages of development is to focus on what not to do. Actively considering what *to do* is equally beneficial and often more reinforcing to us. For example, think about when we started telling people to stop smoking. We did not tell them what to do, just what *not* to do. As a result, some people who smoked assumed the habit of using chewing tobacco. The point about the harmful effects of tobacco was lost in the focus on what to stop. The incorporation of reflection on a regular basis, however, allows us to move from a narrow thinking of what not to do to the broader thinking about possibilities and what fits with our values.

Reflection occurs through a variety of formats. The cognitive and emotional benefits of writing down our thoughts are well known. Thus, journaling, also known as reflective journaling, is a method to support self-confidence, critical thinking, and resilience (Horton et al., 2021). Journals allow you to retrace your thinking and to see improvements in your thinking actions over time.

Because journaling is an individual exercise, you have flexibility to write in your journal at any time. You may choose a simple notebook or an e-journal. You might also choose from a variety of guided journals that contain focused themes and questions designed to help direct your thinking. Writing in a journal may feel unnatural at first. Box 7.2 describes basic considerations for an individual who is just beginning to journal.

Regardless of the way that you choose to practice reflection, by committing time and energy to this practice you allow yourself an opportunity to grow in clarity around your own beliefs and values and your philosophies about nursing and the core of leadership. You become more adept at integrating the person you are into the professional role of nurse and leader. Reflection is a foundational skill needed to move each of us along the path from individual thought leader to nursing thought leader. Think about it!

BOX 7.2 Tips for Creating a Personal Journal

1. Determine whether you are going to use a hard copy journal or whether you are going to do this electronically.
2. Consider finding a space that is comfortable—a place where you can concentrate.
3. Create an entry as soon as possible after an important event so you can remember details, including how you felt.
4. Write in the first person—it is your journal. And don't worry about spelling, etc. Be sure to use abbreviations that are clear to you.
5. Focus on lessons learned. After you make an entry, you need to answer two questions: So what? and What if? "So what" asks whether this was life-changing (or practice-changing) and what you will do. "What if" addresses the idea of alternative thinking so you consider different contexts, players, outcomes, and other ideas.

> **EXERCISE 7.4** Conduct an Internet search about methods and tools for reflection or reflective practice. Explore what resources are available. What strategy for reflection made sense to you? Consider how routine reflective practice might be used to enhance your individual leadership ability.

Emotional Intelligence

For years, we have focused on test scores, the most common being intelligence tests. Those tests, such as the GRE (Graduate Record Examination) or SAT (Scholastic Assessment Test), are typically used to determine a person's ability to be successful in a graduate program or undergraduate program, respectively. Emotional intelligence (EI, or EQ as it is known by some) tests or assessments, however, are typically used by an individual, and to a lesser extent by an organization, to understand what aptitude people have in understanding themselves and others. Furthermore, EI can improve—thus, it is a flexible view of your ability to relate to self and others (Bradberry, n.d.).

Emotional intelligence can be defined as understanding and managing our own emotions with the added social awareness of discerning the emotions of others. Knowing how to identify and use emotions to guide personal behavior and engagement with others is essential for effective followers and leaders. The core elements of EI, as described in the now classic work, *Emotional Intelligence 2.0* (Bradberry & Greaves, 2009), consist of understanding and then managing yourself (you) and social awareness and how to manage relationships (others). Why is this important to know? Several answers are possible; one of the most important is that people with better EI scores are viewed as more successful. EI is viewed as the basis for numerous skills we use every day as humans, nurses, and leaders. EI is the "single biggest predictor of performance in the workplace and the strongest driver of leadership and personal excellence" (p. 21). Although some of us, at least at some point in our careers, may deny interest in being a leader, who of us would not want to be our personal best? Therefore, knowing one's EI would be of great value. The even better news about EI is that it can be improved.

Being self-aware does not require a process of psychoanalysis. Rather, self-awareness refers to our ability to consider who we are as people. What would we say we do well? What makes us respond with a proverbial "knee jerk" response? What makes us feel confident? Thinking about our "good" and "bad" insights and responses is not geared to categorizing ourselves. It is geared to helping us understand who we are and what we do.

Self-management requires that we act independently for ourselves to strengthen those things we do well and to alter our approach to things we do not do so well. Although we may appreciate someone else pointing out something we need to do differently, our real source of making change is within us. Just knowing how we are is insufficient. We need to determine whether we are going to adjust or whether we want to maintain our current state. This aspect of EI is really about aligning ourselves with our goals and sometimes delaying certain actions or satisfactions to advance toward our goals.

Social awareness now turns the awareness toward others. Gaining the perspective of another person is what that person lacks and what is critically important to working with others. Our observational and listening skills predispose us to being capable of determining what others are experiencing.

Relationship management pulls the first aspects (understanding and managing self and social awareness) together so that you can be effective at responding to people, being clear in expressing your personal assessment of a situation, and creating connections with others that allow you together to be more effective in the work you need to do. Being able to know yourself and others and then manage your own personal reactions allows you to direct energy toward managing a relationship. While nursing requires technical competency, EI adds a skill required of today's clinicians. Further, research supports how the relationship between EI and mindfulness as a protective factor for healthcare professionals (see the Research Perspective).

> **EXERCISE 7.5** Conduct an Internet search using the term *emotional intelligence assessments*. What types of assessments are available? Did they identify reliability and validity information? What was the cost range? Were any that seemed useful available online? What could you do with the results of such an assessment?

> **EXERCISE 7.6** Go to *https://hbr.org/2015/06/quiz-yourself-do-you-lead-with-emotional-intelligence* and complete this online assessment of your EI. Print or save your results. What did you learn about yourself?

RESEARCH PERSPECTIVE

Resource: Jimenez-Picon, N., Romero-Martin, M., Ponce-Blandon, J. A., Ramirez-Baena, L., Palomo-Lara, J. C., & Gomez-Salgado, J. (2021). The relationship between mindfulness and emotional intelligence as a protective factor for healthcare professionals: A systematic review. *International Journal of Environmental Research and Public Health*, 18, 5491. https://doi.org/10.3390/ijerph.18105491.

Using the Joanna Briggs Institute criteria, the researchers performed a systematic review of the literature spanning the years 2010 and 2020. The inclusion criteria were—the article was published in English or Spanish, a quantitative methodology was used, the study population was healthcare professionals or students; and the focus was related to mindfulness and emotional intelligence. Ten studies met the criteria and showed a positive relationship between mindfulness and EI. Additionally, the researchers found an increase in personal resilience who had undergone mindfulness training, and as a result have been able to reduce emotional exhaustion, increase their commitment to their work and improve their performance when facing challenge at work (p. 10 of 14).

Implications for Practice

Practicing mindfulness enhances the potential for emotional intelligence and limits the potential impact of emotional exhaustion. Based on the strains placed on health care today, serious consideration should be given to supporting the benefits of mindfulness practices as a strategy to aid in developing and strengthening healthcare professionals' ability to enhance their emotional intelligence and lessen their chances of emotional exhaustion.

Moral Courage

As a leader or effective follower, having the ability to speak up or provide input and/or feedback is a skill that requires courage. Speaking up for or against issues within the team requires taking a moral stand. This type of courage can also be called moral courage. Moral courage is defined as "standing up for what is right" (Rainer & Schneider, 2020, p. 349). Leaders and effective followers have an obligation to be aware and take ownership of their professional values to make ethical decisions when the need to speak up arises regardless of the fear of rejection or ridicule by their peers (Gibson, 2019). Rainer and Schneider (2020, p. 349) stated that nurses not speaking up is concerning for three reasons:

- Nurses not speaking up can result in patient harm.
- Nurses are in a key position to speak up for patients.
- Nursing as a profession has a strong moral and ethical imperative for patient advocacy.

Healthcare organizations should strive to create an environment where leaders and effective followers feel empowered to speak up, putting their principles into action. As partners within healthcare teams, supporting the discussion of concerns and confronting issues head on is a courageous act.

EXERCISE 7.7 You are the nurse in an emergency department. You are taking care of a patient who is having a right-sided myocardial infarction (MI). The provider orders metoprolol 5 mg IVP × 3 doses. Incorporating your knowledge about right sided MIs and the contraindications of metoprolol, you confirm the order with the provider. The provider insists that the order is correct. Would you have the courage to speak up and advocate for your patient's safety and well-being? What would you say as an effective follower? What would you say as a leader? Are they different?

Strengths

One of the most widely used self-assessment tools is StrengthsFinder 2.0 (Rath, 2007). Because it has been used worldwide, in numerous cultures, and across all sorts of personal characteristics, this is one of the most tested tools to help people determine their talents for developing strengths. The Research Perspective provides greater detail about the analyses of this tool. If you complete this assessment by yourself, you are given your top five strengths, or talents, out of the possible 34 themes. If you complete this assessment with others, you can identify how various themes contribute to the whole of a project or a relationship. Imagine if everyone in your group were deliberative, which is one of the 34 themes. This theme is described as careful, private, and cautious. What would the work look like? Likely, few timelines would be met and very little would be accomplished. However, what was done would have withstood multiple tests of thinking. Now, imagine that everyone in your group were competitive. This group would be great to enter into tournaments

RESEARCH PERSPECTIVE

Resource: Echevarria, I. M., Patterson, B. J., & Krouse, A. (2017). Predictors of transformational leadership of nurse managers. *Journal of Nursing Management 25*, 167–175.

This study utilized a predictive correlation design to explore relationships between education, leadership experience, and emotional intelligence as predictors of transformational leadership in 148 nurse managers from various healthcare settings. Transformational leadership is one of several positive relationship styles that incorporate elements of EI. Consistent with previous research, this study found that EI was a strong predictor of transformational leadership. The findings were also consistent with an American Nurses Association position paper supporting EI as a required nurse manager skill.

Implications for Practice
EI is not just a good idea. It is important for nurses who desire a formal leadership role. Nursing leadership job descriptions may include EI as a required skill, supporting the need for ongoing self-reflection and education.

to represent your organization. However, because they are so driven by the need to compete, these individuals might dim others' prospects of participating. In addition, we might wonder whether they could ever really reach agreement on a course of action or whether their competitiveness kept them focused on making their own individual points. Fortunately, this tool provides your top five strengths rather than only focusing on one. The authors point out that we can develop any of the strengths. However, our natural tendency is to respond in any given situation with just one of our strengths.

The key with strengths is to capitalize on those that are *your* talents and to surround yourself with people with other talents that "fill in" the total set of talents needed to accomplish work. No single strength is better than another except as it relates to some specific activity and goal. You always must meet the minimum performance expectations for any position in your career. How you will be deemed successful, however, typically derives from practicing and honing your talents so that they become great assets. Leaders need to help their followers develop their talents to their best potential. As a result, their followers are focusing on what is positive about themselves and not on what is not among their best talents.

EXERCISE 7.8 Conduct an Internet search using the term *personal strengths assessments*. What types of assessments are available? Did they identify reliability and validity information? What was the cost range? Were any that seemed useful available online? What could you do with the results of such an assessment?

BECOMING AN AUTHENTIC LEADER

Earlier, we discussed various leadership theories and models, some of which tend to be more applicable in situations in which a person holds a formal title (see Chapter 1). To begin a solid advancement in leadership, one of the most direct models is that developed by George (2003). That model is authentic leadership. Although developing leadership competence is a lifelong journey, being authentic is a good introduction to thinking of oneself as a leader.

Authentic leadership (Raso, 2019) focuses on building honest relationships by remaining true to personal values and honoring all relationships (think of Ruiz's statement about being impeccable with your word). How those relationships are formed may be artificial—you are assigned to an organizational task, know none of the people, and have a time frame to accomplish specific goals. In other words, at this point, you are not an organized whole; you are a group. Valuing what each person brings helps others develop trust in you and increases your potential for trusting the others in the group (think of Ruiz's statement about not making assumptions). Exploring with each other what values you hold, how you see the assigned task unfolding, and who has what strengths and talents to contribute to the task are examples of how to build a cohesive team. Yet if we are not authentic in our approach, trust will be at a minimum.

Being truthful and open is critical to developing as an authentic leader. As George (2003, p. 11) said when he created this view of leadership, "It's being yourself; being the person you were created to be." He goes on to contrast this view of leadership with the idea of creating an image of what a leader is. Thus, no matter what list of characteristics you might read, if they are not the real you, trying to adopt

TABLE 7.2   **Behaviors and Developments of Leading Authentically**

Dimensions	Corresponding Developments
Purpose	Passion
Values	Behavior
Heart	Compassion
Relationships	Connectedness
Self-discipline	Consistency

Data from George, B. (2003). Authentic leadership: Rediscovering the secrets to creating lasting value. San Francisco, CA: Jossey Bass.

those only makes you look fake. That does not mean you should not explore those characteristics or styles. It simply means you will not look as genuine in leading as you would if you are being the real you. Being the real you, however, is built on a true caring for others and a desire to help everyone maximize talents so that any group effort is as powerful as possible. As an example, being an authentic leader relies on having a true passion for people and the work in which they engage. Being able to respond to situations in an authentic manner promotes people's personal values. Although this may seem somewhat concerning because some people do not necessarily have values that fit a mission or task, authenticity quickly filters people into those who can achieve a particular goal and those who cannot.

George (2003) developed the concept of authentic leadership having five dimensions: purpose, values, heart, relationships, and self-discipline. The corresponding developments are passion, behavior, compassion, connectedness, and consistency, as Table 7.2 illustrates. Think, as an example, of someone who does not have real compassion. We say that person does not have heart or that person's heart is not in the work.

If all we developed as a skill was awareness of self, think of the potential for further explorations of who we are and the actions we could take to be more—for our patients and ourselves.

National Academy of Medicine: Future of Nursing 2020–2030

Nurses have always contributed to the health and well-being of the populations they serve by advocating for improved outcomes. The report conducted by the National Academy of Medicine (formerly known as the Institute of Medicine [IOM]) and the Robert Wood Johnson Foundation (RWJF) expanded the reach of nursing practice to assist with the need from the public for healthcare. This initiative included ideas such as nurses practicing to the full extent of their training and education and becoming full partners with physicians and other healthcare professionals in redesigning healthcare to provide improved access and promote health equity (Flaubert et al., 2021).

This initiative expands the view of the development of effective followership. Educated and well-trained professionals in nursing with limited experience can feel the weight of the hierarchy ladder on their shoulders. Becoming an effective follower in a learning institution and workforce organization elevates your position by acknowledging your strengths among your team. Ultimately, your voice is given merit—increasing your ability to speak up and be heard. The National Academy of Medicine calls for the nursing workforce to partner with providers and other healthcare professionals. This partnership changes the clinical ladder to a clinical roundtable where nurses and providers can listen and engage in discussions to address the social determinants of health and health inequities facing communities today.

Quintuple Aim

Nurses in leader or effective follower roles are expected to fulfill the expectations of the Quintuple Aim. The Institute for Healthcare Improvement (IHI) developed the Triple Aim in 2008 (Berwick et al., 2008). The Triple Aim's ultimate goal is to improve the health of the communities in which each healthcare organization serves (Bodenheimer & Sinsky, 2014). The specific actions necessary to meet the goal included the following:
- Enhancing patient experience
- Improving population health
- Reducing costs

The aims were expanded to include another: to decrease the incidence of healthcare provider burnout (Bodenheimer & Sinsky, 2014). Guiding healthcare professionals to achieve the Quintuple Aim will help achieve the goal of improved health while keeping the providers engaged and decreasing turnover through improving the work life of care providers. The addition of the fifth aim, advancing health equity, reflects the concern for the inequities in health care (IHI, 2022).

The importance of achieving the Quintuple Aim can be emphasized with the engagement of the leader–follower relationship. The outcomes from promoting the leader–follower relationship can be seen in Table 7.3.

TABLE 7.3 How Leaders and Effective Followers Achieve the Quintuple Aim

Quintuple Aim Guidelines	Leader	Effective Follower	Outcomes
1. Enhancing patient experience	Sets the tone on the unit Trusts in the follower's instincts Listens actively to concerns Guides decision-making Creates trust	Sees the practical Identifies risks Voices concerns Advocates actively for patients Grows and learns Builds trust	Decreases errors Improves quality of care Improves patient outcomes Engages patients
2. Improving population health	Provides an environment that advocates for high-quality care delivery Uses open communication Encourages participation	Delivers high-quality care to every patient Educates the patient and family Gains the patient's trust to ask questions	Informs populations of patients to return to their communities healthier and more engaged
3. Reducing costs	Promotes a more productive team	Commits to increasing productivity	Reduces waste from nonproductive leaders and followers
4. Improving the work life of care providers	Reduces stress by trusting followers Delegates tasks effectively without overloading followers	Reduces stress by increasing autonomy Commits to the organization Feels accomplished and important because the follower has a voice	Reduces turnover Increases retention Increases production Results in an effective unit
5. Advancing health equity	Creates plans for services to address inequities	Identifies inequities in care for population served	Results in outcomes comparable across differing groups

CONCLUSION

No matter where you are in your leadership trajectory, being complacent is not an option. Seeking new insights, using established tools (such as journaling), and wanting to do one's best and what is right are lifelong habits that allow each of us to develop our full potential. If leadership is a journey expressed as a skill, each of us has the potential to contribute to the needed changes in healthcare by starting with a solid knowledge of and value for who we are and what we can become.

THE SOLUTION

I decided to report this issue to the manager of our unit and to advocate for the purchase of hospital-grade thermometers for every room while removing the generic thermometers from our stock room. When I brought the issue to my manager, she was hesitant at first to make a sweeping change. In an effort to demonstrate how widespread the issue was, I asked for several other nurses to begin using both thermometers to measure infant temperatures. Within days, they all started to report the same results—the generic thermometers were contributing to unnecessary interventions in our infants. With this evidence at the table, my manager agreed to remove the generic thermometers and required the use of the hospital-grade ones, eventually purchasing larger quantities so that all nurses could have one during their shift.

While it can be intimidating to be the first one to speak up, I always tell myself that as a nurse, I am my patient's advocate. In many cases, our insights can lead to better processes and safer environments for our patients.

Would this be a suitable approach for you? Why?

Amy McCarthy

REFLECTIONS

Taking on the role of the effective follower and leader is a continuous task. It involves all of the characteristics described in this chapter, including active listening, open communication, trusting your own knowledge and instincts, and have the courage to speak up and voice any questions or concerns you may have in any situation. How effective are you in each role?

What are one or two first steps you can take to ensure you are developing as an effective follower and leader? What do you need to learn about yourself? How do you think others perceive you as an effective follower and leader? How will you intentionally use reflection to enhance your leadership competence to be the best nurse possible?

BEST PRACTICES FOR EFFECTIVE FOLLOWING AND LEADING

- Participate in self-assessments and reflect on the results.
- Know that the journey to effective following and leading is a journey rich with discovery of self and others.

TIPS FOR EFFECTIVE FOLLOWING AND LEADING

- Stay up-to-date on evidence-based care.
- Engage in open communication.
- Take an active role within your organization.
- Practice reflection daily
- Allow what you learn from your reflections to guide your next steps
- Trust in your knowledge and instincts.
- Do not be afraid to ask questions.
- Have the courage to voice any concerns

REFERENCES

Alegbeleye, I. D., & Kaufman, E. K. (2020). Relationship between middle managers' transformational leadership and effective followership behaviors in organizations. *Journal of Leadership Studies*, *13*(4), 6–19. https://doi.org/10.1002/jls.21673.

Berwick, D., Nolan, T., & Whittington, J. (2008). The triple aim: Care, cost, and quality. *Health Affiliate*, *27*(3), 759–769.

Bodenheimer, T., & Sinsky, C. (2014). From Triple to Quadruple Aim: Care of the patient requires care of the provider. *Annals of Family Medicine*, *12*(6), 573–576. https://doi.org/10.1370/afm.1713.

Bradberry, R. (n.d.). Emotional Intelligence—EQ. Retrieved from http://www.forbes.com/sites/travisbradberry/2014/01/09/emotional-intelligence/#4cf302463ecb.

Bradberry, R., & Greaves, J. (2009). *Emotional Intelligence 2.0*. San Diego, CA: TalentSmart.

Chaleff, I. (2017). In praise of followership style assessments. *Journal of Leadership Studies*, *10*(3), 45–48. https://doi.org/10.1002/jls.21490.

Echevarria, I. M., Patterson, B. J., & Krouse, A. (2017). Predictors of transformational leadership of nurse managers. *Journal of Nursing Management*, *25*, 167–175. https://doi.org/10.1111/jonm.12452.

Falls, A., & Allen, S. (2020). Leader-to-follower transitions: Flexibility and awareness. *Journal of Leadership Studies*, *14*(2), 24–37. https://doi.org/10.1002/jls.21696.

Flaubert, J. L., Le Menestrel, S., Williams, D. R., & Wakefield, M. K. (Eds.). (2021). *The future of nursing 2020–2030: Charting a path to achieve health equity*. Washington, DC: National Academies Press.

George, B. (2003). *Authentic leadership: Rediscovering the secrets to creating lasting value*. San Francisco: Jossey-Bass.

Gibson, E. (2019). Longitudinal learning plan for developing moral courage. *Teaching and Learning in Nursing*, *14*(2), 122–124.

Heard, C. P. (2018). Informal leadership in the clinical setting: Occupational therapist perspectives. AOTA Annual Conference & Expo, April 19–22, 2018, Salt Lake City, Utah. *American Journal of Occupational Therapy*, *72*(4), 1. https://doi.org/10.5014/ajot.2018.72S1-PO4018.

Horton, A. G., Gibson, K. B., & Curington, A. B. (2021). Exploring reflective journaling as a learning tool: An interdisciplinary approach. *Archives of Psychiatric Nursing*, *35*(2), 195–199. https://doi.org/10.1016/j.apnu.2020.09.009.

Institute for Healthcare Improvement (IHI). (2022). *Triple aim for populations*. http://www.ihi.org/Topics/TripleAim.

Kouzes, J. M., & Posner, B. Z. (2017). *The leadership challenge: How to make extraordinary things happen in organizations*. San Francisco: Jossey-Bass.

Malak, R. (2016). A concept analysis of "Follower" within the context of professional nursing. *Nursing Forum, 51*(4), 286–294. https://doi.org/10.1111/nuf.12158.

Rainer, J. B., & Schneider, J. K. (2020). Testing a model of speaking up in nursing. *The Journal of Nursing Administration, 10*(6), 349–354. https://doi.org/10.1097/NNA.0000000000000896.

Raso, R. (2019). Be you! Authentic leadership. *Nursing Management, 50*(5), 18–25. https://doi.org/10.1097/01.NUMA.0000557619.96942.50.

Rath, T. (2007). *StrengthsFinder 2.0*. New York: Gallup Press.

Rosler, G. (2018). Your journey to authentic leadership. *American Nurse Today, 13*(2), 40–41. https://www.myamericannurse.com/journey-authentic-leadership/.

Ruiz, D. M. (1997). *The Four Agreements: A practical guide to personal freedom*. White Plains, NY: Peter Pauper Press.

Schön, D. A. (1983). *The reflective practitioner*. New York: Basic Books.

Varpio, L., & Teunissen, P. (2021). Leadership in interprofessional healthcare teams: Empowering knotworking with leadership. *Medical Teacher, 43*(1), 32–37. https://doi.org/10.1080/0142159X.2020.1791318.

Watters, D., Smith, K., Tobin, S., & Beasley, S. (2019). Follow the leader: Followership and its relevance for surgeons. *ANZ Journal of Surgery, 89*(5), 589–593. https://doi.org/10.1111/ans.14912.

8

Communication and Conflict

Victoria N. Folse

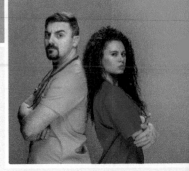

ANTICIPATED LEARNING OUTCOMES

- Describe behaviors and techniques that affect communication among members of the healthcare team.
- Evaluate effective communication techniques to improve patient and team outcomes.
- Assess the nature and sources of perceived and actual conflict to be more effective in communicating and resolving future conflict.
- Determine which of the five approaches to conflict is the most appropriate in potential and actual situations.
- Identify conflict management techniques that will prevent lateral violence and bullying from occurring.

KEY TERMS

accommodating
avoiding
bullying
bystander intervention
collaborating
competing
compromising
conflict

handoff communication
horizontal violence
incivility
interpersonal conflict
interprofessional communication
intrapersonal conflict
lateral violence
mediation

negotiating
organizational conflict
situation, background, assessment, and recommendation (SBAR)
volatility, uncertainty, complexity, and ambiguity (VUCA)

THE CHALLENGE

Patients with a spinal cord injury often have wounds from pressure injuries or from trauma, like a motor vehicle accident, shooting, or stabbing. My preceptor taught me the importance of changing these dressings daily, or as ordered by the primary care provider, in order to prevent infection of the wound and osteomyelitis. One day, I was receiving report from a nurse about a patient with multiple gunshot wounds. I asked if the dressings were changed and she confirmed they were. I noticed that they were also charted as "changed." The day was so busy, and I had not yet assessed the dressings for drainage or assured they had not become loose, in which case we would change the dressings again. Toward the end of the day,

the patient asked me if I was going to change the dressings, since they have not been changed today. Confused, I told him the previous nurse said she had changed them. The patient denied it and, as I looked at his dressings, they were initialed by a different nurse and had the previous date written on them reflecting when they were last changed. I was upset that the previous nurse did not tell the truth about not changing the dressings that day and was concerned the patient's care had been compromised.
What would you do if you were this nurse?

Elia Nava, RN, BSN
Registered Nurse 2, 22nd floor Spinal Cord Injury
Shirley Ryan AbilityLab, Chicago, IL

INTRODUCTION

In today's complex practice environment, communicating effectively and resolving conflict are more important than ever to provide optimal patient care and to consistently meet the six competencies identified by Quality and Safety Education for Nurses (QSEN): patient-centered care, teamwork and collaboration, evidence-based practice, quality improvement, safety, and informatics (QSEN Institute, n.d.). To achieve these competencies and to reduce the likelihood of miscommunication that leads to healthcare errors, nurses must effectively communicate with patients and families, nurse colleagues, and other members of the healthcare team. The Literature Perspective of a concept analysis describes how effective communication promotes high-quality nursing care, positive patient outcomes, and patient and nurse satisfaction (Afriyie, 2020).

Interprofessional communication is effective when healthcare providers communicate with each other and with patients and their families in an open, collaborative, and respectful manner. Conflict is a disagreement in values or beliefs within oneself or between people that causes harm or has the potential to cause harm. Conflict is a catalyst for change and has the ability to produce either detrimental or beneficial effects. Conflict, when used positively, can stimulate stagnant teams and increase productivity. If properly understood and managed, conflict can lead to positive outcomes and practice environments. If it is left unattended, it can have a negative impact on both the individual and the organization. Good leadership—combined with positive team dynamics, effective communication, and successful conflict management practices—promotes shared problem solving and acceptance of change (Fowler & Robbins, 2021). In professional practice environments, unresolved conflict and miscommunication among nurses is a significant issue resulting in job dissatisfaction, absenteeism, and turnover. Effective healthcare team communication may strengthen nurses' engagement within their organizations and improve nurse retention. Patient satisfaction is lower in hospitals in which nurses are frustrated and burned out, which signals a problem with quality of care (White et al., 2019). Communication and conflict management are two key competencies of professional practice, as identified by the American Association of Colleges of Nursing (AACN, 2021), and they need to be mastered to be an effective leader.

Successful organizations are proactive in anticipating the need for interprofessional education about communication, conflict resolution, and teamwork—they enact innovative and integrated conflict resolution strategies and communication programs. Structured shadowing and cross-training across interprofessional departments may lead to improved teamwork and communication between units, which improves patient safety (Sarver et al., 2020). Conflict should not be avoided; it can be a strategic tool when leveraged appropriately to promote teamwork and collaboration (Fowler & Robbins, 2021). Some of the first authors on organizational conflict (e.g., Blake & Mouton, 1964; Deutsch, 1973) claimed that a complete resolution of conflict might, in fact, be undesirable because conflict also stimulates growth, creativity, and change. Seminal work on the concept of organizational conflict management suggested that conflict was necessary to achieve organizational goals and cohesiveness of employees, facilitate organizational change, and contribute to creative problem solving and mutual understanding. Moderate levels of conflict contribute to the quality of ideas generated and foster cohesiveness among team members, contributing to an organization's success. An organization without conflict is characterized by no change. In contrast, an optimal level of conflict will generate creativity, a problem-solving atmosphere, a strong team spirit, and motivation of its workers. Conflict in an interdisciplinary team can result in better patient care when collaborative treatment decisions are based on carefully examined and combined expertise. Nursing leaders must focus on healthy work environments to promote effective communication in stressful situations to promote successful teamwork and increase patient safety. Positive patient and staff outcomes are associated with a leader who exhibits communication competence. For example, nurses' intent to stay and their job satisfaction are impacted by a consistent and systematic method to provide praise and recognize accomplishments (Fowler & Robbins, 2021).

The complexity of the healthcare environment compounds the impact that ineffective communication, caregiver stress, and unresolved conflict have on patient safety. Conflict is inherent in clinical environments in which nursing responsibilities are driven by patient needs that are complex and frequently changing and in practice settings in which nurses have multiple professional roles. Healthcare providers are exposed to high stress levels from increased demands on a limited and aging workforce, a decrease in available resources, a more acutely ill and underinsured patient population, and a profound period of change in the practice environment. Interventions aimed at promoting nurses' psychological well-being can promote a better practice environment, improved patient safety, and better nursing outcomes (Lee et al., 2019). Conflict among healthcare providers is inevitable and is compounded by employee diversity, high patient-to-nurse ratios, pressure to make timely decisions, and status differences. Nurses employed in better care environments report more positive job experiences and fewer concerns about quality care (White et al., 2019). Interprofessional collaboration has been characterized by effective communication and is a key factor in reducing error and improving patient outcomes. Further, being competent in using communication technology and systems within any given organization is important to facilitate effective communication and promote patient safety. Moreover, hospitals with good nurse–physician relationships are associated with better nurse and patient outcomes, making collaboration and conflict resolution among nurses and physicians crucial in promoting quality of care outcomes.

An important factor in the successful management of stress and conflict is a better understanding of its context within the practice environment. The diversity of people involved in healthcare may stimulate conflict, but the shared goal of meeting patient care needs provides a solid foundation for conflict resolution. Because nursing remains a predominately female profession, this may contribute to the use of avoidance and accommodation as primary conflict handling strategies. The stereotypical self-sacrificing behavior seen in avoidance and accommodation is strongly supported by the altruistic nature of nursing. Avoidance may be appropriate during times of high stress; however, when overused, avoidance threatens the well-being of nurses and retention within the discipline. To illustrate, a correlation exists for nurses who experience job stress and emotional exhaustion and who use avoidance to handle conflict (Lee et al., 2019).

EFFECTIVE COMMUNICATION WITHIN HEALTHCARE SETTINGS

Effective communication between a healthcare provider and other members of the healthcare team promotes optimal patient outcomes. Equally important is making certain that the communication occurring between healthcare providers and patients and their families ensures quality care and patient safety and satisfaction. When communicating with populations who speak different primary languages, using language-interpreting services enhances communication with patients and their families, reduces health disparities, and promotes safe nursing care (Boruff, 2020). Although the communication within healthcare settings is often complex and chaotic, understanding the basic principles of the communication process is essential (Fig. 8.1). The Joint Commission (TJC, 2020) recognizes that breakdown in communication is the root cause of sentinel events, which are unexpected occurrences that result in death

---

EXERCISE 8.1 Access The Joint Commission website (https://www.jointcommission.org/standards_information/npsgs.aspx) for the current National Patient Safety Goals. Identify how each goal is affected by communication.

LITERATURE PERSPECTIVE

Resource: Afriyie, D. (2020). Effective communication between nurses and patients: An evolutionary concept analysis. *British Journal of Community Nursing, 25*(9), 438–445.

Communication is a complex phenomenon and is an essential element of building trust as well as promoting clinical reasoning and advancing the nursing process to individualize care. Effective communication is bidirectional; both the nurse and patient must work together to achieve their desired outcomes, including the patient's satisfaction with care and the nurse's ability to provide the best care. Effective communication promotes high-quality nursing care, positive patient outcomes, and patient and nurse satisfaction.

Implications for Practice
Effective communication is a key component of nursing practice and must be prioritized in nursing education and practice. It must be intentional in nature and can be improved through direct actions taken by the nurse. Engaging nurses in professional education and offering continuing education training focused on communication skills will empower them to communicate effectively with their patients.

Sender [Encode] → Message → Receiver [Decode]
FEEDBACK [Roles reverse in typical communication exchanges.]

Fig. 8.1 Basic communication model.

or serious injury. Communication when the patient is handed over from one provider to another or from one setting to another is especially problematic. Not surprisingly, each of the National Patient Safety Goals (see TJC for the current goals, https://www.jointcommission.org/standards_information/npsgs.aspx) is directly or indirectly related to communication.

Because adverse patient outcomes commonly are a result of communication failures, TJC's National Patient Safety Goals added standardization of handoff communication, the verbal and written exchange of pertinent information during transitions of care. Handoff communication occurs during nurse change-of-shift reports, transfer of patients between units or facilities, and reports between departments and between disciplines. Effective communication is also important when nurses are describing changes in a patient's condition to other members of the healthcare team. Common language for communicating critical information, such as during huddles or rounding, can help prevent misunderstandings. Bedside handoffs have the added benefit of increasing direct patient contact, increasing the possibility of patient participation, and enhancing patient safety (Malfait et al., 2018). Healthcare providers need to allow sufficient time to ask and respond to questions. Reading back information also helps identify any miscommunication and ensures that the information received is accurate. Intimidating and disruptive behaviors affect communication and must not be tolerated in healthcare settings because both employee satisfaction and patient safety can be affected.

Conflicts and miscommunication between nurses and other healthcare providers, including physicians, may be intensified because of the overlapping nature of their professional domains and lack of clarification between roles. Differences in nursing and medical school training have caused differences between nurses and physicians in communication styles and approaches to handling conflict (Vandergoot et al., 2018). Differences in power can also affect communication and create conflict. While effective communication between nurses and physicians is essential, communication between nurses and unlicensed assistive personnel is also foundational for good patient outcomes (Campbell et al., 2019).

Use of common language, such as SBAR, when communicating critical information helps prevent misunderstandings and promotes a culture of quality and safety. SBAR, which stands for situation, background, assessment, and recommendation (Institute for Healthcare Improvement, 2021), has become a best practice for standardizing communication between healthcare providers. Research suggests that if nursing students modified SBAR to ISBAR to include an introduction, the consistent practice with this standardized communication approach could improve communication with healthcare providers, which would lead to reduced threats to patient safety and improve patient care (Foronda et al., 2021). The fast pace, frequent interruptions, and stress present in healthcare settings interfere with effective communication (Rhudy et al., 2019). The term VUCA describes today's healthcare environment: volatility, uncertainty, complexity, and ambiguity. Each of these elements increases the potential for miscommunication. Clear, complete, and accurate communication among healthcare providers directly affects the quality and safety of care. Nurses have a responsibility to provide quality care; thus, they must serve in leadership roles to ensure effective communication and conflict resolution.

TYPES OF CONFLICT

The recognition that conflict is a part of everyday life suggests that mastering conflict management strategies is essential for overall well-being and personal and professional growth. A need exists to determine the type of conflict present in a specific situation because the more accurately conflict is defined, the more likely it will be resolved. Conflict occurs in three broad categories: intrapersonal, interpersonal, and organizational. A combination of types can also be present in any given conflict.

Intrapersonal conflict occurs within a person when confronted with the need to think or act in a way that seems at odds with one's sense of self. Questions often arise that create a conflict over priorities, ethical standards, and values. When a nurse decides what to do about the future, conflicts arise between personal and professional priorities—for example, "Do I want to accept the job in the city with more cultural opportunities or remain in my hometown and be close to my family?". Some issues present a conflict over comfortably maintaining the status quo—for example, "I know my newest charge nurse likes the autonomy of working nights. Do I really want to ask him to move to days to become a preceptor?". Taking risks to confront people when needed can produce intrapersonal conflict and, because it involves other people, may lead to interpersonal conflict—for example, "Would recommending a change in practice that I learned about at a recent conference jeopardize unit governance?". Many nurses expressed this type of conflict during the COVID-19 pandemic in 2020. Standards of care deteriorated for many reasons and nurses experienced unprecedented levels of conflict, resulting in burnout, turnover, and staffing gaps (Business Wire, 2021).

Interpersonal conflict is the most common type of conflict. It transpires between and among patients, family members, nurses, physicians, and members of other departments. Conflicts occur that focus on a difference of opinion, priority, or approach with others. A manager may be called upon to assist two nurses in resolving a scheduling conflict or issues surrounding patient assignments. Members of healthcare teams often have disputes over the best way to treat particular patient concerns or disagreements over how much information is necessary for patients and families to have about their illness. Yet, interpersonal conflict can serve as the impetus for needed change and can strengthen the practice setting.

Organizational conflict arises when discord exists about policies and procedures, personnel codes of conduct, or accepted norms of behavior and patterns of communication. Some organizational conflict is related to hierarchical structure and role differentiation among employees. Nurse managers, as well as their staff, often become embattled in institution-wide conflict concerning staffing patterns and how they affect the quality of care. Complex ethical and moral dilemmas often arise when profitable services are increased and unprofitable ones are downsized or even eliminated.

A major source of organizational conflict stems from strategies that promote more participation and autonomy of direct care nurses. Increasingly, nurses are charged with balancing direct patient care with active involvement in the institutional initiatives surrounding quality patient care. A growing number of standards set by TJC target improving communication and conflict management. Specifically, TJC requires that healthcare organizations have a code of conduct that defines acceptable and inappropriate behaviors and that leaders create and implement a process for managing intimidating and disruptive behaviors that undermine a culture of safety. Standards pertaining to medical staff also include interpersonal skills and professionalism (TJC, 2020). The Magnet Recognition Program® of the American Nurses Credentialing Center (ANCC) identifies effective interdisciplinary relationships as one of the 14 Forces of Magnetism necessary for Magnet® designation (American Nurses Credentialing Center, n.d.). Specifically, collaborative working relationships within and among the disciplines are valued, demonstrated through mutual respect, and result in meaningful contributions in the achievement of shared clinical outcomes. Magnet® hospitals must have conflict management strategies in place and use them effectively when indicated. The following are examples of "forces" contained within the 5 Model Components that are particularly germane to communication and conflict in the practice environment:

- Organizational structure (nurses' involvement in shared decision-making)
- Management style (nursing leaders who create an environment that supports participation, encourage and value feedback, and demonstrate effective communication with staff)
- Personnel policies and programs (efforts to promote nurse work–life balance)
- Image of nursing (nurses effectively influencing system-wide processes)
- Autonomy (nurses' inclusion in governance, leading to job satisfaction, personal fulfillment, and organization success)

EXERCISE 8.2 Recall a situation in which conflict between or among two or more people was apparent. Describe verbal and nonverbal communication and how each person responded. What was the outcome? Was the conflict resolved? Was anything left unresolved?

Before moving further ahead in discussing conflict, we might want to think about how easily conflicts occur. Misunderstandings occur frequently because of diminished hearing, different meanings attributed to words, different accents or languages, cultural or even regional meanings of words, potential or actual religious meanings to words, and probably countless other factors. The Theory Box provides one option for considering a way to manage conflict from a cultural perspective.

THEORY BOX

Cultural Brokering in Conflict Management

Key Contributor	Key Ideas	Application to Practice
Jezewski (1995): Evolution of a Grounded Theory: Conflict Resolution through Culture Brokering	Twelve attributes of a cultural broker in health care were identified. The purpose of cultural brokering is resolution of conflict and is defined as "bridging, linking or mediating between groups or persons of different cultural systems for the purpose of reducing conflict or producing change." (p. 20)	This theory can be applied to prevent conflict, as in when a nurse suspects a patient misperceives information or to correct misspoken information, as in when a nurse manager misstates a policy and another nurse provides the correct information to a staff member.

STAGES OF CONFLICT

The classic view of conflict is that it proceeds through four stages: frustration, conceptualization, action, and outcomes (Thomas, 1992). The ability to resolve conflicts productively depends on understanding this process (Fig. 8.2) and successfully addressing thoughts, feelings, and behaviors that form barriers to resolution. As one navigates through the stages of conflict, moving into a subsequent stage may lead to a return to and change in a previous stage (Fig. 8.3). To illustrate, the evening shift of a cardiac step-down unit has been asked to pilot a new hand-off protocol for the next 6 weeks, which stimulates intense emotions because the unit is already inadequately staffed (frustration). Two nurses on the unit interpret this conflict as a battle for control with the nurse educator; a third nurse thinks it is all about professional standards (conceptualization). A nurse leader/manager facilitates a discussion with the three nurses (action). They listen to the concerns and present evidence about the potential effectiveness of the new hand-off protocol. All agree that the real conflict comes from a difference in goals or priorities (new conceptualization), which leads to less negative emotion and ends with a much clearer understanding of all of the issues (diminished frustration). The nurses agree to pilot the hand-off protocol after their ideas have been incorporated into the plan (outcome).

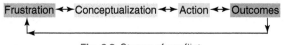

Fig. 8.2 Stages of conflict.

Frustration

When people or groups perceive that their goals may be blocked, frustration results. This frustration may escalate into stronger emotions, such as anger and deep resignation. For example, a nurse may perceive that a postoperative patient is noncompliant or uncooperative, when, in reality, the patient is afraid or has a different set of priorities at the start from those of the nurse. At the same time, the patient may view the nurse as controlling and uncaring because the nurse repeatedly asks whether the patient has used his incentive spirometer as instructed. When such frustrations occur, it is a cue to stop and clarify the nature and cause of the differences.

Similarly, frustration intensified during the COVID-19 pandemic because so little could be controlled and threats to personal safety were amplified. Initially, that frustration centered around the lack of personal protective equipment. Later, that frustration related to inadequate staffing levels in many organizations and disruptions in the practice environment due to so many temporary personnel.

Conceptualization

Conflict arises when different interpretations of a situation occur, including a different emphasis on what is important and what is not, and different thoughts about what should occur next. All involved develop an idea of what the conflict is about, and their views may or may not be accurate. Conclusions may be instant or developed over time. Everyone involved has an individual interpretation of what the conflict is and why it is occurring. Most often, these interpretations

Conflict Concept Analysis

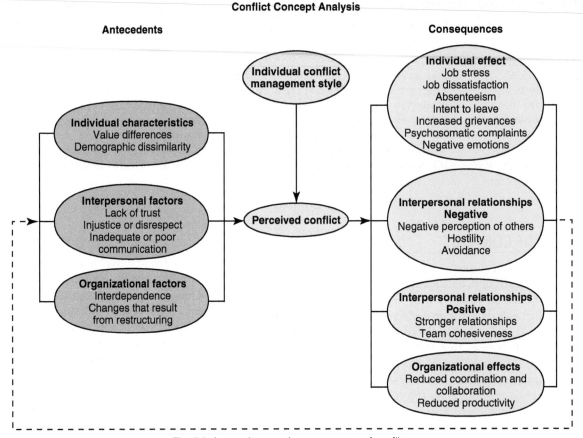

Fig. 8.3 Antecedents and consequences of conflict.

are dissimilar and involve the person's own perspective, which is based on personal values, beliefs, and culture.

Regardless of its accuracy, conceptualization forms the basis for everyone's reactions to the frustration. The way that individuals perceive and define the conflict has a great deal of influence on the approach to resolution and subsequent outcomes. For example, within the same conflict situation, some individuals may see a conflict between a nurse manager and a direct care nurse as insubordination on the part of the latter and become angry at the threat to the leader's role. Others may view it as trivial complaining, may voice criticism (e.g., "We've been over this new protocol already; why can't you just adopt the change?"), and withdraw from the situation. Such differences in conceptualizing the issue block its resolution. Thus, each person must clarify "the conflict as I see it" and "how it makes me respond" before all of the people involved can define the conflict, develop a shared conceptualization, and resolve their differences. The following are questions to consider:

- What is the nature of our differences?
- What are the reasons for those differences?
- Does our leader endorse ideas or behaviors that add to or diminish the conflict?
- Do I need to be mentored by someone, even if that individual is outside my own department or work area, to successfully resolve this conflict?

Action

A behavioral response to a conflict follows the conceptualization. This may include seeking clarification about how another person views the conflict, collecting additional information that informs the issue, or engaging in dialog about the issue. As actions are taken to resolve the conflict, the way that some or all parties conceptualize the conflict may change. Successful resolution often stems from identifying a common goal that unites (e.g., quality patient care, good working relations). People are always taking some action regarding the conflict, even if that action is avoiding dealing with it, deliberately delaying action, or choosing to do nothing. The longer ineffective actions continue, though, the more likely people will experience frustration, resistance, or even hostility. The more the actions appropriately match the nature of the conflict, the more likely the conflict will be resolved with desirable results.

Outcomes

Tangible and intangible consequences result from the actions taken and have significant implications for the work setting. Consequences include (1) the conflict being resolved with a revised approach, (2) stagnation of any current movement, or (3) no future movement.

Constructive conflict results in successful resolution, leading to the following outcomes:

- Growth occurs.
- Problems are resolved.
- Groups are unified.
- Productivity is increased.
- Commitment is increased.

Unsatisfactory resolution is typically destructive and results in the following:

- Negativity, resistance, and increased frustration inhibit movement.
- Resolutions diminish or are absent.
- Groups divide, and relationships weaken.
- Productivity decreases.
- Satisfaction decreases.

Assessing the degree of conflict resolution is useful for improving individual and group skills in resolutions, including more effective communication. Two general outcomes are considered when assessing the degree to which a conflict has been resolved: (1) the degree to which important goals were achieved and (2) the nature of the subsequent relationships among those involved (Box 8.1).

BOX 8.1 General Outcomes in Conflict Management

Assessing the Degree of Conflict Management

I. Quality of decisions
   A. How creative are planned solutions?
   B. How practical and realistic are they?
   C. How well were intended goals achieved?
   D. What surprising results were achieved?
II. Quality of relationships
   A. How much understanding has been created?
   B. How willing are people to work together?
   C. How much mutual respect, empathy, concern, and cooperation have been generated?

Modified from Hurst, J., & Kinney, M. (1989). *Empowering self and others*. Toledo, OH: University of Toledo.

CATEGORIES OF CONFLICT

Categorizing a conflict can further define an appropriate course of action for resolution. Conflicts arise from discrepancies in four areas: facts, goals, approaches, and values. Sources of fact-based conflicts are external written sources and include job descriptions, hospital policies, standards of nursing practice, and TJC mandates. Objective data can be provided to resolve a disagreement generated by discrepancies in information. Goal conflicts often arise from competing priorities (e.g., desire to empower employees vs. control through micromanagement). Frequently, a common goal (e.g., quality patient care) can be identified and used to frame conflict resolution. Even when all agree on a common goal, different ideas about the best approach to achieve that goal may produce conflict. For example, if the unit goal is to reduce costs by 10%, one leader may target overtime hours and another may eliminate the budget for continuing education. Values, opinions, and beliefs are much more personal; thus, they generate disagreements that can be threatening and adversarial. Because values are subjective, value-based conflicts often remain unresolved. Therefore, a need to find a way for competing values to coexist is necessary for effective communication and conflict management.

MODES OF CONFLICT MANAGEMENT

Understanding the way the healthcare providers respond to conflict is an essential first step in identifying effective strategies to help nurses constructively handle conflicts in the practice environment. Five classic approaches can be used in conflict resolution: avoiding, accommodating, competing, compromising, and collaborating (Thomas & Kilman, 1974, 2002). These approaches can be viewed within two dimensions: assertiveness (satisfying one's own concerns) and cooperativeness (satisfying the concerns of others). Most people tend to employ a combined set of actions that are appropriately assertive and cooperative, depending on the nature of the conflict situation (Thomas, 1992). See the conflict self-assessment in Box 8.2.

EXERCISE 8.3 Self-assessment of preferred conflict-handling modes is important. As you read and answer the 30-item conflict survey in Box 8.2, think of how you respond to conflict in professional situations. After completing the survey, tally and reflect on your scores for each of the five approaches. Consider the following questions:

- Which approach do you prefer? Which do you use least?
- What determines whether you respond in a particular manner?
- Considering the reoccurring types of conflicts you have, what are the strengths and weaknesses of your preferred conflict-handling styles?
- Have others offered you feedback about your approach to conflict?

Throughout the rest of this section are descriptions of each approach and related self-assessment and commitment-to-action activities. Use your totals from Box 8.2 to stimulate your thinking about how you do and how you could handle conflict at work. Most important, consider whether your pattern of frequency tends to be consistent or inconsistent with the types of conflicts you face. That is, does your way of dealing with conflict tend to match the situations in which that approach is most useful?

As you read the rest of this section, use this pattern of scores and your reflections to examine the appropriate uses of each approach, assess your use of each approach more extensively, and commit to new behaviors to increase your future effectiveness.

Avoiding

Avoiding, or withdrawing, is very unassertive and uncooperative, because people who avoid neither pursue their own needs, goals, or concerns immediately nor assist others to pursue theirs. Avoidance as a conflict management style ensures that conflict is only postponed, and conflict has a tendency to escalate in intensity when ignored. That is not to say that all conflict must be addressed immediately; some issues require considerable reflection and action should be delayed. The positive side of withdrawing may be postponing an issue until a better time or simply walking away from a "no-win" situation (Box 8.3). The self-assessment in Box 8.4 will help you recognize your own avoidance behaviors and use them more effectively.

Accommodating

When accommodating, people neglect their own needs, goals, and concerns (unassertive) while trying to satisfy those of others (cooperative). This approach has an element of being self-sacrificing and simply obeying orders or serving other people. For example, a coworker requests that you cover her weekends during her children's holiday break. You had hoped to visit friends from college, but you know how important it is for her to have more time with her family, so you agree. Box 8.5 lists some appropriate uses of accommodation.

Individuals who frequently use accommodation may feel disappointment and resentment because they "get nothing in return." This is a built-in by-product of the overuse of this approach. The self-assessment in Box 8.6 asks you to examine your current use of accommodation and challenges you to think of new ways to use it more effectively.

Competing

When competing, people pursue their own needs and goals at the expense of others. Sometimes, people use whatever power, creativeness, or strategies that are available to "win." Competing may also take the form of standing up for your rights or defending important principles, as when opposition to mandatory overtime is voiced (Box 8.7).

People whose primary mode of addressing conflict is through competition often react by feeling threatened, acting defensively or aggressively, or even resorting to

BOX 8.2   Conflict Self-Assessment

Directions: Read each of the following statements. Assess yourself in terms of how often you tend to act similarly during conflict at work. Place the number of the most appropriate response in the blank in front of each statement. Put *1* if the behavior is never typical of how you act during a conflict, *2* if it is seldom typical, *3* if it is occasionally typical, *4* if it is frequently typical, or *5* if it is very typical of how you act during conflict.

_____ 1. Create new possibilities to address all important concerns.
_____ 2. Persuade others to see it and/or do it my way.
_____ 3. Work out some sort of give-and-take agreement.
_____ 4. Let other people have their way.
_____ 5. Wait and let the conflict take care of itself.
_____ 6. Find ways that everyone can win.
_____ 7. Use whatever power I have to get what I want.
_____ 8. Find an agreeable compromise among people involved.
_____ 9. Give in so others get what they think is important.
_____ 10. Withdraw from the situation.
_____ 11. Cooperate assertively until everyone's needs are met.
_____ 12. Compete until I either win or lose.
_____ 13. Engage in "give a little and get a little" bargaining.
_____ 14. Let others' needs be met more than my own needs.
_____ 15. Avoid taking any action for as long as I can.
_____ 16. Partner with others to find the most inclusive solution.
_____ 17. Put my foot down assertively for a quick solution.
_____ 18. Negotiate for what all sides value and can live without.
_____ 19. Agree to what others want to create harmony.
_____ 20. Keep as far away from others involved as possible.
_____ 21. Stick with it to get everyone's highest priorities.
_____ 22. Argue and debate over the best way.
_____ 23. Create some middle position everyone agrees to.
_____ 24. Put my priorities below those of other people.
_____ 25. Hope the issue does not come up.
_____ 26. Collaborate with others to achieve our goals together.
_____ 27. Compete with others for scarce resources.
_____ 28. Emphasize compromise and trade-offs.
_____ 29. Cool things down by letting others do it their way.
_____ 30. Change the subject to avoid the fighting.

Conflict Self-Assessment Scoring

Look at the numbers you placed in the blanks on the conflict assessment. Write the number you placed in each blank on the appropriate line below. Add up your total for each column and enter that total on the appropriate line. The greater your total is for each approach, the more often you tend to use that approach when conflict occurs at work. The lower the score is, the less often you tend to use that approach when conflict occurs at work.

Collaborating	Competing	Compromising	Accommodating	Avoiding
1. _____	2. _____	3. _____	4. _____	5. _____
6. _____	7. _____	8. _____	9. _____	10. _____
11. _____	12. _____	13. _____	14. _____	15. _____
16. _____	17. _____	18. _____	19. _____	20. _____
21. _____	22. _____	23. _____	24. _____	25. _____
26. _____	27. _____	28. _____	29. _____	30. _____
Total _____	Total _____	Total _____	Total _____	Total _____

From Hurst, J. B. (1993). *Conflict self-assessment.* Toledo, OH: Human Resource Development Center, University of Toledo.

BOX 8.3   Appropriate Uses for the Avoiding Approach

1. When facing trivial and/or temporary issues, or when other far more important issues are pressing
2. When there is no chance to obtain what one wants or needs, or when others could resolve the conflict more efficiently and effectively
3. When the potential negative results of initiating and acting on a conflict are much greater than the benefits of its resolution
4. When people need to "cool down," distance themselves, or gather more information

BOX 8.4   Avoidance: Self-Assessment and Commitment to Action

If you tend to use avoidance often, ask yourself the following questions:
1. Do people have difficulty getting my input and understanding my view?
2. Do I block cooperative efforts to resolve issues?
3. Am I distancing myself from significant others?
4. Are important issues being left unidentified and unresolved?

If you seldom use avoidance, ask yourself the following questions:
1. Do I find myself overwhelmed by a large number of conflicts and a need to say "no"?
2. Do I assert myself even when things do not matter that much? Do others view me as an aggressor?
3. Do I lack a clear view of what my priorities are?
4. Do I stir up conflicts and fights?

Commitment to Action
What two new behaviors would increase your effective use of avoidance?
1.
2.

BOX 8.5   Appropriate Uses of Accommodation

1. When other people's ideas and solutions appear to be better or when you have made a mistake
2. When the issue is far more important to the other person or people than it is to you
3. When you see that accommodating now "builds up some important credits" for later issues
4. When you are outmatched and/or losing anyway; when continued competition would only damage the relationships and productivity of the group and jeopardize accomplishing major purpose(s)
5. When preserving harmonious relationships and avoiding defensiveness and hostility are very important
6. When letting others learn from their mistakes and/or increased responsibility is possible without severe damage

BOX 8.6   Accommodation: Self-Assessment and Commitment to Action

If you use accommodation often, ask yourself the following questions:
1. Do I feel that my needs, goals, concerns, and ideas are not being attended to by others?
2. Am I depriving myself of influence, recognition, and respect?
3. When I am in charge, is "discipline" lax?
4. Do I think people are using me?

If you seldom use accommodation, ask yourself the following questions:
1. Am I building goodwill with others during conflict?
2. Do I admit when I have made a mistake?
3. Do I know when to give in or do I assert myself at all costs?
4. Am I viewed as unreasonable or insensitive?

Commitment to Action
What two new behaviors would increase your effective use of accommodation?
1.
2.

cruelty in the form of cutting remarks, deliberate gossip, or hurtful innuendo. Competition within work groups can generate ill will, favor a win-lose stance, and commit people to a stalemate. Such behaviors force people into a corner from which there is no easy or graceful exit. Use Box 8.8 to help you learn to use competing more effectively.

Compromising

Compromising involves both assertiveness and cooperation on the part of everyone and requires maturity and confidence. Negotiating is a learned skill that is

BOX 8.7   Appropriate Uses of Competing

1. When quick, decisive action is necessary
2. When important, unpopular action needs to be taken or when trade-offs may result in long-range, continued conflict
3. When an individual or group is right about issues that are vital to group welfare
4. When others have taken advantage of an individual's or group's noncompetitive behavior and now are mobilized to compete about an important topic

BOX 8.9   Appropriate Uses of Compromise

1. When two powerful sides are committed strongly to perceived mutually exclusive goals
2. When temporary solutions to complex issues need to be implemented
3. When conflicting goals are "moderately important" and not worth a major confrontation
4. When time pressures people to expedite a workable solution
5. When collaborating and competing fail

BOX 8.8   Competing: Self-Assessment and Commitment to Action

If you use competing often, ask yourself the following questions:
1. Am I surrounded by people who agree with me all the time and who avoid confronting me?
2. Are others afraid to share themselves and their needs for growth with me?
3. Am I out to win at all costs? If so, what are the costs and benefits of competing?
4. What are people saying about me when I am not around?

If you seldom compete, ask yourself the following questions:
1. How often do I avoid taking a strong stand and then feel a sense of powerlessness?
2. Do I avoid taking a stand so that I can escape risk?
3. Am I fearful and unassertive to the point that important decisions are delayed and people suffer?

Commitment to Action
What two new behaviors would increase your effective use of competition?
1.
2.

developed over time. A give-and-take relationship leads to conflict resolution, with the result that each person can meet one's most important priorities as much of the time as possible. Compromise is very often the exchange of concessions, as it creates a middle ground. This is the preferred means of conflict resolution during union negotiations, in which each side is appeased to

some degree. In this mode, nobody gets everything, but a sense of energy exists that is necessary to build important relationships and teams.

Negotiation and compromise are valued approaches. They are chosen when less accommodating or avoiding is appropriate (Box 8.9). Compromising is a blend of both assertive and cooperative behaviors, although it calls for less finely honed skills for each behavior than does collaborating. Compromise supports a balance of power between self and others in the workplace. The compromising mode is a common conflict-handling mode used in nurse–physician interactions. A need exists to strengthen a healthy professional alliance that relies on collaborative practice to ensure favorable patient outcomes. Effective communication with other members of the healthcare team positively influences teamwork and staff satisfaction and improves quality of patient care and safety.

Negotiating is more like trading—for example, "You can have this if I can have that" as in "I will chair the unit council task force on improving morale if you send me to the hospital's leadership training classes next week so I can have the skills I need to be effective." Compromise is one of the most effective behaviors used by nurse leaders because it supports a balance of power between themselves and others in the work setting. The self-assessment in Box 8.10 will help you become more aware of your own use of negotiation and compromise and improve it.

Collaborating

Collaborating, although the most time-consuming approach, is the most creative stance. It is both assertive and cooperative, because people work creatively

BOX 8.10   Negotiation and Compromise Self-Assessment and Commitment to Action

If you tend to use negotiation often, ask yourself the following questions:
1. Do I ignore large, important issues while trying to work out creative, practical compromises?
2. Is there a "gamesmanship" in my negotiations?
3. Am I sincerely committed to compromise or negotiated solutions?

If you seldom use negotiation, ask yourself the following questions:
1. Do I find it difficult to make concessions?
2. Am I often engaged in strong disagreements or do I withdraw when I see no way to get out?
3. Do I feel embarrassed, sensitive, self-conscious, or pressured to negotiate, compromise, and bargain?

Commitment to Action
What two new behaviors would increase your compromising effectiveness?
1.
2.

BOX 8.11   Appropriate Uses for Collaboration

1. When seeking creative, integrative solutions in which both sides' goals and needs are important, thus developing group commitment and a consensual decision
2. When learning and growing through cooperative problem solving, resulting in greater understanding and empathy
3. When identifying, sharing, and merging vastly different viewpoints
4. When being honest about and working through difficult emotional issues that interfere with morale, productivity, and growth

BOX 8.12   Collaboration Self-Assessment and Commitment to Action

If you tend to collaborate often, ask yourself the following questions:
1. Do I spend valuable group time and energy on issues that do not warrant or deserve it?
2. Do I postpone needed action to get consensus and avoid making key decisions?
3. When I initiate collaboration, do others respond in a genuine way, or are there hidden agendas, unspoken hostility, and/or manipulation in the group?

If you seldom collaborate, ask yourself the following questions:
1. Do I ignore opportunities to cooperate, take risks, and creatively confront conflict?
2. Do I tend to be pessimistic, distrusting, withdrawing, and/or competitive?
3. Am I involving others in important decisions, eliciting commitment, and empowering them?

Commitment to Action
What two new behaviors would increase your collaboration effectiveness?
1.
2.

and openly to find the solution that most fully satisfies all important concerns and goals to be achieved. Collaboration involves analyzing situations and defining the conflict at a higher level where shared goals are identified and commitment to working together is generated (Box 8.11). Collaboration demonstrates relationship-centered approaches with patients and with others because both parties are concerned with their relationship with the other person, not just with the issue at hand. When nurses use cooperative conflict management approaches, decision-making becomes a collective process in which action plans are mutually understood and implemented. An organizational culture that supports collaborative communication and behavior among nurses and other members of the team is needed to merge the unique strengths of all professions into opportunities to improve patient outcomes. For example, when nurses and physicians work together, they can collaborate by asking, "What is the best thing we can do for the patient and family right now?" and "How does each of us fit into the plan of care to meet their needs?" This requires discussion about the plan, how it will be accomplished, and who will make what contributions toward its achievement and proposed outcomes. Use the self-assessment in Box 8.12 to determine your own use of collaboration.

At the onset of conflict, involved collaborating individuals can carefully analyze situations to identify the nature and reasons for conflict and choose an appropriate approach. For example, a conflict arises when a direct care nurse and a charge nurse on a psychiatric unit disagree about how to handle a patient's complaints about the direct care nurse's delay in responding to the patient's requests. At the point that they reach agreement that it is the direct care nurse's responsibility and decision to make, collaboration has occurred. The charge nurse might say, "I didn't realize your plan of care was to respond to the patient at predetermined intervals or that you told the patient that you would check on her every 30 minutes. I can now inform the patient that I know about and support your approach." Or the direct care nurse and the charge nurse might talk and subsequently agree that the direct care nurse is too emotionally involved with the patient's problems and that it may be time for her to withdraw from providing the care and enlist the support of another nurse, even temporarily. Discussion can result in collaboration aimed at allowing the direct care nurse to withdraw appropriately. Another less desirable choice could be to compete and let the winner's position stand—for example, "I'm in charge; I'm going to assign another nurse to this patient to preserve our patient satisfaction scores" or "I know what is best for this patient; I took care of her during her past two admissions."

DIFFERENCES IN CONFLICT-HANDLING STYLES AMONG NURSES

An increased emphasis has been placed on effective communication and appropriate conflict management styles in healthcare. Avoidance and accommodation are often the predominant choices for direct care nurses, and the prevalent style for nurse managers is frequently compromise despite the benefits placed on collaboration as an effective strategy for conflict management. Nursing students and new graduates may be unprepared to handle conflict in the practice environment and may experience a number of barriers, such as fear of causing conflict (Vandergoot et al., 2018). Speaking up as a patient advocate is difficult for novice nurses. This highlights the need to develop delegation strategies, including conflict-handling skills, to adapt to the evolving professional role. A prevalent conflict management style for nursing students and new nurses is avoidance and accommodation. Nurses who successfully manage disruptive workplace conflict reported a deliberate approach that included delaying confrontation, approaching the colleague calmly, and acknowledging the colleague's point of view. Nurses may need to adapt communication and conflict management strategies to respond to diverse patient populations and the unique mix of interprofessional colleagues. See the Research Perspective, which describes early-career hospital nurses' experiences with verbal abuse in the workplace.

RESEARCH PERSPECTIVE

Resource: Cho, H., Pavek, K., & Steege, L. (2020). Workplace verbal abuse, nurse-reported quality of care and patient safety outcomes among early-career hospital nurses. *Journal of Nursing Management, 28,* 1250–1258.

The differences between early-career nurses' verbal abuse experiences and the relationship to patient care quality and safety outcomes were examined. Nurses' gender and age and the type of unit on which they work predispose early-career nurses to verbal abuse, including yelling and cursing at work. Male nurses reported more verbal abuse from patients and families than female nurses. Nurses in their 20s reported more verbal abuse from physicians than older nurses, while nurses in their 30s reported more incivility from disciplines other than nurses in their 20s. Nurses working on step-down units and on general units reported more verbal abuse than those working in intensive care units. Early-career nurses who experienced verbal abuse reported lower ratings of quality of care and patient safety, regardless of age, perpetrator, or unit.

Implications for Practice

Managing verbal abuse is important to promote a safe and healthy workplace and, in turn, improve patient quality and safety. Leaders should monitor unit culture and schedule regular meetings with new graduate nurses and early-career nurses to discuss any concerns about bullying, lateral violence, or incivility. Nurse managers can collaborate with other leadership structures such as unit councils to implement changes in the practice environment to reinforce a zero-tolerance culture and provide bystander intervention training. Education about how to effectively confront workplace disruptions should begin in nursing school and continue into orientation and nurse residency programs.

THE ROLE OF THE LEADER

Encouraging positive working relationships among healthcare providers requires effective conflict management as part of a healthy working environment. The role of the nurse leader is to create a practice environment that fosters open communication and collaborative practices for achieving mutual goals that enable nurses to use constructive approaches to conflict management. Specifically, leaders must adopt a strategic proactive approach that aligns conflict management approaches with the overall mission of the organization. The training of nurse managers as conflict coaches shows promise in creating a positive practice environment when integrated with other conflict intervention processes. By modeling open communication and acknowledging each team member's viewpoint, the nurse manager can coach staff to independently and effectively resolve future conflicts themselves.

With the aging workforce and current nursing shortage, practice environments must be designed to retain nurses and prevent premature departure from the discipline. How to preserve the wisdom that experienced nurses have is a critical challenge. Moreover, nurse leaders need to help challenge the stereotypical gender behavioral expectations and self-esteem issues frequently associated with a female-dominated profession and model effective management and leadership styles. One way to promote a positive work setting is to promote conflict prevention and ensure conflict management. The Literature Perspective highlights the results of an integrative review of publications about teamwork, delegation, and communication among registered nurses and nursing assistants. Nurse leaders must provide the best example of advocacy and empowerment to their staff by coaching newer nurses to think strategically about a mode of conflict handling that is appropriate for the situation. Poor communication often creates conflict that jeopardizes patient safety, whereas inadequate leadership appears to be a contributing factor to adverse patient outcomes. Nurse managers need to support their staff's use of effective conflict management strategies by modeling open and honest communication, including staffing decision-making, and securing resources whenever possible that meet the staff's needs in delivering quality care. Providing education about conflict management could empower

LITERATURE PERSPECTIVE

Resource: Campbell, A. R., Layne, D., Scott, E., & Wei, H. (2019). Interventions to promote teamwork, delegation and communication among registered nurses and nursing assistants: An integrated review. *Journal of Nursing Management, 28,* 1465–1472.

An integrative review of publications focusing on interventions to promote teamwork, delegation, and communication among registered nurses (RN) and unlicensed assistive personnel (UAP) revealed strategies to strenghten the RN-UAP dyad to promote patient safety and positive patient and staff outcomes. Of the seven articles included in the review, four measured patient outcomes, including patient falls, hospital-acquired pressure injuries, and patient satisfaction. With improved RN-UAP relations, three studies reported decreased falls, two described increased patient satisfaction, and one reported a reduction in hospital-acquired pressure injuries. Five of the studies reflected improved teamwork and communication and two studies reported improved job satisfaction. Team building is essential for enhancing team unity, improving communication, and building mutual respect and trust. The organizational impact of ineffective communication and negative conflict management includes reduced productivity and ineffective teamwork, which can lead to adverse patient outcomes. The need to build a foundation of trust and respect and to engage in effective communication was evident across all studies.

Implications for Practice

Although emphasis is frequently placed on improving nurse–physician relations, the need to foster effective relationships between registered nurses and nursing assistants is also essential. Providing quality patient care requires collaborative working relationships punctuated by effective communication and conflict resolution. Interprofessional handoffs or rounding could include unlicensed nursing personnel to promote teamwork. Healthcare leaders must model effective communication, conflict management, and appropriate delegation to promote an organizational culture of quality and safety. Nursing leaders should focus educational efforts on nursing care that requires RN-UAP coordination, including turning, ambulating, feeding, hygiene, emotional support, documentation, and surveillance.

nurses to use these newly acquired skills in negotiation and creative problem-solving techniques. One example is nurse leaders using an interprofessional education program designed by the Department of Defense and the Agency for Healthcare Research and Quality (AHRQ) called *TeamSTEPPS* to reduce stress and conflict because it focuses on evidence-based strategies to enhance teamwork and communication (AHRQ, 2018). Healthcare providers do not always voice concerns about patients and often avoid conflict in clinical settings.

EXERCISE 8.4 Review the educational program TeamSTEPPS. Identify two strategies you can incorporate into your practice. State your rationale for selecting those and create an action plan to incorporate those strategies into your practice.

Healthcare leaders and managers who promote effective conflict resolution skills and who discourage the use of avoidance as a strategy have the potential to reduce employee stress and burnout as well as promote higher job satisfaction. Effective conflict resolution enhances team performance, increases patient safety, and improves patient outcomes (Fowler & Robbins, 2021).

Nurse conflict, stress, burnout, and turnover must be reduced to positively transition new graduate nurses into the workforce and retain experienced nurses. Organizations must support nurses by reducing role stress through reasonable workloads, clear expectations, and providing opportunities to be mentored, including in communication and conflict resolution (Hallaran et al., 2021). The nature of the differences, underlying reasons, importance of the issue, strength of feelings, and commitment to shared goals all have to be considered when selecting an approach to resolving conflict. Preferred and previously effective approaches can be considered, but they need to match the situation. Sometimes, a third party may be introduced into a conflict so that mediation can occur. Mediation is a learned skill for which advanced training or certification is available. Principled negotiation can produce mutually acceptable agreements in every type of conflict. The method involves separating the people from the problem; focusing on interests, not positions; inventing options for mutual gain; and

insisting on using objective criteria. The mediator is usually an impartial person who assists each party in the conflict to better hear and understand the other. In society, for example, much focus is on who can control whom and on who is the "winner." The successful individual involved in conflict resolution and negotiation often moves beyond avoidance, accommodation, and compromise. In nursing practice, added difficulty occurs in negotiating conflicts when at least one of the parties is on an unequal or uneven playing field. This disadvantage is made even worse when the other party to the conflict does not even acknowledge the disparities involved.

MANAGING INCIVILITY, LATERAL VIOLENCE, AND BULLYING

An expression of conflict may be incivility, lateral violence, or bullying. In nursing, they are prevalent in all settings. Incivility is one or more rude, discourteous, or disrespectful actions, which can range from gossiping to refusing to assist a coworker. A significant source of interpersonal conflict in the workplace stems from lateral violence—aggressive and destructive behavior or psychological harassment of nurses against each other. Nurses are particularly vulnerable because lateral or horizontal violence involves conflictual behaviors among individuals who consider themselves peers with equal power—but with little power within the system. Bullying is closely related to lateral or horizontal violence; however, a real or perceived power differential between the instigator and recipient must be present in bullying. Bullying (defined as repeated, unwanted harmful actions intended to humiliate, offend, and cause distress in the recipient) is a very serious issue that threatens patient safety, nurse safety, and the nursing profession as a whole.

Understanding the sources of intraprofessional conflict in the practice environment is essential. Nurses are in positions to identify and intervene on the part of their colleagues when they see or experience horizontal violence or bullying, which is referred to as bystander intervention in the workplace. With increased awareness and sensitivity, nurses may be better able to monitor themselves and to assist their peers to recognize when they are participating in negative behaviors. Identifying and understanding particular incidences (e.g., heavy workload, short staffing) when nurses are most vulnerable and apt to engage in negative behavior and establishing performance expectations has the potential to reduce lateral violence in the workplace (Crawford et al., 2019). Incorporating workplace civility in nursing orientation programs and modeling professional behaviors provides a foundation to promote a healthy work culture. Nursing students and new graduates often lack the confidence and skill set to prevent interpersonal conflict and must rely on experienced nurse leaders to reduce the likelihood of incivility, horizontal violence, or bullying. The actions of nurse leaders will determine not only the future of professional nursing practice but also how the public views the nursing profession (Crawford et al., 2019). Nurse educators have a similar responsibility to develop nursing curricula that educate and encourage dialogue about incivility and horizontal violence to increase awareness, communication, and conflict resolution skills.

In hostile work environments, the ability to provide quality patient care is compromised. TJC (2020) acknowledges that unresolved conflict and disruptive behavior adversely affect safety and quality of care. The vulnerability of newly licensed nurses as they are socialized within the nursing workforce and deal with interpersonal conflicts is a significant challenge (Cho et al., 2020). Lateral violence affects newly licensed nurses' job satisfaction and stress. It also affects their perception of whether to remain in their current position and in the profession. Similarly, nursing students are particularly vulnerable to lateral violence and bullying in the transition to becoming a nurse. This could lead to nursing students questioning their long-held belief that nurses are caring and supportive professionals and can negatively affect quality of care and patient safety outcomes (Cho et al., 2020).

Lateral violence may be a response to the practice environment, in which ineffective leadership may exacerbate the problem. Incivility and disruptive behavior that intimidates others and affects morale or staff turnover can be harmful to patient care. It mandates that organizations have a code of conduct defining acceptable, disruptive, and inappropriate behaviors and that leaders create and implement a process for managing these conflictual situations. Ignoring the importance of informal communication and informal social networks can be detrimental to employee satisfaction, patient outcomes, and organizational goal attainment. Managing the rumor mill, the grapevine, or the gossip chain will assist in decreasing incivility and improve the work environment (Prestia, 2021). One-on-one conflict resolution must be encouraged, but a mechanism for confidential reporting is also necessary. Training on conflict management that includes how to recognize and defend against lateral violence is necessary to ensure a positive professional practice environment. Senior-level leaders and nurse managers are responsible for ensuring that appropriate policies are in place to confront negative workplace behaviors, including lateral violence and bullying. The ANA Position Statement on Incivility, Bullying, and Workplace Violence (American Nurses Association, 2015) remains relevant today. It states that the nursing profession will not tolerate violence of any type from any source and directs nurses and nurse leaders to collaborate to create a culture of respect.

EXERCISE 8.5 Consider a conflict you would describe as "ongoing" in a clinical setting. Talk to some people who have been around for a while to get their historical perspective on this issue. Then, consider the following questions:
- What are their positions and years of experience?
- How are resources, time, and personnel wasted on mismanaging this issue?
- What blocks the effective management of this issue?
- What currently aids in its management?
- What new things and actions would add to its management in the future?

CONCLUSION

Communication is impossible to avoid. Even when we say nothing, we are communicating. The complexity of healthcare and its delivery have created specific approaches to safeguard how information is transmitted to prevent, as much as possible, harm occurring to patients.

Conflict is inevitable within healthcare environments. The major issue of miscommunication and unresolved conflict in nursing is that patients could suffer. Knowing how to respond appropriately in conflictual situations helps the entire healthcare team focus on quality and safety rather than disagreements and disruptions.

Unresolved conflict in the professional practice environment results in negative outcomes for nurses and other healthcare professionals, organizations, and patients.

Incivility, bullying, and lateral violence are toxic to the profession through the negative impact on the retention of staff and on detrimental outcomes for patients. Registered nurses must work in an effective and collaborative manner with other members of the healthcare team to enhance retention and eliminate incivility, lateral violence, and bullying from the workplace. Incivility, bullying, lateral violence, and all forms of disruptive behaviors have a negative effect on the retention of nursing staff and the quality and safety of patient care. Nurses must enhance their knowledge and skills in managing conflict, communicating clearly, and promoting workplace policies to eliminate bullying and lateral violence. Nurse leaders must eliminate hostile work environments, workplace intimidation, reality shock for new graduates, and the acceptance of inappropriate professional interactions.

THE SOLUTION

I apologized to the patient about not having the dressings changed earlier and changed them immediately. I was really upset that this had happened. I knew this was not right, for both the patient's quality of care and the dishonesty from the nurse. I did not want to be the nurse who points out other's mistakes or who created conflict. I knew I had to speak up, because not only was this not the first time this happened with that nurse, but also because we need to prevent this from happening again because it affects patients' quality of care. I spoke with the charge nurse about the situation, and I was relieved when she said she was ecstatic about me speaking up about this, since not many new graduate nurses would feel comfortable doing so. I felt proud of myself for communicating these concerns. I felt heard and understood, and I realized that it does not matter that you are a new graduate nurse; if you see something wrong, you have to say something, because in the end you are your patient's advocate.

Would this be a suitable approach for you? Why?

Elia Nava

REFLECTIONS

How will you use the material from this chapter to promote effective communication and reduce conflict with the patients for whom you provide care as well as with interprofessional coworkers? How do healthcare environments compound the complexity of communication and contribute to conflict? Write a one-page summary including specific examples with an emphasis on how you can be more effective in managing conflict.

BEST PRACTICES

Civil work environments promote patient safety and favorable patient and staff outcomes. Because communication is such a critical element in patient care, all members of the interprofessional team must employ effective strategies and speak up when care can be compromised. Effective communication contributes to positive patient care.

TIPS FOR EFFECTIVE COMMUNICATION AND ADDRESSING CONFLICT

- Develop common language for critical information for handoff communications and communication of changes in a patient's condition.
- Use a communication tool such as SBAR to standardize communication.
- Use a standardized format for change-of-shift report and handoff communication.
- Use a standardized format for report when patients are transferred to other units or facilities.
- Provide the opportunity for questions and confirmation of understanding of communication.
- Have face-to-face communication when possible.
- Read back all healthcare provider orders or other pertinent information.
- Create a culture of patient safety that has zero tolerance for intimidating and disruptive behavior.
- Work in interprofessional teams to develop common language.

- Develop skills in assertive communication and conflict management.
- Recognize that conflict is a necessary and beneficial process typically marked by frustration, different conceptualizations, a variety of approaches to resolving it, and ongoing outcomes.
- Assess the work environment to see what behaviors are endorsed and fostered by the leaders. Determine whether these behaviors are worthy of imitation.
- Determine any similarities and differences in facts, goals, methods, and values in sorting out the different conceptualizations of a conflict situation.

- Assess the degree of conflict resolution by asking questions about the quality of the decisions (e.g., creativity, practicality, achievement of goals, breakthrough results) and the quality of the relationships (e.g., understanding, willingness to work together, mutual respect, cooperation).
- Remind yourself of your preferences for resolving conflict (e.g., which of the five approaches do you not use often enough and which do you overuse?) and assess each situation to match the best approach for that type of conflict regardless of which is your favorite approach.
- Assist others around you in assessing conflict situations and determining how they can best approach them.

REFERENCES

Afriyie, D. (2020). Effective communication between nurses and patients: An evolutionary concept analysis. *British Journal of Community Nursing, 25*(9), 438–445.

Agency for Healthcare Research and Quality (AHRQ). (2018). *TeamSTEPPS 2.0.* Retrieved from https://www.ahrq.gov/teamstepps/instructor/index.html.

American Association of Colleges of Nursing (AACN). (2021). *The Essentials: Core Competencies for Professional Nursing Education.* Washington, DC: Author.

American Nurses Association (ANA). (2015). *ANA Position Statement on Incivility, Bullying, and Workplace Violence.* Retrieved from https://www.nursingworld.org/practice-policy/nursing-excellence/official-position-statements/id/incivility-bullying-and-workplace-violence/.

American Nurses Credentialing Center (ANCC). (n.d.). *Magnet model: Creating a Magnet culture.* Retrieved from https://www.nursingworld.org/organizational-programs/magnet/magnet-model/.

Blake, R. R., & Mouton, J. S. (1964). *Solving costly organization conflict.* San Francisco: Jossey-Bass.

Boruff, R. (2020). Preparing nursing students for enhanced communication with minority populations via simulation. *Clinical Simulation in Nursing, 45*(2), 47–49.

Business Wire. (2021). *New Press Ganey findings show healthcare safety scores fell amid the pandemic.* Retrieved from https://www.businesswire.com/news/home/20211021005658/en/New-Press-Ganey-Findings-Show-Healthcare-Safety-Scores-Fell-Amid-the-Pandemic#.YXKXVH8aZRE.linkedin.

Campbell, A. R., Layne, D., Scott, E., & Wei, H. (2019). Interventions to promote teamwork, delegation and communication among registered nurses and nursing assistants: An integrated review. *Journal of Nursing Management, 28*(7), 1465–1472.

Cho, H., Pavek, K., & Steege, L. (2020). Workplace verbal abuse, nurse-reported quality of care and patient safety outcomes among early-career hospital nurses. *Journal of Nursing Management, 28*(6), 1250–1258.

Crawford, C. L., Chu, F., Judson, L. H., Cuenca, E., Jadalla, A. A., Tze-Polo, L., Kawar, L. N., Runnels, C., & Garvida, R. (2019). An integrative review of nurse-to-nurse incivility, hostility, and workplace violence: A GPS for nurse leaders. *Nursing Administration Quarterly, 43*(2), 138–156.

Deutsch, M. (1973). *The resolution of conflict: Constructive and destructive processes.* New Haven, CT: Yale University Press.

Foronda, C. L., Barroso, S., Yeh, V. J., Gattamorta, K. A., & Bauman, E. B. (2021). A rubric to measure nurse-to-physician communication: A pilot study. *Clinical Simulation in Nursing, 50*(1), 38–42.

Fowler, K. R., & Robbins, L. K. (2021). Nurse manager communication and outcomes for nursing: An integrative review. *Journal of Nursing Management, 29*(6), 1486–1495.

Hallaran, A. J., Edge, D. S., Almost, J., & Tregunno, D. (2021). New registered nurse transition to the workforce and intention to leave: Testing a theoretical model. *Canadian Journal of Nursing Research, 53*(4), 384–396.

Hurst, J. B. (1993). *Conflict self-assessment.* Toledo, OH: Human Resource Development Center, University of Toledo.

Hurst, J., & Kinney, M. (1989). *Empowering self and others.* Toledo, OH: University of Toledo.

Institute for Healthcare Improvement (IHI). (2021). *SBAR Tool: Situation-Background-Assessment-Recommendation.* Retrieved from http://www.ihi.org/resources/Pages/Tools/SBARToolkit.aspx.

Jezewski, M. A. (1995). Evolution of a grounded theory: Conflict resolution through culture brokering. *Advances in Nursing Science, 17*(3), 14–30.

Lee, T. S., Tzeng, W. C., & Chiang, H. H. (2019). Impact of coping strategies on nurses' well-being and practice. *Journal of Nursing Scholarship, 51*(2), 195–204.

Malfait, S., Van Hecke, A., Van Biesen, W., & Eeckloo, K. (2018). Do bedside handovers reduce handover duration? An observational study with implications for evidence-based practice. *Worldviews on Evidence-Based Nursing, 15*(2), 432–439.

Prestia, A. S. (2021). Informal communication: Coexisting with the grapevine. *Nurse Leader, 19*(5), 489–492.

QSEN Institute. (n.d.). *QSEN competencies*. Retrieved from http://qsen.org/competencies/pre-licensure-ksas/.

Rhudy, L. M., Johnson, M. R., Krecke, C. A., Keigley, D. S., Schnell, S. J., Maxson, P. M., McGill, S. M., & Warfield, K. T. (2019). Change-of-shift nursing handoff interruptions: Implications for practice. *Worldviews on Evidence-Based Nursing, 16*(5), 362–370.

Sarver, W. L., Seabold, K., & Kline, M. (2020). Shadowing to improve teamwork and communication: A potential strategy for surge staffing. *Nurse Leader, 18*(6), 597–603.

The Joint Commission (TJC). (2020). *Sentinel Event Data Summary*. Retrieved from https://www.jointcommission.org/sentinel_event_statistics_quarterly/.

Thomas, K. W. (1992). Conflict and conflict management: Reflections and update. *Journal of Organizational Behavior, 13*(3), 265–274.

Thomas, K. W., & Kilmann, R. H. (1974). *Thomas-Kilmann conflict mode instrument*. Tuxedo, NY: Xicom.

Thomas, K. W., & Kilmann, R. H. (2002). *Thomas-Kilmann conflict mode instrument* (revised edition). Mountain View, CA: CPP, Inc.

Vandergoot, S., Sarris, A., Kirby, N., & Ward, H. (2018). Exploring undergraduate students' attitudes toward interprofessional learning, motivation-to-learn, and perceived impact of learning conflict resolution skills. *Journal of Interprofessional Care, 32*(2), 211–219.

White, E. M., Aiken, L. H., & McHugh, M. D. (2019). Registered nurse burnout, job dissatisfaction, and missed care in nursing homes. *Journal of American Geriatric Society, 67*(10), 2065–2071.

9

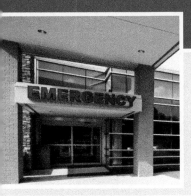

Healthcare Organizations and Structures

Kristin K. Benton and Nina Almasy

ANTICIPATED LEARNING OUTCOMES

- Analyze the characteristics of different healthcare organizations.
- Classify healthcare organizations by major types.
- Analyze economic, social, and demographic forces that drive the development of healthcare organizations.

- Compare and contrast opportunities for nurse leaders and managers during the evolution of healthcare organizations.

KEY TERMS

accountable care organization
accreditation
care coordination
consolidated systems
deeming authority
fee-for-service
for-profit organization
horizontal integration
independent practice associations (IPAs)

managed care
medical home
networks
preferred provider organizations (PPOs)
primary care
private nonprofit (or not-for-profit) organization
public institution
secondary care

social determinants of health (SDOH)
teaching institution
tertiary care
third-party payers
value-based payment
vertical integration

THE CHALLENGE

Now, more than ever, America is faced with a lack of affordable housing and decreased capacity of housing assistance programs. These challenges have led to the increasing rise in persons experiencing homelessness. A lack of affordable healthcare can also lead to higher utilization and system costs due to inappropriate use of the emergency department instead of connecting individuals with primary preventive care.

As an example, a 42-year-old male who was recently hospitalized with recurrent rectal bleeding and anemia. After a complete physical assessment, the gentleman stated he had been homeless for the past five years and never planned for that to happen. Due to unforeseen circumstances and a divorce, he ended up living on the streets. He now calls the street his home. He has been unable to work due to his criminal background history. With further conversation, he begins to explain about his family and being disconnected from them for the last 10 years. He shares that he drinks a liter of vodka almost daily. He does not have a medical home for primary care and does not believe it is necessary. He is now being admitted to the hospital. As the case manager on the accepting unit, I was responsible for creating a discharge plan for him.

What do you think you would do if you were this nurse?

Veronica Buitron-Camacho, MSN, RN
Director of Medical Management, Central Health, Austin, TX

INTRODUCTION

Organizations are collections of individuals brought together in a defined environment to achieve a set of predetermined objectives. Healthcare organizations are systems composed of people, institutions, and resources designed to address the healthcare needs of a target population. Economic, social, and demographic factors affect the purpose and structuring of the system, which, in turn, interact with the mission, philosophy, and structure of healthcare organizations.

Healthcare organizations provide two general types of services: illness care (restorative) and wellness care (preventive). Illness care services help the sick and injured. Wellness care services promote better health as well as illness and accident prevention. In the past, most organizations (e.g., hospitals, clinics, public health departments, community-based organizations, and physicians' offices) focused their attention on illness services. However, economic, social, and demographic dynamics have stimulated the development of organizations designed to achieve the Institute for Healthcare Improvement's Quintuple Aim. The purpose of the Quintuple Aim is to improve the patient experience of care, improve population health, reduce the per capita cost of care, improve the experience of administering care for providers, and improved health equity. Contemporary organizations must optimize care delivery to focus on the full spectrum of health, especially wellness and prevention, to meet consumers' needs in more effective ways.

Opportunities exist for nurses in roles as designers of these restructured organizations and as healthcare leaders and managers within the organizations. For example, nurses today take a much more active and independent role in providing and coordinating patient care than in the past. Similarly, as population numbers increase, we should anticipate new roles for nurses within the healthcare system. An increased focus on quality improvement, outcomes measurement, and benchmarking demands that organizations evaluate their practices and make appropriate improvements, including those related to the organization's culture and the role of nurses within the organization. The skills needed for quality improvement, outcome measurement, and benchmarking are certainly within the skill set for nurses, as defined by the 2020 American Association of Colleges of Nursing (AACN) Essentials (AACN, 2020). Being able to apply knowledge about systems is critical to working effectively across the continuum of care.

Nurses practice in many different types of healthcare organizations. Nursing roles develop in response to the same social, cultural, economic, legislative, and demographic factors that shape the organizations in which they work. Nurses must answer the call to lead, whether it be at the frontline or management or administrative level within an organization. As the largest group of healthcare professionals providing direct and indirect care services to individuals, families, and communities, nurses have an obligation to be involved in the development and evaluation of healthcare, social, regulatory, and economic policies that shape healthcare organizations.

CHARACTERISTICS AND TYPES OF ORGANIZATIONS

Responding to the rapidly changing nature of the economic, social, and demographic environment at the national, state, and local level, the U.S. healthcare system, and the organizations within the system, are in a continual state of flux. Organizations either anticipate or respond to these environmental changes and can be classified in a variety of ways. Some classifications include the type of institution, type of services provided, length of services offered, ownership structure, teaching status, and accreditation status. An overview of how these classifications distinguish organizations follows.

Institutional Providers

Acute care hospitals, long-term care facilities, and rehabilitation facilities have traditionally been classified as institutional providers. Major characteristics that differentiate institutional providers as well as other healthcare organizations are (1) types of services provided, (2) length of direct care services provided, (3) ownership, (4) teaching status, and (5) accreditation status.

Types of Services Provided

The type of services offered is a characteristic used to differentiate institutional providers. Services can be classified as either general or specialty care. Facilities that provide specialty care offer a limited scope of services, such as those targeted to specific disease entities or patient populations. Examples of specialty care facilities are those providing psychiatric care, cardiac care, burn care, children's care, women's and infants' care, and oncology care. Alternatively, facilities such as general hospitals provide a wide range of services to multiple segments of the population.

Length of Direct Care Services Provided

Another characteristic that is used to differentiate healthcare organizations is the duration of the care provided. According to the American Hospital Association (AHA, 2021) most hospitals are acute care facilities, giving short-term, episodic care. Acute care hospitals provide inpatient care and other related services for short-term medical conditions. Chronic care or long-term facilities provide services for patients who require care for extended periods, in excess of 30 days. Many institutions expand their scope of services through community partnerships not only to provide acute healthcare services

but also to address risk factors for chronic disease, such as obesity and tobacco use. The term *healthcare network* refers to interconnected units that either are owned by the institution or have cooperative agreements with other institutions to provide a full spectrum of wellness and illness services. The spectrum of care services provided is typically described as primary care (first-access care), secondary care (disease-restorative care), and tertiary care (rehabilitative or long-term care). Table 9.1 describes the continuum of care and the units of healthcare organizations that provide services in the three phases of the continuum.

TABLE 9.1   Continuum of Healthcare Organizations

Type of Care	Purpose	Organization or Unit Providing Services
Primary	• Entry into system • Health promotion • Disease prevention • Chronic care • Treatment of temporary nonincapacitating conditions	• Ambulatory care centers • Physicians' offices • Preferred provider organizations • Nursing centers • Independent provider organizations • Health maintenance organizations • School health clinics
Secondary	• Prevention of disease complications	• Home health care • Ambulatory care centers • Acute care hospitals • Freestanding emergency departments • Nursing centers
Tertiary	• Rehabilitation • Long-term care	• Home health care • Long-term care facilities • Hospice care • Rehabilitation centers • Skilled nursing facilities • Assisted-living facilities

EXERCISE 9.1 Consider the experience of a patient in your community who was healthy until being diagnosed with cardiovascular disease at age 52. Despite initial interventions, the patient suffers a myocardial infarction 2 years later. Over the next 20 years, the patient develops chronic heart failure that after specialty interventions, requires continuing chronic care. Reflect on the spectrum of care services to explain how this patient's care was delivered. Search online to identify the specific services in your community that would meet this patient's needs. Table 9.1 provides examples of primary, secondary, and tertiary care services.

Ownership

Ownership is another characteristic used to classify healthcare organizations. Ownership establishes the organization's legal, business, and mission-related imperatives. Healthcare organizations have three basic ownership forms: public, private nonprofit, and for profit. Public institutions provide health services to individuals under the support and/or direction of local, state, or federal government. These organizations answer directly to the sponsoring government agency or boards and are indirectly responsible to elected officials and taxpayers who support them. Examples of these service recipients at the federal level are veterans, members of the military, Native Americans, and inmates of correctional facilities. State-supported organizations may be health service teaching facilities, chronic care facilities, and correctional facilities.

Locally supported facilities include county-supported and city-supported facilities. Table 9.2 shows how several common healthcare organizations are classified.

Private nonprofit (or not-for-profit) organizations—often referred to as *voluntary agencies*—are controlled by voluntary boards or trustees and provide care regardless of a patient's ability to pay. In these organizations, excess revenue over expenses is redirected into the organization for maintenance and growth rather than returned as dividends to stockholders. Historically, nonprofit organizations have been exempt from paying taxes because they commit to providing an important community service. The owners of such organizations include churches, communities, industries, and special interest groups such as the Shriners. Ascension Health, based in St. Louis, Missouri, is one of the largest nonprofit healthcare organizations with a presence in 19 states and the District of Columbia (Ascension, 2022). The ownership influences how organizations are structured, what services they provide, and which patients they serve.

For-profit organizations are also referred to as *proprietary* or *investor-owned organizations*. These organizations operate with the specific intent of earning a profit by providing healthcare services to individuals who can afford to pay for these services. HCA Healthcare is an example of a for-profit organization.

Organizations in the healthcare space may also provide health care coverage. These public or private insurers are known as third-party payers.

Accountable care organizations (ACOs) emerged as a result of the Patient Protection and Affordable Care

TABLE 9.2   Characteristics and Types of Healthcare Organizations

Healthcare Organization	Type	Services	Ownership	Financing	Teaching Status	Multiunit
Veterans Administration	Institution	General	Federal	NP	Y	Y
Academic Medical Center	Institution	General	Private	NP	Y	Y
Community General	Institution	General	Private	NP	N	Y
Public Hospital	Institution	General	County	NP	Y	N
Shriners Burn Hospitals	Institution	Specialty	Private	NP	N	N
Prepaid Health Plan	HMO	General	Private	NP-P	N	N
Public Health Department	Community	General	State	NP	N	N
Women's and Infants' Project	Community	Specialty	State	NP	N	N
Long-Term Care Corporation	Institution	Long term	Private	NP	N	Y
Visiting Nurses Association	Community	Specialty	Private	NP	N	N

HMO, Health maintenance organization; *N,* no; *NP,* nonprofit; *P,* profit; *Y,* yes.

Act of 2010 as a mechanism to meet the challenges of value-based payment models. ACOs aim to coordinate care and chronic disease management and improve the overall quality of care provided to Medicare patients. ACOs are designed as seamless healthcare delivery systems that bring together physicians, hospitals, and other caregivers focused on improving the health of individuals and communities while decreasing costs. These person-centered organizations are designed for the healthcare team and patients to be true partners in caring. Participation in the program is voluntary, and payments to ACOs are tied to achieving explicit healthcare quality goals and outcomes. The Medicare Shared Savings Program is the most prevalent ACO program. Several quality measures are used to determine the percentage of savings that is captured by an ACO. These quality measures are organized in four domains: patient–caregiver experience of care, care coordination/patient safety, preventive health, and at-risk population health. Nurses at all levels of the organization are vital to achieve these quality measures as we move from volume to value-based care (National Advisory on Nurse Education and Practice, 2019).

Ownership can affect efficiency and quality. Although hospital ownership is defined legally, significant differences are found within the three sectors related to teaching status, location, bed size, and corporate affiliation. For-profit hospitals are typically nonteaching, suburban facilities with a small to medium bed capacity and have the ability to access group purchasing cooperatives that lower nonsalary expenses. For-profit hospitals tend to have higher hospital charges and lower wage and salary costs that most likely represent an aggressive approach to maximizing return on investment.

Teaching Status

Teaching status is a characteristic that can differentiate healthcare organizations. The term teaching institution is applied to academic health centers (those directly affiliated with a school of medicine and at least one other health profession school) and affiliated teaching hospitals (those that provide only the clinical portion of a medical school teaching program). Although care is usually more costly at teaching hospitals than at nonteaching hospitals, teaching hospitals are generally able to offer access to state-of-the-art technology and researchers. While teaching hospitals have been described as having higher costs of patient care, some research suggests that there is some research suggesting that long-term teaching

hospital costs may be the same or even lower than those of nonteaching hospitals when the cost of readmissions and post–acute care are considered (Burke et al., 2019).

Historically, teaching hospitals have received some government reimbursement to cover the additional costs associated with the teaching process. Maintaining a teaching program places a financial burden on hospitals relative to the direct cost of the program and the indirect cost of the inefficiencies surrounding the training process. These inefficiencies include (1) salaries of physicians who supervise students' care delivery and participate in educational programs such as teaching rounds and seminars, (2) duplicated tests or procedures, and (3) delays in processing patients related to the teaching process. Because of the additional costs, few for-profit hospitals sponsor teaching programs. Teaching hospitals are usually located close to their affiliated academic institution. They tend to be larger and located in more urban and economically disadvantaged areas than their nonteaching counterparts.

> **EXERCISE 9.2** Building on the healthcare services you explored in Exercise 9.1, identify the financial and teaching status for each care setting.

Accreditation Status

Another characteristic that can be used to distinguish one organization from another is whether a healthcare organization has been accredited by an external body as having the structure and processes necessary to provide high-quality care. Private organizations play significant roles in establishing standards and ensuring care delivery compliance with standards by accrediting healthcare organizations. Examples are the American Nurses Credentialing Center (ANCC), The Joint Commission (TJC) and the National Committee for Quality Assurance (NCQA). The ANCC offers a voluntary Magnet Recognition Program® that reflects a commitment to nursing excellence in providing high-quality healthcare. TJC provides accreditation programs for ambulatory care, behavioral healthcare, acute care and critical access hospitals, laboratory services, long-term care, and hospital-based surgery. The NCQA is a nonprofit organization that accredits, certifies, and recognizes a wide variety of healthcare organizations, services, and providers. More information on accrediting organizations is provided in the Accrediting Bodies section later in this chapter.

RESEARCH PERSPECTIVE

Resource: Spaulding, A., Hamadi, H., Moody, L., Lentz, L., Liu, X., & Wu, Y. (2020). Do Magnet®-designated hospitals perform better on Medicare's Value-Based Purchasing Program? *JONA: The Journal of Nursing Administration, 50*(7/8), 395–401.

The Magnet Recognition Program® offers a mechanism to indicate the strength and quality of nursing care. However, this study was the first to explore whether or not Magnet®-designated hospitals perform better on Medicare's Value-Based Purchasing Program. Using a cross-sectional study design, value-based purchasing scores of 2686 acute general hospitals inclusive of all 50 U.S. states were analyzed. A number of other statistically significant associations were found. Magnet®-designated hospitals were associated with higher scores for total performance, process of care, and patient experience of care, but lower efficiency of care scores.

Implications for Practice

This study demonstrated that Magnet® designation is associated with improved outcomes as measured by the Medicare Value-Based Purchasing Program. While Magnet®-designated hospitals scored lower in efficiency of care, it is logical to infer that quality care may not be the most efficient care. For example, nurse staffing tends to be more robust in Magnet®-designated hospitals. Nurse leaders can use the findings and discussion from this study to advocate for hospitals to strive toward Magnet® designation citing the positive associations demonstrated with Magnet® designation compared with those hospitals without it.

Consolidated Systems and Networks

Healthcare organizations are being organized into consolidated systems through both the formation of for-profit or not-for-profit multihospital systems and the development of networks of independently owned and operated healthcare organizations. Consolidated systems tend to be organized along five levels. The first level includes the large national hospital companies, most of which are investor owned. The second level involves large voluntary affiliated systems, which provide members with access to capital, political power, management expertise, joint venture opportunities, and links to health insurance services or, as in Canada, to a national healthcare coverage program. The third level involves regional hospital systems that cover a defined geographic area, such as an area of a state. The fourth level involves metropolitan-based systems. The fifth level is composed of the special-interest groups that own and operate units organized along religious lines, teaching interests, or related special interests that drive their activities. This level often crosses over the regional, metropolitan, and national levels already described. Through the creation of multiunit systems, an organization has greater marketing, policy, and contracting potential.

In recent years, the number of partnerships among healthcare organizations increased in response to the shift from a model driven by quantity of care to one driven by quality, person-centered, value-based care to address population health. Joint ventures are arrangements between two unrelated entities to provide a new or existing service while sharing economic risks and rewards. For example, a hospital system might enter into a joint venture partnership with an existing insurance provider to create a new network product. Although the insurance provider holds the authority to offer the insurance, the financial risks and gains of the new network product are shared among the partners. Theoretically, this sharing of risk and savings encourages cooperation to keep costs controlled and innovate to meet the requirements of a value-based payment model.

Ambulatory-Based Organizations

Many health services are provided on an ambulatory basis. The organizational setting for much of this care has been the group practice or private physician's office. Prepaid group practice plans, referred to as *managed care systems*, combine care delivery with financing and provide comprehensive services for a fixed prepaid fee. A goal of these services is to reduce the cost of expensive acute hospital care by focusing on out-of-hospital preventive care and illness follow-up care.

Since the opening of the first retail clinic in 2001 in Minnesota, the number of retail clinics and their utilization have increased dramatically. For example, CVS currently operates over 1,100 MinuteClinic® locations across the United States with plans to expand services offered in 2021. Retail clinics aim to offer convenient care access to patients in retail stores with the goal of increasing store retail business. Although some traditional physician practice–based clinics have expanded access through more flexible scheduling, retail clinics offer walk-in services where patients shop after work and school, including weekends. Retail clinics may offer primary prevention care, health screening and testing, and chronic disease care. Although concerns that sporadic use of retail clinics might contribute to the fragmentation of patient care, patient use continues to grow.

Group practice plans take various forms. One form has a centralized administration that directs and pays salaries for physician practice, for example, health maintenance organizations (HMOs). The HMO is a configuration of healthcare agencies that provide basic and supplemental health maintenance and treatment services to voluntary enrollees who prepay a fixed periodic fee without regard to the amount of services used. To be federally qualified, an HMO company must offer inpatient and outpatient services, treatment and referral for drug and alcohol problems, laboratory and radiology services, preventive dental services for children younger than 12 years, and preventive healthcare services in addition to physician services.

An HMO plan aims to coordinate all patient care services through an approved primary care provider who belongs to a provider network. Patients are most often required to obtain referrals from the primary care provider to see a specialist, such as a surgeon. If patients opt to see an out-of-network provider, the HMO will not provide the same level of coverage offered by in-network providers; in some cases, the patient may be responsible for paying 100% of the costs. Although an HMO may limit a patient's choice of providers, patients are usually not required to file individual claims to cover services provided in network.

Independent practice associations (IPAs), also known as professional associations (PAs), are a form of group practice in which physicians in private offices are paid on a fee-for-service basis by a prepaid plan to deliver care to enrolled members. Preferred provider organizations (PPOs) operate similarly to IPAs; contracts are developed with private practice physicians, but fees are discounted from their usual and customary charges. In return, physicians are guaranteed prompt payment.

Advanced practice registered nurses' leadership in managing patient care in group practices has contributed greatly to their success. Increasing evidence shows that nurse-run clinics as well as ambulatory care centers can succeed whether they are integrated within a larger medical complex or physically and administratively

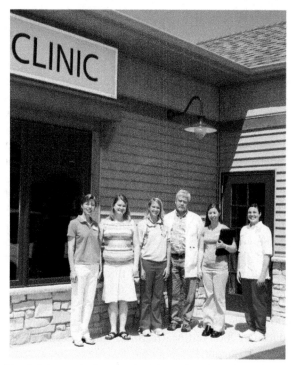

Fig. 9.1 Increasingly, care is delivered through freestanding clinics or community- or hospital-affiliated services.

separate organizations. Examples of freestanding organizations include surgicenters, urgent care centers, imaging centers, and primary care centers (Fig. 9.1).

Other Organizations

Although hospitals, nursing homes, health departments, visiting nurse services, and private clinics have made up the traditional primary service delivery organizations, the critical role being played by other organizations that may be freestanding or units of hospitals or other community organizations cannot be ignored. These include community service organizations, subacute facilities, home health agencies, long-term care facilities, and hospices. In addition, nurse-owned/nurse-organized services and self-help voluntary organizations contribute to the overall service provision.

Community Services

Community services, including public health departments, are focused on the health of the community rather than that of the individual. The historical focus of these organizations has been on control of infectious agents and provision of preventive services under the auspices of public health departments. Local, state, and federal governments allocate funds to health departments to provide a variety of necessary health services. Monies are allocated also for environmental services (e.g., ensuring that food services meet established standards) and for health resources (e.g., reproductive care, safe sex promotion, and breast cancer screening programs). Local health departments have been provided some autonomy in determining how to use funds that are not assigned to categorical programs.

Funding provides for personal health services that include maternal care and childcare, care for communicable diseases such as acquired immunodeficiency syndrome (AIDS) and tuberculosis, services for children with birth defects, mental health care, and investigation of epidemiology and emergent threats, including pandemics and bioterrorism. The COVID-19 (coronavirus disease 2019) pandemic of 2020 thrust public health into the spotlight as the need for preventive strategy education, local testing, treatment, and vaccination became paramount.

School health programs whose funds are also allocated to them by local, state, and federal governments traditionally have been organized to control infectious disease outbreaks; to identify and coordinate care for students with conditions that impact learning; to treat on-site injuries and illnesses; and to provide basic health education programs. Increasingly, schools are being seen as primary care sites for children.

Day care centers offer services for both adults and children in the community. Day care centers for older adults can provide social interaction, exercise, nutritious meals, and stimulating activities with nurse supervision. These programs give respite to family caregivers and allow adult children the opportunity to work during the day while their parent is being cared for in a safe environment. Day care centers for medically complex children also provide respite to parents while offering children social, cognitive, and emotional stimulation in a safe setting overseen by nurses. This community service helps prevent caregiver burnout and long-term institutionalization by allowing individuals to remain living in their communities.

Visiting nurse associations, which are voluntary organizations, have provided a large amount of the follow-up care for patients after hospitalization and for newborns and their mothers. Some are organized by cities, and others serve entire regions. Some operate for profit; others do not.

Subacute Facilities

As hospitals began to discharge patients earlier in their recuperation, the subacute facility, also known as a *long-term acute care (LTAC) hospital*, emerged as a health-care organization. Initially, many of these facilities were former nursing homes refurbished with the high-tech equipment necessary to deal with patients who have just come out of surgery or who are still acutely ill and have complex medical needs. Today, many are newly built centers or new businesses that have taken over existing clinical facilities.

Home Health Organizations

Home health organizations have numerous configurations; they may be freestanding or owned by a hospital and may be for-profit or not-for-profit organizations. Professional nurses often lead the care team in home health and provide expertise in assessing patients' self-care competencies, designing a plan of care to promote patient independence and coordinate the personnel and material resources needed. Home care agencies staffed appropriately with adequate numbers of professional nurses have the potential to keep older adults, those with disabilities, and persons with chronic illnesses comfortable and safe at home.

Long-Term Care and Residential Facilities

Long-term care (LTC) facilities may also be known as *skilled nursing facilities*. These organizations provide long-term rehabilitation and professional nursing services. In residential facilities, no skilled care is provided, but individuals are offered safe environments in a home-like setting designed to honor the dignity of each person.

Hospice and Palliative Care

The concept of hospice and palliative care was launched at St. Christopher Hospice in London. Hospices can be located on inpatient nursing units, such as the kind commonly found in Canada, the United Kingdom, and Australia, or in the home or residential centers in the community. Hospice care focuses on confirming rather than denying the reality of death and, thus, provides care that ensures dignity and comfort.

Since its launch in the 1980s, palliative care expanded dramatically to meet the unique needs of patients experiencing chronic illness who may not qualify for hospice coverage. Palliative care offers patients of all ages the option of seeking continuing care—symptom control for serious illnesses concurrently with other treatments. Members of a palliative care team, usually comprising a physician, nurse, social worker, and chaplain, work together to address the physical, social, cultural, and spiritual needs of patients and families who are coping with a serious illness.

Most hospitals adopted palliative care after TJC's advanced certification program for hospitals that provide quality palliative care. Palliative care has been found to increase patient satisfaction and quality of life (Neville & Laramee, 2020).

Nurse-Owned and Nurse-Organized Services

Nursing centers, which are nurse-owned and nurse-operated places where care is provided by nurses, are another form of community-based organizations. Many nursing centers are administered by schools of nursing and serve as a base for faculty practice and research along with clinical experience for students. Others are owned and operated by groups of nurses. These centers have a variety of missions. Some focus on care for specific populations, such as people who are experiencing homelessness, or on care for people with sexually transmitted infections. Others have taken responsibility for university health services. Some have assumed responsibility for school health programs in the community, and others operate employee wellness programs, hospices, and home care services.

Self-Help and Peer Assistance Voluntary Organizations

Other organizations are the self-help/self-care and peer assistance voluntary organizations. These organizations also come in various forms. They are often composed of and directed by peers who are consumers of healthcare services. Their purpose is most often to enable patients to provide support to each other and raise community consciousness about the nature of a specific health condition. Grief support groups and Alcoholics Anonymous are two examples. Community geriatric organizations, frequently sponsored by healthcare organizations and offering multiple services for promoting wellness and rehabilitation, are increasing rapidly.

> **EXERCISE 9.3** Search your community for existing self-help and voluntary organizations. Document your findings regarding the services they provide and their accessibility. Can you determine whether nurses are playing leadership or frontline roles in those organizations and what functions are incorporated into existing nursing roles?

Supportive and Ancillary Organizations

Organizations involved in the direct provision of healthcare are supported by a number of others whose operations have a significant effect on provider organizations, as well as on the overall performance of the health system. These include regulatory organizations; accrediting bodies; third-party financing organizations; pharmaceutical and medical equipment supply corporations; and various professional, educational, and training organizations.

Regulatory Organizations

Regulatory organizations set standards for the operation of healthcare organizations, ensure compliance with federal and state regulations developed by governmental administrative agencies, and investigate and make judgments regarding complaints brought by consumers of the services and the public. They approve organizations for licensure as providers of healthcare. Healthcare organizations are regulated by a number of different federal, state, and local agencies to protect the health and safety of the patients and communities they serve. A number of different regulatory agencies monitor functions in healthcare organizations. These include the Centers for Medicare & Medicaid Services (CMS), the U.S. Food and Drug Administration (FDA), the Occupational Safety and Health Administration (OSHA), the U.S. Equal Employment Opportunity Commission (EEO), and state licensing boards for various health professions. Regardless of the type of organization in which they work, nurses are often involved in these processes. Therefore, all nurses need to be familiar with the regulations that affect their organization.

Established in 1965, Medicare is the country's largest and most influential health insurance program, providing healthcare funding for more than 55 million individuals. This makes the federal government the primary payer of healthcare costs in the United States. The Medicare program is not limited to individuals age 65 years or older. Persons with certain permanent illnesses, such as end-stage renal disease, also receive

Medicare health benefits. Because of the size of the Medicare market, the federal government serves as the leading regulator of healthcare services in the United States.

Medicare is organized into four parts that recipients may choose from. Medicare Part A, also known as hospital insurance, covers inpatient hospital stays, skilled nursing facility stays, hospice care, and some home health care. Medicare Part B, also known as medical insurance, covers some physicians' services, outpatient care, medical supplies, and primary prevention care. Medicare Part C, or Medicare Advantage Plans, offers recipients the option to enroll in a health plan offered by a private company that contracts with Medicare to coordinate and cover services offered by Parts A and B, often including prescription drug coverage. Medicare Part D covers prescription drug coverage associated with Medicare Parts A and B and most Part C Medicare Advantage Plans.

Medicaid offers government-funded coverage to eligible low-income adults, children, pregnant women, older adults, and people with disabilities. In contrast to Medicare, Medicaid is administered by states, under federal requirements, and is funded by state and federal funding. A state may opt in or opt out to receive federal funding associated with a particular requirement. Families with children dependents who do not meet the income-related eligibility requirement to receive Medicaid but who still cannot afford private coverage may be eligible to receive coverage through the Children's Health Insurance Plan (CHIP), a joint state and federally funded program.

The CMS administers the Medicare and Medicaid programs. Participation in these programs is regulated by a complex set of rules outlined in a lengthy set of guidelines—the Conditions of Participation (CoP). These guidelines are established to improve quality and protect the health and safety of Medicare and Medicaid beneficiaries by specifying the requirements that organizations must meet to be eligible to receive Medicare and Medicaid reimbursement.

To be in compliance with the CoP, healthcare organizations must meet certain quality assessment and performance improvement requirements. Through its Quality Improvement Organization program (formerly called *Peer Review*), the CMS contracts with one organization in each state (typically the state's department of health) to work with healthcare organizations to improve the quality, efficiency, and effectiveness of care provided in that state to Medicare beneficiaries. The CMS provides a financial incentive for hospitals to report quality data. These data are used to establish minimum quality standards for healthcare facilities and by patients to help them make decisions about where to seek healthcare. The program is designed to ensure that healthcare organizations systematically examine the quality of care provided and that they use the data obtained to develop and implement projects that improve quality, enhance patient safety, and reduce medical errors. To help reach these quality goals, the CMS sponsors the Medicare Quality Improvement Community (MedQIC). The MedQIC website contains information and tools to support healthcare providers and organizations in creating community-based approaches to quality improvement.

Nurses are actively involved in CMS patient safety and quality improvement processes. The level of their participation may be as participants in facility-based quality or utilization management activities or they may be involved as case managers. Nurse case managers can serve in a number of different roles, but they frequently serve as the organization's interface with the physician. In this role, these case managers routinely monitor for appropriate physician documentation of medical necessity and other required CoP elements. In the ambulatory or acute care setting, nurses in the role of case managers typically work with physician advisors to ensure that patient care follows recognized standards and facilitates patient flow to the appropriate setting for care.

Nurses also play key roles in developing, implementing, and evaluating the review processes of these regulatory agencies. As members of healthcare organizations providing both direct and indirect services to patients and as members of or advisors to regulatory agencies, baccalaureate- and graduate-prepared nurses in roles of direct care nurse and nurse managers have active roles in monitoring and improving quality as well as establishing standards and ensuring that organizations comply with standards.

EXERCISE 9.4 Choose a facility at which you recently completed a clinical rotation. Which regulatory organizations oversee that facility? What are the implications of regulatory oversight for the nurse in the frontline, manager, and administrative leadership roles at this facility?

Accrediting Bodies

Accreditation refers to the approval, recognition, or certification by an official review board that an organization has met certain standards. The CMS is responsible for the enforcement of its standards through its certification activities. For a healthcare organization to participate in and receive payment from either Medicare or Medicaid, the organization must be certified as complying with the CoP. One way in which an organization can be recognized as complying with the CoP is through a survey process conducted by a state agency on behalf of the CMS. Alternatively, an organization can be surveyed and accredited by a national accrediting body holding "deeming authority" for the CMS. To obtain deeming authority, an accreditation organization must undergo a comprehensive evaluation by the CMS to ensure that the standards of the accrediting organization are at least as rigorous as CMS standards. (See Table 9.3 for a list of organizations with deeming authority.) Healthcare organizations accredited by an organization with CMS deeming authority are therefore deemed as meeting Medicare and Medicaid certification requirements.

Acute care healthcare organizations commonly seek accreditation by the American Osteopathic Association (AOA), The Joint Commission (TJC), or Det Norske Veritas Germanischer Lloyd Healthcare, Inc. (DNV GL Healthcare). These organizations have been granted deeming authority by the CMS. The AOA is a professional association specifically for osteopathic healthcare organizations. The Joint Commission is an independent, not-for-profit organization that accredits more than 22,000 healthcare organizations in the United States and internationally. The mission of TJC is to continuously improve the safety and quality of care provided to the public through the provision of healthcare accreditation and related services that support improvement of performance in healthcare organizations. DNV GL Healthcare received deeming authority in 2008. Its mission is to accredit organizations that demonstrate high performance and continuous improvement of healthcare quality and safety.

Third-Party Financing Organizations

Organizations that provide financing for healthcare comprise another subset of supportive and ancillary organizations. As noted earlier, the government, through the CMS, finances a large portion of the population healthcare and represents the largest third-party

TABLE 9.3 Accrediting Organizations With Deeming Authority for Centers for Medicare & Medicaid Services

Accrediting Organization	Program Types
Accreditation Association for Ambulatory Health Care (AAAHC)	ASCs
Accreditation Association for Hospitals and Health Systems/Health Facilities Accreditation Program (AAHHS/HFAP)	ASCs, CAH, Hospitals
Accreditation Commission for Health Care, Inc (ACHC)	ESRD Facilities, HHA, Hospice
American Association for Accreditation of Ambulatory Surgery Facilities (AAAASF)	ASCs, OPTs, RHCs
Center for Improvement in Healthcare Quality (CIHQ)	Hospitals
Community Health Accreditation Program (CHAP)	HHAs, hospice
Det Norske Veritas Germanischer Lloyd Healthcare, Inc. (DNV GL)	CAH, Hospital, Psychiatric Hospital
National Dialysis Accreditation Commission (NDAC)	ESRD Facilities
The Compliance Team (TCT)	Program Types: RHC
The Joint Commission (TJC)	ASC, CAH, HHA, Hospice, Hospital, Psychiatric Hospitals

ASC, Ambulatory surgery center; *CAH,* critical access hospital; *HHA,* home health agency; *OPT,* outpatient physical therapy; *RHC,* rural health clinics.
Retrieved from Centers for Medicare and Medicaid Services (2020). CMS-Approved Accrediting Organizations. https://www.cms.gov/Medicare/Provider-Enrollment-and-Certification/SurveyCertificationGenInfo/Downloads/Accrediting-Organization-Contacts-for-Prospective-Clients-.pdf

organization involved in healthcare provision. Private health insurance carriers, which account for most of the remaining financing, are composed of not-for-profit and for-profit components. Commercial insurance companies represent the private sector.

Third-party financing organizations have a major effect on the actual delivery of healthcare. They do so by identifying those procedures, tests, services, or drugs that will be covered under their healthcare insurance programs.

Pharmaceutical and Medical Equipment Supply Organizations

Healthcare expenditures that are allocated to drugs and medical equipment are increasing. Nurses in direct care, manager, and leadership roles are primary decision makers of these products. They play a significant role in healthcare organizations in setting standards for safe and efficient products that meet both consumers' and organizations' needs in a cost-effective manner. Supply organizations often seek nurses as customers and as participants in market surveys for the design of new products, services, and marketing techniques. Examples of the roles that nurses play can be seen by studying organizations that employ nurses to design new products and market them through production and distribution of a newsletter and ongoing continuing education presentations.

INTEGRATION

As the healthcare industry faces continuing and increasing pressure to improve patient safety as well as to be efficient and effective, healthcare organizations are entering into a number of different organizational relationships, such as ACOs. Organizations can come together to form affiliations, consortiums, and consolidations that result in multihospital systems and/or multiorganizational arrangements. When organizations that provide similar services come together, the arrangement is referred to as horizontal integration. An example of horizontal integration is a group of acute care facilities that come together to provide coverage for an expanded region. When organizations align to provide a full array or continuum of services, the arrangement is referred to as vertical integration. Organizations brought together in a vertical integration might include an acute care facility, a rehabilitation facility, a home care agency, an ambulatory clinic, and a hospice. Benefits attributed to vertical integration include enhanced coordination of services, efficiency, and customer services. Fig. 9.2 illustrates these approaches to integration.

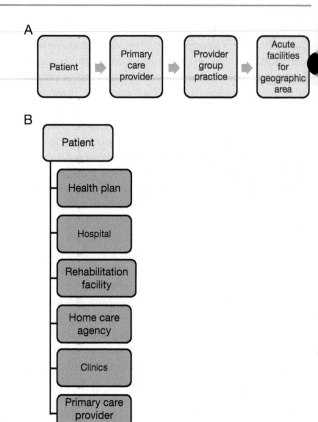

Fig. 9.2 Horizontal (A) and vertical (B) integration of healthcare organizations.

ACQUISITIONS AND MERGERS

The economic forces of capitated payments and managed care have caused healthcare organizations to reorganize, restructure, and reengineer to decrease waste and economic inefficiency. Many organizations are forming multi-institutional alliances that integrate healthcare systems under a common organizational infrastructure. These alliances are accomplished through acquisitions or mergers. Acquisitions involve one organization directly buying another. Mergers involve combining two or more organizations and their assets to form a new entity. As an example, CVS Health merged with the Aetna insurance carrier in 2018. Mergers can also happen within organizations as departments or patient care units are joined together. The health of an organization's culture is a primary factor in predicting whether or not a merger and acquisition will be successful (Chesley, 2020). Nurses in all levels of an organization undergoing such a change must anticipate the challenges of integrating two or more organizational cultures.

Economic, social, and demographic factors provide the input for future development and act as major forces driving the evolution of healthcare organizations.

Economic Factors

Overall economic conditions as well as decisions surrounding the financing of health care have shaped the supply, configuration, and distribution of healthcare organizations and substantially changed the provision of healthcare in the United States. The radical restructuring of the healthcare system required to reduce the continuing escalation of economic resources into the system and to make health care accessible to all citizens will necessitate ongoing changes in healthcare organizations. Nurses have great potential to be engaged with more services and to revamp the approach to care.

U.S. healthcare spending grew 4.6% and reached 17.7% of the gross domestic product in 2019 according to the CMS (2020). In 2020, the COVID-19 pandemic introduced unprecedented economic challenges to the healthcare system. Hospital costs of treating patients with COVID-19, the costs of additional staffing and personal protective equipment, as well as lost revenue due to cancelled routine procedures and surgeries were estimated at over $200 billion in just the four-month period from March to June 2020 (AHA, 2020).

The complexity of controlling costs remains a major driver of change in the healthcare system. Nurses have a major role to play in demonstrating that access to care and quality management are essential components of cost control. With the increasing involvement of industry, business management techniques will assume greater emphasis in healthcare organizations. Nurses will need to lead efforts to redesign roles and restructure healthcare organizations. Nurse leaders, managers, and followers will need to advocate for change and economic policies that will enhance the quality and safety of patient care while achieving cost-effectiveness (American Association of Colleges of Nursing, 2020). The increasing focus on preparing registered nurses at the levels of master's degrees and doctoral degrees reflects the clear need for practicing nurses, nurse managers, and nurse administrators to be able to work efficiently and effectively in a constantly changing healthcare environment.

A study by Disch & Finis (2022) based on the literature and interviews of thought leaders advocates for a major restructuring of how we approach health care delivery and nurses' contributions to that delivery. Our current approaches are outdated in terms of the complexity of what we do and the contributions we make. Capturing those data are critical.

Social Factors

Increasing consumer attention to disease prevention and promotion of healthful lifestyles is redefining relationships of healthcare organizations and their patients. Consumers are becoming increasingly active in care planning, implementation, and evaluation and are seeking increased participation with their providers. Demands will be made of healthcare organizations for more personal, responsive, and coordinated care. As such, development of strategies that allow patients to become empowered controllers of their own health status is essential. Responsive structural changes in service delivery will be needed to maintain congruence, with new missions and philosophies developed in response to cultural demands and social changes. Continuous evaluation will be needed to assess cost and quality outcomes related to these changes. Maintaining focus on the quality of care provided as well as access to care will be required so that bottom-line costs do not overshadow quality care provisions. Nursing's history of work with the development of person-centered interactive strategies places nurses in a position to assume leadership roles in this area of organizational development.

Demographic Factors

Geographic dispersion, regional access to care, incomes of the population, aging of the population, and immigration trends are among the demographic factors influencing the design of healthcare organizations. Changing economic and demographic characteristics of many communities are resulting in a larger number of uninsured and underinsured individuals. Geographic isolation often limits access to necessary health services and impedes recruitment of healthcare personnel. Community-based rural health networks that provide primary care links to urban health centers for teaching, consultation, personnel sharing, and the provision of high-tech services are one solution for meeting needs in rural areas. Federal and state funding, which includes incentives for healthcare personnel to work in rural areas, is another approach. Strategic planning by nursing is critical to address community needs.

A major influence exerted on healthcare organizations comes from the aging of the population.

According to U.S. Census data, all of the Baby Boomer generation will reach the age of 65 by 2030. The population segment older than 80 years is also increasing. Although the entire segment of this population does not necessarily have dependency needs, a need exists for more long-term beds, supportive housing, and community programs. To meet the needs of older adults, new healthcare organizations will continue to evolve and will be evaluated and restructured based on findings. New roles for nurses as leaders and managers of the care of older adults are evolving. An example is the role of advanced practice registered nurses to direct the care of patients who have become members of geriatric care organizations such as retirement centers.

According to the World Health Organization (2021), social determinants of health (SDOH) are the conditions in which people are born, grow, live, work, and age. Understanding how these conditions impact both the social and physical health of a population is key to understanding SDOH. Because SDOH influence the health of a community, they also influence what is needed from healthcare organizations. Many healthcare systems integrate addressing SDOH for the populations they serve. For example, federal law requires healthcare organizations to perform community health needs assessments every three years to inform what services must be prioritized in their communities. Nurses have expertise in community health and may be called upon to play a leadership role in these assessments. Nurse leaders can also help forge partnerships between the community and healthcare organizations.

THEORETICAL PERSPECTIVES

Two major theories apply to the functioning and productivity of most healthcare organizations. One is that organizations evolve in an orderly and holistic manner (systems theory). The other is that change is disruptive and not orderly (chaos theory).

Systems Theory

Systems theory attempts to explain complex systems holistically. Each component or part of the system has an effect on the entire system. Systems can be either closed (self-contained) or open (interacting with both internal and external forces). The healthcare system is composed of decision makers, policy makers, groups of people, and organizations that influence how care is delivered (Cordon, 2013). The actions of each of these groups have an effect on the system as a whole. For example, a decision to change the way nursing care is delivered will have an effect across the organization. Systems theorists focus on the interplay among the system components within a framework of (1) inputs—resources such as people, money, or materials; (2) throughputs—the processes that produce a product from the inputs; and (3) outputs—the product of inputs and throughputs.

The theoretical concepts of systems theory have been applied to nursing and to organizations. Systems theory presents an explanation of organizational evolution similar to biological evolution. A model of systems theory can explain the process of healthcare organization evolution (Fig. 9.3). The survival of the organization, as portrayed

---

LITERATURE PERSPECTIVE

Resource: Weston, M. J., Pham, B. H., & Zuckerman, D. (2020). Building community well-being by leveraging the economic impact of health systems. *Nursing Administration Quarterly, 44*(3), 215–220.

Evidence suggests that health outcomes are more influenced by SDOH than by access to healthcare. If healthcare systems are to improve health outcomes of the populations they serve, SDOH must be addressed. This article presents the practice of hospitals and healthcare systems becoming anchor institutions missioned to improve the economic status of local communities by hiring, purchasing, and investing within the community. These intentional practices leverage the financial strength of the healthcare system to lessen disparities that can negatively affect health outcomes. For example,

seeking to hire and train residents of zip codes with high unemployment rates can set the conditions for long-term economic improvements. Resources, publications, and toolkits are available through the Healthcare Anchor Network, a consortium of hospitals and systems that serve as anchor institutions.

Implications for Practice
Nurses understand how SDOH impact the health of communities. Nurses are the most trusted profession, with strong communication and relationship-building skills, making them well positioned to forge positive relationships between healthcare systems and local communities to improve health outcomes outside of the facility walls as well as within.

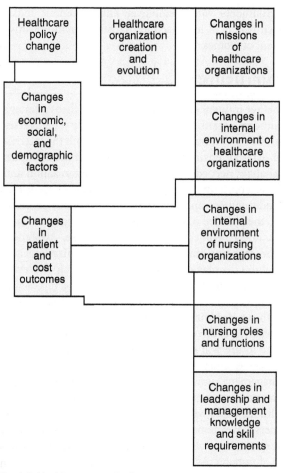

Fig. 9.3 Healthcare organizations as open systems.

throughout this chapter, depends on its evolutionary response to changing environmental forces; it is seen as an open system. The response to environmental changes brings about internal changes, which produce changes that alter environmental conditions. The changes in the environment, in turn, act to bring about changes in the internal operating conditions of the organization.

This open-systems approach to organizational development and effectiveness emphasizes a continual process of adaptation of healthcare organizations to external driving forces and a response to the adaptations by the external environment, which generates continuing inputs for further healthcare organization development. This open system is in contrast to a closed-system approach that views a system as being sufficient unto itself and, thus, untouched by what happens around it.

Chaos Theory

Unfortunately, healthcare as an industry is not always as predictable and orderly as systems theorists would have us believe. In contrast to the somewhat orderly universe described in systems theory, in which an organization can be viewed in terms of a linear, cause-and-effect model, chaos theory sees the universe as filled with unpredictable and random events (Hawking, 1998). According to the proponents of chaos theory, organizations must be self-organizing and adapt readily to change to survive. Therefore, organizations must accept that change is inevitable and unrelenting. When one embraces the tenets of chaos theory, one gives up on any attempt to create a permanent organizational structure. Using creativity and flexibility, successful leaders will be those who can tolerate ambiguity, take risks, and experiment with new ideas in response to each day's unique situation or environment. They will not rest on a successful transition or organizational model because they know the environment that it flourished in is fleeting. The successful nurse leaders will be those individuals who are committed to lifelong learning and problem solving. The Theory Box notes key elements of systems and chaos theories.

THEORY BOX		
Theory/Contributor	**Key Ideas**	**Application to Practice**
Von Bertalanffy (1968) Systems Theory	Comprised of four elements (structure, technology, people, and environment) Viewed as inputs, throughputs, and outputs Closed systems: self-contained Open systems: interacting with internal and external forces	Consideration of how the hospital interacts with the community (open system)
Lorenz (1972) Chaos Theory	Requires organizations to be self-organizing and adaptive to survive Unpredictable and random events Constant change and instability	Nurses leaving organizations where they were long-term employees to join staffing agencies

NURSING ROLE AND FUNCTION CHANGES

Leadership and management roles for nurses are proliferating in healthcare organizations that are developing or evolving in response to environmental driving forces. With a focus on primary care and population health, the proportion of nursing positions in the community is increasing, as are various care management positions, clinical nurse leaders, and advanced practice registered nurses. Filling these roles requires knowledge and skills to coordinate the care of patients or communities with the many other disciplines and organizational units providing the continuum of care. Our society needs nurses who can engage in the political process of policy development, coordinate care across disciplines and settings, use conflict management techniques to create win-win situations for patients and providers in resolving the healthcare system's delivery problems, and use business savvy to market and prepare financial and organizational plans for the delivery of cost-effective care.

Economic, social, and demographic changes are not limited to patients and communities. These shifts are affecting the workplace as well. To be effective, nurse managers and leaders need to consider how these phenomena affect the workplace in the same way they consider when to address the needs of their patients and the communities they serve. The fourth aim of the Quintuple Aim is to enhance the joy and meaning in the work of healthcare (Grant et al., 2020). Nurse leaders must focus not only on patient needs but also on staff well-being—and their own. Establishing healthy work environments where employee engagement is maximized results in increased job satisfaction and positive patient outcomes.

CONCLUSION

Whether influenced by systems or chaos theory, today's healthcare organizations are in a dynamic state. Nurses must be continuously alert to assessing both the internal and external environment for forces that act as inputs to changes needed in their healthcare organization and for the effects of changes that are made. These forces include policies and regulations that impact or influence the practice of nursing and health disparities and, thus, affect people's access to nursing care. Awareness of the changing status of healthcare organizations and the ability to play a leading role in creating and evaluating adaptation in response to changing forces will be central functions of nurse leaders and managers in healthcare organizations. Due to the rapidity of change in healthcare, the need to evaluate system effectiveness in the future will require more energy than it does today. Nurses must develop a foundation of leadership and management knowledge that they can build on through a planned program of continuing education. Even in tumultuous times within the healthcare industry, nursing leaders have demonstrated their ability to strengthen the quality of both their organizations and the practice of nursing. As healthcare organizations continue to undergo transformation, tomorrow's nurses—whether leaders, managers, or frontline caregivers—need to carry these lessons forward.

THE SOLUTION

As the RN case manager, I completed a comprehensive assessment of the patient. He requested that I reach out to his sister, which I did. His sister validated she has been estranged from her brother for quite some time but would be willing to talk to him now that he is having medical issues. I confirmed the patient did not have a primary care provider and is now willing to connect with one but needs help. After researching local clinic systems, I helped schedule a hospital follow-up appointment and provided the patient with a bus pass so he could attend his appointment. After a three-day hospital stay, the patient communicated his readiness to stop drinking. I consulted with the unit social worker to connect him with local entities that could assist him in navigating treatment options. I received a telephone call from the patient's sister stating she would allow him to stay with her for a short period of time. The social worker also provided him with a list of homeless shelters in the area should things not work out with his sister.

An important aspect to caring for a homeless individual is to determine the eligibility criteria for existing programs within the residing county. This will facilitate connecting him to primary care, post-acute services, durable medical equipment, and specialty care.

It is imperative for the nurse to address other social determinants of health, as they significantly impact the patient's ability to follow up with outpatient care providers.

THE SOLUTION—cont'd

Homeless patients are predisposed to poor outcomes due to poor and unstable living conditions as well as food insecurity. These patients tend to have limited resources, which also makes it difficult to purchase and store medications safely. Lack of transportation makes it difficult for patients to attend appointments and seek follow-up care. In this particular challenge, the patient was provided bus passes to attend his follow-up care appointment. Addressing social determinants of health is crucial in addressing care from a holistic perspective.

In this challenge, the patient had a home to discharge to, but if he had not, he would have been predisposed to unhealthy and toxic living conditions as well as unsafe living environments that pose threats, robbery, and assault. Depending on the state and county in which patients reside, housing options may be very limited to scarce. Existing guidelines and criteria can make placement challenging. For example, an individual with substance use history and/or a criminal background may be restricted from public housing. Homeless individuals are at increased risk of having negative encounters with the criminal justice system.

Regardless of the discharging facility or institution the patient may be leaving, discharge planning should include a multidisciplinary team to successfully transition the patient back into the community. This challenge illustrates the need for nurses practicing in acute care settings to be knowledgeable about resources both within the system of their practice setting and in the local community. Would this be a suitable approach for you? Why?

Veronica Buitron-Camacho

REFLECTIONS

As a nurse, you will have the opportunity to practice in collaboration with several types of healthcare organizations. Based on what you have learned about the ownership, governance, structure, and quality focus of contemporary healthcare organizations, with which type of organization in your community do you believe you would prefer to practice? What rationale do you have for that decision?

BEST PRACTICES

Nurses can participate in designing and restructuring decision making within their healthcare delivery systems by serving in nontraditional roles and on organizational committees. Nurses can promote an openness to exploring the introduction of best practices to the practice setting. Because organizational structures, types of services, populations served and oversight by regulatory and accreditation bodies differ, providing insight about the distinctiveness of a specific organization during orientation can enhance new nurses' transition to practice.

TIPS FOR HEALTHCARE ORGANIZATIONS

Leaders can

- Leverage existing partnerships with community organizations and nurse leaders of other systems.
- Seek opportunities to mentor nurses with leadership potential and interest in learning more about the healthcare organization.
- Develop communication systems that provide information on patients receiving services at various points of care in the organization as systems are integrated.

Managers can

- Share with nurses the connections between direct patient care and the organizational mission and strategic plan to empower nurses to engage in the decision-making process.
- Foster a healthy and psychologically safe working environment within units to achieve optimal patient care outcomes.
- Provide opportunities for nurses on the unit to explore leadership and management functions.

Followers can

- Stay abreast of local healthcare industry news to gain an understanding of how the systems and organizational structures are changing.

- Share ideas during team meetings about how your organization can achieve the fifth aim of the Quintuple Aim to increase joy and meaning in healthcare.

REFERENCES

Ascension. (2022). Ascension. Retrieved February 21, 2022 from https://healthcare.ascension.org.

American Association of Colleges of Nursing (AACN). (2020). *The essentials: Core competencies for professional nursing education. AACN draft essentials document [November 5, 2020].* Retrieved from https://www.aacnnursing.org/Portals/42/Downloads/Essentials/Essentials-Draft-Document.pdf.

American Hospital Association (AHA). (2021). Fast facts on US hospitals, 2021. https://www.aha.org/infographics/2020-07-24-fast-facts-infographics.

American Hospital Association (AHA). (2020). *Hospitals and health systems face unprecedented financial pressures due to COVID-19.* Retrieved January 15, 2022 from https://www.aha.org/guidesreports/2020-05-05-hospitals-and-health-systems-face-unprecedented-financial-pressures-due.

Burke, L. G., Khullar, D., Zheng, J., Frakt, A. B., Orav, E. J., & Jha, A. K. (2019). Comparison of costs of care for Medicare patients hospitalized in teaching and nonteaching hospitals. *JAMA Network Open, 2*(6), e195229. https://doi.org/10.1001/jamanetworkopen.2019.5229.

Centers for Medicare & Medicaid Services (CMS). (2020). *National health expenditure data: Historical.* Retrieved January 15, 2022 from https://www.cms.gov/Research-Statistics-Data-and-Systems/Statistics-Trends-and-Reports/NationalHealthExpendData/NationalHealthAccountsHistorical.

Chesley, C. G. (2020). Merging cultures: Organizational culture and leadership in a health system merger. *Journal of Healthcare Management, 65*(2), 135–149. https://doi.org/10.1097/JHM-D-18-00213.

Cordon, P. (2013). System theories: An overview of various system theories and its application in healthcare. *American Journal of Systems Science, 2*(1), 13–22. https://doi:10.5923/j.ajss.20130201.03.

Disch, J., & Finis, N. (2022). Rethinking nursing productivity: A review of the literature and interviews with thought leaders. *Nursing Economics, 40*(2), 59–71.

Grant, S., Davidson, J., Manges, K., Dermenchyan, A., Wilson, E., & Dowdell, E. (2020). Creating healthful work environments to deliver on the quadruple aim: A call to action. *The Journal of Nursing Administration, 50*(6), 314–321. https://doi.org/10.1097/NNA.0000000000000891.

Hawking, S. (1998). *A brief history of time.* London: Bantam Press.

Lorenz, E. N. (December 29, 1972). Does the flap of a butterfly's wings in Brazil set off a tornado in Texas? American Association for the Advancement of Science. 139th Meeting, Washington, DC.

National Advisory Council on Nurse Education and Practice. (2019). *Promoting nursing leadership in the transition to value-based care: Fifteenth report to the Secretary of Health and Human Services and the US Congress.* https://www.hrsa.gov/sites/default/files/hrsa/advisory-committees/nursing/reports/2019-fifteenthreport.pdf.

Neville, B., & Laramee, A. (2020). Understanding palliative care: A nursing perspective. *Vermont Nurse Connection, 23*(3), 12–13. https://d3ms3kxrsap50t.cloudfront.net/uploads/publication/pdf/2075/Vermont_Nurse_Connection_7_20.pdf.

Von Bertalanffy, L. (1968). *General systems theory: Foundations, development, applications.* New York: George Braziller.

World Health Organization (WHO). (2021). *Social determinants of health.* https://www.who.int/health-topics/social-determinants-of-health#tab=tab_1.

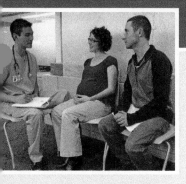

10

Person-Centered Care

Margarete Lieb Zalon

ANTICIPATED LEARNING OUTCOMES

- Describe the evolution of person-centered care as a focal point in healthcare delivery.
- Describe factors that affect the importance of person-centered interactions within the healthcare system.
- Evaluate the impact of effective person-centered care in fostering patient engagement.
- Appraise the major responsibilities of nursing in relation to the promotion of person-centered care.

KEY TERMS

advocate
big data
care coordination
careful nursing
cultural and linguistic
   competence
healthcare provider

Internet of Everything
Internet of Things
motivational interviewing
patient-centered care
patient-centered medical home
   (PCMH)
patient engagement

patient satisfaction
people-centred
personal health literacy
person-centered care
organizational health literacy

THE CHALLENGE

Everything we do is about caring—for our patients, our health plan members, our family of physicians and employees, and our communities. It is this *purpose* that galvanizes our patient-centered care approach in every segment of our organization. Nursing, throughout the health system, embraces the importance of a person-centered approach and commits to the ProvenExperience, a program that offers refunds to patients whose expectations weren't met based on kindness and compassion. Geisinger has a strong history of delivering high-quality, innovative care and patient-centered care; nursing is the heart of Geisinger's commitment to person-centered care.

I received an email from a nurse whose husband had recently been hospitalized for two days detailing her concerns about inconsistencies between the medications listed on the computer-generated discharge instructions and discharge prescriptions. Although the nurse indicated that the medical and nursing staff were clear about the changes to be made to the prescriptions, she was concerned about the discrepancies, pointing out that it would be confusing for her husband and for the average person, and potentially dangerous. The first error was noticed by an astute home care nurse who asked why a new prescription was not on the discharge summary, yet product information had been provided. The wife also observed

(Continued)

that a new medication and new as-needed medication were not listed in the discharge medications. There was no heading labeled for new medications. Dosage changes for two medications were not listed. Three medications remained with the same dosage and one medication was discontinued, all of which were correct on the instructions. Thus, for four out of eight medications on the discharge summary did not match the discharge prescriptions, a 50% error rate. The concern was that if both documents (discharge summary and prescriptions) were computer-generated, they should be the same. The patient's wife was concerned about the vulnerability of patients when being discharged to home or transferred to another healthcare facility.

What would you do if you were this nurse?

Angelo Venditti, DNP MBA, RN, NEA-BC, FACHE
Formerly Chief Nursing Officer, Northeast Region, Geisinger Health System, Wilkes-Barre, PA

INTRODUCTION

Had nurses wanted to create the perfect example of what person-centered care looked like, we would have capitalized on the COVID-19 pandemic in 2020 as that example. Amidst all of the tragedy surrounding the care issues from vaccinations through the final moments of life, we saw nurses focused on the person. The examples in the COVID-19 units in hospitals were simply breathtaking. Nurses engaged patients' families restricted from physical presence with their loved ones, arranging for families to talk with their loved ones before they were intubated, or holding an electronic tablet device while families said their good byes to patients dying in a room with tubes, machines, a tablet—and a nurse. Families entrusted their loved ones to us and we performed at the top of our ethical responsibilities, professional competencies. This is the embodiment of person-centered care.

Person-centered care in healthcare delivery refers to the primacy of patients' needs and perspectives in all encounters between patients, their families, and the people important to them with healthcare providers and all aspects of the healthcare system. It indicates that an individual's values and preferences guide all aspects of healthcare, that patients and the people important to them and their providers are involved in a dynamic relationship, and that this collaboration informs decision-making (American Geriatrics Society, 2016) (see Box 10.1). Person-centered care is distinguished from patient-centered care in that the latter is focused on the person in a patient role within the context of a healthcare system. According to Eklund et al. (2019), the main goal for patient-centered care is a functional life, whereas for person-centered care, it is a meaningful life. Principles guiding person-centered care include (1) treating people with dignity, compassion, and respect; (2) coordination of care; (3) personalization of

> **BOX 10.1   Essential Elements of Person-Centered Care**
>
> - An individualized, goal-oriented care plan based on the person's preferences
> - Ongoing review of the person's goals and care plan
> - Care supported by an interprofessional team in which the person is an integral team member
> - One primary or lead point of contact on the healthcare team
> - Active coordination among all healthcare and supportive service providers
> - Continual information sharing and integrated communication
> - Education and training for providers and, when appropriate, the person and those important to the person
> - Performance measurement and quality improvement using feedback from the person and caregivers

From American Geriatrics Society Expert Panel on Person-Centered Care. (2016). Person-centered care: A definition and essential elements. *Journal of the American Geriatrics Society, 64*(1), 15–18.

care; and (4) support of people to develop their strengths and abilities (Health Foundation, 2014) (Fig. 10.1).

Hildegard Peplau was the first nurse after Florence Nightingale to focus on theory, developing her theory of interpersonal relations that focused on how the nurse's relationship with the patient was central to nursing practice. Subsequently, person-centered care was popularized in the 1960s by Carl Rogers, a psychotherapist, who also focused on the primacy of the person in interpersonal relationships. His work is an example of the theoretical basis for person-centered care and is illustrated in the Theory Box.

Later, the term was expanded to care for people with dementia to counteract dehumanizing relationships

THEORY BOX

Humanistic Psychology

Theory	Key Ideas	Application to Practice
Person-centered theory is humanistic, existential, and phenomenological and is based on 19 propositions.	Nurses must be aware that individuals experience the world from a centric perspective. Self-concept is a core element.	Because most of the ways people behave are related to satisfying personal needs, nurses need to attend to the way in which people behave. Experiences inconsistent with the view of self may be seen as threats and may pose threatening situations clinically.

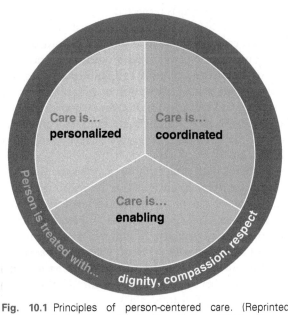

Fig. 10.1 Principles of person-centered care. (Reprinted with permission from Health Foundation. (2014). *Person-centred care made simple: What everyone should know about person-centred care. Quick Guide.* https://www.health.org.uk/publications/person-centred-care-made-simple.)

with caregivers (Evardsson et al., 2010). The impetus for person-centered care in the United States is derived from the landmark report, *Crossing the Quality Chasm* (2001) issued by the Institute of Medicine (IOM; now the National Academy of Medicine [NAM]). The report indicated that one of the six aims for improvement in the healthcare system was *patient-centered care*, "providing care that is respectful of and responsive to individual patient preferences, needs and values, and ensuring that patient values guide all clinical decisions" (IOM, 2001, p. 3). A systematic review of research on person-centered care interventions for older people in non-hospital settings indicated that there were four critical interrelated

themes for their implementation: (1) knowing and confirming the patient as a person, (2) a jointly developed an individualized health plan, (3) interprofessional team work and collaboration involving the older person and family, and (4) creating a supportive environment for care delivery (Ebrahimi et al., 2021).

Person-centered care can be extended to a systems perspective to address the strains on health systems with people living longer and the burden of disease across the world. The World Health Organization (WHO) developed a framework on "Integrated People-Centred Health Services" (IPCHS), which focuses on "people and communities, not diseases at the centre of health systems and empowering people to take charge of their own health" (WHO, 2021). Five interrelated strategies that can be used to match priorities, capabilities, and resources for its member countries include (1) engaging and empowering people and communities, (2) strengthening governance and accountability, (3) reorienting the model of care, (4) coordinating services within and across sectors, and (5) creating an enabling environment (WHO, 2021).

Nurses set the tone for effective communication by providing the foundation for person-centered care. Because nurses are the healthcare providers who spend the most time with the patient and their traditional focus has been on the patient's problems as the patient experiences them, nurses are in an ideal position to lead initiatives designed to deliver person-centered care.

Leaders in healthcare organizations recognize that their facilities are not as person-centered as they might be—that is, they have been built and organized in a manner that best serves the organization and not the recipients of care and their families. Care is compartmentalized, with each department having specialized functions. Patients are transported between departments to receive services. They risk loss of privacy, excessive exposure, increased discomfort and fatigue during transfers, and long periods of waiting. On an average day, a seriously ill patient in a hospital may have encounters with 50 or more staff members. This approach is not person centered and can be very disruptive for patients. One initiative to address this is the contribution of the American Academy of Nursing (AAN) to the American Board of Internal Medicine's Choosing Wisely® campaign, recommending that nurses not disturb patients during sleep unless specifically warranted by their condition (AAN, 2018). Nurses are often confronted with competing goals of providing adequate opportunity for rest and sleep and monitoring patients for clinical deterioration (Hope et al., 2018). They face challenges in addressing a complex array of physiological, psychological, psychosocial, sensory, and environmental factors (Reuter-Rice et al., 2020); demands for adherence to protocols; minimizing protocols; and a lack of guidance for sleep-promoting interventions. Sleep disruptions in critical care settings, hospital units, long-term care settings, and the home are all areas where nurses can make a difference with interventions designed to enhance sleep and/or diminish disruptions. These interventions may be as simple as grouping tasks together, such as taking vital signs at the same time that medication is administered or when answering a call light. Nurse leaders should be alert to these kinds of opportunities to focus on patients' needs in improving care in their practice settings.

Services provided to patients should be comfortable, pleasant, and as effective as possible. Meeting the emotional, psychosocial, and spiritual needs of the patient is important. Care should be technologically advanced but also compassionate, addressing what matters to patients.

EXERCISE 10.1   List five examples of practices or situations in your nursing setting that could be more person centered—for example, patients being asked to repeat information several times to different healthcare team members and referring to patients by their conditions. For each practice, identify at least two strategies to make it more person centered. One strategy should focus on what direct care nurses can do to immediately address the situation. Another strategy should focus on what nurse leaders can do to improve the delivery system so that the change can be embedded in practice.

HISTORY OF PERSON-CENTERED CARE IN NURSING

Nursing has a long history of priding itself on the provision of *patient-centered care*. Now, as the focus on care evolves to a broader perspective, the term being used is *person-centered care*. That term is reflective of a shifting focus of care that moves beyond an individual episode of illness or a single encounter with a healthcare provider in a clinical setting to a focus on how individuals (families, communities, or populations) respond to illness while their autonomy is respected.

Nursing's history of being focused on person-centered care is embodied in the profession's definition of nursing: "Nursing is the protection, promotion, and optimization of health and abilities, prevention of illness and injury, alleviation of suffering through diagnosis and treatment of human response, and advocacy in the care of individuals, families, communities and populations" (American Nurses Association [ANA], 2010).

The ANA definition of nursing, or a variation of it, is almost universally included in the registered nurse (RN) practice acts of the states and territories of the United States. The *Code of Ethics for Nurses* declares that the "nurse's primary commitment is to the recipients of nursing health services" with the expectation that the nurse involves patients in planning for care (ANA, 2015, p. 5). Involving patients in their care and in making decisions is a key feature of person-centered care. It demonstrates respect for persons and their right to self-determination. Integral to person-centered care is the relationship that nurses have with patients, their families, and/or their significant others; the value of caring as an element of that relationship; and how nursing's holistic approach enhances person-centered care.

Person-centered care is identified as a domain, a "broad distinguishable area of competence" for nursing practice in *The Essentials: Core Competencies for Professional Nursing Education*, by the American Association of Colleges of Nursing (AACN, 2021). In this context, person-centered care "focuses on the individual within multiple complicated contexts, including family and/or important others. Person-centered care is holistic, individualized, just, respectful, compassionate, coordinated, evidence-based, and developmentally appropriate" (AACN, 2021, p. 10).

BIASES IMPACTING PERSON-CENTERED CARE

Being person centered requires a conscious effort to address attitudes and biases that may creep into our care and everyday language out of habit. While we teach that patients and their families/caregivers/support persons should be treated with respect and dignity, this may not occur consistently in all practice settings. Person-first is the motto for how to think about addressing the people for whom we provide care. As an example, we could say the "patient who had a mastectomy" rather than the "mastectomy in room 502." The choice of descriptors for patients will subtly convey our attitudes and may influence our care. While we may gather data that quantifies or standardizes certain observations, we must not lose sight of the individual and how that person experiences health problems and the delivery of care. Words matter in the use of patient descriptors. Bias inherent in the use of certain terms—such as "frequent flyer," "drug-seeking," "non-compliant," or "addict," among others—can result in blaming the patient, inadequate assessment, delays in care, misdiagnoses, limiting access to care, and harm to the patient (Valdez, 2021). See Table 10.1 for an illustration of how person-first documentation can replace documentation that may reflect unconscious biases. While this table contains a specific example for documentation, Raney et al. (2021) suggest being mindful when communicating by asking whether the language (a) casts blame, (b) reinforces stereotypes, (c) includes extraneous information, (d) includes pejorative language, or (e) is something you would want the patient or family to read.

We all need healthcare—friends, neighbors, families, people like us, and people very different from us. We need to recognize that people are diverse culturally, ethnically, socially, physically, and psychologically. The patients we encounter may be better consumers of healthcare than they were in the past by accessing healthcare information from a variety of sources. They can access their own test results and schedule appointments. Healthcare organizations are working hard to engage patients in their own healthcare through various means, including the use of patient portals, so that they can monitor key indicators and communicate with their healthcare providers. However, these portals may not be consistently used by patients, who may have providers from different healthcare systems, and thus, multiple patient portals which do not interface with one another.

TABLE 10.1   Creating a Person-Centered Culture Through Language

Traditional Documentation	Person-Centered Documentation
This 74-year old diabetic female was admitted complaining of chest pain. She has been morbidly obese for the last 10 years. Her Hba1C is 9.0 due to noncompliance with medication regimen. She consented to a cardiac catheterization but is now refusing to go for the procedure that was scheduled for 2 PM. She has been uncooperative with efforts to make preparations. She keeps on demanding her lunch tray despite being told she needs to remain NPO for the procedure.	Mrs. Smith is a 74-year-old female who has had diabetes for 20 years and weighs 550 lbs. She was admitted this morning because of 3 chest pain episodes unrelieved by nitroglycerin. She has not been taking her medications, which include metformin, metoprolol, and atorvastatin because her daughter hasn't had time to get her prescriptions filled. She signed the consent for a cardiac catheterization but is now afraid to go because someone told her she is too heavy for the table in the cath lab.

PERSON-CENTERED CARE—WHY NOW?

Person-centered care has captured the interest of healthcare professionals as an overarching strategy to improve health and transform the delivery of health care and is considered a "burgeoning social movement and a mission statement for modern health care" (Sakallaris et al., 2016). This innovation comes at a time of an increased burden of chronic disease around the world. Chronic illness accounted for 71% of global mortality in 2016, reflecting inadequate progress in addressing and controlling noncommunicable diseases (WHO, 2020). The WHO global targets include reducing cardiovascular disease, chronic respiratory diseases, alcohol and addresses tobacco use, obesity, diabetes, hypertension, and insufficient physical activity with the recognition that people who have noncommunicable diseases such as these are disproportionately impacted by COVID-19. Achieving these global targets requires not only a concerted effort by healthcare professionals, healthcare organizations, and the implementation of sound health-care policy but also the involvement of the most important person, the recipient of healthcare.

Person-centered care means that people are equal partners with their healthcare providers in planning and implementing their care and evaluating the outcomes of that care. Healthcare provider relationships with patients have changed. Physicians' typical modes of practice have moved from a single, private enterprise to multigroup practices that also include nurse practitioners, certified nurse-midwives, certified registered nurse anesthetists, clinical nurse specialists, RN first assistants, physician assistants, and other healthcare professionals. Some group practices are incorporated into integrated service models that include health maintenance organizations (HMOs), managed care programs, physician-hospital organizations, accountable care organizations, and patient-centered medical homes (PCMHs).

The nature of these practice settings has changed relationships that patients have with healthcare providers. When patients visit a group practice, they might not have the option of selecting a specific healthcare provider with whom they can have a personal relationship. Insurers have increasingly restricted provider networks. Rural healthcare consumers have seen local hospitals closed or purchased by large healthcare systems, resulting in the need to develop relationships with new healthcare providers. Additionally, as a result of the COVID-19 pandemic, many rural hospitals closed and many providers left their professions—at least temporarily. As a result, people may experience fewer options for service and longer delays in securing even basic services. This is especially true after the upheaval in healthcare in 2021, with multiple resignations in various professions, including nursing.

Patients new to a healthcare system may not know how to navigate it. Others may change their insurance to save money, resulting in a change in healthcare providers. Sometimes, these changes are made by an employer or other group plan rather than by the patient. Access to health insurance does not necessarily mean that people will take advantage of the available services. Parents in a young family may ensure that their children receive needed care and immunizations but forgo obtaining preventive healthcare for themselves. Transportation and time off to access health services

may be a concern. Patients may feel insecure in unfamiliar circumstances, even if they are receiving excellent care. Patients may no longer know their healthcare providers as they did in the past and providers may be less familiar with their patients, resulting in decreased opportunities for the development of mutual respect, trust, and continuity of care. Fear of divulging highly personal information to someone who is now seen as a stranger only increases the risk of receiving subpar healthcare.

Many hospitals use hospitalists instead of patients' own primary care providers, making care coordination after discharge more challenging. In a systematic review, the rate of medication error or unintentional medication discrepancy was nearly 50% in adult and elderly patients discharged from hospitals, with adverse drug events impacting nearly 20% (Alqenae et al., 2020) as illustrated in the Challenge. Prior to the COVID-19 pandemic, medical errors were found to be the third leading cause of death (Makary & Daniel, 2016). Patients themselves report that breakdowns in care are associated with perceived harm; of those who experienced a breakdown, 38% had not spoken with a hospital staff member (Fisher et al., 2020). This, in turn, creates stressors for patients and their caregivers.

The Healthy People 2030 goals include an increased and overarching focus on social determinants of health, which comprises economic stability, education access and quality, healthcare access and quality, neighborhood and built environment, and social and community context (Office of Disease Prevention and Health Promotion [ODPHP], 2021). The myriad factors described here together create significant pressures to improve care as it is experienced by individuals, families, groups, and populations. As a result, the emphasis on person-centered care by providers is more important than ever. Efforts have been made to reduce costs by changing reimbursement mechanisms to provide incentives to improve the efficiency and effectiveness of care. A number of programs are in place to provide support for patients seeking healthcare services and to incentivize healthcare organizations to make specific improvements in services. Examples of these efforts are listed in Table 10.2. Additionally, a study reported in the journal BMC Public Health can broaden our view of social determinants, as the Research Perspective shows.

TABLE 10.2 Examples of Incentive Programs Designed to Improve Care Efficiency and Effectiveness

Enabling Legislation	Program	Key Features
Patient Protection and Affordable Care Act of 2010	Hospital Readmission Reduction Program (HRRP)	Examines 30-day hospital readmissions for patients with myocardial infarction, heart failure, pneumonia, coronary artery bypass graft surgery, chronic obstructive pulmonary disease (COPD), and total hip and knee replacements.
	Hospital-Acquired Condition Reduction Program (HACRP)	Reduces payment for conditions such as pressure injuries when acquired after admission.
	Hospital Value-Based Purchasing (HVBP)	Medicare payments are adjusted to reward providers for quality of care provided.
Deficit Reduction Act of 2005	Hospital-Acquired Conditions (Present on Admission Indicator)	Hospitals do not receive additional payment for selected conditions when they were not present on admission.
Medicare Access and Children's Health Insurance Program (CHIP) Reauthorization Act (MACRA) of 2015	Quality Payment Program Merit-based Incentive Payment System (MIPS) Advanced Alternative Payment Models (APMs)	Rewards healthcare providers for administering coordinated, comprehensive, and higher-quality care.

Source: Centers for Medicare & Medicaid Services (CMS), www.cms.gov.

RESEARCH PERSPECTIVE

Resource: Ziaei, S., & Hammarström, A. (2021). What social determinants outside paid work are related to development of mental health during life? An integrative review of results from the Northern Swedish Cohort. *BMC Public Health, 21*(1), 2190.

This integrative review examined both work and outside paid work and the effects on mental health of an individual in a 27-year prospective cohort study in Sweden. Twenty-seven papers were included in this review using Bronfenbrenner's Ecological Systems Theory, consisting of five concentric, mutually influential layers, to identify key themes. Class structure and gender issues playing out at the macro level can affect all levels and manifest as mental illness in individuals over the life course. Although Sweden is generally considered an egalitarian society, class structures such as access to employment, neighborhoods, and resources, and gender relations, including its power

structures, have a significant impact at the macro level. Likewise, factors impacting mental health during adolescence have long-term effects throughout the life course.

Implications for Practice

Nurses need to consider a broad perspective of what helps shape personhood. People are affected at various levels and in various ways that have not been universally studied and that have the ability to affect people later in life. Mental health issues are prevalent in societies throughout the world. This review illustrates the lasting impact of social determinants of mental health, where people are "born, grown, live, work and age." The calls for nurses and the profession to take on a greater role in addressing the social determinants of health in the *Future of Nursing 2020–2030: Charting a Path to Achieve Health Equity* report (National Academies, 2021) are supported by research.

INITIATIVES TO DELIVER PERSON-CENTERED CARE

Increased emphasis on person-centered care has been facilitated by the efforts to optimize the performance of healthcare systems by improving the experience of care

(which includes quality and satisfaction) and improving population health while reducing cost, otherwise designated the "Triple Aim" by the Institute for Healthcare Improvement (IHI, 2022a). Bodenheimer and Sinsky (2014) make the case for expanding the Triple Aim to the "Quintuple Aim" with the inclusion of a focus on improving the work life of healthcare providers to improve outcomes. This is consistent with the historic work established by the Magnet Recognition Program® of the American Nurses Credentialing Center. Improved outcomes can be achieved by promoting positive engagement of the workforce, changes in reimbursement for healthcare services and initiatives that affect the delivery of person-centered care include the development of innovative models of care, transitional care models, the use of PCMHs, and the use of big data. The expansion to the Quiptuple Aim (Nundy et al., 2022) by the addition of advancing health equity further supports the goals of person-centered care.

A number of person-centered care models have been developed for use in home, and community-based settings and acute care (Sillner et al., 2021). For example, innovative models of care have been developed to fulfill specialized needs for healthcare and to address system problems—for example, a company providing pediatric day health services for children with complex healthcare needs or another composed of nurse practitioners providing pediatric urgent care after pediatrician offices are closed. The AAN's Edgerunner program highlights nurse-developed innovative models of care with demonstrated improved health outcomes. As an example, the Family and Birth Center in the Developing Families Center uses a midwifery–nurse practitioner model for care and has demonstrated success in lowering preterm birth in a Black community (AAN, 2021a). Another Edgerunner program focuses on aging adults, including those with Alzheimer's and related diseases (AAN, 2021b). The program specifically targeted Latino and Haitian families with culturally tailored interventions. During the COVID-19 pandemic, the program incorporated telehealth into its services and expanded its offerings to provide behavioral and mental health services.

Care delivery models have various strengths and weaknesses with regard to the extent to which they support the delivery of person-centered care. Care delivery is influenced by staffing, skill mix (numbers of RNs, licensed practical/vocational nurses [LP/VN], certified nursing assistants [CNAs], and other staff members), setting, and the support of organizational leadership. Person-centered care has strong roots in the development of care models for individuals with dementia. Various features of these models are included in programs such as Eden

Alternative, Wellspring, and Greenhouse (Fazio et al., 2018). Thus, the delivery model in and of itself may not be the key factor influencing the adoption of person-centered care (see Table 10.3).

EXERCISE 10.2 Describe the model of nursing care delivery in your practice site and determine whether the model resembles any of those listed in Table 10.3. How does the skill mix (composition of RNs, LPNs/LVNs, CNAs, and others) influence the delivery models? What strategies are in place or necessary to ensure that the delivery model retains a person-centered approach?

The patient-centered medical home (PCMH) is a delivery model that facilitates care integration across settings. Features of PCMHs include comprehensive care, patient-centered care, coordination, accessibility, and quality and safety (Agency for Healthcare Research and Quality, 2021). Because the Patient Protection and Affordable Care Act (ACA) has provisions supporting their development, PCMHs have proliferated across the country. PCMHs might better be called *healthcare homes* to focus on the primacy of the individual and demonstrate respect for the individual's autonomy. Some healthcare systems have created teams of individuals, often led by a nurse, who are charged with addressing patient concerns related to the experience of care. Nurses are well suited to be team members and leaders of PCMHs because of their holistic approach and ability to establish positive relationships with their patients. The addition of 20 million more people with insurance across the country as a result of the ACA has resulted in policy discussions related to preparing RNs to assume a more substantial role in primary care settings that is in greater alignment with their educational preparation (Flinter et al., 2017). Thus, it is likely that RNs will assume more responsibilities in these settings and more responsibilities for ensuring a person-centered approach.

The use of technology, including the Internet of Things (IoT)—meaning the interconnectedness of various devices with a computer embedded in ordinary objects we use every day, such as smartphones, sensors, self-monitoring devices, and electronic health records—has changed the way people interact with the healthcare system. Technology has also changed how healthcare providers interact with patients, their families, groups, and communities. Smart home devices

TABLE 10.3 **Nursing Care Delivery Models**

Model/Synonyms	Key Features	Typical Settings
Case Method/Total Patient Care	Nurse manages all of the care for a single patient.	Critical care Hospice
Functional	Staff members, RNs, LPNs/LVNs, CNAs perform the same tasks for a large group of patients. Charge nurse coordinates care.	Emergency or short-staffing situations
Team	RN team leader supervises team members who may be RNs or other staff members.	Settings with heavy use of unlicensed or ancillary staff (e.g., long-term care)
Modular/District	Modification of team nursing that groups patient assignments by geographic location.	Acute care
Primary	Primary nurse (RN) responsible for a patient(s) for an entire episode (e.g., hospitalization) of care.	Acute care Rehabilitation Home care
Primary/Partnership; Co-Primary; Patient-focused Care	RN paired with an assistant to provide care for a group of patients.	Acute care Ambulatory care
Differentiated Practice	Baccalaureate-prepared nurse supervises nurses with other levels of preparation.	Acute care
Case Management	RN coordinates care across units or system to address the needs of complex patients.	Specialized resource for staff
Nurse Navigator	Expert nurses guide patients in making informed decision in collaboration with a multidisciplinary team.	Oncology
Transitional Care Model	Nurse-led program to facilitate transition of patients with chronic illnesses from hospital to home. Involves interdisciplinary leadership.	Home care

can be used to support successful aging in place (Choi et al., 2020). Further transformation is taking place with the Internet of Everything (IoE), which goes beyond the connectivity of things to the connectivity among people, data, processes, and devices. Healthcare data that are being collected are continuously analyzed and improvements in provision of care are made based on the information garnered from those data. People are using self-monitoring technologies, such as physical activity monitors, and smart watches that can recognize atrial fibrillation. Smart watches have a variety of features, including accelerometers, gyroscopes, pressure sensors, cameras (image sensors), global positioning system (GPS), and other sensors that facilitate monitoring of physiologic data. Smartphones can be used to detect voice changes that might be indicative of mental distress. Changing behavior requires more than

monitoring; social processes (e.g., social media) guided by a healthcare professional can be used to foster change (Arigo & Butryn, 2019). Thus, new roles for nurses and other professionals will emerge that integrate the use of data with improved self-care, management of illness, and health promotion.

Increasingly competitive healthcare markets experience greater application of data sharing and access to electronic health records. The use of advanced analytic tools to identify trends and provide decision-making support is occurring as a result. "Big data" analytics, using very large patient data sets generated by healthcare systems, are being used to harness huge amounts of information to analyze trends and gain new insights into the nature of illness, behaviors, and the processes of care. New services are being created that include self-monitoring with technology in the home, videoconferencing, text messaging and instant messaging with healthcare providers and clinical staff, and the proliferation of walk-in clinics staffed by nurse practitioners at convenient locations, such as schools and stores. The COVID-19 pandemic accelerated the use of telehealth services, particularly for those who were at high risk for contracting the virus. Many of these telehealth services continue beyond the pandemic.

These changes require healthcare organization leaders to focus on building relationships with patients who are more knowledgeable and demanding. Nurses, because of their unique perspective and focus on a holistic approach, can play an important role in helping organizations to become more person centered.

CHALLENGES IN THE DELIVERY OF PERSON-CENTERED CARE

Healthcare organizations face numerous challenges in making their care processes more person centered. These include health literacy, diversity, patient satisfaction, and access to care.

Health Literacy

People rely on information from a variety of sources to make healthcare decisions. The relationships that consumers develop with their healthcare providers, including nurses, are important in helping them navigate the healthcare system (Fig. 10.2). Understanding consumers' health-literacy needs goes beyond reading ability assessment. Factors ranging from global aging and climate change to medical and technologic advances influence people's ability to access health information. We know

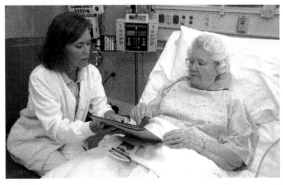

Fig. 10.2 Education empowers consumers to exercise self-determination.

that people with low health literacy are less likely to get preventive health care. When they do enter the healthcare system, they are sicker and have more complex needs. Thus, promoting health literacy involves education, consideration of the context, and sociocultural factors (Fig. 10.2).

However, nearly half of American adults—that is, 90 million people—have difficulty in understanding and using health information (IOM, 2004). While this estimate has not been revised in many years, health literacy is an integral component of person-centered care. *Healthy People 2030*, including health literacy for the first time in its framework, differentiates personal health literacy from organizational health literacy by shifting the focus to people's ability to use health information and making informed decisions as well as the incorporation of a public health perspective and the obligations of organizations to address health literacy (ODPHP, 2021). Personal health literacy is the "degree to which individuals have the ability to find, understand, and use information and services to inform health-related decisions and actions for themselves and others, and organizational health literacy is the degree to which organizations equitably enable individuals to find, understand, and use information and services to inform health-related decisions and actions for themselves and others" (ODPHP, 2021). Health literacy includes reading and understanding text, using quantitative information, being able to speak and listen effectively, using technology, and understanding health and disease. More people from populations with traditionally higher rates of low health literacy received health insurance coverage with the implementation of the ACA. With the ACA's focus on population health by requiring healthcare organizations to complete community needs assessments every three years, efforts to address health literacy have become increasingly important.

Efforts must be made to improve consumer health literacy. One strategy is to foster the development of healthcare-literate organizations. Making an organization healthcare literate requires making health literacy integral to its mission, not only focusing on written materials and spoken communication but also making it easy to navigate the organization and including representatives of the population served in the design of health information and services (Brach, 2017).

BOX 10.2 *Healthy People 2030* Health Literacy Objectives

1. Increase the proportion of adults whose health care provider checked their understanding.
2. Decrease the proportion of adults who report poor communication with their health care provider.
3. Increase the proportion of adults whose health care providers involved them in decisions as much as they wanted.
4. Increase the proportion of people who say their online medical record is easy to understand.
5. Increase the proportion of adults with limited English proficiency who say their providers explain things clearly.
6. Increase the health literacy of the population.

Source: Office of Disease Prevention and Health Promotion. (2021). Health literacy in *Healthy People 2030*. https://health.gov/our-work/national-health-initiatives/healthy-people/healthy-people-2030/health-literacy-healthy-people-2030.

Healthcare systems focusing on health literacy support people in understanding information about their health and how to use their services. See Box 10.2 for *Healthy People 2030*'s health literacy objectives.

A particular challenge is the public's use of Internet and/or social media sources for their health information. People may not have been educated about how to differentiate reputable sources from those that does not spread disinformation. In addition, people may not understand the basis for changing recommendations or they may misinterpret information from credible sources. It is important to assess patients' understanding of their illness and their sources of information. Social media have contributed to the spread of confusion. Addressing accurate information and disinformation is now a competency that will increasingly become part of the nurse's repertoire in health teaching.

EXERCISE 10.3 Locate the mission statement for a healthcare organization in your community. What does the organization state about the commitment to its community? Is there any statement about making it easier for people to navigate, understand, or use services to manage their health? Do you and your colleagues consistently ask patients about their plans for following instructions?

Diversity

Nursing practice involves interacting with consumers who are culturally, economically, and socially diverse. Diversity encompasses more than differences in nationality or ethnicity and may include a variety of ways that patients are different from their healthcare providers. Nurses are responsible for assisting patients in accessing and participating in the healthcare system; they also ensure that patients are treated fairly and equitably. Some patients enter the healthcare system much like immigrants entering a foreign country. Patients who enter a system with a set of values, beliefs, and a language unlike their own may experience culture shock. Patients who speak little or no English and those who have low health literacy are vulnerable to poor health outcomes. Nurses need to recognize the culture of their work setting, realizing that it may differ markedly from the culture of the patient, and move beyond ethnocentrism to provide culturally competent care.

Race and ethnicity as factors in influencing the delivery of healthcare and the quality of health outcomes are a serious concern. Some healthcare providers may erroneously assume that members of a particular group have the same beliefs, attitudes, and values about health, when, in fact, extraordinary diversity exists within ethnic groups. The U.S. Census Bureau predicts that by 2040, more than half the US population will be composed of ethnic minorities. As of 2019, 22% of U.S. residents aged 5 years and older speak a language other than English at home (Statista, 2021).

Diversity refers to race, ethnicity, age, gender, socioeconomic status, religion, sexual orientation, physical characteristics, disabilities, and viewpoints. Thus, cultural competence will play an increasingly important role in the relationships that nurses have with patients, families, and communities. An organization that creates a culture of mutual respect, recognizing the contributions of all of its employees, thereby addressing the fourth aim of the Quintuple Aim of improving employee work life, will be much more effective in providing culturally competent healthcare.

The classic and widely used definition of cultural and linguistic competence means bringing together congruent attitudes, behaviors, and policies within an organization in such a way that allows people to work effectively in cross-cultural situations (Cross et al., 1989). Being culturally and linguistically competent involves understanding a culture and the community, and respecting its values, beliefs, and practices. The National Standards for Culturally and Linguistically Appropriate Services (CLAS) in Health and Health Care focuses on services being responsive to diverse cultural health beliefs and practices, preferred languages, health literacy, and other communication needs (Office of Minority Health, n.d.a). The CLAS includes standards for cultural competence, language access, and organizational support (Office of Minority Health, n.d.a). When CLAS are provided, they have the potential to reduce health disparities and achieve health equity (Office of Minority Health, n.d.b).

Patients often hesitate in asking for help with language skills. Some healthcare agencies include an assessment of a patient's ability to learn, but the lack of guidelines regarding language, reading ability, and/or educational attainment may hinder nurses' efforts to institute tailored teaching interventions. The U.S. Census language-screening questions can be used. Individuals are asked if a language other than English is spoken at home. If the answer is "yes," they are asked to rate how well they speak English: very well, well, not well, or not at all (U.S. Census Bureau, n.d.). The median hospital length of stay was shorter when units identified language or cultural needs of patients upon admission than when these were identified upon discharge (Schiaffino et al., 2020). The authors of the study further concluded that there is limited understanding of culturally competent care in many hospitals. Some patients who speak English as their primary language may have equally challenging difficulties because of their limited grasp of standard English, which is what healthcare providers commonly use. Nurse managers can make a commitment to culturally and linguistically appropriate care highly visible to their staff by advocating for ongoing education to meet the unique needs of their patient population and access language services for patients with limited English proficiency.

> **EXERCISE 10.4** A patient does not speak English and is a member of an immigrant group that is not well represented in your community. Using the CLAS standards, identify four strategies that a culturally competent nurse can use to ensure that the patient receives high-quality care.

Patient Satisfaction

Patient satisfaction, or how satisfied people are with the healthcare they receive, has become increasingly important because it is used to gauge a person's experience of care, an important component of person-centered care. A person's relationships with healthcare providers and healthcare organizations are routinely and systematically evaluated, particularly as pay-for-performance models of care are implemented. Nurses spend a great deal of time with patients and their families. These encounters are generally personal and intensely meaningful. Nurses are in a distinct position to influence and promote positive relationships. The nurse manager can set the tone for effective patient–staff interactions that are centered on the patient.

Understanding how patients determine their satisfaction can only enhance the abilities of nurse leaders and followers in their efforts to improve relationships to impact health outcomes. Patient satisfaction ratings, along with measurable healthcare outcomes, are important data used by healthcare organizations to improve quality care and maintain a competitive edge. Nurses, because of their 24-hour accountability for patient care, are integral to attaining high patient satisfaction ratings. Standard-setting organizations, such as the National Quality Forum (NQF), have patient satisfaction questions included in their outcome measures designed to assess the patient experience of care. The Centers for Medicare & Medicaid (CMS) and the Agency for Healthcare Research and Quality (AHRQ) developed a tool, the Hospital Consumer Assessment of Healthcare Providers and Systems (HCAHPS), which measures patient perceptions of the quality of hospital care. A hospital's HCAHPS performance is included in the calculation of its Medicare reimbursement as part of the Hospital Value-Based Purchasing (VBP) Program (CMS, 2019).

Much of a patient's satisfaction with care is dependent on the nursing care that is received. In addition to questions that are related to nursing, the HCAHPS includes questions related to physician care, staff responsiveness, communications about medicines, and discharge and care transition. HCAHPS reports are available on Medicare's Hospital Compare website (*https://www.medicare.gov/care-compare/*), allowing the public to make meaningful comparisons and creating incentives for hospitals to improve quality.

Comparative data for Medicare- and Medicaid-certified nursing homes are available on the Nursing Home Compare website. Despite the availability of publicly reported data, patients and their families also go to websites such as YELP for information about hospitals and patient experiences. Researchers have found that consumer ratings of patient satisfaction on YELP are positively and significantly correlated with patient experience ratings derived from the HCAPHS hospital surveys (Chakraborty & Church, 2020). Nurses can go to YELP to get a preview of patient concerns before the release of the annual HCAPHS scores, providing the opportunity to take early corrective action. Because measuring patient satisfaction is an evolving science, nurses do not always accurately gauge what factors are most important to patients. Satisfaction measures are often skewed in a positive direction, with scores clustered at the top of the scale. Sometimes, these factors make it difficult to interpret results and make improvements. The use of multiple sources of information has the potential to enhance decision-making about needed improvement.

> **EXERCISE 10.5** Go to the HCAHPS Survey website (*https://hcahpsonline.org/globalassets/hcahps/survey-instruments/mail/effective-july-1-2020-and-forward-discharges/2020_survey-instruments_english_mail.pdf*) and identify which questions are affected by (1) nursing care, (2) good team communication, (3) care coordination, and (4) effective transition to home or another care setting. Go to the Hospital Compare website (*https://www.medicare.gov/care-compare/*) to examine a hospital's HCAHPS scores and discuss the implications of the results for person-centered care. Determine whether the organization's ratings on YELP are similar or different.

Nurses have a responsibility to exercise critical thinking and decision-making skills with respect to patient satisfaction with nursing care. For example, patients who have had major surgery may not want to cough and deep breathe because it is painful; yet, we know that failure to do so can result in pneumonia. Nurses are responsible for (1) advocating for their patients, (2) ensuring adequate pain relief, (3) correcting patient misconceptions, and (4) implementing pain management strategies consistent with established standards. This may be more complicated as concerns are raised about appropriate pain management in the context of preventing opioid use disorders. Patient satisfaction ratings may be low if nurses have not attended to the "hotel amenities," commonly referred to as *customer services*.

Nurses may become frustrated because they want to focus on delivering high-quality nursing care. The use of patient satisfaction measures and similar tools illustrate how important it is for nurses to explain their roles and the purpose of the care being provided.

Reviewing and analyzing patient satisfaction survey ratings are invaluable tools. Managers need to share the results of such surveys with their staff, examine the context of the results, and plan with their staff members as to how meaningful improvements can be made.

Because patient satisfaction ratings are publicly available and they affect the financial status of the organization, some healthcare organizations use scripting to provide standardized responses for rounding and other events. Some nurses dislike these scripts because they limit critical thinking and professional judgment and make them feel like they are being treated as incompetent. Others indicate that scripting provides consistency and assurance to patients by providing tools for handling difficult situations. The key is that the communication affect cannot sound as if a script is being read or the value of the messages is lost. If nurses find scripts unacceptable, managers should encourage reviewing the core messages and using their own words that are not offensive and sound sincere. Strategies used to enhance person-centered care can also positively affect patient satisfaction ratings. These include keeping patients at the front and center of decision-making processes by (a) including first and last names, and position title with introductions, (b) asking patients about their most important concerns, (c) discussing approaches to care with patients, (d) informing the patient on what can be expected for the day, (e) incorporating patient values and cultural preferences into care, and (f) including patients in the handoff processes, such as bedside reports and transition-of-care processes.

Access to Care

Access to care is an important component of person-centered care. Care cannot be person centered if people don't have access to care or if they struggle to get the care that is needed. Access to healthcare includes (1) coverage, having entry to the healthcare system; (2) access to a usual source of care, including screening and preventive services; (3) being able to get healthcare when needed, and (4) having culturally competent and qualified healthcare providers (AHRQ, n.d.). The Health Innovation Network (n.d.) indicates that if people are at the center of care, they will receive care when needed.

Significant healthcare disparities (systematic differences in health between social groups) U.S. Health and Human Services, Health Resources and Services Administration [HRSA], Office of Health Equity, 2020) are manifest in numerous ways across the United States. Health inequities refer to inequalities that are unfair, unjust, or unavoidable that can be addressed through policy (HRSA, 2020). For example, Black and Latina/Latino populations are less likely to have employer-sponsored health insurance, and people with Medicaid insurance may use facilities that are under-resourced. Interventions that can be used to reduce disparities include team care, patient navigation, cultural tailoring, collaboration with families and community members, interactive skills-based training, and increasing the diversity of the healthcare workforce. These interventions are all focused on improving the nature of healthcare delivery, particularly relationships with patients and their families.

A major concern in the delivery of healthcare is unequal treatment because of racial-cultural discrimination. Historically, minorities and women were significantly underrepresented in health-related research, resulting in less information for decision-making. Consequently, federal legislation requires researchers to include women, children, and racial/ethnic minorities in their proposals.

People who are uninsured or underinsured due to lack of economic means or whose citizenship or entry status is undocumented are often vulnerable, sometimes even powerless, in the healthcare delivery system. These people may be denied access to care or, if they achieve access, they may not receive equal care. Heart disease in women often goes unrecognized because of different symptom presentation and a lack of follow-up testing. Blacks may not be offered the same treatment options as Whites, resulting in care delays and worse outcomes. As the implementation of the ACA unfolded, states that did not expand Medicaid under the ACA had the highest rates of uninsured and poverty in the country. By 2019, states that did not expand Medicaid coverage had nearly double the rate of uninsured than those states that did expand Medicaid coverage (15.5% vs. 8.3%) (Garfield et al., 2021). Although the ACA expanded the availability of preventive services, a comparison of their use before and after the implementation of the ACA indicates modest increases, and disparities still exist (Abdus, 2021).

Another access to care issue is the plight of some 57 million people who live in rural areas across the United States. Travel to reach a healthcare provider or hospital

> **EXERCISE 10.6** You are the charge nurse on a unit. A Black nurse who has worked on the unit for 20 years comes to you very upset, telling you that the husband of a patient told her to get out of the room, that he didn't want any Blacks taking care of his wife. How would you handle this situation? Do patients have a right to refuse care from certain staff members? What resources are available to you to address this issue?

may take several hours for people living in rural communities. A rural hospital might not have the specialty services that are available in urban areas. More importantly, rural hospitals have been closing and many more are at risk of closure, particularly in states that have not expanded Medicaid. This is because these hospitals may be in more financial difficulty because of the costs of uncompensated care. If a hospital closes, other associated services may close as well, such as pharmacies and home health agencies.

A foundational principle for *Healthy People 2030* is the elimination of health disparities and achieving health equity (ODPHP, 2021). Strategies to enhance access to care include the use of technology such as videoconferencing and access to patient portals where individuals can track their own health information. Many adults use technology to track their own health indicators or that of a loved one. Broadband Internet access is a significant issue for rural communities across America. Furthermore, individuals with low health literacy are less likely to use fitness and nutrition applications, activity trackers, and patient portals. This digital divide has been exacerbated with hospitalizations due to COVID-19 when patients are separated from their families for extended periods of time. People who are older or Hispanic are less likely to use telehealth video visits (Rodriguez et al., 2021). These patterns of access to technology and health information also affect the nature of the relationship between patients and their healthcare providers, including nurses.

Nurses are positioned to be guardians of the rights of individuals and their families; thus, they can address issues of cultural, ethnic, and racial sensitivity. They are alert to circumstances that may prevent a successful outcome for the patient and can intervene on the patient's behalf. While nurses are often the advocates for patients and their families receiving their care with regard to access to service, they also need to identify and address specific policy issues related to access to healthcare in the communities in which they live and practice.

EXERCISE 10.7 You are a nurse in a busy gynecological-obstetrical practice. You notice that a young woman who appears to be Hispanic has been waiting for some time to be addressed by the receptionist. An older White woman walks up to the desk, and the receptionist immediately addresses her. As it turns out, the older woman, a nurse, was the mother-in-law of the younger woman and had just been parking her car. She was accompanying her daughter-in-law to the office for her first prenatal visit. She raises a concern with the nurse that the staff will not treat her daughter-in-law professionally. Consider what you might say to the young woman and her mother-in-law and what you would do if you were this nurse. How would you address the issue with the receptionist?

PATIENT ENGAGEMENT

Healthcare organizations, including healthcare systems and insurers, use a variety of strategies to improve health outcomes, services, and the experience of care. Foremost in the repertoire of initiatives is focusing on patient engagement. Patient engagement is defined as "patients, families, their representatives, and health professionals working in active partnership at various levels across the healthcare system—direct care, organizational design and governance, and policymaking—to improve health and healthcare" (Carman & Workman, 2017, p. 25). Efforts to increase patient engagement can be made at the direct care, organizational, and policy levels. This is illustrated in the continuum for patient engagement framework in Figure 10.3. Nurses are well

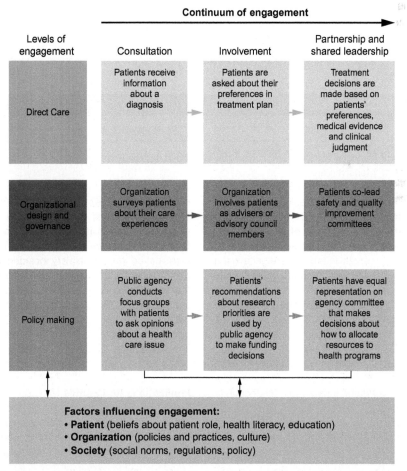

Fig. 10.3 Continuum of patient engagement. (From Carman, K. L., & Workman, T. A. (2017). Engaging patients and consumers in research evidence: Applying the conceptual model of patient and family engagement. *Patient Education and Counseling, 100*(1), 25–29.)

prepared to implement strategies that foster patient engagement because they are educated in establishing productive relationships with patients and their families, seeing them as at the center of care and as partners in managing their health.

When patients are engaged, they are empowered to take an active role in the management of their health. The Literature Perspective describes innovative strategies adopted to maintain and foster parental engagement for neonates hospitalized during the COVID-19 pandemic. Additionally, the benefits of healthcare services are listed in the Engagement Behavior Framework outlined in Box 10.3 (Center for Advancing Health, 2010). The broad range of behaviors identified provides nurses with a roadmap for implementing a wide range of strategies to engage patients and their families at multiple points of contact within the healthcare system. These slightly different perspectives on patient engagement all illustrate the key role that nurses can have in putting patients (and their families) at the center of their care and partnering with them in efforts to improve their health.

BOX 10.3   Engagement Behavior Framework

1. Find good health care.
2. Communicate with health professionals.
3. Organize health care.
4. Pay for health care.
5. Make good treatment decisions.
6. Participate in treatment.
7. Promote health.
8. Get preventive health care.
9. Plan for the end of life.
10. Seek health knowledge.

From Center for Advancing Health (2010). *Engagement behavior framework.* https://silo.tips/download/a-new-definition-of-patient-engagement.

EXERCISE 10.8   Select one of the behaviors in the Engagement Behavior Framework in Box 10.3. Identify at least three activities indicating that individuals and their families are able to achieve the behavior.

LITERATURE PERSPECTIVE

Resource: Duff, J., Curnen, K., Reed, A., & Kranz, C. (2021). Engaging parents of hospitalized neonates during a pandemic. *Journal of Neonatal Nursing, 27*(3), 185–187.

Nurses in a neonatal intensive care unit had adopted a variety of strategies considered best practices to engage parents in the care of their complex, fragile neonates and promote family bonding. Strategies that include allowing families to be present, the provision of education and support, and frequent communication are an expected standard of practice in neonatal intensive care units in the United States and across the world that are widely implemented. With the advent of COVID-19, this facility had to revise visitation policies to help reduce its transmission and minimize the risks to patients, families, and staff. Caregivers were limited to one person for each patient in each 24-hour period with few exceptions.

Core concepts related to patient- and family-focused care included (a) treating every patient and family with dignity and respect, (b) sharing information, (c) encouraging participation in care and decision-making, and (d) collaborating actively in care delivery processes. Innovations designed to treat patients with dignity and respect focused on the use of virtual interventions. Virtual visits were facilitated with the use of iPads. These were also used by family members to talk, read, sing, or otherwise interact with their infant. Angel Eye cameras were used to allow parents and other caregivers to view their infant or chat with those present in the room. Parents were provided a phone line for recording messages that would be played for the infant on a "Story Bear." Communication was changed to a virtual format. Virtual parent hours were substituted for parent support groups. Staff also provided short presentations on timely topics. The nursing staff rounded virtually with the parents daily. Facetime and Skype were used for these activities. Encouraging parent participation in care delivery included involvement in the use of tools for the delivery of music guided by a music therapist. Photo albums were provided to highlight important milestones. Group discharge classes were conducted with appropriate physical distancing. The staff collaborated with parent and family advisory councils about the implementation of changes, particularly with those necessitated by state and national recommendations.

Implications for Practice
Patient engagement, in this example of parent/caregivers, is a multifaceted, evolving process that required the input of a variety of team members and necessitated flexibility in the context of changing circumstances. Nurses and nurse managers have expertise in a variety of patient- and family-centered strategies that can be adapted for successful patient engagement.

KEY FEATURES IN THE DELIVERY OF PERSON-CENTERED CARE

Central to the delivery of person-centered care is the development of trusting relationships. This trust allows nurses to demonstrate accountability for care delivery. Nurses are readily able to develop trusting relationships. They use the nursing process in focusing care on patients' needs and advance knowledge through research focused on patient needs. Nurses are also ideally suited for facilitating care coordination as patients interact with different segments of the healthcare system. The public holds nurses in high regard, viewing them as knowledgeable, worthy of respect, concerned for others, honest, caring, confidential, friendly, hardworking, and especially trustworthy. Nurses have for 20 years topped the list in the Gallup poll of the public's ratings of honesty and ethical standards of various professions, with a great majority of Americans (81%) believing that nurses' honesty and ethical standards are "high" or "very high" (Saad, 2022). Trusting relationships require that nurses be sensitive to the needs of patients. These relationships should extend to ways that nurses work together as a team. Nurse leaders and managers can facilitate a culture that fosters trusting working relationships.

Nursing diagnoses, interventions, and outcomes comprise standardized nursing terminologies that provide additional support for the distinctive role of nurses in the delivery of person-centered care as members of a collaborative, multidisciplinary team. Standardized nursing terminologies are unique in that they describe a patient's current needs irrespective of a medical diagnosis. For example, although an individual may have a medical diagnosis of type 2 diabetes mellitus, determining that a patient has a *lack of knowledge of medication regimen* (an International Classification for Nursing Practice® term [International Council of Nurses, 2022]) facilitates the development of an individualized goal-oriented care plan based on the patient's preferences. With only knowing the medical diagnosis, the patient may be at home, needing guidance about diabetes self-management, or may be in the hospital with hyperosmolar hyperglycemia nonketotic coma. Nursing diagnoses support the identification of patient outcomes and the implementation of nursing interventions. Including standardized international nursing terminologies (noting that many are evidence based) in electronic health records is key to providing a more precise understanding of what exactly is happening with patients and their progress in meeting their goals for healthcare. Some nursing diagnoses may

be totally unrelated to the medical diagnosis and yet may be a main cause of concern in daily living. Without documenting the nursing diagnosis, the person may not receive the assistance needed to address that concern.

Likewise, nursing research largely focuses on persons, families, groups and communities, responses to illness, and the testing of interventions to promote health and prevent disease to support the practice of nursing. Nurses focus on systematically analyzing the evidence from numerous research studies to provide a more solid foundation for practice (see Chapter 6).

Nurses face numerous challenges in the delivery of person-centered care. Patients going home may not understand their discharge plans. Nurses in acute care settings may have limited time to provide complex discharge instructions. Because of reimbursement constraints, home health nurses may not be permitted to make the necessary number of visits to enable patients to successfully manage a chronic illness. Discharge from the hospital is just one of the many types of transitions of care that create additional vulnerabilities for high-risk patients. RNs and advanced practice registered nurses (APRNs) are in ideal positions to provide person-centered care through the oversight of healthcare delivery and facilitation of communication when patients transition across systems. A strategy promoted by the Institute for Healthcare Improvement's campaign to foster patient-centered care is to ask the question, "What matters to you?" (IHI, 2022b). The responses to this question about personal goals then needs to be translated into professional actions (Olsen et al., 2020).

Professional Practice to Address Challenges

Numerous strategies can be used by nurses to deliver person-centered care. A professional practice model such as the Careful Nursing Philosophy and Professional Practice Model (Careful Nursing) is a useful guide for nurse leaders because it is centered on the patient as a unitary or holistic person. Careful Nursing practice is guided by three philosophical principles: the nature and inherent dignity of the human person, Infinite Transcendent Reality in life processes, and health as human flourishing (Meehan, 2020). The *Code of Ethics for Nurses* specifies that respect for the inherent dignity, worth, and unique attributes and human rights of every person is a fundamental principle underlying nursing practice (ANA, 2015). As human persons, we have unique biophysical and psychospiritual characteristics. The Infinite Transcendent Reality principle is concerned with nurses' spirituality and how awareness of one's own spirituality can strengthen nursing practice by acting with calmness and kindness. This, in turn, facilitates nurses' abilities to protect people from harm, foster healing and health, or foster a peaceful death. Health is conceptualized as human flourishing and is key to achieving full human potential. The professional practice model is composed of four dimensions: (1) the therapeutic milieu, (2) practice competence and excellence, (3) management of practice and influence in health systems, and (4) professional authority (Meehan, 2020).

Operational concepts underpin each of these dimensions to illustrate how each of the dimensions is translated into care for individuals, their families, and communities. Although all of nursing care can be described as person-centered care, strategies used by nurses related to safe and restorative physical surroundings, health education, trustworthy collaboration, and visibility are illustrated in Figure 10.4. Nurses need to be deliberative about taking actions that are person centered. Providing safe and restorative surroundings, a component of a therapeutic milieu, can be enhanced by frontline nurse and nurse leader advocacy for individuals and their families.

The definition of nursing includes advocacy in the care of individuals, families, communities, and populations. Nurses, in accordance with the *Code of Ethics for Nurses*, have the responsibility to promote, advocate, and protect the health, safety, and rights of patients (ANA, 2015). Advocacy as an expectation for nurses is further reflected in its addition as a professional practice standard in nursing (ANA, 2021). An advocate is one who does the following:

- Defends or promotes the rights of others
- Changes systems to meet the needs of others
- Empowers and promotes self-determination in others
- Promotes autonomy of diverse cultures and social groups
- Ensures respect, equity, and dignity for others

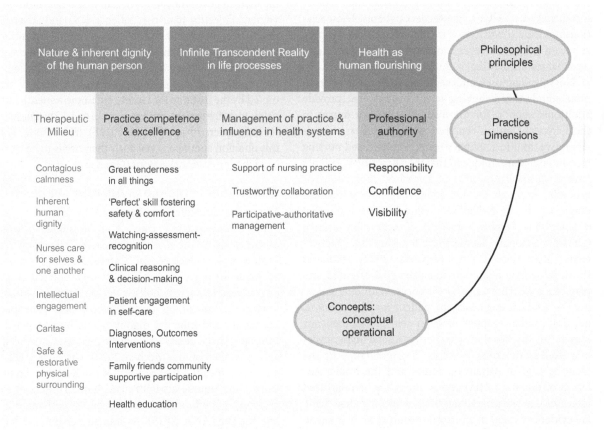

Fig. 10.4 Careful Nursing philosophical principles, and practice dimensions with their concepts.© (From Meehan, T. C. (2020). *Careful nursing philosophy and professional practice model.* http://www.carefulnursing.ie/go/overview/summary.)

Advocacy requires the nurse to perceive and be comfortable with conflict and then mediate, negotiate, clarify, explain, and intervene. The nurse can be a liaison between and among individuals, their families, and the healthcare system by interpreting the processes and procedures of the healthcare organization. The advocacy role also includes negotiating changes when patients and families differ in their values and beliefs. One way to advocate for patients is to allow them to make choices and participate in their care in accordance with their preferences.

Safety as a Strategy for Person-Centered Care

Future nurses and nurse leaders are being prepared under the umbrella of the Quality and Safety Education for Nurses (QSEN) initiative to gain necessary knowledge, skills, and attitudes (KSAs) to improve quality and safety for patients. This approach is expanded to include systems thinking, which is illustrated in Table 10.4 (Dolansky & Moore, 2013). Additional work by Lyle-Edrosolo and Waxman (2016) demonstrated QSEN's

TABLE 10.4   Continuous Systems Thinking for QSEN Domains

QSEN Competency	Personal Effort/ Individual Care	⟵⟶		Systems Thinking/ System Care
Patient-Centered Care	Document the presence and extent of my patients' pain.	Use common definitions, terms, and rating scales in documenting my patients' pain.	Formulate pain management plans with my patients, their families, and other healthcare professionals.	Participate in medical record reviews of our unit's pain management documentation.
Evidence-Based Practice	Differentiate clinical opinion from research and evidence summaries.	Discuss conflicting evidence in the literature with my colleagues.	Question the rationale for routine care approaches on my unit that are not evidence based.	Participate in writing unit-level standards of practice that are evidence based.
Teamwork and Collaboration	Ensure that my patients are ready for discharge by making sure they have their prescriptions.	Formulate discharge plan with my patients, their families, and other healthcare professionals.	Solicit input from other team members to improve my team performance.	Participate in improving the discharge process through team meetings to structure communication during a patient's hospital stay.
Safety	Wash my hands at the appropriate times in the care of my patients.	Get patients and families to participate in the campaign to reduce infection by washing hands.	Observe other nurses' handwashing technique and provide feedback.	Study the workarounds on my unit and create a cause-and-effect diagram to summarize why nurses do not wash their hands.
Quality Improvement	Ensure that I care for central lines using evidence-based practice.	Have a peer watch my central line dressing change so that I can improve my performance.	Review the data for our unit's central line infection rates.	Participate in a quality improvement project to improve compliance with central line bundle on our unit.
Informatics	Protect the confidentiality of my patients' protected health information in the electronic health record (EHR).	Attend in-service training updates to learn about new laws regarding health information protection.	Help design patient information flyers describing the patients' and families' rights to confidentiality of information in the EHR.	Participate in an agency-wide committee to update the agency EHR system.

Reprinted with permission from Dolansky, M. A., & Moore, S. M. (2013). Quality and Safety Education for Nurses (QSEN): The key is systems thinking. *OJIN: The Online Journal of Issues in Nursing*, 18(3):1.

alignment with The Joint Commission criteria for accreditation and the American Nurses Credentialing Center Magnet® Standards, indicating that QSEN can be used as a framework for ensuring that the nursing workforce is prepared to address quality and safety. In a survey examining patient-centered care, competency, and safety, nurses who had had high participation in patient safety activities had higher scores in patient-centered competencies and safety climate (Hwang et al., 2019). Promoting safety involves advocacy: nurses speaking up about safety issues and nurse leaders creating environments that encourage staff to speak up about safety issues. Conducting timeouts in the operating room to ensure that the right procedure is being done on the right patient and empowering nurses to speak up about breaches in infection control during central-line insertion procedures are just two examples of how opportunities for nurses to speak up and be advocates can be structurally embedded in institutional policies. Similarly, using evidence to change nursing practice is necessary for excellence in nursing by obtaining designation as a Magnet® facility.

More challenging are situations in which the policies may not be so clear, or in where no policy exists. An unsafe situation can never be person centered. Here, the nurse must act as an advocate to promote safety to support the delivery of person-centered care. Understanding nursing's role and that all nurses are leaders regardless of whether one has a formal title in a managerial role is critical to providing a person-centered environment. Historically, one of the worst public health crises in the country occurred when health department officials in Nevada found that up to 63,000 patients had a potential exposure to hepatitis C because of poor infection control practices at a chain of endoscopy clinics (Leary & Diers, 2013). Despite the poor infection control practices over an extended time period, only one nurse complained to authorities. Although this example clearly had major implications for many people, day-to-day opportunities for nurses in direct care to promote safety may be subtle, requiring a more nuanced and strategic approach to promote a safe environment. The COVID-19 pandemic and the stresses associated with heavy workloads, lack of personal protective equipment (PPE) and emotional exhaustion resulted in more nurses speaking out about working conditions. However, these efforts have not been without risks to employment (O'Neill, 2021). Part of the response of the "Great Resignation" in 2021 is attributed to nurses being willing to resign their current positions to earn respect and be more fairly compensated.

Safety requires a commitment from the leadership of an organization to not only "talk safety, but walk safety" in its visons, goals, and action. Such visions, goals, and actions increase the likelihood of transparency in examining safety events and establishing partnerships with patients and their families (Mayer & Hatlie, 2020). Leadership commitment to safety includes the involvement of community members and seeking input from staff members. Hospitals are establishing advisory councils focused on quality and safety; they include members of the community on these councils and their boards. A safety culture involves open communication, where nurses feel safe in reporting issues and concerns. Processes for reporting deviations in safety need to be reliable, consistent, and fair. This means that expectations for processes need to be well understood. One hospital desiring to increase reports of safety issues asked nurses providing direct care to identify behaviors of the senior leadership that would help in promoting a safety culture. Communication, access, and visibility were identified (O'Connor & Carlson, 2016). Subsequently, after a concerted effort to act upon the clinical nurses' recommendations, the number of risk and near-risk safety reports were increased, enabling the leaders to make changes to improve safety.

Health Education

Health education, as a component of practice competence and excellence, can be enhanced with the use of motivational interviewing. Teaching is a core role of RNs and APRNs regardless of the setting. Motivational interviewing (MI) is an evidence-based strategy that has become an essential tool in the repertoire of the savvy nurse and nurse leader. MI is consistent with person-centered care because it provides patients with the opportunity to become involved in their care while recognizing and affirming their autonomy in making choices. Health education needs to move beyond just providing patients and their families with information. MI can be used any time people need help with making lifestyle changes.

The central feature of MI is using intrinsic motivation to change behavior. Intrinsic motivation refers to what is rewarding to the individual. For example, losing weight may be important to a mother because it will make it easier to engage in activities with her children. This is consistent with person-centered care in that it focuses behavioral change on what is most important to individuals and their

BOX 10.4 **Questions to Ask in Motivational Interviewing**

1. Why would you want to make this change?
2. How might you go about it in order to succeed?
3. What are the three best reasons for you to do it?
4. How important is it for you to make this change and why?
5. So, what do you think you will do?

Source: Rollnick, S., Miller, W. R., & Butler, C. (2013). *Motivational interviewing: Helping people change in health care* (3rd ed., p. 11). New York: Guilford Press.

families. MI was first developed as a brief person-centered counseling strategy to help people make behavioral changes when dealing with drug and alcohol addictions. It subsequently was expanded to include helping people manage chronic conditions. MI includes four processes: engaging, focusing, evoking a patient's own motivation, and planning (Rollnick et al., 2013). Core communication strategies include asking the person to set goals, informing the person about options and what might be helpful, listening to what the person wants, and offering help in accordance with the person's wishes (Rollnick et al., 2013) (Box 10.4). MI has been demonstrated to be an effective strategy used by nurses for behavioral change in a wide variety of populations. Some healthcare organizations and insurers employ nurse coaches who have received extensive training in MI and are also clinical experts in the care of specific high-risk populations.

Care Coordination

Care coordination also provides opportunities for advocacy. Care coordination "involves deliberately organizing patient care activities and sharing information among all of the participants concerned with a patient's care to achieve safer and more effective care. This means that the patient's needs and preferences are known ahead of time and communicated at the right time to the right people, and that this information is used to provide safe, appropriate, and effective care to the patient" (AHRQ, 2018).

Care coordination is an important factor in the delivery of quality care that requires a strong relationship between the nurse and patient. Frontline nurses and nurse leaders can facilitate care coordination by working with case managers and members of the multidisciplinary healthcare team. Nurses in care coordinator roles are influential advocates for vulnerable populations who are at high risk for subpar or no care in a complicated healthcare system. These groups typically include those who receive no care and need it the most, such as persons who are homeless, uninsured, or underinsured; persons who have opioid-use disorders addictions; children living in poverty; migrant workers; and people with acquired immunodeficiency syndrome (AIDS). Some healthcare organizations capitalize on the care coordination abilities of nurses by creating "navigator" or case management roles designed to assist patients with accessing the resources of a healthcare system or complex decision needs. Effective use of RNs in all practice settings can result in better care coordination, quality, safety, and efficiency, thus enhancing the delivery of person-centered care.

Professional Authority

Professional authority refers to nurses being experts in the delivery of care taking responsibility for care and ownership of nursing practice. One strategy is for frontline nurses to give voice to their actions by being visible in explaining who they are and what they are doing, reflecting the authority they have over their practice. This term does not mean being authoritative with patients. Rather, it means nurses describing who they are and what they are doing that reflects the knowledge, competencies, and compassion that are critical to nursing practice. Instead of being silent and working behind the scenes, nurses need to give voice to their practice, explaining the value of the care that is provided (e.g., encouraging coughing and deep breathing to prevent pneumonia). Being silent about what we do as nurses means that the fourth aim of the Quintuple Aims, improving the work life of healthcare providers, will never be recognized as important for nurses. Part of creating value is documented in the second *Future of Nursing* report (National Academies, 2021). Substantive contributions of nursing to the outcomes of patient care are not minimized and include taking responsibility for one's actions and describing one's actions in a manner that reflects the expertise of the nurse. Frontline nurses can do this every day as they explain the assessments and interventions that will be provided.

Some nurses are reluctant to use their last names in their encounters with patients, turning over their badges so that their names are not revealed. Additionally, some organizations show first names and title only and the last name is on a less visible portion of the badge. From the perspective of the person receiving care, this can be perceived as impersonal, rude, or dangerous, because the nurse may be performing a skill that requires intimacy and personal knowledge. Identifying oneself to patients is a first step in treating them with dignity and respect. Providing our first and last names and our title to people with whom we interact in the healthcare system signals that we are willing to be accountable for our actions and take responsibility for following up with concerns while providing needed reassurance. However, the extended experience of the COVID-19 pandemic has placed additional stressors on patients, their families, nurses, other healthcare professionals, and support staff. The increase in verbal and physical violence experienced by nurses during the pandemic has no doubt created anxiety and impacted the nature of nurse–patient relationships. Sensible nurses exercise sound judgment about what to disclose and to whom, even with the desire to be as open as possible.

EXERCISE 10.9 Examine a healthcare organization's newsletter, website, or other media outlet. Are nurses' contributions to care highlighted? Are the full names of nurses, their credentials, and roles included in stories? How does this compare with stories about other healthcare professionals?

Describing nursing care to clearly communicate that nurses are knowledgeable and skillful is important in giving voice to nurses' authority. Although patients may think that the nurse is just idly chatting about the weather or television programs in a patient room, they may not understand that the nurse has monitored intravenous fluids, checked outputs of catheters and drains, and assessed for evidence of dyspnea, all in the space of a few minutes. In a clinic setting, the patient may not realize that the nurse has determined whether additional teaching is necessary or whether a new symptom needs to be brought to a healthcare provider's attention. Similarly, in the home, as the nurse walks from the door to wherever the person is, the nurse assesses for safety and health hazards and general living conditions while having a general conversation. See Box 10.5 for strategies to enhance the visibility of nursing practice.

Nurse leaders can enhance professional authority by increasing the visibility of nursing practice through active participation at policy tables, where decisions are made about healthcare both within an organization and in the community. Nurses must actively contribute to decisions

---

BOX 10.5   Giving Visibility to Nursing Practice

1. Provide a complete introduction to patients, including full name, your role, and purpose of the interaction.
2. Ask the patient about the patient's most important concerns.
3. Explain why you are doing assessments, the results of assessments, and the purpose of related interventions.
4. Describe how your interventions will affect outcomes for your patients.
5. Link your interventions to nursing research and/or evidence-based practice.
6. Describe how the judgments you make require consultation or discussion with other health professionals rather than just indicating you are "ask the physician."
7. Regularly participate in team rounds to communicate important findings and patient concerns.
8. Ask patients and families if they have anything additional to share on team rounds.
9. Follow up on patient concerns and communicate the plan for follow-up to patients and/or their families.
10. Validate with patients that their concerns have been addressed.
11. Include patients and families when planning for transitions of care.

---

being made about nursing practice, patient care, and its documentation using standardized nursing terminologies. Nurses should not be just a token representative of nursing in a policy-making group, whose only role is to implement policies developed by others. Rather, nurses should be experts whose contributions are valued by the organization. Frontline nurses can begin their involvement in policy by volunteering to be on a healthcare agency's committee, joining a professional association, or volunteering for a community organization. These provide valuable experience in articulating the viewpoints of nurses and collaborating with members of other healthcare disciplines and representatives of the community.

Nurse leaders can broaden their circle of involvement and improve the health of communities by volunteering to join a board. Nurse leaders bring not only their experiences in person-centered care but also their expertise in communication, quality improvement, patient engagement, and decision-making, which demonstrates the value of nursing to the mission of healthcare organizations. Nurses can join a national effort to increase the number of nurses on boards, the Nurses on Boards

Coalition (NOBC), which is designed to improve the health of communities (NOBC, 2021). Although joining a hospital board may seem daunting, joining the board of a local affiliate of a national healthcare organization or the board of a local affiliate of a professional association provides an opportunity to demonstrate the nursing perspective and the value of person-centered care. Board service provides the opportunity to learn about the kinds of support services that may be offered to people in the community while having the opportunity to increase nursing's visibility by sharing information about nurses and how nursing care improves health.

EXERCISE 10.10 Find out whether a nurse is on the board of a local hospital. Is there a nurse on the board of the city or county health department? Ask a nurse leader about the leader's involvement in committees, community boards, or professional associations and what strategies are used to focus on person-centered approaches to the delivery of services. Ask a direct care nurse about community involvement.

SYNTHESIS AND APPLICATION

Understanding paradigm shifts in health care and the need to be responsive to the needs of individuals, families, groups, communities, and populations will position nurses to fully participate in shaping healthcare in the future.

Nurse leaders influence the quality of care delivered by frontline staff, setting the tone for the implementation of the organization's mission and focus on the delivery of person-centered care. They must believe in and model a philosophy of care that is focused on the person.

Nurse leaders are in a distinct position to not only model a person-centered approach for their staff but also to find solutions that enhance the quality of care. This can be accomplished by understanding the types of problems and their nature as experienced by patients and their families as well as the barriers faced by frontline nurses in delivering person-centered care. Being successful in facilitating the delivery of person-centered care requires openness and flexibility.

CONCLUSION

Healthcare is changing rapidly, resulting in changes in the roles of frontline nurses and nurse leaders. The movement of healthcare into the home, community, clinic, and myriad outpatient settings has placed a new perspective on how to scale up for the volume of care while maintaining quality. Harnessing the motivations of patients and their families to engage them in the self-management of their health has the potential to enhance outcomes while reducing costs. Nurses, with their holistic approach and focus on the person and the person's needs, are a pivotal and powerful resource in the delivery of healthcare. Likewise, providing frontline nurses with the support and tools to engage in advocacy early in their careers has the potential to reap rewards as they apply the competencies learned in direct care to more complex situations and leadership roles.

THE SOLUTION

Recognizing the concern posed as a patient safety concern, the nurse leader must leverage multiple resources in the pursuit of a patient-centered resolution. First, we connected the patient and family with our patient advocate to establish a consistent, single point of contact. Once the patient advocate contacted the patient's wife for a discussion, we leveraged the nursing process to evaluate the concern. We gathered the appropriate team members from various departments—including information technology, physicians, pharmacists, and direct care nurses—to assess the concerns and provide an explanation for the outcome. One of the most important diagnoses to make is whether the identified issue was caused by failure of a process or failure to follow an established process. In this specific case, the team determined the root cause to be a process failure. With that in mind, a workflow redesign was undertaken inclusive of redesign of the electronic medical record to enable reliable flow of information from order to discharge instructions to prescription. Although the resolution of the concern was primarily tactical and workflow, maintaining an open line of communication while the health system navigated the resolution process was important. This was accomplished by first acknowledging the concern and then closing the loop with the patient by sharing details about the problem's resolution.

Would this be a suitable approach for you? Why?

Angelo Venditti

▮ REFLECTIONS

Think of a recent challenging interaction with a patient and/or a family member. What might you do differently to enhance person-centered care the next time that you encounter a similar situation?

Identify one action that you took to advocate for a patient at an individual level. What actions can you take to translate that advocacy to promoting a safe environment at the systems level?

▮ BEST PRACTICES

The single best practice is to start with the patient in mind, talk about the patient before the diagnosis and consider the patient's perspective before taking action, using strategies such as motivational interviewing enhances your effect.

1. Treat people with dignity and respect.
2. Focus on developing a trusting relationship with patients.
3. Introduce yourself to patients and include your role, what will be included in their care, and what can be expected during the course of the day/encounter.
4. Ask patients about their most important concerns.

5. Use standardized and person-centered terminology when documenting care and communicating with other healthcare professionals.
6. Examine your organization's commitment to the CLAS standards in the delivery of culturally and linguistically competent care.
7. Provide the next healthcare professional with the necessary information about what is required for care coordination, follow-up, or transition to a new setting.
8. Foster motivation and belief in the importance of everyone and the value of each person's contribution to care.

REFERENCES

Abdus, S. (2021). Trends in differences across subgroups of adults in preventive services utilization. *Medical Care, 59*(12), 1059–1066. https://doi.org/10.1097/MLR.0000000000001634.

Agency for Healthcare Research and Quality (AHRQ). (2018). *Care coordination.* Retrieved from https://www.ahrq.gov/ncepcr/care/coordination.html.

Agency for Healthcare Research and Quality (AHRQ). (n.d.). *Topic: Access to care.* Retrieved from https://www.ahrq.gov/topics/access-care.html.

Agency for Healthcare Research and Quality (AHRQ). (2021). *Defining the PCMH.* Retrieved from https://pcmh.ahrq.gov/page/defining-pcmh.

Alqenae, F. A., Steinke, D., & Keers, R. N. (2020). Prevalence and nature of medication errors and medication-related harm following discharge from hospital to community settings: A systematic review. *Drug Safety, 43*(6), 517–537. https://doi.org/10.1007/s40264-020-00918-3.

American Academy of Nursing (AAN). (2018). *Twenty-five things nurses and patients should question.* Retrieved from https://www.choosingwisely.org/societies/american-academy-of-nursing/.

American Academy of Nursing (AAN). (2021a). *Family and Birth Center in the Developing Families Center.* Retrieved from https://www.aannet.org/initiatives/edge-runners/profiles/edge-runners-family-health-and-birth-center-in-the-developing-families-center.

American Academy of Nursing (AAN). (2021b). *A caring science model of specialized dementia care for transforming practice and advancing health equity.* Retrieved from https://www.aannet.org/initiatives/edge-runners/profiles/caring-science-model-of-specialized-dementia-care.

American Association of Colleges of Nursing (AACN). (2021). *The essentials: Core competencies for professional nursing education.* Retrieved from https://www.aacnnursing.org/Portals/42/AcademicNursing/pdf/Essentials-2021.pdf.

American Geriatrics Society Expert Panel on Person-Centered Care. (2016). Person-centered care: A definition and essential elements. *Journal of the American Geriatrics Society, 64*(1), 15–18. https://doi.org/10.1111/jgs.13866.

American Nurses Association (ANA). (2015). *Code of Ethics for Nurses with interpretive statements.* Retrieved from https://www.nursingworld.org/practice-policy/nursing-excellence/ethics/code-of-ethics-for-nurses/.

American Nurses Association (ANA). (2021). *Nursing: Scope and standards of practice* (4th ed.). Silver Spring, MD: Author.

American Nurses Association (ANA). (2010). *Nursing's social policy statement* (2nd ed.). Author.

Arigo, D., & Butryn, M. L. (2019). Prospective relations between social comparison orientation and weight loss outcomes. *Behavioral Medicine, 45*(3), 249–254. https://doi.org/10.1080/08964289.2018.1481010.

Bodenheimer, T., & Sinsky, C. (2014). From Triple to Quadruple Aim: Care of the patient requires care of the provider. *Annals of Family Medicine, 12*(6), 573–576. https://doi.org/10.1370/afm.1713.

Brach, C. (2017). The journey to become a health literate organization: A snapshot of health system improvement. *Studies in Health Technology and Informatics, 240,* 203–237. https://doi.org/10.3233/978-1-61499-79-790-0-203.

Carman, K. L., & Workman, T. A. (2017). Engaging patients and consumers in research evidence: Applying the conceptual model of patient and family engagement. *Patient Education and Counseling, 100*(1), 25–29. https://doi.org/10.1016/j.pec.2016.07.009.

Center for Advancing Health. (2010). *Engagement behavior framework.* Retrieved from https://silo.tips/download/a-new-definition-of-patient-engagement.

Centers for Medicare and Medicaid Services (CMS). (2019). *HCAHPS fact sheet.* Retrieved from https://www.hcahpsonline.org/globalassets/hcahps/facts/hcahps_fact_sheet_october_2019.pdf.

Chakraborty, S. & Church, E. M. (2020). Social media hospital ratings and HCAHPS survey scores. *Journal of Health Organization and Management, 34*(2), 162–172. https://doi.org/10.1108/JHOM-08-2019-0234.

Choi, Y. K., Thompson, H. J., & Demiris, G. (2020). Use of an Internet-of-Things smart home system for healthy aging in older adults in residential settings: Pilot feasibility study. *JMIR Aging, 3*(2), e21964. https://doi.org/10.2196/21964.

Cross, T., Bazron, B., Dennis, K., & Isaacs, M. (1989). *Towards a culturally competent system of care (Volume I).* Washington, DC: Georgetown University Center for Child and Human Development, CASSP Technical Assistance Center.

Dolansky, M. A., & Moore, S. M. (2013). Quality and Safety Education for Nurses (QSEN): The key is systems thinking. *OJIN: The Online Journal of Issues in Nursing, 18*(3), 1. https://doi.org/10.3912/OJIN.Vol18No03Man01.

Duff, J., Curnen, K., Reed, A., & Kranz, C. (2021). Engaging parents of hospitalized neonates during a pandemic. *Journal of Neonatal Nursing, 27*(3), 185–187. https://doi.org/10.1016/j.jnn.2020.11.013.

Ebrahimi, Z., Patel, H., Wijk, H., Ekman, I., & Olaya-Contreras, P. (2021). A systematic review on implementation of person-centered care interventions for older people in out-of-hospital settings. *Geriatric Nursing, 42*(1), 213–224. https://doi.org/10.1016/j.gerinurse.2020.08.004.

Eklund, J. H., Holmström, I. K., Kumlin, T., Kaminsky, E., Skoglund, K., Höglander, J., Sundler, A. J., Condén, E., & Meranius, M. S. (2019). "Same same or different?" A review of reviews of person-centered and patient-centered care. *Patient Education and Counseling, 102*(1), 3–11. https://doi.org/10.1016/j.pec.2018.08.029.

Evardsson, D., Fetherstonhaugh, D., Nay, R., & Gibson, S. (2010). Development and initial testing of the Person-centered Care Assessment Tool (P-CAT). *International Psychogeriatrics, 22*(1), 101–108. https://doi.org/10.1017/S1041610209990688.

Fazio, S., Pace, D., Flinner, J., & Kallmyer, B. (2018). The fundamentals of person-centered care for individuals with dementia. *The Gerontologist, 58*(suppl_1), S10–S19. https://doi.org/10.1093/geront/gnx122.

Fisher, K. A., Smith, K. M., Gallagher, T. H., Huang, J. C., & Mazor, K. M. (2020). We want to know—A mixed methods evaluation of a comprehensive program designed to detect and address patient-reported breakdowns in care. *Joint Commission Journal on Quality and Patient Safety, 46*(5), 261–269. https://doi.org/10.1016/j.jcjq.2020.01.008.

Flinter, M., Hsu, C., Cromp, D., Ladden, M. D., & Wagner, E. H. (2017). Registered nurses in primary care: Emerging new roles and contributions to team-based care in high-performing practices. *The Journal of Ambulatory Care Management, 40*(4), 287–296. https://doi.org/10.1097/JAC.0000000000000193.

Garfield, R., Orgara, K., & Damico, A. (2021, January 21). *The coverage gap: Uninsured poor adults in states that did not expand Medicaid. Issue Brief. Medicaid. Kaiser Family Foundation.* Retrieved from https://www.kff.org/medicaid/issue-brief/the-coverage-gap-uninsured-poor-adults-in-states-that-do-not-expand-medicaid/.

Health Foundation. (2014). Person-centred care made simple: *What everyone should know about person-centred care.* In *Quick Guide.* Retrieved from https://www.health.org.uk/publications/person-centred-care-made-simple.

Health Innovation Network. (n.d.). *What is person-centred care and why is it important?* https://healthinnovationnetwork.com/wp-content/uploads/2016/07/What_is_person-centred_care_HIN_Final_Version_21.5.14.pdf.

Hope, J., Recio-Saucedo, A., Fogg, C., Griffiths, P., Smith, G. B., Westwood, G., & Schmidt, P. E. (2018). A fundamental conflict of care: Nurses' accounts of balancing patients' sleep with taking vital sign observations at night. *Journal of Clinical Nursing, 27*(9-10), 1860–1871. https://doi.org/10.1111/jocn.14234.

Hwang, J. I., Kim, S. W., & Chin, H. J. (2019). Patient participation in patient safety and its relationships with nurses' patient-centered care competency, teamwork, and safety climate. *Asian Nursing Research, 13*(2), 130–136. https://doi.org/10.1016/j.anr.2019.03.001.

Institute for Healthcare Improvement (IHI). (2022a). *The IHI Triple Aim.* Retrieved from http://www.ihi.org/Engage/Initiatives/TripleAim/Pages/default.aspx.

Institute for Healthcare Improvement (IHI). (2022b). *The power of four words. "What matters to you?".* Retrieved from http://www.ihi.org/Topics/WhatMatters/.

Institute of Medicine. (2001). *Crossing the quality chasm: A new health system for the 21st century.* The National Academies Press. https://doi.org/10.17226/10027.

Institute of Medicine (IOM). (2004). *Health literacy: A prescription to end confusion.* The National Academies Press.

International Council of Nurses. (2022). *About ICNP.* Retrieved from https://www.icn.ch/what-we-do/projects/ehealth-icnptm/about-icnp.

Leary, E., & Diers, D. (2013). The silence of the unblown whistle: The Nevada hepatitis C public health crisis. *Yale Journal of Biology and Medicine, 86*(1), 79–87.

Lyle-Edrosolo, G., & Waxman, K. (2016). Aligning healthcare safety and quality competencies: Quality and Safety Education for Nurses (QSEN), The Joint Commission, and American Nurses Credentialing Center (ANCC) Magnet® Standards crosswalk. *Nurse Leader, 14*(1), 70–75. https://doi-org.ezp.scranton.edu/10.1016/j.mnl.2015.08.005.

Makary, M. A., & Daniel, M. (2016). Medical error—the third leading cause of death in the US. *BMJ, 353*, i2139. https://doi.org/10.1136/bmj.i2139.

Mayer, D. B., & Hatlie, M. J. (2020). Commentary: Leadership and a true culture of patient safety. *American Journal of Medical Quality, 35*(5), 427–428. https://doi.org/10.1177/1062860620943484.

Meehan, T. C. (2020). *Careful nursing: Philosophy and professional practice model.* Retrieved from http://www.careful-nursing.ie/go/overview/summary.

National Academies of Science, Engineering, and Medicine. (2021). *The future of nursing 2020–2030: Charting a path to achieve health equity.* Washington, DC: The National Academies Press. https://doi.org/10.17226/25982.

O'Neill, N. (2021). Recognizing the importance of whistleblowers in healthcare. *Nursing, 51*(4), 54–56. https://doi.org/10.1097/01.NURSE.0000736912.14380.65.

Nundy, S., Cooper, L., Mate, K. (2022). The Quintuple Aim for healthcare improvement: A new imperative to advance health equity. *JAMA, 327*(6), 521–522.

Nurses on Boards Coalition. (2021). *To improve the health of communities and the nation.* Retrieved from https://www.nursesonboardscoalition.org.

O'Connor, S., & Carlson, E. (2016). Safety culture and senior leadership behavior: Using negative safety ratings to align clinical staff and senior leadership. *Journal of Nursing Administration, 46*(4), 215–220. https://doi.org/10.1097/NNA.0000000000000330.

Office of Disease Prevention and Health Promotion (ODPHP). (2021). *Health literacy in Healthy People 2030.* Retrieved from https://health.gov/our-work/national-health-initiatives/healthy-people/healthy-people-2030/health-literacy-healthy-people-2030.

Office of Minority Health (OMH). (n. d. a). *National standards for culturally and linguistically appropriate services (CLAS) in health and health care.* Retrieved from https://thinkculturalhealth.hhs.gov/assets/pdfs/EnhancedNationalCLAS-Standards.pdf.

Office of Minority Health (OMH). (n. d. b). *What is CLAS?* Retrieved from https://thinkculturalhealth.hhs.gov/clas/what-is-clas.

Olsen, C. F., Debesay, J., Bergland, A., Bye, A., & Langaas, A. G. (2020). What matters when asking, "what matters to you?" - perceptions and experiences of health care providers on involving older people in transitional care. *BMC Health Services Research, 20*(1), 317. https://doi.org/10.1186/s12913-020-05150-4.

Raney, J., Pal, R., Lee, T., Saenz, S. R., Bhushan, D., Leahy, P., Johnson, C., Kapphahn, C., Gisondi, M. A., & Hoang, K. (2021). Words matter: An antibias workshop for health care professionals to reduce stigmatizing language. *MedEdPORTAL: The Journal of Teaching and Learning Resources, 17*, 11115. https://doi.org/10.15766/mep_2374-8265.11115.

Reuter-Rice, K., McMurray, M. G., Christoferson, E., Yeager, H., & Wiggins, B. (2020). Sleep in the intensive care unit: biological, environmental, and pharmacologic implications for nurses. *Critical Care Nursing Clinics of North America, 32*(2), 191–201. https://doi.org/10.1016/j.cnc.2020.02.002.

Rodriguez, J. A., Betancourt, J. R., Sequist, T. D., & Ganguli, I. (2021). Differences in the use of telephone and video telemedicine visits during the COVID-19 pandemic. *The American Journal of Managed care, 27*(1), 21–26. https://doi.org/10.37765/ajmc.2021.88573.

Rollnick, S., Miller, W. R., & Butler, C. (2013). *Motivational interviewing in health care* (3rd ed.). New York: Guilford Press.

Saad, L. (2022, January 12). Military brass, judges among professions at new image lows. In *Gallup.* Retrieved from https://news.gallup.com/poll/388649/military-brass-judges-among-professions-new-image-lows.aspx.

Sakallaris, B. R., Miller, W. L., Saper, R., Kreitzer, M. J., & Jonas, W. (2016). Meeting the challenge of a more person-centered future for US healthcare. *Global Advances in Health and Medicine, 5*(1), 51–60. https://doi.org/10.7453/gahmj.2015.085.

Schiaffino, M. K., Ruiz, M., Yakuta, M., Contreras, A., Akhavan, S., Prince, B., & Weech-Maldonado, R. (2020). Culturally and linguistically appropriate hospital services reduce Medicare length of stay. *Ethnicity & Disease, 30*(4), 603–610. https://doi.org/10.18865/ed.30.4.603.

Sillner, A. Y., Madrigal, C., & Behrens, L. (2021). Person-centered gerontological nursing: An overview across care settings. *Journal of Gerontological Nursing, 47*(2), 7–12. https://doi.org/10.3928/00989134-20210107-02.

Statista. (2021). Percentage of population in the United States speaking a language other than English at home in 2019, by state. Retrieved from https://www.statista.com/statistics/312940/share-of-us-population-speaking-a-language-other-than-english-at-home-by-state/.

U. S. Census Bureau. (n. d.). American Community Survey. *Why we ask questions about language spoken at home.* Retrieved from https://www.census.gov/acs/www/about/why-we-ask-each-question/language/.

U.S. Health and Human Services, Health Resources and Services Administration (HRSA), Office of Health Equity. (2020). *Health equity report 2019–2020. Special feature on housing and health inequalities.* https://www.hrsa.gov/sites/default/files/hrsa/health-equity/HRSA-health-equity-report-printer.pdf.

Valdez, A. (2021). Words matter: Labelling, bias and stigma in nursing. *Journal of Advanced Nursing, 77*(11), e33–e35. https://doi.org/10.1111/jan.14967.

World Health Organization. (2020). *World Health Statistics 2020. Monitoring health for the SDGs.* Retrieved from https://apps.who.int/iris/bitstream/handle/10665/332070/9789240005105-eng.pdf.

World Health Organization (WHO). (2021). *Framework on Integrated People-Centred Health Services.* Retrieved from https://www.who.int/teams/integrated-health-services/clinical-services-and-systems/service-organizations-and-integration.

Ziaei, S., & Hammarström, A. (2021). What social determinants outside paid work are related to development of mental health during life? An integrative review of results from the Northern Swedish Cohort. *BMC Public Health, 21*(1), 2190. https://doi.org/10.1186/s12889-021-12143-3.

11

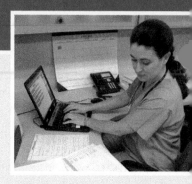

Staffing and Scheduling

Susan Sportsman

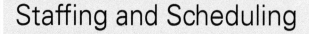

THE CHALLENGE

The inpatient general surgical units of a large regional medical center have a total of 54 beds, and the surgical trauma intensive care unit (STICU) has 16 beds. The organization was faced with severe capacity constraints as it prepared to begin a master site facility plan that would result in an additional 120 beds over the next 3 years. The lack of a step-down unit for surgical patients was a particular void in service. The coronary care unit (CCU), medical intensive care unit (MICU), and cardiovascular intensive care unit (CVICU) all have step-down units to which they can transfer patients and free up beds for truly critical patients. Beds that were already filled with general surgery patients were targeted to be the step-down unit for the STICU.

The challenge to develop the surgical step-down unit included the identification of the appropriate number of step-down beds needed by considering the volume of

patients in the STICU that could be transferred to the surgical step-down unit. Admission and discharge criteria for this step-down unit needed to be developed and approved by the medical staff. New equipment needs also had to be identified. The staff competencies necessary to provide appropriate care to these patients had to be considered and education plans developed. In addition, a staffing plan had to be outlined. Communication to the nursing staff was critical—some feared that they would lose their jobs because the critical care staff would assume their positions.

What would you do if you were this nurse?

Mary Ellen Bonczek, BSN, RN, MPA, NEA-BC
Senior Vice President and Chief Nurse Executive, New Hanover
Regional Medical Center, Wilmington, North, Carolina

INTRODUCTION

A key role of the nurse manager in a healthcare organization is to ensure that sufficient nurses are available to provide the care needed by patients. However, given the emphasis on cost control, managing expenses associated with the number of nurses on a unit at any given time is also the responsibility of the nurse manager. Because nursing salaries constitute some of the major drivers of labor costs in a healthcare organization, nurse managers are increasingly challenged to tightly manage both staffing and scheduling within their assigned cost centers.

THE STAFFING PROCESS

Staffing is a comprehensive, dynamic process necessary to ensure that patients receive optimal levels of care. It aligns patient needs, nurse abilities, workload, technology, collaboration with other disciplines, the culture of the work environment, and many other factors to maintain the safety of clients. Managing the staffing process in order to ensure patient safety and quality of care is one of the competency domains identified in *The Essentials: Core Competencies for Professional Nursing Education* required by the American Association of Colleges of Nursing (AACN, 2021).

In general, staffing may be either fixed or flexible. Fixed staffing models are built on a set number of nurses for a particular unit or shift. The result of this

approach is an unalterable nurse-to-patient staffing ratio. Frequent changes within a patient care environment (e.g., changes in severity of patient conditions, volume, or procedural requirements) are not considered.

A fixed staffing pattern presents a one-size-fits-all approach that does not address the variations in staffing needs on a shift-to-shift basis. Flexible staffing considers these variations. While a flexible staffing plan is more responsive to the complex healthcare environment, it is also more difficult to develop.

Staffing may be either centralized or decentralized. With centralized staffing, one department is responsible for staffing in all units, including call-in staff, call-off staff, and float staff. With decentralized staffing, unit leaders (e.g., nurse managers and charge nurses) determine the level of staffing needed before and during the shift. The centralized approach takes advantage of all of the nursing resources available for the organization and reduces the burden of staffing for unit leaders. On the other hand, the unit leaders are more familiar with the needs of their units and which available nurses have the background and expertise to care for patients specific for their unit, perhaps making decentralized staffing more desirable.

Developing a Staffing Budget

When developing a staffing budget to determine the staffing needs for a certain time period, nurse managers must consider services offered on the unit as well as organizational plans to provide new or expanded clinical services. For example, a manager of an inpatient surgical unit must consider the potential effect of offering a new surgical procedure to the community. What projections have been made for this market? What is the expected length of stay for patients undergoing this new procedure? What are the national standards for care for this type of patient? A nurse manager will use this information to project added staff to manage these changes in service. Conversely, nurse managers must also be aware of any organizational plans to end an existing service that their unit supports. If a nurse manager in a home care setting knows that reimbursement for a certain procedure in the home has declined to the point that this service must be discontinued, allowances for fewer required staffing resources in the coming year must be made.

To develop an adequate staffing or personnel budget, the amount of work performed by a nursing unit, or cost center, is referred to as its workload. Workload is measured in terms of the unit of service (UOS) defined by the cost center.

Units of service (UOS) are productivity targets, such as nursing hours per patient day (HPPD) or hours per visit for emergency departments or clinics. The UOS multiplied by the volume for a clinical area determines the number of staff needed in each period. The formula can be adjusted for total paid staff or just for those required for the delivery of direct patient care.

Nurse managers must understand the nature of the work in their area of responsibility to define the units of service that will be used as their workload statistic and to forecast, or project, the volume of work that will be performed by their cost center during the upcoming year.

Calculation of Full-Time Equivalents

Nurse managers use the unit's forecasted workload to calculate the number of full-time equivalents (FTEs) needed to construct the unit's overall staffing plan. The distinction between an employee in a position and an FTE (fully, including the method of calculation) is important. To achieve a balanced staffing plan, nurse managers must determine the correct combination of full-time and part-time positions needed. Nurse managers must also consider the effect of productive and

nonproductive hours when projecting the FTE needs of the unit. Productive hours are the paid hours that are worked on the unit. Productive hours can be further defined as *direct* or *indirect*.

Benefit time includes those hours paid to an employee for vacation, holiday, personal, or sick time and, in some organizations, for an employee attending orientation or continuing-education activities. In most practice settings, nurses must be replaced when they are off duty and accessing their paid benefit for time off. Nurse managers must be aware of the average benefit hours required for their unit or they will understate their FTE needs. This requires nurse managers to consider carefully how to allocate their budgeted FTEs into full-time and part-time positions to meet the staffing requirements for the unit when a portion of the staff is taking paid time off. In addition, looking at the number of employees being paid for any specific day may not reflect the number providing care.

Thus, the nurse manager's role must include competencies in finances, information technology, and automation of staffing and scheduling programs. If healthcare organizations follow the approach of some businesses to increase jobs by creating more part-time positions, major implications for staffing scheduling will need to be considered.

Impact of Staffing on Patient Outcomes

A significant amount of research has been done in the United States and internationally to evaluate links among nursing staffing, workloads, skill mix, and patient outcomes. Adequate nursing care has been associated with a decrease in falls, medication errors, hospital-acquired infections, and mortality rates, as well as enhanced nurse retention and job satisfaction plus improved patient satisfaction in acute care hospitals and nursing homes. Table 11.1 provides an overview of selected research over the last 20-plus years that evaluates the impact of staffing on patient outcomes.

Research has also focused on whether greater nurse engagement in organizational decision-making is associated with improved patient outcomes. Carthon et al. (2019) describe a study that explores nurse engagement in hospital affairs, patient-to-nurse staffing ratios, and nurse reports of patient safety. This study found that

TABLE 11.1 Previous Research Related to Nurse Staffing

Category	Research Finding	Resource
Nurse Education	Using Pennsylvania nurse survey and patient discharge data from 1999 and 2006, the researchers found that a 10-point increase in the percentage of nurses holding a baccalaureate degree in nursing within a hospital was associated with an average reduction of 2.12 deaths for every 1000 patients; for a subset of patients with complications, they found an average reduction of 7.47 deaths per 1000 patients. They estimated that if all 134 hospitals in the study had increased the percentage of their nurses with baccalaureate degrees by 10 points during the study's time period, some 500 deaths among general, orthopedic, and vascular surgery patients might have been prevented.	**Aiken, L. (2012)**. Patient safety, satisfaction, and quality of hospital care: Cross sectional surveys of nurses and patients in 12 countries in Europe and the United States. *British Medical Journal 344*, e1717.
	In 2010, the IOM (now the National Academy of Medicine) recommended an increase in the proportion of nurses with a baccalaureate degree to 80% by 2020. Other recommendations included: "(1) level of clinical experience (i.e., novice to expert), (2) experience with the population services, (3) competency with technology and clinical interventions, (4) language capabilities and cultural competency, and (5) organizational experience."	Institute of Medicine (IOM). (2010). *The future of nursing: Leading change, advancing health.* Washington, DC: National Academies Press.
Overtime	A survey of 80% of nurses working 12-hour shifts in four states reported satisfaction with the scheduling practices at their hospital. When nurses worked more than 13 hours per shift, patient dissatisfaction increased. Nurses working shifts of 10 hours or longer were up to 2.5 times more likely than nurses working shorter shifts to experience burnout and job dissatisfaction and expressed an intent to leave the job.	Stimpfel, A., Sloane, D., & Aiken, L. (2012). The longer the shifts for hospital nurses, the higher the levels of burnout and patient dissatisfaction. *Health Affairs*, 31(11), 2501–2509.
	Literature review found a strong relationship between working long hours and adverse outcomes.	Bae, S. H., & Fabry, D. (2014). Effects of nurse overtime and long hours worked on nursing and patients' outcomes. *Nursing Outlook, 62*(2), 138–156.
Nurse Fatigue	Specific Recommendations for Employers • Involve nurses in designing work schedules that implement a "regular and predictable schedule that allows nurses to plan." • Stop using mandatory overtime. • Encourage "frequent, uninterrupted rest breaks during work shifts." • Adopt official policies that give RNs the "right to accept or reject a work assignment. Policies should indicate that there will be no retaliation or negative consequences for rejecting the assignment." • Encourage nurses to be proactive about managing their health and rest. • Specific Recommendations for Nurses • Work no more than 40 hours in a 7-day period and limit work shifts to 12 hours in a 24-hour period, including on-call hours worked.	American Nurses Association (ANA). (2014). *Addressing nurse fatigue to promote safety and health: Joint responsibilities of registered nurses and employers to reduce risk.* https://www.nursingworld.org/practice-policy/nursing-excellence/official-position-statements/id/addressing-nurse-fatigue-to-promote-safety-and-health/

nurses who reported the opportunity to participate in policy decisions were considered most engaged. Nurses who reported the opportunity to serve on hospital internal governance committees were considered moderately engaged. Nurses who reported the opportunity to serve on nursing committees were considered somewhat engaged. Nurses who indicated that none of these opportunities were available in their hospital were considered least engaged. Nurse leaders should make a conscious effort to engage direct care nurses in organizational decision-making, not only for professional development of the nurse but also for the safety and well-being of the patient.

The research by Carthon et al. (2019) found, consistent with earlier research, increased medical errors and threats to patient safety when staffing is inadequate. In this study, nurses consistently reported patient safety concerns, including patient information falling through the "cracks" when nurses assumed high patient workloads. Increased investments in nurse staffing may increase nurses' ability to detect patient safety threats and intervene when they occur. Unfortunately, efforts to improve patients' safety may not be feasible due to financial concerns. In addition, in times of crisis, such as a pandemic, poor staffing becomes even more problematic.

Nursing staffing is also a concern in nursing homes and other long-term care facilities. Federal regulations require facilities to have sufficient nursing staff with the appropriate competencies and skill sets to ensure residence safety and attain the highest possible level of well-being. The regulations require enough registered nurses (RNs), licensed vocational nurses/licensed practical nurses (LVNs/LPNs), and certified nursing assistants (CNAs) on a 24-hour basis to provide nursing care to all residents, including a charge nurse on each shift. At a minimum, adequate staffing includes the following conditions:

- An RN must be present for at least 8 consecutive hours a day, 7 days a week, and a designated RN must serve as the director of nursing on a full-time basis. The director of nursing may serve as a charge nurse only when the facility has an average daily occupancy of 60 or fewer residents.

- Nursing homes are required to post daily nursing staffing information, including the total number of staff and the actual hours worked by nursing staff by shift. Facilities must also ensure that nursing staff have the competency and skill sets to care for residents (Harrington et al., 2020).

Inadequate staffing levels can have devastating consequences on patient safety. For example, California nursing homes with high rates of COVID-19 infections reported 25% lower RN staffing than facilities that had lower rates of COVID-19 infections.

The fatigue and burnout that nursing staff in all healthcare environments have experienced throughout the COVID-19 pandemic has resulted in an escalation of staff shortages throughout the healthcare delivery system in the United States. These shortages will require new and innovative approaches to developing staffing as well as a changed emphasis on recruitment and retention.

Theoretical Framework for Nursing Staffing

Corresponding with the research to determine the impact of appropriate staffing, particularly in acute care hospitals, nurse theorists have also been developing theoretical frameworks to support the practical application of nurse staffing in acute hospitals. For example, Cavell proposed the Nursing Intellectual Capital (NIC) Theory in 2009. This theoretical framework specific for nursing is derived from the Intellectual Capital Theory developed in business and accounting, which illustrates a relationship among knowledge at all levels in the organization. As an increase in individual, group, and organizational knowledge occurs, performance improves. This increase in knowledge can occur because of organizational investment in learning and/or in hiring and retaining qualified employees. This increase in knowledge is spread using social networks within the organization (Covell & Sidani, 2013).

The Nursing Intellectual Capital theory, a middle-range theory, explores the relationship between nursing staffing, nursing knowledge, and variables within the work environment and their influence on patient and organizational outcomes (Cavell, 2009). The Theory Box defines the concepts in this framework.

THEORY BOX

Concepts in Nursing Intellectual Capital (NIC) Theory

NIC Theory Concepts	Definition
Nursing Intellectual Capital	Nursing knowledge translated into nursing and organizational performance
Nursing Performance	Improvement in patient outcomes, reduced adverse events
Organizational Performance	Improvement in organizational outcomes, such as cost-related outcomes associated with recruitment and retention
Nursing Human Capital	Knowledge, skills, and experience of RNs, including: • Academic preparation • Specialty certification status • Hours of continuing education attended • Professional experience • Unit tenure • Clinical specialty experience
Nursing Structural Capital	Structural resources that contain nursing knowledge used to support RNs in applying their knowledge and skills to patient care. Operationalized as: • Availability of practice guidelines, care maps and protocols • Information technology for diagnostic purposes • Portable computerized devices for obtaining information
Nursing Capital Investment	Employer support for nursing continued professional development, including: • Financial assistance for RNs to attend professional development activities • Paid and unpaid time off for formal or informal education purposes • Availability of replacements for RNs away from unit to learn • Availability of clinical educators or consultants to assist with clinical decision-making as well as further knowledge and skill development
Nursing Human Capital Depletion	Limited nursing staffing (supply and mix of RNs) operationalized by: • Hours per patient per day • Skill mix • Registered nurse to patient ratios

Adapted from Covell, C., & Sidani, S. (2013). Nursing intellectual therory: Implications for research and practice. OJIN: The Online Journal of Issues in Nursing, 18(2).

The NIC Theory was critiqued by Williams as part of a dissertation from Ferris State University (Williams, 2019). This critique found that despite the recognition that the NIC Theory meets much of the criteria for an effective theoretical framework and can be easily operationalized in a healthcare system, the theory has not been evaluated in a sufficient number of research studies. Williams recommends that this theory should be used in empirical research in order to be helpful, particularly for nursing administration.

Models for Nurse Staffing

Many methods have been described in the literature for determining the number of nurses who should be available to care for patients at any given time. These approaches are generally classified into several broad types, although the distinction between these approaches is less absolute than it may appear when the models are compared. In addition, terminology varies.

While the research examining the association between nurse staffing and patient outcomes is significant, there is a lack of consensus on what staffing levels are acceptable in different situations and how to plan for them. Nursing managers must decide how many nursing staff to employ and how many nursing staff to deploy each shift. These are separate but interrelated decisions, which rely on being able to quantify nursing workload. Two nurse staffing models are commonly used to determine the number of nurses required to care for patients at any given time.

Nurse–Patient Ratios

The nurse–patient ratio approach assigns a minimum or fixed number of nursing staff per occupied bed. This approach assumes that all patients have similar requirements for care and that the average is stable across patient groups. Needs can largely be anticipated and met with a set roster. These approaches tend to set a minimum level with an explicit or implied expectation that any additional staffing requirements may be deployed when demand increases (Savillea et al., 2019).

In 1999, California passed legislation to mandate specific nurse–patient ratios, which was fully implemented in 2004. This law required that a nurse must care for no more than Aiken et al. (2010):

- Six patients in a psychiatric unit
- Five patients in a medical-surgical unit
- Four pediatric patients
- Three patients in a labor and delivery unit
- Two patients in intensive care units (ICUs)

In an important, and now classic, evaluation of the nurse–patient ratio policy, Aiken et al. (2010) examined the effects of California's 2004 minimum nurse–patient staff ratio mandate for acute care facilities by comparing patient outcome data and hospital staffing information at hospitals in California, New Jersey, and Pennsylvania. According to the nurse survey, 88% of the California nurses working in a medical-surgical area reported caring for only five patients per shift, as required by the California law. In contrast, only 33% of the Pennsylvania nurses surveyed and 19% of those surveyed in New Jersey reported being responsible for five or fewer patients. California nurses cared for two fewer patients than nurses in New Jersey and 1.7 fewer patients than nurses in Pennsylvania (Aiken et al., 2010).

The California nurse–patient ratio had been in effect for 20 years when COVID-19 infections surged in California in 2020. The spike in hospitalizations from COVID-19 led California governor Gavin Newsom to relax this law after California had exhausted strategies to improve its nursing staffing capacity amid the pandemic, including asking the federal government to send medical personnel and working with staffing agencies to contract travel nurses. As a result, by December 2020, 170 hospitals had implemented new ratios. California's pandemic ratios allow ICU nurses to care for three patients instead of two, emergency department and telemetry nurses can care for six patients instead of four, and medical-surgical patients are permitted to care for seven patients instead of five. In December of 2020, some nurses expressed concern that the revised ratios may remain in place after the COVID-19 pandemic has been resolved (Carbajal, 2020). As this concern grew in 2021, discussion of legislation to return to the previous California nurse–patient ratio has surfaced despite the ongoing influence of the pandemic and subsequent numbers of nurses in the state leaving the acute care setting or the profession altogether.

Alternative to the Nurse–Patient Ratio Staffing

For the last 20-plus years, there has been much discussion regarding the effectiveness of nurse–patient ratios over other staffing models. Labor unions that represent nurses have focused on the nurse–patient ratio approach as the best method to capture the necessary workforce on a unit. In contrast, the American Nurses Association (ANA) has opted to support the *nurse staffing committee* as the approach to ensure safe staffing. In addition, the ANA has articulated principles for ensuring safe staffing. Fig. 11.1 provides a graphic of the third edition of the ANA Principles for Safe Staffing and Box 11.1 defines the components of the five principles.

For almost a decade, the ANA has advocated for passage of a Registered Nurse Safe Staffing Act in the U.S. Congress. Typically, the Safe Staffing for Nurse and Patient Safety Act submitted to both the U.S. Senate and U.S. House of Representatives during each legislative session is based on the ANA Safe Staffing Principles and requires Medicare-participating hospitals to form committees composed of at least 55% direct care nurses to create and implement unit-specific nurse-to-patient ratio staffing plans. This staffing approach benefits patients, RNs, and hospitals by decreasing adverse health events, nurse turnover, and costly hospitalization. Unfortunately, none of these bills, including the Nurse Staffing Standards for Hospital Patient Safety and Quality Care Act of 2021, had passed yet as of June 2021 (Davis, 2021). Despite the lack of success in passing this federal legislation, many states—including California, Connecticut, Illinois, Massachusetts, Minnesota, Nevada, New Jersey, New York, Ohio, Oregon, Rhode Island, Texas, Vermont, Washington, and Illinois—currently address nurse staffing in hospitals through either law or regulations.

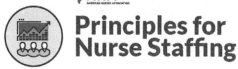

Principles for Nurse Staffing

Nurse staffing is an asset to ever-evolving health care systems. Appropriate nurse staffing, with sufficient numbers of nurses, improves the health of the populations. Nurses at all levels within a health care system must have a substantive and active role in staffing decisions.

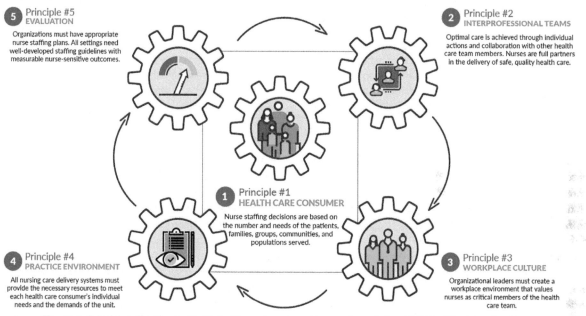

5 Principle #5
EVALUATION

Organizations must have appropriate nurse staffing plans. All settings need well-developed staffing guidelines with measurable nurse-sensitive outcomes.

2 Principle #2
INTERPROFESSIONAL TEAMS

Optimal care is achieved through individual actions and collaboration with other health care team members. Nurses are full partners in the delivery of safe, quality health care.

1 Principle #1
HEALTH CARE CONSUMER

Nurse staffing decisions are based on the number and needs of the patients, families, groups, communities, and populations served.

4 Principle #4
PRACTICE ENVIRONMENT

All nursing care delivery systems must provide the necessary resources to meet each health care consumer's individual needs and the demands of the unit.

3 Principle #3
WORKPLACE CULTURE

Organizational leaders must create a workplace environment that values nurses as critical members of the health care team.

Fig. 11.1 Principles for Nurse Staffing. (From American Nurses Association [2022]. *Principles for Nurse Staffing*. https://www.nursingworld.org/~4a51bc/globalassets/practiceandpolicy/nurse-staffing/staffing-principles-infographic.pdf).

BOX 11.1 American Association of Critical-Care Nursing (AACN) Principles for Developing Transformational Staffing

1. Nurses are essential to the successful delivery of healthcare.
2. Nurses constitute the largest body of healthcare practitioners and provide more direct care than any other profession. Nurses assess, develop, deliver, and optimize plans of care. They are a linchpin of the hospital healthcare team. Nurses make unique and vital contributions to optimal patient outcomes, higher patient and family satisfaction, and lower morbidity and mortality.
3. Appropriate nurse staffing is crucial for optimal patient care.
4. Appropriate staffing ensures the effective match between patient and family needs and nurse knowledge, skills, and abilities. Evidence confirms that the likelihood of serious complications or death increases when fewer registered nurses are assigned to care for patients. A substantial body of evidence indicates better patient outcomes occur when registered nurses provide a higher proportion of care hours in healthy work environments.
5. Appropriate staffing is inextricably linked to healthy work environments.
6. Healthy work environments are safe, healing, humane, and respectful of the rights, responsibilities, needs, and contributions of all people—including patients, their families, nurses, and other healthcare professionals. Studies show that investing solely in staffing resources in the absence of a healthy work environment is ineffective.
7. Higher nurse job satisfaction, which leads to lower staff turnover, is closely tied to appropriate staffing.

(Continued)

BOX 11.1   American Association of Critical-Care Nursing (AACN) Principles for Developing Transformational Staffing—cont'd

8. Nurses can experience intense stress when staffing resources do not meet patient care demands. Inadequate staffing contributes to nurse dissatisfaction, burnout, compassion fatigue, and turnover.

9. Collaboration between hospital administrators and the professional nursing staff to achieve appropriate staffing can contribute to less turnover, improved quality of care, greater patient/family satisfaction, increased hospital financial viability, and decreased patient costs.

10. The creation of appropriate staffing plans requires a nimble, comprehensive approach. The conditions of critically ill patients fluctuate rapidly and continuously.

Because of this, it is imperative that nurse staffing decisions go beyond fixed nurse-to-patient ratios.

11. Appropriate staffing requires nurses to be involved in all aspects of staffing, from planning to evaluation. It aligns patient needs, complexity, and acuity with nurse knowledge, skills, and abilities. It also considers numerous human and technological factors and the health of the work environment.

12. Appropriate staffing requires flexible systems and tools, dynamic scheduling options, and influential, educated leaders accountable for the outcomes of staffing decisions.

From American Association of Critical Care Nurses. (2018). *AACN guiding principles for appropriate staffing.* https://www.aacn.org/policy-and-advocacy/guiding-principles-for-staffing.

EXERCISE 11.1 Consider the nurse–patient ratio and the nurse staffing committee approach. Which models of staffing have you participated in? Which approach seems the most effective for providing nursing coverage in the acute care setting? Which seems most satisfactory for nurses? Why do you think that one or the other approach is more attractive to healthcare administrators, policy makers, and legislators?

In addition to state regulations, other groups such as accrediting bodies and professional organizations have proposed guidelines for safe staffing standards. For example, in 2018, the American Association of Critical Care Nurses (AACN) developed principles for staffing for critical care areas in hospitals. The principles are based on the organization's belief that "there is no one-size-fits-all answer, and the staffing challenge has defied systemic solutions" (AACN, 2018). To this end, the organization has identified principles for staffing, outlined in Table 11.2.

The Joint Commission (TJC), whose purpose is to support performance improvement in healthcare organizations through standards and a survey accreditation process, requires that adequate nurse staffing be present to meet the care, treatment, and service needs of the patients. TJC is not prescriptive as to what constitutes "adequate" staffing. However, in response to increasing public concerns about patient care safety and quality, TJC correlates an organization's clinical outcome data

with its staffing patterns to determine the effectiveness of the overall staffing plan.

During the accreditation process of TJC, the surveyor reviews the staffing plans developed by the nurse manager for any obvious staffing deficiencies—for example, a shift or series of shifts in which the unit staffing plan was not met. The surveyor also interviews direct care nurses outside of the presence of nurse managers to inquire about their perceptions of the units' staffing adequacy. Surveyors may review the staffing effectiveness data for that unit as it compares with any variations from the staffing plan to identify quality-of-care concerns. Nurse managers are well advised to prepare a balanced staffing plan that supports a unit's unique patient care needs and the scrutiny of the survey process of TJC. They also should post this staffing plan and the compliance reports for staff to see on a routine basis. In some states, this posting is required.

Tools to Estimate the Number of Nurses Needed

Patient Classification Systems

The acuity or severity of patients' conditions—influenced by their age, primary diagnosis, comorbidities, severity of illness, treatment stage, socioeconomic status, ability to provide self-care, anticipated length of stay, and family or caregivers to be included in patient education and care planning—is a key component in determining the staffing required for safe care. However, the dynamic nature of patient care often makes it difficult to quantify the care

TABLE 11.2   Definition of Components of the 2019 ANA Staffing Principles

Components of Staffing Principles	Definitions
Consumer	Nurse staffing decisions are based on the number and needs of the individual healthcare consumer, families, groups, communities, and populations served. Consideration must be given to the elements affecting care at the level of the individual practice setting. Each setting should have staffing guidelines based on patient safety indicators and clinical and administrative/operational outcomes specific to that area. Sufficient resources and pathways for care coordination and health education for the patient/healthcare consumer and/or family should be readily available.
Interprofessional Team	Specific needs of populations served should determine the appropriate clinical competencies required of the registered nurses practicing in an area. This includes specifying appropriate credentials and qualifications of registered nurse staff and ensuring that registered nurses are permitted to practice to the full extent of their education, training, scope of practice, and licensure. Staffing plans should use skills of experienced nurses, providing time and resources for mentoring, precepting, and skill development. Regular monitoring of specified indicators— such as nurse satisfaction, burnout, turnover and retention, and workplace injuries—can help ensure that staffing outcomes are evaluated and adjusted.
Work Culture	Balance of quality and safety with the overall expenditure of nursing resources and associated costs is needed to achieve best practices and optimal care outcomes. Healthcare leaders and organizations must create a workplace environment that values registered nurses and other employees as critical members of the healthcare team. Policies should support the ability of registered nurses to practice to the full extent of their license, education, scope of practice, and documented competence. Leaders should recognize that in addition to appropriate nurse staffing, agencies must provide sufficient interprofessional support and ancillary services and sufficient orientation and preparation of nursing staff. Creation of a culture of values that supports respect, trust, collaboration, and interprofessional healthcare team building help cultivate loyalty and, ultimately, retention. The increased complexity of today's healthcare environment requires availability of enhanced support in ethical decision-making for all aspects of care planning and care delivery.
Practice Environment	Staffing includes structures and processes that affect the safety of patients and nurses. Registered nurses have a professional obligation to report unsafe conditions or inappropriate staffing that adversely impacts safe, quality care, and they have the right to do so without reprisal. Registered nurses should be provided with a professional nursing practice environment in which they have control over nursing practice and have autonomy in their workplace. Policies on length of shifts, management of meals and rest periods, and overtime should be in place to ensure the health, well-being, and stamina of nurses and prevent fatigue-related errors. Mandatory overtime is an unacceptable solution to achieve appropriate nurse staffing.
Evaluation	Staffing plans must be adjustable to reflect changes in evidence and outcomes, care scenarios, and the needs of the population served, all of which can vary from hour to hour, shift to shift, and day to day. Evaluation of any staffing system should include examination of environmental factors affecting the healthcare consumers' safety and outcomes in addition to the evaluation of nurse-specific indicators such as work-related staff illness and injury rates, turnover/ vacancy/retention rates, and levels of healthcare consumer satisfaction and nurse satisfaction. When evaluating nurse staffing costs, the organization should always consider the cost of adverse outcomes when staffing is inappropriate as well as the variability in costs related to staffing and assignment patterns, skill mix, and wages of nurses and nursing personnel related to experience. The allocation of identified costs of nursing care in patient billing records and reimbursement requests makes visible the value of nurses and nursing services.

From https://www.nursingworld.org/practice-policy/nurse-staffing/staffing-principles/.

needs of patients at any given time. Patient classification systems, used primarily in acute care settings, were developed to give nurse managers the tools and language to describe the acuity of patients on their unit. More seriously ill patients receive higher classification scores, indicating that more nursing resources are required to provide patient care. Acuity was determined by either preexisting categories, such as diagnostic groups or classifications based on levels of acuity. This acuity is determined via the timed-task approach, in which a detailed care plan consists of tasks assigned a recommended length. Alternatively, a standard care protocol may be used. Nurse managers use the classification data to adjust the unit's staffing plan for a given time or to quantify acuity trends over longer periods as they forecast their staffing needs during the budget process (Savillea et al., 2019).

Two basic types of patient classification systems exist: prototype and factor. A prototype evaluation system, an older approach to evaluating patient characteristics, is considered both subjective and descriptive. Patients are classified into broad categories, which are used to predict patient care needs. The relative intensity measures (RIMs) system often used in nursing homes is a prototype system. This system classifies patient care needs based on their diagnosis-related group (DRG). The data are then fed to an electronic decision support system that integrates clinical and financial information.

A factor evaluation system is considered more objective than a prototype evaluation system. It gives each task, thought process, and patient care activity a time or rating. These associations are then summed to determine the hours of direct care required or they are weighted for each patient.

Typically, if two patient classification systems are used for staffing decisions, organizations use a combination of the two. Some patient types with a single healthcare focus, such as maternal deliveries or outpatient surgical patients, would be appropriately classified with a prototype system. Patients with more complex care needs and a less predictable disease course, such as those with pneumonia or stroke, are more appropriately evaluated with a factor system.

Numerous potential problems exist with patient classification systems. The issue most often raised by administrators relates to the questionable reliability and validity of the data collected through a self-reporting mechanism of the nurses. In short, is the nurse evaluation accurate or is there an attempt to "game the system" to get more staff? Another concern with patient classification data relates to the inability of the organization to meet the prescribed staffing levels outlined by the patient classification system.

Concern over the accuracy of biased data and the inability to meet prescribed staffing levels outlined by the patient classification systems has caused many healthcare organizations to abandon patient classification as a mechanism for determining appropriate staffing levels. Staff morale is at risk when acuity models indicate that one level is necessary and the organization cannot increase staffing to meet those needs. Likewise, staff morale is at risk without acuity models when it is clear to staff that patient needs exceed care capacity.

> **EXERCISE 11.2** Administrators worry that they risk potential liability if they do not follow the staffing recommendations of the patient classification system or the nursing staffing committee. If the recommendation indicates that six caregivers are needed for the upcoming shift but the organization can provide only five caregivers, what are the potential consequences for the organization if an adverse event occurs?

Budget-Based Staffing

Budget-based staffing requires the staffing plan for the year be developed in concert with the personnel budget. Together, the nursing leadership and the personnel department project the number of nursing HPPD that will be needed annually. The number of HPPD is based on historical data and evaluated against national benchmarks from nursing units with similar characteristics.

Nursing hours includes various components: direct care hours, indirect care hours, and fixed hours. Direct care hours represent the hours worked by nursing staff assigned to a unit who have direct patient care responsibilities for greater than 50% of the shift in activities. These activities may include medication administration and nursing treatments; admissions, discharge, and transfer activities; patient teaching and communication; coordination of patient care and nursing rounds; documentation time; and treatment planning. This type of staff is counted in the staffing matrix, which is a tool to assist in deciding what level of each staff group (RN, LPN/LVN, CNA) is needed based on the patient census. Direct care providers are replaced if they call in sick and the hours worked are charged to the unit cost center (Watkins, 2020).

Indirect care hours are those hours that unit-based staff worked on or off the unit/department. This includes in-service education time, orientation hours, staff meeting time, committee meeting time or work, shared governance meetings or activities, and unit-related project work, such as quality assurance/quality improvement (QA/QI) and standards development. Fixed hours are those hours required to support the department activity or volume, such as management staff, or unit-based educators. Additional hours that must be considered include productive hours (hours worked) and nonpaid but not worked. When nurses benefits cover nonworking hours, such as vacation, holiday, Family Medical Leave Act, jury duty and educational professional leave, the time paid is referred to as Nonproductive hours. (Watkins, 2020).

These hours are calculated and then compared with the budget established at the beginning of the year. If the hours are higher than identified in the budget during a particular time, the nurse manager is expected to reduce staffing later in the time period to meet the set budget. Such an approach works when the needs of patients on the unit ebb, resulting in fewer nursing hours spent. When the census and needs of the patients remains high throughout the budget period, the unit may go over budget. As a result, the nurse manager must negotiate with other hospital leaders to ensure sufficient staffing.

WHY SAFE STAFFING MATTERS

Organizational policies and clear expectations communicated to staff are essential to manage high and low volume as well as changes in acuity. Proposed personnel budgets and staffing plans that cannot flex up or down when patient acuity or volumes change put the nurse manager in a position in which patient safety may not be maintained and financial obligations cannot be met. In addition, mechanisms must be in place and internally publicized to allow staff to ask for additional help as needed. Patient, staff, and physician satisfaction; service and care improvement; and patient safety improvement are all outcomes of a solid staffing plan. Nurse managers are obligated to consider these variables when preparing the personnel budget.

Despite the varying efforts over the years to ensure safe staffing, external factors often influence the availability of nurses. Buerhaus (2021) notes that there are often "background nursing shortages" in various loca-

tions that occur when external forces alter either the demand or supply of nurses. Despite the inconvenience these shortages bring, they almost always resolve and do not become permanent. However, national factors may make the shortages in healthcare organizations particularly severe. For example, retirement of Baby Boomer nurses, increased acuity of patients in hospitals and nursing homes, making it difficult for novice nurses to replace seasoned RNs, and the increasing number of RNs leaving the bedside to become nurse practitioners or work in other advanced practice roles have had an impact. This environment became worse when the COVID-19 pandemic escalated and nurses in hospitals and nursing homes were faced with increasing pressure to care for incredibly ill patients under frightening circumstances. While this emergency has encouraged interest in nursing as a career, many nurses working in healthcare, suffering from stress and burnout, have left the healthcare environment completely or taken jobs in nonacute environments. The entire country is suffering from the resulting nursing shortage.

The 2020–2021 pandemic painted a negative picture of the healthcare system and demonstrated gaps in care delivery. Buerhaus (2021) suggests that "hospital, nurses, thought leaders and policymakers must consider ways to fix current and long-standing problems together, rethinking and planning for improving patient care in a post-COVID world." Such plans must include innovative ways to recruit and employ nurses to care for patients.

COMPLEX FACTORS IN HEALTH CARE INFLUENCING PATIENT OUTCOMES

The effectiveness of nurse staffing on patient outcomes is not only influenced by inadequate staffing itself but also by related issues such as missed care and patient conditions such as hospital-acquired infections.

Missed Care

Missed nursing care means that care is delayed, partially completed, or not completed at all. Missed care is problematic, as it is associated with poor patient care experiences and health outcomes as well as nurse ethical distress and burnout. Several studies have demonstrated that missed nursing care processes in hospitals are both prevalent and portend certain patient outcomes, including higher occurrence of infections and falls, new-onset delirium, pneumonia, medication variances and increased length of stay, delayed discharge, and increased pain and discomfort. This significant amount of nursing care processes missed in hospitals spans all nursing care responsibilities, including assessment (44%), interventions and basic care (73%), and planning (71%) (Lake et al., 2020).

Hessels, Paliwal, Weaver, Siddiqui, and Wurmser (2019), in a cross-sectional study focused on missed nursing care and four types of adverse events, found that the majority of nurses reported missing some aspect of nursing care, including ambulation, patient turning, feeding and nutrition. These "misses" were typically when nurses engaged in patient assessment, education, and evaluation. This finding validates findings from previous studies on missed care (Hessells et al., 2019).

Similarly, over a 10-year period, Lake et al. (2020) analyzed survey data from approximately 24,000 nurses in 2006 and 15,000 in 2017 from 458 hospitals in four large and geographically diverse states to demonstrate how change to a more supportive work environment and improved staffing led to less missed care, regardless of the hospital characteristics and technological capability. A total of 67% of nurses surveyed in 2006 and 75% in 2016 reported missing one or more care activities on their shift. Out of the 14 activities that encompass fundamental nursing responsibilities, nurses missed on average 2.4 necessary activities in 2006 and 2.6 in 2017. However, in hospitals that reported a more supportive work environment during this period, 11% fewer nurses missed care compared with hospitals with "less" supportive environments. In summary, the frequency of missed care decreased substantially in hospitals that improved their work environment but changed only slightly in hospitals with improved staffing (Lake et al., 2020)

Hospital-Acquired Conditions

Hospital-acquired conditions (HACs) represent a failure of the hospital system to provide safe care. To reduce the rates of HACs and improve patient safety, the Hospital-Acquired Condition Reduction Program (HACRP) was established by the Affordable Care Act in 2013. Under this pay-for-performance program, 25% of hospitals with the highest rates of HACs were penalized with a 1% reduction in Medicare payment rates for inpatient care by the Centers for Medicare & Medicaid Services (CMS). Box 11.2 identifies the specific conditions included in the HACRP program.

The *AHRQ National Scorecard on Hospital-Acquired Conditions: Final Results for 2014 through 2017* by the Agency for Healthcare Research and Quality documents progress toward achieving the goal of reducing HACs. This report showed that, from 2014 to 2017, HACs fell

---

BOX 11.2   Hospital-Acquired Conditions

- Foreign object retained after surgery
- Air embolism
- Blood incompatibility
- Stage III and Stage IV pressure ulcers
- Falls and trauma
  - Fractures
  - Dislocations
  - Intracranial Injuries
  - Crushing Injuries
  - Burn
  - Other Injuries
- Manifestations of poor glycemic control
  - Diabetic ketoacidosis
  - Nonketoic hyperosmolar coma
  - Hyperglycemic coma
  - Secondary diabetes with ketoacidosis
  - Secondary diabetes with hyperosmolarity
- Catheter-associated urinary tract infection (CAUTI)
- Vascular catheter-associated infection

- Surgical site infection mediastinitis following coronary artery bypass graft (CABG)
- Surgical site infection following bariatric surgery for obesity
  - Laparoscopic gastric bypass
  - Gastroenterostomy
  - Laparoscopic gastric restrictive surgery
- Surgical site infection following orthopedic procedures
  - Spine
  - Neck
  - Shoulder
  - Elbow
- Surgical site infection following cardiac implantable electron device (CIED)
- Deep vein thrombosis (DVT) or pulmonary embolism (PE) following certain orthopedic procedures
  - Total knee replacement
  - Hip replacement
- Iatrogenic pneumothorax with venous catheterization

Data from Agency for Healthcare Research and Quality (AHRQ). (2020). *AHRQ national scorecard on hospital-acquired conditions.* https://www.ahrq.gov/sites/default/files/wysiwyg/professionals/quality-patient-safety/pfp/Updated-hacreportFInal2017data.pdf.

by 13%, saving about 20,700 lives and about $7.7 billion in healthcare costs (AHRQ, 2020).

Other analyses do not agree with the result of the AHRQ final report. Researchers from the University of Michigan Institute for Healthcare Policy and Innovation state that their research indicates that the HACRP has not been effective. They note that the use of data-based measures to evaluate care leading to patient safety were not helpful in improving patient outcomes. They cite two main reasons for the lack of success: (1) inaccurate, unreliable assessment of hospital acquired conditions; and (2) poor risk adjustment, leading to disproportionate penalties for teaching hospitals and hospitals caring for more patients with socioeconomic disadvantages. These researchers suggest various policy strategies to improve the effectiveness of the HACRP.

National Database of Nursing Quality Indicators as Evidence of Staffing Effectiveness

Even prior to the institution of the HACRP as part of the Patient Protection and Affordable Care Act in 2013, nursing developed an approach to determine the impact of appropriate nurse staffing upon patient safety. A vital component in evaluating the effectiveness of staffing is having a process and structure to ensure that the measurement of outcomes is similar enough so that results can be compared across studies. The National Database of Nursing Quality Indicators (NDNQI) provides an opportunity to monitor staffing effectiveness in a specific nursing service or unit. The NDNQI, a program developed by the ANA and now operated by the Press Ganey Company, provides a benchmarking report comparing "like" participating organizations and units around the country. This database provides quarterly and annual reporting of structure, process, and outcome indicators to evaluate "nursing-sensitive" measures at the unit level. The NDNQI was built on the 1994 ANA Patient Safety and Quality Initiative. This initiative involved a series of pilot studies across the United States to identify nurse-sensitive indicators to use in evaluating patient care quality.

The NDNQI is a comprehensive, national nursing database that provides hospitals with nursing unit–level comparison on 18 quality indicators that can be used in quality improvement plans to prevent adverse events and improve patient outcomes, such as patient mortality. More than 2000 U.S. hospitals, including 95% of Magnet®-recognized facilities (see Chapter 5 for more information on Magnet® status), participate in the NDNQI program to measure nursing quality, improve

---

RESEARCH PERSPECTIVE

Source: Van, T., Annis, A. M., Matheos, Y., Robinson, C., Duffy, S., Yu-Fang, L., Taylor, B. A., Krein, S., Sullivan, S. C., & Sales, A. (2020) Nurse staffing and healthcare-associated infections in a national healthcare system that implemented a nurse staffing directive: Multi-level interrupted time series analyses. *International Journal of Nursing Studies*, 104, 103531.

A growing body of literature suggests that nurse staffing levels, using nurse–patient ratios, nursing staffing committees, patient classification systems, and minimum staffing levels, are associated with several inpatient health outcomes such as length of stay, quality of care, and mortality. The United States Veterans Health Administration introduced a staffing policy nationwide. This approach was designed to project the number of full-time equivalent nursing staff. The approach engaged front-line nursing staff in the process of data collection and analysis as well as unit decision-making about future staffing. The Staffing Methodology Directive outlined a multistep process to project the number of full-time equivalent employees for nursing personnel and nursing hours per patient day required for safe and effective care.

As a result of implementing the Staffing Methodology Directive, inpatient units in the Veterans Health Administration, on average, experienced increases in their nursing hours per patient day over the course of the study. This trend was not significantly different before versus after the introduction of the new staffing methodology. However, increases in staffing were associated with lower infection rates postimplementation.

Conclusions

Widespread interest in data-driven staffing models highlights the importance of continued development and research of best practices of nurse staffing to support current changes and advancements in the healthcare system. Future evaluations should include further exploration of appropriate measures of nurse staffing and examination of the impact on patient health outcomes.

Implications for Practice

As hospitals implement various approaches to staffing, evaluating the approach by assessing its impact on various indicators of staffing effectiveness is important.

nurse satisfaction, strengthen the nursing work environment, assess staffing levels, and improve reimbursement under current pay-for-performance policies.

Nursing-sensitive structure, process, and outcomes measures monitor relationships between quality indicators and outcomes. Hospitals can benchmark (or compare) their own data against other similar hospitals and participate in the ongoing research on nurse-sensitive data.

Box 11.3 outlines the nurse-sensitive indicators included in the NDNQI project. The comparison of like units is important because patient acuity and activity, patient care goals, clinical tasks, role expectations, team relations, and social milieu vary by unit and affect patient outcomes. The measures included in the NDNQI can be important in making staffing decisions when the accumulated evidence underlying these measures is included.

LITERATURE PERSPECTIVE

Source: Spano-Szekely, L., Winkler, A., Waters, C., Dealmeida, S., Brandt, K., Williamson, M., Blum, C., Gasper, L., & Wright, F. (2019). Individualized fall prevention program in an acute care setting: An evidence-based practice improvement. *Journal of Nursing Care Quality, 34*(2), 127–132.

This article describes the work of staff of a 245-bed hospital in revising a patient fall prevention as its patient safety priority. The baseline fall rate was 3.21, higher than the NDNQI's median fall rate of 2.91. Using an evidence-based practice improvement model, an interprofessional fall prevention team evaluated the fall program currently in place. A clinical practice guideline with seven key practices guided the development of an individualized program.

Interventions to address fall risks and an algorithm to identify interventions were used. These interventions included mobility assessment, purposeful hourly rounding, and video monitoring for confused and other fall-risk patients.

These interventions resulted in a fall rate decreasing a 1.14 fall rate. The program also reported an expense reduction based on decreased sitter usage.

Implications for Practice
The use of standardized data in a quality improvement process provides evidence of the current situation, allowing clinicians to set specific goals for improvement. Use of subsequent data can provide evidence of improvement in the process under consideration,

BOX 11.3   Nurse-Sensitive Indicators

- Nursing hours per patient day
  - Registered nurses
  - Licensed vocational nurses/licensed practical nurses (LVNs/LPNs)
  - Unlicensed assistive personnel
- Patient falls, with and without injury
  - Injury level
- Pediatric pain assessment, intervention, reassessment (AIR) cycle
- Pediatric peripheral intravenous infiltration rate
- Pressure ulcers prevalence
  - Hospital acquired
  - Unit acquired
  - Community acquired
- Psychiatric physical/sexual assault rate
- Restraint prevalence
- RN education/certification
- RN satisfaction survey options
  - Job satisfaction scales
  - Job satisfaction scales–short form
  - Practice Environment Scale (PES)
- Skill mix: percent of total nursing hours supplied by agency staff
  - RNs
  - LVN/LPN
- Voluntary nurse turnover
- Nurse vacancy rate
- Healthcare-associated infection
  - Catheter-associated urinary tract infection (CAUTI)
  - Central line–associated bloodstream infection (CLABSI)
  - Ventilator-associated pneumonia (VAP)

From Montalvo, I. (2007). *National Database of Nursing Quality Indicators® (NDNQI®). OJIN: The Online Journal of Issues in Nursing, 12*(3). https://ojin.nursingworld.org/MainMenuCategories/ANAMarketplace/ANAPeriodicals/OJIN/TableofContents/Volume122007/No3Sept07/NursingQualityIndicators.aspx.

Nurse Overtime

Nurse overtime has a significant impact on patient outcomes. *Requiring* staff to stay on duty after their shift ends to fill staffing vacancies is called mandatory overtime. Mandatory overtime has become a major negotiating point for nurses in unionized settings, and some state nurses' associations that use workplace advocacy strategies to improve the work environment in their states have developed legislation that prohibits mandatory overtime. The ANA and other nursing organizations oppose mandatory overtime because it is seen as a risk to both patients and nurses.

In contrast, *requesting* staff to stay on duty after their shift ends to fill staffing vacancies is simply called overtime. This differs from mandatory overtime because staff experience no employment consequences when they refuse to work overtime. In addition, in each week, nurses may work in more than one employment setting as a means of increasing their income. Although this practice is an individual decision, tired and overworked nurses are more likely to have compromised clinical judgment abilities and technical skills because of fatigue. As part of the solution to these negative consequences, the ANA recommends legislation to limit the number of hours that nurses are *required* to work. However, individual nurses must consider their responsibilities for patient safety when voluntarily working overtime.

EXERCISE 11.3 Review a healthcare organization's policies on overtime. Is mandatory overtime covered in the policy? If so, the consequences for failing to work mandatory overtime when requested to do so by a supervisor should be outlined in the policy. How would you respond to a nurse manager who required you to stay on the job after your shift was over? Develop a list of questions you might ask on a job interview relating to use of overtime in the organization. What does the state board of nursing in your state allow regarding mandatory overtime? As a nurse manager, how would you respond to a staffing shortage without mandatory overtime as an option? Develop a list of strategies for eliminating mandatory overtime if it exists.

SUPPLEMENTAL (AGENCY OR CONTRACT) STAFF AND FLOAT POOLS

Many nurses choose to work for staffing agencies. They may be hired by a nursing unit as an independent contractor for a shift, a week, or longer. Advantages of working for an agency are higher hourly rates of pay, diversity in work assignments, exposure to a variety of work teams, and the ability to travel. Organizations may use supplemental staff to fill temporary staff vacancies. Despite the response to an unexpected vacancy, nurse managers must consider the potential negative aspects of depending on supplemental staff to meet the unit's staffing plan. Patients should be unable to distinguish short-term, supplemental staff from unit staff. In addition, the ability to provide that level of orientation to supplemental agency or contract staff is often difficult.

A specific type of supplemental staffing agency is the traveling nurse agency. These organizations provide skilled nurses in short-term assignments, typically 3 months in length, for hospitals that have short-term staffing needs. These nurses are compensated far more than the "home" nurses and the total cost to the healthcare system for both the nurse who is traveling and the agency is significant. This approach has been used during the COVID-19 pandemic; nurses in the armed services have been deployed to civilian hospitals as well to help during this extraordinary health crisis.

Another strategy that may be used to fill unanticipated staff vacancies involves "floating" nurses from one clinical unit to another. In practice, the use of float nurses may be effective if the nurses are deployed from a centralized flexible staffing pool and they have the competencies to work on the unit to which they are assigned. Those who are willing to work as float nurses are generally experienced and maintain a broad range of clinical competencies. They often receive added compensation for their willingness to be flexible and to float to a variety of units on short notice.

When an organization does not have the flexibility of a staffing pool, the organization may expect nurses to float across clinical units to fill vacancies. To ensure patient safety and nurse satisfaction, the organization must develop a policy regarding the reassignment of the staff to clinically similar units. If direct care nurses are asked to be reassigned to an area outside of their sphere of clinical competence, they should be asked to support only basic care needs and not assume a complete and independent assignment. This practice should be used only on an emergency basis or with the nurse's agreement, because being required to float is often a "dissatisfier" for nurses and potentially a concern for patient safety.

ORGANIZATIONAL FACTORS THAT AFFECT STAFFING PLANS

Organizational factors include issues such as types of clinical units and the duration of the shift that nurses work as well as the extent to which shifts are rotated. These factors are typically addressed in the structure and philosophy of the nursing service department, organizational staffing policies, organizational supports, and services offered.

Structure and Philosophy of the Nursing Services Department

A nursing philosophy statement outlines the vision, values, and beliefs about the practice of nursing and the provision of patient care within the organization. The philosophy statement is used to guide the daily practice of nursing in the various nursing units. Nurse managers must propose a staffing plan and personnel budget that allow consistency between the written philosophy statement and the observable practice of nursing on their units. Nurses feel demoralized when they cannot comply with their nursing philosophy statement or professional values because of problems associated with consistently inadequate staffing. The philosophy statement also guides the establishment of the overall structure of the nursing service department and the staffing models that are used within the organization. The staffing model adopted by the organization plays a key role in determining the mix of professional and assistive staff needed to provide patient care.

Organizational Support Systems

A critical variable that affects the development of the nursing personnel budget is the presence or absence of organizational systems that support the nurse in providing care. If the organization has recognized the need to keep the professional nurse at the bedside, support systems to allow that to happen will be evident Examples of support systems that enhance the nurse's ability to remain on the unit and provide direct care to patients include transporter services, clerical support services, and hospitality services.

However, professional nurses often work in organizations that require them to function in the role of a multipurpose worker, particularly in acute or long-term care. Because nurses in these settings are generally available 24 hours a day, 7 days a week, they may be required to provide services for other professionals who provide more limited hours of care to patients. Competent or knowledgeable nurse managers identify what costs are being incurred in the unit because of the absence of adequate organizational support systems and develop strategies to put those systems into place or justify the budget accordingly.

SCHEDULING

Scheduling is a function of implementing the staffing plan by assigning unit personnel to work specific hours and specific days of the week. Scheduling depends on the historical census in a particular unit, as well as its anticipated volume. Schedules may be developed 1 to 3 months in advance, although scheduling for holidays may be developed 6 to 12 months before the holiday. Although the development of a schedule is generally the responsibility of the nurse manager, direct care nurses can influence the schedule through the unit's shared governance or staffing committees.

The nurse manager is often challenged to take the FTEs that are allotted through the personnel budget, distribute them appropriately, and create a master schedule for the unit that also meets each employee's personal and professional needs. Although completely satisfying each individual staff member is not always possible, a schedule can usually be created that is both fair and balanced from the employee's perspective while still meeting patient care needs. Creating a flexible schedule with a variety of scheduling options that leads to work schedule stability for each employee is one mechanism likely to retain staff that is within the control of nurse managers.

Constructing the Schedule

Mechanisms are typically in place within an organization for staff to use in requesting days off and to know when the final schedule will be posted. In addition, most organizations have written policies and procedures that must be followed by nurse managers to ensure compliance with state and federal labor laws relative to scheduling. These policies also aid managers in making scheduling decisions that will be perceived as fair and equitable by all employees. Schedules are usually constructed for a predetermined block of time based on organizational policy—for example, weekly, biweekly, or monthly—typically using the staffing matrix for each unit. The unit schedule may be prepared in a decentralized fashion by nurse managers or by unit staff through a self-scheduling method. In some organizations, centralized staffing coordinators may oversee all of the schedules prepared for the patient care units. Each method of schedule preparation has pros and cons.

Decentralized Scheduling

One decentralized method for preparing the schedule involves nurse managers developing the schedule in isolation from all other units. In this model, the nurse managers approve all schedule changes and spend time on a regular basis drafting the staff schedule, considering only the staffing needs of the unit. In other decentralized models, managers do the preliminary work on schedules and then submit them to a centralized staffing office for review and for the addition of any needed supplemental staff. The advantage of a decentralized model is that the accountability for submitting a schedule in alignment with the established staffing plan rests with managers. These individuals are ultimately the ones responsible for maintaining unit productivity in line with the personnel budget; thus, the incentive to manage the schedule tightly is strong. The negative aspect of this decentralized method is the inability of any individual nurse manager to know the "big picture" related to staffing across multiple patient care units. Requests for time off are approved in isolation from all other units; a real potential with this model is that each manager's decisions at the unit level will be felt in aggregate as a "staffing shortage" across multiple units.

Staff Self-Scheduling

A self-scheduling process has the potential to promote staff autonomy and to increase staff accountability. In addition, team communication, problem-solving, and negotiating skills can be enhanced through the self-scheduling process. Successful self-scheduling is achieved when everyone's personal schedule is balanced with the unit's patient care needs. Self-scheduling has become more complicated in the wake of care delivery changes and the decentralization of many activities to the individual patient care units. The professional nursing staff cannot work in isolation from other care members when creating a schedule. Assessing the readiness of support staff to participate in this type of initiative is critical, as resource utilization and cost containment continue to be major focal points of concern. Self-scheduling or flexible scheduling needs to be responsibly managed. Although personal needs of the staff are important to meet, the patient care needs on the unit are the paramount focus for building a schedule. Unit standards for a staffing plan are established. Then, a negotiated schedule that results in meeting the needs of staff and patients is the expected and ultimate outcome.

Centralized Scheduling

One benefit to centralized scheduling is that the staffing coordinator is usually aware of the abilities, qualifications, and availability of supplemental personnel who may be needed to complete the schedule. In many organizations, the centralized staffing coordinator is also aware of each unit's personnel budget and any constraints it may impose on the schedule. On the other hand, a disadvantage to centralized staffing is the limited knowledge of the coordinator relative to changing patient acuity needs or other patient-related activities on the unit. Developing a mechanism for the centralized staffing coordinator to share unit-specific knowledge with the respective nurse manager can resolve this disadvantage satisfactorily.

Many organizations have invested in computer software designed to create optimal schedules based on the approved staffing plans for individual units. The centralized staffing coordinator maintains the integrity of the computerized databank for each unit; enters schedule variances daily; generates planning sheets, drafts, and final schedules; and runs any specialized productivity reports requested by nurse managers. Nurse managers review the initial schedule created by the computer, make necessary modifications, and approve the final schedule.

Variables Affecting Staffing Schedules

Nurse managers must consider many variables to create a fair and balanced schedule for their unit; examples of anticipated variables are found in Box 11.4.

BOX 11.4   Anticipated Scheduling Variables

- Hours of operation
- Shift rotations
- Weekend rotations
- Approved benefit time for the schedule period—for example, vacations and holidays
- Approved leaves of absence/short-term disability
- Approved seminar, orientation, and continuing education time
- Scheduled meetings for the schedule period
- Current filled positions and current staffing vacancies
- Number of part-time employees

BOX 11.5   Formulas for Calculating Volume Statistics

Assume that a 20-bed medical-surgical unit (*capacity statistic*) accrued 566 patient days in June (*volume statistic*). Of these patients, 98 were discharged during the month.

Average Daily Census (ADC) on this unit is 18.9
Formula: Patient days for a given time period divided by the number of days in the time period
  1. 30 days in June
  2. 566 patient days/30 days = ADC of 18.9

Average length of stay for June is 5.8
Formula: Number of patient days divided by the number of discharges
  566 patient days/98 patient discharges = 5.8 (rounded)

Percentage of occupancy for June is 95%
Formula: Daily patient census (rounded) divided by the number of beds in the unit
  19 patients in a 20-bed unit
  19 patients/20 beds = 95% occupancy

Unanticipated variables can complicate the best-prepared schedule. When faced with call-ins for illness, compassion leaves, jury duty, or an emergent need for a leave of absence (LOA), nurse managers must attempt to fill a shift vacancy on short notice. Requesting staff to add hours over their planned commitment, floating staff from another unit or securing someone from a staffing pool, contracting with agency nursing staff, and seeking overtime are examples of strategies that nurse managers may be compelled to use to ensure safe staffing of their units. However, as discussed, many potential negative consequences are associated with using these strategies.

EXERCISE 11.4 Suppose that you are going on a job interview. Considering your personal preferred work schedule, what scheduling practices would be most satisfying to you and might lead you to accept employment with the organization? What scheduling practices might cause you to look elsewhere for a job? Develop a list of questions to ask your potential employer regarding scheduling practices in the organization.

EVALUATING UNIT STAFFING AND PRODUCTIVITY

Nurse managers are increasingly being pressed to justify their staffing decisions to their staff, senior management, and accrediting agencies. The unit activity or production report, which provides a variety of measures of unit workload, can be helpful in such justification. In addition, a review of the extent to which the actual staffing over a specific period matches the staffing plan, particularly coupled with various outcomes over the same period, gives a picture of the productivity and effectiveness of the unit. Although the format of these reports may vary, the kinds of information typically available to nurse managers in an activity report are included in Box 11.5.

In the inpatient setting, the average daily census (ADC) is one measure considered by nurse managers to project the potential workload of the unit. The ADC is a simple measure of the average number of patients being cared for in the available beds on the unit trended over a specific period. The formula for calculating the ADC is found in Box 11.5. If a unit's ADC is trending upward, the nurse manager should propose additional personnel to manage this increase in patient volume. If the ADC is trending downward, the nurse manager should propose the need for fewer resources to manage this downward census trend. In the acute care setting, a unit's ADC can be extremely volatile based on the patterns of admissions, transfers, and discharges on the unit. In a long-term care setting, however, the unit's ADC may be very stable over prolonged periods. Nurse managers may note census trends based on a particular shift, the day of the week, or the season of the year. The addition of new physicians, the creation of innovative programs or services, and many other variables may also affect a unit's ADC. Increased admissions and discharges staffing demands. Nurse managers must maintain a strong grasp on these measures of workload to prepare an adequate staffing plan for their unit.

As reimbursement dollars have decreased, so have lengths of stay. However, the cost of treating the patient has not decreased as dramatically, because patient acuity is greater. Essentially, hospitals need to provide more care in less time for fewer dollars with the same, if not better, outcomes. For this reason, as a unit's average length of stay (ALOS) trends downward, the need for staffing resources may not change substantially, or it may climb. The formula for calculating the ALOS is found in Box 11.5.

Another way of assessing a unit's activity level is to calculate the percentage of occupancy. The unit's occupancy rate can be calculated for a specific shift, daily, or as a monthly or annual statistic. The formula for calculating the percentage of occupancy is found in Box 11.5. Nurse managers use the percentage of occupancy to develop the unit's staffing plan (Fig. 11.2). Optimal occupancy rates may vary by practice setting. In a long-term care facility, the organization would desire 100% occupancy rates. However, in an acute care facility, 85% occupancy rates would ensure the best potential for patient throughput.

The measures just mentioned provide the nurse manager with an understanding of the number of patients who have been admitted to the unit over a period of time. The nurse is then charged with matching the needs of these patients with the appropriate number of staff members. Managers have positions and subsequent budgeted nursing salary dollars in the personnel budget based on the estimated units of service that will be provided in the unit. If managers can provide more care to more patients while spending the same or fewer salary dollars, they have increased their unit productivity. Conversely, if the same or more salary dollars are spent to provide less care to fewer patients, managers have decreased their unit productivity.

Nursing productivity is a formula-driven calculation. UOS multiplied by the volume (patient days or emergency department visits) equals hours available to create direct productive staffing plans. Those hours multiplied by a nonproductive factor (e.g., 1.12) to account for paid time off equals the total hours available for the staffing plan. Getting a ratio of patients to RN is essential. This is then applied to the total hours available, and the support structure (nursing assistants or unit clerks) can be built accordingly. Patient type, scope of service, and acuity and/or classification of the patient are all factors correlated with patient outcomes that drive staffing decisions. Meeting these productivity standards is important to ensure the financial well-being of the organization. However, if the safety needs of the patients are put at risk to achieve this productivity level, the consequences are harmful to patients, staff, and the organization.

Calculating nursing productivity is challenging for nurse managers because it is difficult to quantify the efficiency and effectiveness of individual nurses providing care to patients. Individual nurses can vary greatly in their critical-thinking abilities, their skill levels, and their ability to make timely and accurate decisions that affect patient outcomes.

Variance Between Projected and Actual Staff

Organizations can use labor cost or a straight FTE model for comparison of actual with projected staff. Labor cost per unit of service is a simple measure that compares budgeted salary costs per budgeted volume of service (productivity target) with actual salary costs per actual volume of service (productivity performance). This measure requires managers to staff according to their staffing plan because the plan reflects the approved personnel budget. Box 11.6 shows an analysis of labor

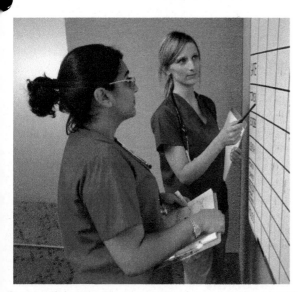

Fig. 11.2 Calculating the percentage of occupancy is essential when developing a unit's staffing plan.

BOX 11.6   Analysis of Labor Costs Per Unit of Service

A manager of a cardiac telemetry unit proposes the following in the personnel budget. These are the unit's productivity targets:

Total patient days: 5840
- ADC = 16
- Staffing plan for ADC of 16
  - Day shift: 3 RNs and 3 UNP (50% RN skill mix)
  - Evening shift: 3 RNs and 3 UNP (50% RN skill mix)
  - Night shift: 3 RNs and 1 UNP (75% RN skill mix)

Direct care labor costs are also projected by the manager based on the average RN and UNP salaries for this unit
- Target = $139.32 per patient, or $2229.12 per day

The manager staffs as follows:
- ADC = 16
- Actual staffing for ADC of 16
  - Day shift: 4 RNs and 2 UNP (66% RN skill mix)
  - Evening shift: 4 RNs and 2 UNP (66% RN skill mix)
  - Night shift: 3 RNs (100% RN skill mix)
- Direct labor costs for this day = $145.44 per patient, or $2327.04 per day

The manager has incurred a variance:
- Exceeded target by $6.12 per patient, or $97.92 for the day

ADC, Average daily census; *RN,* registered nurse; *UNP,* unlicensed nursing personnel.

costs per UOS. Typically, nurse managers must evaluate and explain changes in productivity resulting in a difference between the projected staffing plan and the actual schedule, using a variance report. If managers compare the two numbers and the actual productivity performance number is higher than the target, they have spent more money for care than they budgeted. Several variables may cause the labor costs to be higher than anticipated, such as increased overtime, paying bonus pay for regular staff, using costly agency resources, or a higher-than-anticipated amount of indirect education or orientation time.

If managers compare the two numbers and the actual productivity performance number is lower than the target, they have spent less money for care than they budgeted. Managers must also explain this high degree of productivity. One variable that may cause the labor costs to be lower than anticipated is an increased nonprofessional skill mix or consistently understaffing their unit.

Having a productivity performance number that is either higher or lower than that planned does not represent effective management. Assuming that staffing plans were an accurate reflection of the conditions on the specific units, if managers compare the actual productivity performance with their productivity target and the two numbers match, the managers have probably managed effectively. However, given the dynamic nature of patient care, an ongoing evaluation of the conditions on the unit as well as the extent to which proposed staffing levels are reached or exceeded should be monitored on an ongoing basis. Variance reports provide an opportunity for such evaluation.

EXERCISE 13.5 Suppose that you are working in the charge nurse role. One of the staff assigned to collaborate with you becomes ill and must go home suddenly, leaving his designated patient assignment to be assumed by someone else. As a charge nurse, what factors would you consider as you determine how to reassign his work to other nurses? If you were a coworker on the shift instead of the charge nurse, what effective follower behaviors might you demonstrate to support the charge nurse in this situation? Can you identify behaviors of coworkers that would complicate the staffing situation further?

Impact of Leadership on Productivity

Nurse managers must possess staffing and scheduling skills to prepare a staffing plan that balances organizational directives with unit needs for care and services. Nurse managers must spend time each month evaluating their unit's productivity performance. Yet, it is also important that nurse managers improve unit productivity by spending more of their work time coaching and mentoring staff and providing them with clear information and direction related to meeting unit productivity goals. Nurse managers are the chief retention officers and need to perform their duties accordingly.

CONCLUSION

Staffing and scheduling are some of the greatest challenges for a nurse manager. When these functions are performed well, the resulting satisfaction of the unit staff contributes to positive patient outcomes. When they are not performed well, low morale and discontent can result. The manager has various data available to help in planning the staffing patterns for the unit. Success, however, depends on the unit staff and the manager working collaboratively and using effective negotiation strategies to meet the needs for care.

THE SOLUTION

A staff meeting was called to discuss the impact of the transition of several beds for STICU step-down patients on the inpatient general surgery unit. Information was given to all staff regarding the potential size of the step-down unit and the methods for staffing it. Staff members were assured that no jobs would be lost and that appropriate training would be provided to current staff to ensure their competence.

Six beds were determined to be the initial number of step-down beds to be incorporated into the surgical inpatient unit. Staff members engaged in the design of the space from the perspective of identifying which rooms were to be used and what in-room supplies and equipment would be necessary. Continuous pulse oximetry and bedside computers were among the top equipment needs identified.

A staffing plan was established for the step-down unit; staff members on the general surgery unit were first to be offered the positions. The unit's staffing plan was filled with staff members from the general surgical unit as well as a related unit. Educational plans were developed, and the STICU nursing staff members were open and welcoming when the new step-down staff rotated and partnered with the STICU staff in the critical care environment. The new step-down staff completed didactic education and the same STICU nurses provided backup for them when the unit opened.

Continuous discussions were held with the medical staff involved through a champion who was identified within the department of general surgery. Talking points were distributed to the medical staff and the other hospital staff to keep everyone current with the progress. Interdisciplinary teams were developed around the care models and are now engaged in daily patient care conferences to monitor the progress of patients.

The unit has been open for 6 months and is a success. We have no vacant positions, critical care beds are more available, medical staff are pleased with the care delivered, patient satisfaction for this unit is particularly good, and the staff feel accomplished and proud of their contribution to the overall capacity challenge!

Would this be a suitable approach for you? Why?

Mary Ellen Bonczek, BSN, RN, MPA, NEA-BC

REFLECTIONS

The nurse manager's role in staffing and scheduling a nursing unit requires clinical, legal, regulatory, communication, negotiation, and financial competencies to ensure appropriate outcomes. In preparation for the nurse manager role, what skills will you need to develop to be successful? And because roles are fluid, what do you need to know to be effective as a follower?

BEST PRACTICES

- Efforts to increase nurse engagement in units and organizations have the potential to improve patient safety and decrease potential negative outcomes. Focusing on the ANA Staffing Principles will enhance patient safety no matter what staffing model an organization uses to determine the appropriate level of staffing. Further, a culture of safety on a nursing unit reduces the chances of missed care occurring. Staffing and scheduling are complex processes with many variations that affect patient care outcomes. Using critical data, such as the NDNQI Nurse Sensitive Indicators, is needed to effectively and objectively evaluate patient outcomes.

TIPS FOR STAFFING AND SCHEDULING

- Know state laws and voluntary accreditation (professional society and institutional) standards for staffing.
- Evaluate organizational policies for congruence with accreditation and state licensing expectations.
- Integrate ongoing research regarding the impact of numerous factors on patient outcomes into staffing plans.

- Identify current demands for staff and anticipate externally imposed changes, such as services offered and availability of RNs and LPNs/LVNs.
- Value the various responses to short staffing from the manager, staff, and patient perspectives.
- Recognize the complexity of staffing issues and how they relate to staff satisfaction, community perception, budget, and accreditation standards.

REFERENCES

Agency for Healthcare Research and Quality (AHRQ). (2020). *AHRQ national scorecard on hospital-acquired conditions: Final results for 2014 through 2017*. Retrieved from https://www.ahrq.gov/sites/default/files/wysiwyg/professionals/quality-patient-safety/pfp/Updated-hacreportFInal2017data.pdf.

Aiken, L. (2012). Patient safety, satisfaction, and quality of hospital care: Cross sectional surveys of nurses and patients in 12 countries in Europe and the United States. *British Medical Journal, 344*, e1717.

Aiken, L., Sloane, D., Cimiotti, J., Clarke, S., Flynn, L., Seago, J., et al. (2010). Implications of the California nurse staffing mandate for other states. *Health Services Research, 45*(4), 904–921.

American Association of Colleges of Nursing (AACN). (2021). *The essentials: Core Competencies for professional nursing education*. Retrieved from https://www.aacnnursing.org/Portals/42/AcademicNursing/pdf/Essentials-2021.pdf.

American Association of Critical Care Nurses. (2018). *AACN guiding principles for appropriate staffing*. Retrieved from https://www.aacn.org/policy-and-advocacy/guiding-principles-for-staffing.

American Nurses Association (ANA). (2014). *Addressing nurse fatigue to promote safety and health: Joint responsibilities of registered nurses and employers to reduce risk*. Retrieved from https://www.nursingworld.org/practice-policy/nursing-excellence/official-position-statements/id/addressing-nurse-fatigue-to-promote-safety-and-health/.

American Nurses Association (ANA). (2019). *Nurse staffing advocacy*. Retrieved from https://www.nursingworld.org/practice-policy/nurse-staffing/nurse-staffing-advocacy/.

Bae, S. H., & Fabry, D. (2014). Effects of nurse overtime and long hours worked on nursing and patients' outcomes. *Nursing Outlook, 62*(2), 138–156.

Buerhaus, P. (2021). Current nursing shortages could have long-lasting consequences: Time to change our present course. *Nursing Economics, 39*(5), 247–250.

Carbajal, E. (2020). California nurses struggle as nurse-to-patient ratios stretched amid COVID-19 surge. *Becker Hospital Review*. Retrieved from https://www.beckershospitalreview.com/nursing/california-nurses-struggle-as-nurse-to-patient-ratio-stretched-amid-covid-19-surge.html#:~:text=New%20pandemic%20ratios%20allow%20intensive,seven%20patients%20instead%20of%20five.

Carthon, J. M. B., Hatfield, L., Plover, C., Dierkes, A., Davis, L., Hedgeland, T., Sanders, A. M., Visco, F., Holland, S., Ballinghoff, J., Del Guidice, M., & Aiken, L. H. (2019). Association of nurse engagement and nurse staffing on patient safety. *Journal of Nursing Care Quality, 34*(1), 40–46.

Centers for Medicare & Medicaid (CMS). (2020). *Hospital-acquired conditions*. Retrieved from https://cms.gov/Medicare/Medicare-Fee-for-Service-Payment/HospitalAcqCond/Hospital-Acquired_Conditions.

Covell, C., & Sidani, S. (2013). Nursing intellectual theory: Implications for research and practice. *OJIN: The Online Journal of Issues in Nursing, 18*(2).

Davis, C. (2021). Congressional bill seeks to set federal nurse-to-patient staffing requirements. In *Healthleaders*. Retrieved from https://www.healthleadersmedia.com/nursing/congressional-bill-seeks-set-federal-nurse-patient-staffing-requirements.

Harrington, C., Dellefield, M. E., Halifax, E., Flemming, M. L., & Bakerjian, D. (2020). Appropriate nurse staffing levels for U.S. nursing homes. *Health Services Insights, 13*, 1–14.

Hessels, A., Paliwal, M., Weaver, S., Siddiqui, D., Wurmser, T. (2019). Impact of patient safety culture on missed nursing care and adverse patient events. Journal of Nursing Care Quality, 34(4), 287–294.

Institute of Medicine (IOM). (2010). *The future of nursing: Leading change, advancing health*. Washington, DC: National Academies Press.

Lake, E., Riman, K., & Sloane, D. (2020). Improved work environments and staffing lead to less missed care: A panel study. *Nursing Management, 28*(8), 2157–2165.

Montalvo, I. (2007). *National Database of Nursing Quality Indicators® (NDNQI®). OJIN: The. Online Journal of Issues in Nursing, 12*(3). Retrieved from https://ojin.nursing-world.org/MainMenuCategories/ANAMarketplace/ANAPeriodicals/OJIN/TableofContents/Volume122007/No3Sept07/NursingQualityIndicators.aspx.

Savillea, C., Griffiths, P., Ball, J. E., & Monks, T. (2019). How many nurses do we need? A review and discussion of operational research techniques applied to nurse staffing. *International Journal of Nursing Studies, 97*, 7–13.

Spano-Szekely, L., Winkler, A., Waters, C., Dealmeida, S., Brandt, K., Williamson, M., Blum, C., Gasper, L., & Wright, F. (2019). Individualized fall prevention program in an acute care setting: An evidence-based practice improvement. *Journal of Nursing Care Quality, 34*(2), 127–132.

Stimpfel, A., Sloane, D., & Aiken, L. (2012). The longer the shifts for hospital nurses, the higher the levels of burnout and patient dissatisfaction. *Health Affairs, 31*(11), 2501–2509.

Watkins, S. (2020). *Hospital staffing budget development.* Washington State Nursing Association. Retrieved from https://www.aft.org/sites/default/files/hospital_staffing_budget_dev.pdf.

Williams, D. (2019). *Theory of nursing intellectual capital.* Ferris State University. https://deborahwilliams.weebly.com/uploads/5/9/2/5/5925337/nursing_theory_critique_covell.docx.

Van, T., Annis, A. M., Matheos, Y., Robinson, C. H., Duffy, S. A., Yu-Fang, L., Taylor, B. A., Krein, S., Sullivan, S. C., & Sales, A. (2020). Nurse staffing and healthcare-associated infections in a national healthcare system that implemented a nurse staffing directive: Multi-level interrupted time series analyses. *International Journal of Nursing Studies, 104*, 103531.

12

Workforce Engagement Through Collective Action and Governance

R. Coleen Wilson

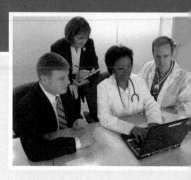

ANTICIPATED LEARNING OUTCOMES

- Evaluate how key characteristics of selected collective action strategies apply in the workplace through professional governance, workplace advocacy, and collective bargaining.

- Evaluate how participation of direct care nurses in decision-making relates to job satisfaction and improved patient outcomes.
- Explain the role of nurse empowerment and engagement in creating healthy work environments.

KEY TERMS

accountability
at-will employee
autonomy
bullying
collective action
collective bargaining
empowerment

engagement
healthy work environment
high reliability
incivility
just culture
organizational justice
ownership of practice

professional governance
responsibility
right to work
union
whistleblower
workplace advocacy

THE CHALLENGE

In 2008, UCLA Health embarked on its journey to institute a shared governance structure within the department of nursing. Unit Practice Councils (UPCs) and its membership were established to represent a specific unit or service population of the main campus hospital (then CHS, now Ronald Reagan), the Resnick Neuropsychiatric Hospital, and the Santa Monica campus hospital. Education was provided to all of the UPC members and unit leadership.

The UPCs were given the charge to complete a unit-based project each year to enhance patient outcomes and/or staff satisfaction. To celebrate and share the work being completed through these UPCs, a *World Café* was

created, in which three to four members of every UPC would be invited to share their work through either a poster or podium presentation. This provided an opportunity to share best practices.

However, in 2016, the organization completed a gap analysis on the current shared governance structures and processes led by a nurse leader. The results of the analysis found that the UPCs varied in practice, process, policy, and outcomes. Some were strong and well supported while others were less engaged. Furthermore, the analysis identified a lack of collaboration and communication between the campuses and even within each hospital.

INTRODUCTION

In 1999, the Institute of Medicine (IOM), currently called the National Academy of Medicine (NAM), published a groundbreaking white paper revealing the prevalence and impact of medical errors, *To Err Is Human: Building a Safer Health System*. At that time, the IOM estimated that medical errors were the eighth leading cause of death, with an estimate of 44,000 to 98,000 deaths based on two studies done in Colorado/Utah and New York (IOM, 2000). The report defined errors as either errors of execution or errors of planning (IOM, 2000). Errors of execution means that the appropriate action was not done correctly, for example, a patient needed a right lower limb amputation and instead received a left lower limb amputation. Errors of planning means that the determination to take an action was incorrect, for example, a patient receives chemotherapy when there is no indication for receiving such.

In 2019, Armstrong and Derek published a white paper through the Armstrong Institute for Patient Safety

and Quality at Johns Hopkins Medicine for the Leapfrog Group. Their study estimated that approximately 150,000 deaths occur annually due to a medical error. In accordance with the Centers for Disease Control and Prevention–National Center for Health Statistics (CDC–NCHS), that would put healthcare errors in a tie with stroke as the fifth leading cause of death (CDC, 2021).

Why is all this important and what does it have to do with workforce engagement? In 2019, Clapper and Ching (2020) completed a systematic review of the main causes of medical errors. They found that the majority of errors were due to deficits in knowledge and skills (practice and clinical reasoning) and problematic attitudes (clinical judgment). While medical errors encompass everything from assessment, diagnosis, prescribing, and treatment, one member of the interdisciplinary team is not solely responsible for the care and outcome of our patients. Every member of the care team has a responsibility and obligation to ensure patient safety. It is the collective action in a healthcare organization that results in quality care or in poor outcomes.

CULTURE AND STRUCTURAL FRAME

Culture

The culture of an organization is important, as it dictates the success or failure of initiatives. Organizations that promote a culture of transparency, trust, and engagement are more likely to embrace safety and change.

High Reliability Organizations

In 2008, The Joint Commission created the Center for Transforming Healthcare with a goal to help organizations on their journey to high reliability and zero harm. The Joint Committee Center for Transforming Healthcare defines high reliability as sustained excellence in quality and safety over all services (2021). To date, healthcare organizations have not fully and consistently reached high reliability. However, many are on the journey toward becoming a high reliability organization (HRO).

When the concept of high reliability was initially described, five key principles were identified as necessary to meet the standard: (1) preoccupation with failure, (2) reluctance to simplify, (3) sensitivity to operations, (4) deference to expertise, and (5) commitment to resilience. Definitions of each characteristic may be found in Table 12.1 (Patient Safety Network, 2019). Veazie et al. (2019) created a logic model that linked the five

TABLE 12.1	**Key Principles of High Reliability**
Characteristic	**Description**
Preoccupation with Failure	Everyone is aware of and thinking about the potential for failure. People understand that new threats emerge regularly from situations that no one imagined could occur. Thus, all personnel actively think about what could go wrong and are alert to small signs of potential problems. The absence of errors or accidents leads not to complacency but to a heightened sense of vigilance for the next possible failure. Near misses are viewed as opportunities to learn about systems issues and potential improvements rather than as evidence of safety.
Reluctance to Simplify	People resist simplifying their understanding of work processes and how and why things succeed or fail in their environment. People in high reliability organizations (HROs) understand that the work is complex and dynamic. They seek underlying rather than surface explanations. While HROs recognize the value of standardization of workflows to reduce variation, they also appreciate the complexity inherent in the number of teams, processes, and relationships involved in conducting daily operations.
Sensitivity to Operations	Based on their understanding of operational complexity, people in HROs strive to maintain a high awareness of operational conditions. This sensitivity is often referred to as "big picture understanding" or "situation awareness." People cultivate an understanding of the context of the current state of their work in relation to the unit or organizational state—i.e., what is going on around them—and how the current state might support or threaten safety.
Deference to Expertise	People in HROs appreciate that the people closest to the work are the most knowledgeable about the work. Thus, people in HROs know that in a crisis or emergency, the person with greatest knowledge of the situation might not be the person with the highest status and seniority. Deference to local and situation expertise results in a spirit of inquiry and de-emphasis on hierarchy in favor of learning as much as possible about potential safety threats. In an HRO, everyone is expected to share concerns with others and the organizational climate is such that all staff members are comfortable speaking up about potential safety problems.
Commitment to Resilience	Commitment to resilience is rooted in the fundamental understanding of the frequently unpredictable nature of system failures. People in HROs assume that the system is at risk for failure, and they practice performing rapid assessments of and responses to challenging situations. Teams cultivate situation assessment and cross monitoring so that they may identify potential safety threats quickly and either respond before safety problems cause harm or mitigate the seriousness of the safety event.

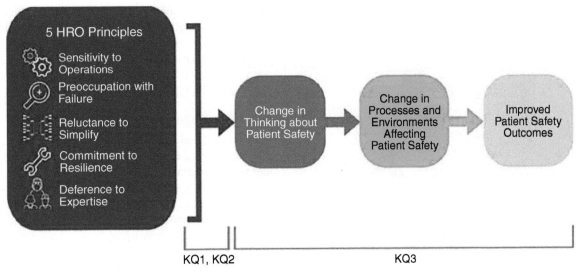

Fig. 12.1 Logic model for high reliability (Veazie et al., 2019; public domain).

principles to the end goal of improved patient safety/ zero harm (Fig. 12.1). This logic model demonstrates the outcomes that can be achieved when organizations focus their efforts on the five key principles of high reliability.

As Veazie et al. (2019) indicated in their logic model, when all five principles are at the forefront of actions and processes, the organization will begin to change thinking in regard to patient safety. People will begin to look at their processes and culture to identify where their current failure points (or almost failure points) are and seek constant improvement. Additionally, they focus on what is going well and why. Having an in-depth understanding of the processes that are successful will help to spread best practices. This will also help to identify practices that have opportunities for improvement *before* an error has been made.

When everyone in an organization is empowered to speak up, question, and challenge the status quo, organizations will achieve the final stage of the logic model for high reliability—improved patient safety outcomes. The journey to high reliability is one that will be never ending for organizations that embark on it. Innovations, research, and changes will always occur to improve patient safety, and high reliability organizations will always promote appreciative inquiry to strive for patient safety and best practices.

The Joint Commission Center for Transforming Healthcare identified three domains of change required to reach high reliability (2021):

1. Leadership committed to the goal of zero harm.
2. An organizational culture of safety in which all staff can speak up about things that would negatively impact the organization.
3. An empowered workforce that employs robust process improvement (RPI) tools to address improvement opportunities and drive significant and lasting change.

Each of these domains is important by itself. Together, they form a process of engagement in dedication to creating an organization that is highly reliable. The second domain is critically important because psychological safety is a major concern for today's workforce.

Culture of safety

In order to achieve zero harm, a culture of safety must be present. Veazie et al. (2019) recommend fostering a culture of safety through strong collaboration, communication, and coordination. In order to develop a culture of safety, a foundation of trust is necessary. Trust allows employees to feel empowered to speak up without a fear of reprisal.

A key measure that has been identified to develop a culture of safety is to create a just culture (American College of Healthcare Executives [ACHE], Institute for Healthcare Improvement [IHI], & Leape Foundation, 2017) (Fig. 12.2). A just culture work environment is preoccupied with failure. Preoccupation with failure focuses on broken processes that may cause harm. A just culture

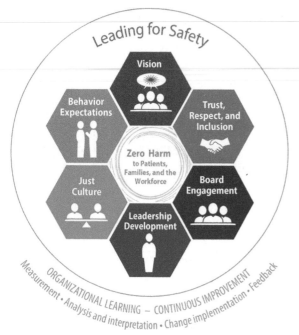

Fig. 12.2 A Culture of Safety: The Six Domains (American College of Healthcare Executives [ACHE], IHI/NPSF Lucian Leape Institute, 2017, p. 5).

focuses on accountability for the organization as well as the individuals within. The goal is to move from a blaming culture to one that is patient/person-centered and works together to find a solution. In a just culture environment, incidents are reviewed and assessed for process issues, human error, at-risk behavior, or reckless behavior.

If a process issue is the root cause of the error, the organization will work on revising the process with end-users to ensure that patient safety is the focus as well as policies and protocols. If human error is the root cause, the organization/leader should support the individual who made the error and identify any system issues that could keep the error from occurring again. If the root cause of the error is an individual's at-risk behavior, the leader will coach and educate the individual to make the person aware of the impact of one's decisions and actions. If the root cause of the error is due to reckless behavior, such as the individual consciously making a decision to do the wrong thing, that person will be held accountable through disciplinary action.

In short, to create a just culture, assumptions should never be made and all events should be investigated thoroughly to identify the cause behind the error. A just culture is not a blame-free environment; rather, it is one in which due process is utilized to ensure that patient and staff safety is the end goal, addressing the true root cause, be it process or people.

HEALTHY WORK ENVIRONMENT

What Are Healthy Work Environments?

Many nurses find that working in an environment that does not match their personal values or expectations creates dissatisfaction and a sense of unfulfillment at their job. Poor job fit is a known contributor to employee turnover. One of the critical factors to evaluate when choosing which organization to work for includes an assessment of the work environment. A healthy work environment is one that supports excellence in nursing practice. Saunders et al. (2021) describe a healthy work environment as a "workplace that is positive, supportive, safe, collaborative, empowering, motivational, collegial, professional, respectful, caring, and satisfying" (p. 2). In 2004, the IOM, now known as the NAM, published a seminal document, *Keeping Patients Safe: Transforming the Work Environment of Nurses*. The report recommended changes to improve patient outcomes based on the understanding that the environment in which nurses work has a profound effect on the safety and quality of care. Since the release of the report, both progress and persistent gaps in improving nurse work environments have resulted.

Healthy work environments are critical in achieving the fourth aim of the Quintuple Aim—improved clinical experience (health and well-being of the care providers). While many aspects impact the health and well-being of care providers (e.g., an increased workload caused by the need to see more patients, budgetary constraints, changes in workflow, and so on), the work environment continues to have the greatest impact on nurses' health and well-being. Through their meta-analysis, Lake et al. (2019) found the nurse work environment to be a powerful driver of quality, safety, and experience outcomes in hospitals. Recent studies indicate that work environments in which nurses believe their physical and psychological safety are a priority have a greater influence than staffing optimization on many of the key indicators of patient safety, quality, satisfaction with care, and reimbursement (Press Ganey, 2016). Hospitals and healthcare systems are beginning to realize that to be competitive in the present consumer-driven, value-based marketplace, they must understand and attend to these environmental influences to achieve their strategic goals.

Workplace stressors that have a negative impact on the healthy work environment can be placed in five categories: staffing shortages, regulatory requirements, disruptive and disrespectful behaviors from patients and families, poor leadership behaviors (lack of authenticity and trust), and a hostile work culture (bullying and incivility) (Grant et al., 2020). As indicated in Box 12.1 (Mento et al., 2020), bullying, incivility, and workplace violence continue to have serious consequences for nurses, the organization, and the community. A review of the literature demonstrates the importance of creating an environment that promotes professionalism, respect, strong communication, and kindness to enhance patient outcomes, prevent errors, and enhance staff engagement and satisfaction (Munro, 2020; Vessey & Williams, 2021; McCright et al., 2019; ANA, 2019; Rehder et al., 2020; Grant et al., 2020; Bowles et al., 2019).

Changing culture starts at the top and must be role modeled by leaders. The American Nurses Credentialing Center is designed to help organizations develop a culture of safety, respect, and excellence through such programs as the Pathway to Excellence® designation. Recommendations to address a culture of safety and a healthy work environment are as follows (McCright et al., 2019, p. 11):

- Develop, maintain, and enforce a zero-tolerance policy for workplace violence, incivility, and bullying.
- Establish a culture of respect and safety that's foundational to the organization's mission, values, and philosophy.
- Ensure staff awareness of workplace violence, incivility, and bullying policies during orientation and then through frequent updates.
- Provide education and practice conflict negotiation/resolution skills.
- Encourage and support self-care, stress reduction and management, fatigue reduction, and resilience training.
- Offer ongoing support for those who've experienced workplace violence.
- Have systems in place that encourage and allow staff to report violence, including verbal abuse, and track and trend all reports.

Nursing leaders have a responsibility to create and maintain healthy work environments. Strong nursing leadership has been highly correlated with positive work environments that have resulted in improved quality of care and nurse retention. Leaders must actively support ensuring zero tolerance for incivility, bullying, and workplace violence. They must address it as soon as it is identified and coach and mentor their staff toward stronger communication skills. However, leaders are not present 24 hours a day. They rely on the informal or shift leaders in the unit to help ensure the expectations for professional, respectful, and kind communication and that behaviors are being met through coaching of their colleagues when issues arise. This, too, can be a challenge due to fear of reprisal, fear of loss of relationship, or simply for a lack of wanting to get involved. As identified by Bowles et al. (2019), many resources and pathways are in place to help lead the way to a healthier work environment. However, engagement is needed from not only leadership to set the tone to change the culture but also the nurses and interdisciplinary team to combat incivility and bullying from a grass roots perspective.

Nurse administrators must monitor the work environment constantly for subtle changes that may lead to

---

BOX 12.1 Negative Impacts of Workplace Violence

For the individual:
- Job dissatisfaction leading to decreased productivity
- Psychological illnesses—such as depression, anxiety, and suicidal ideation—that may lead to drug or alcohol abuse
- Burnout—exhibiting symptoms such as cynicism, emotional exhaustion, decrease in professional self-worth
- Potential of workplace violence leading to nurses leaving the workforce

For the workplace:
- Absences due to work injuries or sick days (costly due to replacement workers or overtime to meet the needs of patient care)
- Frequent absenteeism (decreases continuity and may impact clinical practice)
- Burnout leading to leaving the organization
- Decreased job satisfaction (impacts quality and work environment)

For the community:
- Access to quality health services threatened

job dissatisfaction and burnout. They must also work to help nurses have a sense of empowerment and control over their work environment. By examining factors that affect nurses' job satisfaction, organizations can begin to balance retention, cost containment, and patient outcomes.

Characteristics of Healthy Work Environment
Organizational Justice

Organizations that work to create and maintain healthy work environments have observable common characteristics. One characteristic is organizational justice, which is described as an employee perceiving fairness in practices related to distributive, procedural, interpersonal, and informational dimensions (Mengstie, 2020). Table 12.2 illustrates four types of justice.

Hashish (2020) found that nurses value organizational justice, and organizations that value justice and fairness from the leadership to the bedside have stronger outcomes and healthy work environments. Organizational justice concepts can usually be identified through mission, vision, and value statements that describe the philosophic approach of the organization. Examples of key words that reflect organizational justice include *respect, dignity, fairness, compassion,* and *advocacy.* Organizations that utilize and promote just cultures help to create a healthy work environment. The overall impression of a healthy work environment is a sense of teamwork and community across disciplines that meets organizational goals and promotes job satisfaction.

Leadership and Healthy Work Environment

Another characteristic of a healthy work environment is a strong sense of trust between management and employees. Disruptive behaviors between team members have been linked to increased medical errors and adverse events, reduced quality of care and patient safety, higher mortality rates, and, for the organization, higher staff turnover and lower staff satisfaction (Rehder et al., 2020). Trust is foundational to developing strong relationships between the leader and the staff. To build trust, leaders must be respectful, kind, consistent in practices and commitments, empathetic, and authentic (Sherman, 2019). One of the key components for building trust between a leader and the team is psychological safety. Psychological safety is a key factor in healthy work environments that support staff to speak up about problems or concerns without fear of retaliation (Sherman, 2019; Greene et al., 2020). Nurse leaders play an important role in creating and maintaining the psychological work environment by implementing leadership practices consistent with the psychosocial needs of those who work with them. This includes creating clarity and expectations for behaviors and actions from the leader but also among the team.

During the COVID-19 pandemic, a great deal of mistrust developed in some organizations because the policies changed so rapidly. What was true at the beginning of a shift might be replaced with newer information by the end—change was happening that quickly. This is an extreme example of how critical clear and truthful communication is in maintaining a healthy work environment. However, mistrust can result in times of regular conditions in the wake of lack of clarity in communication from leadership.

> **EXERCISE 12.1**   Identify common characteristics of a healthy work environment. From your perspective, which characteristics do you believe are most important? Would your perspective change in a leadership position?

TABLE 12.2   Four Types of Justice

Type of Justice	Definition of Justice
Distributive Justice	The balance between one's perceived contributions relative to what is received from the organization—for example, salary or promotion is based on skills and contributions.
Procedural Justice	The perceived fairness of the process by which outcomes are derived.
Interpersonal Justice	The perceived quality or extent to which people are treated with dignity and respect.
Informational Justice	Related to transparency and authenticity of information and decision-making.

Zero Tolerance for Workplace Violence, Bullying, and Incivility

[S]ome states have enacted legislation to protect nurses, at least in some settings, from physical violence in the workplace. This is a result of collective action through legislation.

Violence in healthcare, whether from persons external or internal to an organization, has been shown to have negative effects: increased job stress, reduced productive work time, decreased morale, and increased staff turnover. Violence is also linked to both physical and mental health consequences (Chaiwuth et al., 2020; Grant et al., 2020; McCright et al., 2019). Not all healthcare workplace violence is of a physical nature; like any other business, the workplace is subject to intradisciplinary and interdisciplinary incivility or bullying. The ANA *Position Statement: Incivility, Bullying and Workplace Violence* (2015b) describes incivility as one or more rude, discourteous, or disrespectful actions that may or may not have a negative intent behind them. Bullying is "repeated, unwanted harmful actions intended to humiliate, offend and cause distress in the recipient" (ANA, 2015b). Workplace violence impacts nurses, the interdisciplinary team, and patient safety. It led to the creation of the Quintuple Aim—staff well-being (Grant et al., 2020). Incivility and bullying, whether subtle, covert, or overt, affects every nursing setting, from academia to practice (Box 12.2).

Studies report that bullying can result in psychological symptoms in the victims, such as anxiety, sleep problems, depression, burnout, or increased substance use, and can negatively impact job satisfaction and effective engagement (see Box 12.1) (Chaiwuth et al., 2020; Grant et al., 2020; McCright et al., 2019). Any type of violence in healthcare interferes with opimal job performance and has negative effects on the delivery of high-quality patient care (Chaiwuth et al., 2020; Grant et al., 2020; McCright et al., 2019). Ulrich et al. (2019) completed a study with 8080 critical care nurses regarding healthy work environment elements and prevalence of workplace violence. Of the participants, 42% indicated that they do not routinely report incidents of workplace violence. The reasons cited for not reporting were as follows: the RNs did not think anything would be done about the incident, some felt it was not a major issue, and others feared retribution. Workplace violence in nursing is an international issue that has garnered attention and a call to action from not only the American Nurses Association (ANA), The Joint Commission, and the National Institute of

---

BOX 12.2 Range of Bullying Behaviors

Overt
- Aggressive behaviors, such as shouting or threatening harm
- Being accused of making errors made by someone else
- Nonverbal intimidation
- Eye rolling
- Physical harm

Covert
- Being sabotaged
- Having information or resources withheld that affects performance
- Moving the "goal post" in a person's work without informing them
- Giving confusing or inaccurate information
- Being told tasks were urgent when they were not
- Not responding when a response is called for

Subtle
- Being excluded from activities
- Being gossiped about
- Having opinions ignored
- Assigned unreasonable unpleasant or impossible tasks, targets, or deadlines
- Being humiliated at work
- Having key areas of responsibility removed or replaced with trivial or unpleasant tasks
- Having all decisions challenged
- Being manipulated into taking on roles or tasks that were not in the nurse's best interest

---

Occupational Safety and Health (NIOSH) but also from the World Health Organization (WHO). The common message from these organizations is that all members of the profession must be acquainted with the types and degrees of violence and learn how to manage them.

In 2015, the ANA created a Professional Issues Panel on Incivility, Bullying, and Workplace Violence. The panel revised a previous position statement that charges all registered nurses to "create a culture of respect that is free of incivility, bullying and workplace violence" (para 1). The position statement stresses that any form of workplace violence threatens nursing's contract with society (ANA, 2015b) and that any nurse who chooses to ignore or fail to report such violence is perpetuating it. In their Sentinel Event Alert 59, The Joint Commission advocated for organizations to commit to a policy of zero harm to patients and staff in regard to workplace violence (zero tolerance) (The Joint Commission, 2018). Violence is not a part of the profession, and nurses deserve to work in a safe working environment. No organization can completely prevent or eliminate workplace violence. Planning effective programs can dramatically reduce the chances of violence or incivility.

Workplace violence is not an isolated, individual problem. Rather, it is a structural problem rooted in social, economic, organizational, and cultural factors. Consequently, strategic interventions should be developed that attack the problem at its root. This involves all concerned taking into account the organizational, cultural, and gender dimensions of the problem. The ANA and The Joint Commission recommend that every healthcare organization create an infrastructure to identify and alleviate the occurrences and impacts of workplace violence, bullying, and incivility (McCright et al., 2019). This requires sharing a common vision and goals, actively promoting the development of socialization processes, sharing problems, and supporting group problem solving. A clear policy statement should be issued from top management in consultation with stakeholders, recognizing the importance of the fight against workplace violence. The statement should contain a clear definition of violence and an organizational commitment of zero tolerance to any form of violence. Raising awareness about the negative effects of workplace violence can help gain support for planned interventions. The Workplace Civility Index© is a tool that can be used to raise awareness and identify strengths and areas for improvement in regard to the perception of workplace civility (Clark et al., 2018).

Organizations that prioritize a just culture with a healthy work environment for all members of the institution will attain stronger patient outcomes as well as stronger staff safety, leading to a zero harm culture. However, in order for this to occur, organizations must commit fully to a just culture and healthy work environment. This commitment must start at the top. When management role-models positive attitudes and behaviors in the workplace, the entire organization is likely to follow suit. A management style based on openness, communication, and dialogue can greatly contribute to the diffusion and elimination of workplace violence. Particular attention should be paid to new nurses in their transitional year when they are at highest risk for being a target of incivility (Craft et al., 2020).

> **EXERCISE 12.2** Think about your behavior in the workplace. Have you ever acted in a way that could be described as bullying or incivility? How might you guard against such behaviors? Do you think you would confront a coworker participating in bullying? If you were a manager, how would you handle incivility on your unit?

Adoption of Standards for a Healthy Work Environment

Characteristics of healthy work environments discussed earlier are in alignment with the American Association of Critical-Care Nurses (AACN, 2016) standards for establishing and maintaining healthy work environments. The six standards include skilled communication, true collaboration, effective decision-making, appropriate staffing, meaningful recognition, and authentic leadership. The standards recognize the links between the quality of the work environment and its impact on nursing care and practice outcomes (Fig. 12.3). Organizations that adopt these standards and actively seek to improve the work environment are attractive to nurses and generally have positive outcomes, as demonstrated through the Research Perspective.

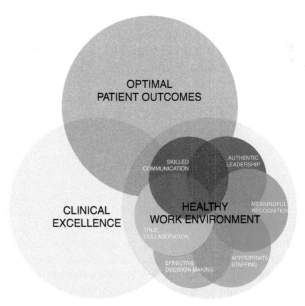

Fig. 12.3 Interdependence of healthy work environment, clinical excellence, and patient outcomes. (From American Association of Critical-Care Nurses. [2016]. *AACN Standards for establishing and sustaining healthy work environments: A journey to excellence* (2nd ed.). Aliso Viejo, CA: Author.)

RESEARCH PERSPECTIVE

Resource: Ulrich, B., Barden, C., Cassidy, L., & Varn-Davis, N. (2019). Critical care nurse work environments 2018: Findings and implications. *Critical Care Nurse, 39*(2), 67–84.

The health of critical care nurse work environments affects patient and nurse outcomes. The results of the 2018 Critical Care Nurse Work Environment Study are reported with comparisons to previous studies and recommendations for continued improvement. The objective was to evaluate the current state of critical care nurse work environments. An online survey was used to collect quantitative and qualitative data for this mixed-methods study. A total of 8080 AACN members and constituents responded to the survey. The results demonstrated that the health of critical care nurse work environments has improved since the previous study in 2013. However, areas of concern and opportunities for improvement still exist. Key findings include documented absence of appropriate staffing by more than 60% of participants; an alarming number of physical and mental well-being issues (198,340 incidents reported by 6017 participants); one-third of the participants expressed intent to leave their current positions in the next 12 months; and evidence of the positive outcomes of implementing the AACN Healthy Work Environment standards.

Implications for Practice
The results of this study provide evidence of the positive relationship between implementation of the AACN Healthy Work Environment standards and the health of critical care nurse work environments, between the health of critical care nurse work environments and job satisfaction, and between job satisfaction and intent of critical care nurses to leave their current positions or stay. This study also demonstrates the need to continue to focus on safer staffing matrices as well as the need to focus on the physical and mental health and well-being of the clinicians.

WORKPLACE ADVOCACY, ENGAGEMENT, AND EMPOWERMENT

Workplace advocacy is an umbrella term that includes an array of activities and strategies undertaken to address the challenges faced by nurses in their practice settings. Healthy workplaces require active participation of all members of the work unit to create conditions in which it is safe to speak up, hazards can be addressed quickly, incivility is addressed, and diversity is supported. Workplace advocacy reflects a framework of mutuality, facilitation, protection, and coordination in which nurses control their own practice and which is consistent with the goals of the nursing profession. Workplace advocacy activities and strategies focus on career development, employment opportunities, terms and conditions of employment, employment rights and protections, control of practice, labor-management relations, occupational health and safety, and employee assistance. The objective of workplace advocacy is to equip nurses to practice in a rapidly changing environment. Workplace advocacy must be practiced by both staff and leaders to be effective. For example, just as the manager needs an awareness of when a staff member is too tired to work, the staff member must also acknowledge that condition and make the decision to decline additional work. This idea can be expanded to include a staff member having an awareness of when the leader is also too tired or stressed to be effective. Proactively addressing such issues improves the workplace and supports nurses, which also benefits patients.

Engagement in the workplace is defined as an employee's commitment to the organization's mission, vision, and values. Engagement contributes to the success of an organization while also enhancing an individual's sense of professional and personal satisfaction. An engaged workforce is critical for minimizing the risks of patient harm by complex healthcare services (Olender et al., 2020). Trust and autonomy are required for engagement in the workplace. Creating a supportive environment in which trust is the core of the work takes effort on the part of all members of the team. Rather than worrying about "am I safe here," all can focus on improving their mutual work. Autonomy, the freedom to make independent decisions consistent within the scope of practice, is also necessary for engagement. When nurses share their individual decisions with each other, they help others move toward more expert practice either through acquiring new knowledge or through challenging the status quo. Autonomy encourages innovation, which may result in processes to improve patient care and reduce cost. Engagement is a critical factor that helps to create a healthy work environment and organizational satisfaction (O'Rourke, 2021). Nurse engagement impacts patient safety and patient outcomes and can promote professional nursing practice (Richey & Waite, 2019).

Engagement is accomplished by leaders who coach and mentor their staff. For example, clinicians experience the positive impact of their actions in their unit-based council as they are building leadership skills such as leading effective meetings, facilitating decision-making, negotiating through conflict, and leading their peers and the council (Hancock & Meadows, 2020). Leadership behaviors that promote an environment focused on trust, support, accountability, creativity, and risk-taking and innovation tend to lead to higher levels of nurse engagement (Richey & Waite, 2019). Successful engagement can be measured by better patient outcomes and satisfaction with the healthcare received as well as by improved nurse job satisfaction and better nurse retention. Engagement requires individual and group action.

EXERCISE 12.3   Investigate how your organization promotes nurse engagement.
- How is engagement measured in this organization?
- Do you believe that the engagement strategies are effective?
- What ideas do you have to improve nurse engagement?

Empowerment in the workplace is defined as sharing power and control through participation in shared decision-making. Empowerment basically translates to supporting nurses and their voice in their own practice. Empowered clinicians are associated with stronger engagement, satisfaction, and a stronger commitment to the organization (Olender et al., 2020). Clinicians develop a sense of empowerment through their personal accountability as well as their participation in the collective work and decision-making through professional governance structures (Porter-O'Grady, 2019). Staff feel empowered when they have the resources and tools to perform their duties, opportunities for advancement, and a sense of autonomy and power within their work setting (Olender et al., 2020). As with engagement, leaders play a critical role in creating the environment to promote empowerment. Engagement and empowerment are linked concepts—you cannot have one without the other. Both promote improved patient outcomes and increased job satisfaction and create a positive work environment for nurses. Box 12.3 demonstrates how professional governance structures and processes enhance engagement and empowerment. Box 12.4 (Oss et al., 2021) identifies the outcomes of professional governance structures.

BOX 12.3   Effects of Professional Governance Structures and Processes

Professional governance structures and processes create an environment that:
- Enhances clinical practice through full ownership and practicing at the top of licensure
- Improves quality, competence, and knowledge
- Creates a culture of accountability and professional obligation
- Models strong shared decision-making

From Porter-O'Grady, T., & Clavelle, J. T. (2020). The structural framework for nursing professional governance: Foundation for empowerment. *Nurse Leader, 18*(2), 181–189.

BOX 12.4   Demonstrated Outcomes of Successful Professional Governance Structures

- Improved patient outcomes and satisfaction
- Improve staff satisfaction and engagement
- Culture of professionalism and accountability

PROFESSIONAL PRACTICE RESPONSIBILITY

Nurses have the right to practice in environments that allow them to act in accordance with professional standards and legally authorized scopes of practice. The nurse practice act of each state governs the scope of nursing practice and guides nurses and protects the public in performing their duties. Nurses are also guided by the ANA's *Code of Ethics with Interpretive Statements* (ANA, 2015a). The *Code of Ethics* speaks to the responsibility and accountability of nurses to be advocates for patients and their families, whether it is intervening on their behalf or working with healthcare organizations through decision-making processes. It also means participating in shaping healthcare policy at the institutional, local, state, or national level. To be able to meet the professional ethical obligations to society, nurses and others must protect the dignity and autonomy of nurses in the workplace. To protect the rights of nurses, the ANA Bill of Rights speaks to several concepts covered in this chapter. The key foci of these rights appear in Box 12.5. This document sets forth seven premises concerning workplace expectations and

BOX 12.5 American Nurses Association Nurses' Bill of Rights

The Bill of Rights is designed to delineate the corollary to statements of responsibilities. The latter can be found in numerous documents: state laws, rules and regulations, position descriptions, and professional standards. With responsibilities, certain rights need to be clear. The American Nurses Association identifies that nurses have certain rights that:

- Meet obligations to society and patients
- Meet professional and legal standards
- Allow for ethical practice
- Facilitate advocacy
- Support fair compensation
- Ensure safety
- Address employment conditions

environments that nurses from across the United States recognize are necessary for sound professional nursing practice. The *Code of Ethics* (2015a) outlines the ethical obligations and duties of every individual who enters the nursing profession and is an expression of nursing's own understanding of its commitment to society. The ethical standards for the profession help nurses determine whether their work environments support ethical practice.

The ANA *Code of Ethics* Provision 6 (ANA, 2015a) states that "the nurse, through individual and collective action, establishes, maintains, and improves the moral environment of the work setting and the conditions of employment, conducive to quality health care."

EXERCISE 10.4 In your most recent clinical experiences, consider the following. How would you as an individual nurse demonstrate that you are meeting this provision? If you assumed the role of a manager or leader, how would you demonstrate meeting the provision?

Ownership of practice is the professional responsibility of a registered nurse to be accountable for one's practice and the impact it has on patient outcomes (Wilson & Galuska, 2020). Nurses who own their practice will be more successful in providing emotionally supportive evidence-based care to their patients. Ownership of

practice comes when nurses have a sense of pride in their work as well as an expectation of themselves to do the right thing (Sherman & Cohn, 2019). Furthermore, they promote a culture of safety by ensuring that their colleagues are practicing to their fullest potential through mentoring and peer-to-peer accountability. Finally, nurses who own their practice tend to be more empowered and engaged, promoting their organizational mission, vision, and values.

Professional Governance

Since the 1980s, many organizations have been putting shared governance structures into place to enhance patient and staff outcomes and satisfaction. Shared governance structures engage and empower nurses in decisions and actions that impact their practice at the bedside (Porter-O'Grady & Clavelle, 2020). Typically, these were done through a council framework (unit-based and/or facility-level councils). However, most shared governance structures tend to remain hierarchal in nature and do not truly support the clinicians to fully own their practice (Porter O'Grady, 2019).

Professional governance builds on the structures of shared governance and emphasizes accountability, shared decision-making, professional obligation, and strong relationships for bedside clinicians (Porter-O'Grady & Clavelle, 2020). A strong professional governance structure and culture creates a foundation for collaboration within and between departments; peer-based relationships through peer accountability and feedback; stronger communication within and throughout the organization; and collective and collaborative decision-making, which enhances a sense of empowerment and professional ownership (Boxes 12.2 and 12.4) (Porter-O'Grady & Clavelle, 2020).

Professional governance derives from a diverse theoretical perspective, as shown in the Theory Box. Nursing lacks a general definition of shared governance. No common understanding of the shared governance concept can be described by a specified theory with precepts and propositions. This has contributed to persistent barriers to progress toward increasing the scientific rigor related to shared governance research and building evidence-based knowledge through its systematic study.

Since at least 2009, Tim Porter-O'Grady, a leader in the development of shared governance models, has described shared governance as a professional practice model based on the principles of partnership, equity, accountability, and ownership (Porter-O'Grady, 2009).

THEORY BOX

Professional Governance: Evolution from Shared Practices to Professional Practices

Key Contributors	Key Idea	Application to Practice
Porter-O'Grady, T., & Clavelle, J. T. (2020). The structural framework for nursing professional governance: Foundation for empowerment. *Nurse Leader, 18*(2), 181–189.	Shared governance focused on structures and processes to engage nurses in decision-making for initiatives that impact their practice. Professional Governance is based on nurse accountability for practice. Professional governance structures embed the requirements of the professional practice within them. They include: • Related knowledge • Education • Practices • Performance • Regulation • Impact The structures allow nurses to control their practice through accountability, quality, competence, and nursing knowledge. Ownership of practice is the foundation of accountability. Professional nurses accept responsibility of the impact of their practice on patient outcomes. Therefore, it is critical to be involved in decisions that impact that practice. In addition to solid structures, positive and appreciative leadership is critical to ensure professional behaviors that are in alignment with organizational goals and outcomes. Appreciative leaders have strong relationships with their teams. They motivate and inspire nurses and create an empowered environment where nurses collaborate with leaders to create a professional practice environment.	By creating structures and processes that elicit professional behaviors, nurses are able to own their practice and are engaged in decision-making that impacts that practice. Patients benefit through better outcomes and nurses benefit as they have a stronger sense of satisfaction and value in the work they do.

Professional governance structures and culture provide a way to empower nurses to manage their professional practice. As Porter-O'Grady and Clavelle (2020) stated, "the shift to professional governance implies membership in a professional community and the assurance that decisions and actions represent the standards of the profession and positively impact intended outcomes" (p. 211). Organizations that foster a professional governance structure and culture have recognized improved nurse retention and job satisfaction by providing nurses an opportunity to get involved. Professional governance provides the platform for empowering nurses in decision-making that impacts their clinical practice, strengthening their ownership of practice and improving

patient outcomes (Medeiros, 2019). In recent years, the idea of shared governance has spread to other disciplines within healthcare and created the opportunity for interprofessional learning and communication about shared issues. This opportunity has allowed nurses to engage in constructive communication across disciplines. The Research Perspective identifies outcomes related to interprofessional shared governance.

At its core, professional governance is shared decision-making. With the complexity of today's healthcare systems, professional governance provides a structure to decentralize decision-making. To achieve decentralization, these structures include the establishment of councils within the organization at the unit

RESEARCH PERSPECTIVE

Resource: Olender, L., Capitulo, K., & Nelson, J. (2020). The impact of interprofessional shared governance and a caring professional practice model on staff's self-report of caring, workplace engagement, and workplace empowerment over time. *Journal of Nursing Administration, 50*(1), 52–58.

The objective of this study was to describe the impact of the implementation of interprofessional shared governance and a caring professional practice model—Relationship-Based Care (RBC)—on the staff's self-report of caring, work engagement, and workplace empowerment over a 4-year time frame. Utilizing Jean Watson's Theory of Human Caring and appreciative inquiry as underlying frameworks, a longitudinal, quantitative study design was employed. Interprofessional focus groups and introductory sessions were offered to inform and engage all personnel within the medical center. Motivated units were identified, professional shared governance council members elected, and unit-specific education provided. Quality improvement initiatives were facilitated within unit councils, and formal leadership programs to enhance project guidance and to support staff empowerment skills for the managers of the units that were up and running were provided. Pre-implementation and post-implementation measurements of staff's caring, workplace engagement, and work empowerment were assessed, compared, and trended across units over time.

Implication for Practice

Shared governance facilitates frontline decision-making at the point of care, where care is provided. Moreover, associated initiatives, such as establishing a communication network to ensure a comprehensive approach to changes, is critical for the success of these councils. The development of a professional practice model and staff involvement with salient quality care initiatives are crucial for high reliability in the provision of quality care. Transitioning from a directive governance model to a professional governance model is a major transformational and cultural change requiring an extended time frame and the support from key stakeholders within the organization.

level and facility level where professional decisions and actions are made and developed that impact the point of service. Every council must have a management representative to mentor and coach staff through the decision-making process as well as ensure that the resources are available for these decisions (Porter O'Grady & Clavelle, 2021). Additionally, professional staff representation on management councils enhances the partnership between leadership and clinicians as well as providing a "locus for the resolution of differences and challenges" that may arise due to the different perspectives from leadership and clinicians (Porter O'Grady & Clavelle, 2020, p. 210).

A reporting and data management structure is necessary to ensure good communication and demonstrate alignment of goals from the bedside to the boardroom. Organizations must be willing to be transparent with their data, especially the data that reflects clinician practice and patient outcomes. Nurses cannot effectively and efficiently identify opportunities for improvement if they do not have unhampered access to the data that reflect their practice. Implementing a professional governance practice model requires leadership and planning to support staff and demonstrate improved outcomes. Working in a professional governance structure improves the flow of information, stimulates innovation, and reinforces the importance of "us" as a total team-based approach.

Effective professional governance strategies include principles and mechanisms for conflict resolution. To have effective conflict resolution, leadership structures should engage nursing staff to provide decision support and input regarding changes in workflow design at the point of care to improve care delivery systems, processes, and work environments. This requires nurses to become adept at conflict resolution, communication, and negotiation to be adequately prepared to address issues that arise.

MAGNET® AND PATHWAY TO EXCELLENCE® RECOGNITION

The American Nurses Credentialing Center (ANCC, 2021) endorses hospitals that achieve nursing excellence and exceptional patient outcomes through the Magnet Recognition Program®. The designation indicates that the organization has characteristics that produce improved patient outcomes, attracts and retains nurses, demonstrates exemplary professional practice, and has transformational leadership and evidence-based practices. Professional governance structures provide the infrastructure to engage and empower clinicians to participate in decisions that will impact not only their practice but patient outcomes as well, thereby enhancing the opportunity of the organization to obtain Magnet® certification.

Through the Magnet® process, hospitals undergo organizational transformation that significantly improves the quality of the nurse work environment. Achieving recognition has also demonstrated marked improvement in patient outcomes and patient satisfaction (Lasater et al., 2019; Rodríguez-García et al., 2020). Additionally, through their systematic review, Rodríguez-García et al. were able to demonstrate positive outcomes for Magnet® organizations through lower mortality rates, lower workplace accidents, and decreased nurse turnover, leading to an increase in revenue and cost savings.

Magnet® hospitals must sustain their standards and demonstrate excellence in patient care outcomes and clinical practice. Magnet® designation is a multi-year commitment; thus, it offers a long-term framework for quality improvement efforts and a means for engaging and motivating staff at all levels. The Magnet® brand and its significance is becoming increasingly well known to the public. There are approximately 523 hospitals in the United States that have achieved ANCC Magnet Recognition® status, greater than 10% of all registered hospitals (Campaign for Action, 2020). A Magnet® environment is identified by nurses feeling valued by the organization, having standardized processes, staff empowerment, strong leadership, a sense of community, and strategic planning that reflects the missions and goals of the organization (AACN, 2016).

The ANCC Pathway to Excellence Program® recognizes healthcare and long-term care organizations for positive practice environments for nurses. To qualify, organizations meet practice standards essential to an ideal nursing practice environment similar to those of the Magnet® program. Pathway® designation can be achieved only if an organization's nurses validate the data and other evidence submitted via an independent, confidential survey. This critical element exemplifies the theme of empowering and supporting nurses' voice. Pathway®-designated organizations demonstrate respect for nursing contributions, support professional development, and nurture optimal practice environments. Organizations may hold Pathway® and Magnet® designations simultaneously.

COLLECTIVE ACTION, COLLECTIVE BARGAINING, AND UNIONIZATION IN NURSING

Collective action is defined as activities that are undertaken by a group of people who have common interests. In 1998, Minarik and Catramabone saw collective participation for nurses as having four main purposes: (1) promote the practice of professional nursing, (2) establish and maintain standards of care, (3) allocate resources effectively and efficiently, and (4) create satisfaction and support in the practice environment. While this work was more than 20 years ago, it is still relevant in our current promotion of practice. When nurses work to achieve Magnet® status, it is the result of collective action. When nurses participate in professional governance activities to impact their clinical practice, it is the result of collective action. When patient care is delivered in hospitals 24 hours per day, it is the result of the collective action of shifts of nurses. When patients transfer from one specialty clinic to another without disruption of care, it is the result of collective action. The collective action of nurses requires a level of independence during the shift and interdependence among shifts and settings and with other healthcare professionals. Nurses learn quickly to rely on their colleagues but have been less comfortable with formal collectives, such as unions. Understanding power and learning how to use it are essential for nurses to influence practice, work environments, and public policies that affect health. Collective action has been and continues to be utilized to move agendas forward through the collective voice of shared values and goals. Organizational governance structures provide the framework for this participation (Porter-O'Grady, 2019). Collective action can result in an empowered and engaged workforce. When large numbers of nurses in a common setting are engaged in the practice environment, the results are impressive: improved work life, reduced nurse turnover, improved relationships with management, improved patient care, and increased patient satisfaction. Collective action is facilitated by leader behaviors that encourage participative decision-making, display confidence in employees, promote autonomy, and promote ownership of their practice and profession (Porter-O'Grady, 2019).

Collective bargaining is a process of negotiations between employers and a group of employees aimed at reaching agreements to regulate working conditions. Collective bargaining agreements usually address salary, working hours, overtime, training, health and safety, and the right to participate in workplace or organizational decision-making that affects, in our case, nursing practice. Although it is possible to engage in collective bargaining without a union, a union model is commonly used when other methods have failed to achieve results. Collective bargaining provides an opportunity for workers to voice their opinion on issues related to their employment and to protect their interest through collective action. In healthcare, unionization allows for negotiation or bargaining from a position of strength that is in the interest of patients, nurses, and the organization. The goal is to prevent conflict and resolve problems with mutual benefit. In negotiation, failing to reach an agreement can lead to decreased organizational productivity, strikes, lock-outs, and deteriorating working relationships between management and labor. While seeking to ensure economic and general welfare for nurses, nurses engaged in collective bargaining also seek to keep the interests of both nurses and patients in balance. In the current healthcare environment, nurses may find themselves struggling with the complexity and bureaucratic nature of the large multihospital or multistate organizations that employ them. This creates an inherent tension between the desire for clinical autonomy and the need to work within organizational structures and policies. The COVID-19 pandemic aggravated many issues that nurses in unions were attempting to resolve. As a result, we saw more headlines focused on union activities, including strikes.

Union or At Will

A union is an organization of workers who have come together to achieve common goals, such as protecting the integrity of the trade; improving safety standards; achieving higher wages and benefits, such as healthcare and retirement; increasing the number of employees an employer assigns to complete the work; and better working conditions. Collaboration and understanding are paramount for both the bargaining nurses and the organizations when there is a disagreement. Both parties need to keep patient safety and quality care at the center of their decisions (Catlin, 2020). Nurses have a legal right to bargain. The ANA has long supported the rights of registered nurses to have the freedom of choice regarding how they engage in their work environments.

The freedom to decide to organize is underscored in the ANA's *Code of Ethics for Nurses with Interpretive Statements* (2015a).

EXERCISE 12.5
- If you were considering employment at a facility that is unionized, what questions might you want to ask?
- What does it mean to sign a union card?
- How might you educate yourself about unions and the collective bargaining process?

Changes in labor laws have had a direct effect on the level of union activity in the healthcare sector (Box 12.6). A 2018 labor statistics report from the U.S. Department of Labor indicates overall union membership of wage and salary workers in the United States is in decline—down from 20.1% in 1983, which is the first year of reporting, to 10.8% in 2020. Union coverage for nurses has not fallen in the same way as it has for the workforce overall. In contrast, the union rate for nurses is approximately 20.4%, steadily increasing year after year (Burger, 2020). In part, nurses' union coverage rates have been more stable because of successful organizing drives, enlisting community support, coverage through social or other electronic media technologies, and the continued growth of healthcare.

The fear of arbitrary discipline and dismissal may be the catalyst for nurses to seek ways to protect themselves from what are perceived to be capricious actions. The discipline structure provided by a union contract treats all employees in the same manner and may decrease the manager's flexibility in designing or selecting discipline (Box 12.7). Managers of at-will employees have greater latitude in selecting disciplinary measures for specific infractions. State and federal laws do provide a level of protection; however, an at-will employee may be terminated at any time for any reason except discrimination. At-will employees, in essence, work at the will of the employer. Nurses in these positions need to know their rights and accountability. Although whistleblower legislation exists, the current environment in health care places the at-will employee who voices concern about the quality of care in a vulnerable position (see Literature Perspective). A new social order in the workplace must be based on a spirit of genuine cooperation between management and nurses.

BOX 12.6   Labor Laws and Unions

The federal role in labor relations is a dynamic, evolving one. The 1935 Wagner Act (National Labor Relations Act) gave employees the right to self-organize and form unions to bargain collectively. Under this law, employees could organize under the terms of the law without fear of being fired for belonging to or participating in a union. The National Labor Relations Board (NLRB) administers the National Labor Relations Act. State laws further define labor law.

Two years later, the American Nurses Association (ANA) included provisions for improving nurses' work and professional lives. The 1947 Taft-Hartley Act placed curbs on some union activity and excluded employees of nonprofit hospitals from coverage. This meant that employees and nurses working in nonprofit organizations did not have protections if they participated in unions. The rationale was that their services were so essential that organizing activities were a threat to the public's interest. The Labor Management Reporting and Disclosure Act of 1959, also known as the Landrum-Griffin Act, provided greater internal democracy within unions. The 1974 amendments to the Taft-Hartley Act removed the exemption of not-for-profit hospitals so that employees of these types of organizations have the same rights as industrial workers to join together and form labor unions; it included a 10-day warning period for the intent to strike or picket as a way to protect the public. This exemption was related to the ANA efforts to endorse collective bargaining. While working to secure collective bargaining protections, the ANA struggled with its role in representing nurses who were part of a union and those who were from right-to-work

states who did not support unionization. The removal of the exemption for not-for-profit hospitals created a frenzy of activity as traditional industrial unions targeted healthcare facilities.

In a 1991 unanimous opinion, the Supreme Court of the United States upheld the NLRB's ruling that provides for RN-only units. This decision was critical for nursing. At stake was the ability of nurses to control nursing practice and the quality of patient care. Employees, including nurses, must be accorded workplace rights and the protection that allows them to practice. Nurses must have the freedom to do what the profession and their licensure status requires them to do.

Labeling all RNs as supervisors is a second challenge to the right of nurses to organize. RNs monitor and assess patients as a part of their professional practice, not as a statutory supervisor within the definition of the National Labor Relations Act. A 1996 NLRB ruling held that RNs were not statutory supervisors and were protected by federal labor law; the decision was upheld in 1997 by the U.S. Court of Appeals for the Ninth Circuit (Nguyen, 1997). However, a 2001 Supreme Court decision (*National Labor Relations Board v. Kentucky River Community Care, Inc.*, 2001) upheld a lower court's decision to classify RNs as supervisors, though this decision was later appealed.

The most current rules governing the union election process can be found at:

National Labor Relations Board, *www.nlrb.gov/*

Basic Guide to the National Labor Relations Act: *www.nlrb.gov/sites/default/files/attachments/basic-page/node-3024/basicguide.pdf.*

BOX 12.7   Due Process

Union contract language requires management to follow "due process" for represented employees. In a *just culture*, a thorough investigation is considered due process. During the investigation, management will determine whether an action is a human error (inadvertent oversight), an at-risk behavior (taking shortcuts), or reckless behavior (knowingly doing the wrong thing). If reckless behavior is identified, management must provide a written statement outlining disciplinary charges, the penalty, and the reasons for the penalty. Management is required to maintain a record of attempts to counsel the employee. Employees have the right to defend themselves against

charges and the opportunity to settle disagreements in a formal grievance hearing. They have the right to have their representative with them during the process. Management must prove that the employee is wrong or in error. Management maintains the record of counseling. The commitment to nursing requires the manager to be clear about the charge. Although all disciplinary charges are important, those directly related to patient care have a more critical dimension. Clarity in describing the situation is important because it affects patient care, the individual nurse, and nurse colleagues. In a nonunion environment, the burden of proof is generally on the employee.

LITERATURE PERSPECTIVE

Resource: Cypher, R. L. (2021). Whistleblowing in healthcare: Allegations to actions. *Journal of Perinatal & Neonatal Nursing, 35*(1), 12–15.

Whistleblowing Protection

Whistleblowing is when an individual reports unethical or illegal practices to the public. In healthcare, this is typically driven by ethical obligations to protect patient safety. In order for the whistleblowing to be investigated, four conditions must be met: (1) the whistleblower must be in a position that qualifies as a whistleblower (current or former employee who has information on wrongdoing), (2) must present and have specific evidence that the individual has no authority to correct the wrongdoing, (3) the whistleblower must have an entity to make the report to, and (4) the entity receiving the report finds it valid. If you believe you are in a position to report illegal or unethical activities, identify what your rights and responsibilities are through your organization. The 1989 Whistleblower Protection Act protects federal workers; however, it does not cover the private sector. Each state has specific laws and there are federal laws that may apply as well. Be informed on what your rights and protections are—look up your organizational policies as well as your state laws. Whistleblowers need to understand the consequences of action and inaction (Cypher, 2021).

Implications for Practice

As mentioned at the beginning of this chapter, medical errors are neck-in-neck with stroke as the fifth leading cause of death. It is imperative that clinicians speak up when they have identified unsafe practices. However, unfortunately, not all organizations are on the journey to high reliability. Therefore, there may come a time when you will have to speak up to protect your patients and/or your community. If the normal channels of communication are ineffective, you are ethically bound to ensure patient safety and may find yourself in the position of a whistleblower. As mentioned earlier, ensure that you are well informed regarding your organizational policies and your state laws.

CONCLUSION

Nurses play a valuable role in the delivery of healthcare. Organizations and leaders who promote and foster a culture of safety will come to be regarded as centers of excellence. Leaders and managers should facilitate nurse input and create a safe space for nurses to voice their opinions and effect change. Healthy workplace environments require the active participation of all members and can be an avenue for organizations to attract the most qualified workforce. Attracting and retaining quality nurses is good for patients and good for healthcare organizations. Improved patient outcomes, lower costs, and increased job satisfaction are possible when nurses participate in decision-making that shapes their practice and creates positive change in the work environment. Engaging and empowering nurses in the workplace through shared professional governance, collective action, and collective bargaining is key.

Professional governance is an ongoing evolving process that requires continuous support and attention from nurses and nurse leaders. Progress and gains may stall over time, requiring support and innovation to be productive. True professional governance must have shared participation in decision-making. Collective action is when nurses work together to create an impact. An understanding of collective action and the roles of leaders and followers can help the individual nurse navigate in today's ever changing and complex healthcare environment. Negotiations may be competitive or collaborative; collaborative negotiations generally have more positive outcomes. Nurses must understand the rules and regulations that apply to workplace and workforce engagement strategies to make informed decisions about where they would like to work. Efforts toward creating a culture of safety and zero harm benefit patients, nurses, interdisciplinary team members, and the organization.

THE SOLUTION

When designing new structures, processes, and cultures, you must engage all stakeholders that will be impacted by the initiative. When the initiative was initially rolled out, we thought we had crossed all the t's and dotted all the i's. While this initiative focused on engaging bedside clinicians, it required the support and leadership of formal nursing leaders (nurse managers, senior directors, Chief Nursing Officers, and the Chief Nurse Executive). The executive leadership team was strongly engaged, but for some of the nurse managers, we were asking for a total change in processes and leadership (moving from an autocratic/authoritarian or laissez-faire leadership style to an authentic/transformational leadership style). Some managers were not clear on the actual concept of shared decision-making. This required educational classes as well as ongoing coaching and mentoring to ensure organizational sustainability.

Even after education and expectations were provided to nursing leaders, the Nurse Executive Council identified that not all Unit Practice Councils (UPCs) were practicing at the same level, as their support system (Unit Leadership) were not consistently coaching, mentoring, and adhering to the expectations initially developed by the Professional Governance Steering Committee. This led a subcommittee of that council to develop specific expectations for the Unit Directors and Clinical Nurse Specialists in regard to their mentorship and support of either UPCs, facility, or system-level councils. To address sustainability and oversight, the subcommittee developed a meeting assessment tool to provide objective data and feedback for the Chair, Co-Chair, UD Mentor and CNS Mentor. The subcommittee is currently working on a process to ensure inter-rater reliability for use of the assessment tool as well as a team to observe the UPCs, facility, and system-level councils in action.

Another challenge encountered was communication of the activities from the councils to the bedside. Initially, the councils utilized a "7×7" approach (no more than seven words in a bullet point and no more than seven bullet points). A separate subcommittee of the Nurse Executive Council was developed for the express purpose of enhancing communication. With feedback from system- and facility-level councils as well as the System Unit Director council, monthly huddle messages were developed with "What you need to do" and What you need to know" (action vs. information). Additionally, the subcommittee has expanded to look at the communication processes for internal (nursing department only), external (UCLA Health) and outside of the organization (through marketing, social media, etc.). One of the opportunities identified is the challenge of ensuring that nurses have the information they need in a timely fashion to be part of the decision-making process.

Three years later, the organization continues to review and revise the processes and structures to enhance the voice of the clinicians in the work that impacts their practice. To ensure that this structure continues to evolve and become stronger, the Nurse Executive Council reviews patient outcomes as well as the outcomes from the staff engagement surveys and challenges practice that does not improve outcomes, engaging the other councils to address the opportunities identified.

Culture change takes approximately 3 to 5 years to effect and recognize the change. Professional governance is more than a structure—it is a culture that promotes leadership, engagement, empowerment, ownership of practice, and improved outcomes. When implementing culture change initiatives, engage all stakeholders early, provide thorough education and expectations, and develop processes to ensure oversight and forward momentum for sustainability of the initiative. Additionally, it is important to be flexible and willing to change and enhance the initiative. What starts out as looking well formed and thought out on paper may look very different in action.

Would this be a suitable approach for you? If so, why?

R. Coleen Wilson, DNP, RN, NEA-BC

REFLECTIONS

How might you become involved in creating a healthier work environment where you are? What changes would you make? What are the most pressing changes to make? Respond in a one-paragraph summary.

BEST PRACTICES

The evidence continues to mount to show that people across various work settings who are engaged perform more effectively. Leaders and managers can put strategies in place to facilitate engagement. Yet, the peer group often is where engagement is initiated and supported on a day-to-day basis. Acting collectively has great influence when we address issues from the standpoint of benefiting patients and promoting retention of well-qualified staff. Focusing on creating a healthy workplace is a positive strategy that benefits staff and patients alike.

TIPS FOR WORKFORCE ENGAGEMENT AND COLLECTIVE ACTION

- Understanding the culture and the organization's approach to any collective action strategy is important for managers and staff.
- Create a list of pros and cons if a decision is being made regarding a unionized approach and include a comparison of various unions, especially in terms of representation of issues currently unresolved.
- Make a personal commitment to stop behaviors that perpetuate incivility or bullying.
- Investigate the AACN Standards for Establishing and Sustaining Healthy Work Environments.

REFERENCES

American Association of Critical-Care Nurses (AACN). (2016). *AACN standards for establishing and sustaining healthy work environments: A journey to excellence* (2nd ed.). Aliso Viejo, CA: American Association of Critical-Care Nurses. Retrieved from https://www.aacn.org/~/media/aacn-website/nursing-excellence/healthy-work-environment/execsum.pdf?la=en.

American College of Healthcare Executives (ACHE), IHI/NPSF Lucian Leape Institute. (2017). *Leading a Culture of Safety: A Blueprint for Success [White paper].* Retrieved from http://www.ihi.org/resources/Pages/Publications/Leading-a-Culture-of-Safety-A-Blueprint-for-Success.aspx.

American Nurses Association (ANA). (2015a). *Code of ethics for nurses with interpretive statements.* Silver Spring, MD: Author.

American Nurses Association (ANA). (2015b). *Position statement: Incivility, bullying and workplace violence.* https://www.nursingworld.org/practice-policy/nursing-excellence/official-position-statements/id/incivility-bullying-and-workplace-violence/.

American Nurses Association (ANA). (2019). Issue Brief. In *Reporting incidents of workplace violence.* Retrieved from https://www.nursingworld.org/globalassets/practiceandpolicy/work-environment/endnurseabuse/endabuse-issue-brief-final.pdf.

American Nurses Credentialing Center (ANCC). (2021). *ANCC Magnet Recognition Program.* https://www.nursingworld.org/organizational-programs/magnet/.

Bowles, J. R., Batcheller, J., Adams, J. M., Zimmermann, D., & Pappas, S. (2019). Nursing's leadership role in advancing professional practice/work environments as part of the Quadruple Aim. *Nursing Administration Quarterly, 43*(2), 157–163.

Burger, C. (2020). Do unions benefit or harm healthcare & nursing industries? In *Registered Nursing.org.* Retrieved from https://www.registerednursing.org/articles/do-unions-benefit-harm-healthcare-nursing.

Campaign for Action. (2020). *Number of hospitals in the United States with Magnet status.* Retrieved from https://campaignforaction.org/resource/number-hospitals-united-states-magnet-status/.

Catlin, A. (2020). Nursing strike, America, 2019: Concept analysis to guide practice. *Nursing Outlook, 68*(4), 468–475. https://doi-org.ezproxy.loyno.edu/10.1016/j.outlook.2020.03.002.

Centers for Disease Control and Prevention (CDC). (2021). *Leading Causes of Death.* Retrieved from https://www.cdc.gov/nchs/fastats/leading-causes-of-death.htm.

Clapper, T. C., & Ching, K. (2020). Debunking the myth that the majority of medical errors are attributed to communication. *Medical Education, 54*(1), 74–81.

Chaiwuth, S., Chanprasit, C., Kaewthummanukul, T., Chareosanti, J., Srisuphan, W., & Stone, T. E. (2020). Prevalence and risk factors of workplace violence among registered nurses in tertiary hospitals. *Pacific Rim International Journal of Nursing Research, 24*(4), 538–552.

Clark, C. M., Barbosa-Leiker, C., & Sattler, V. (2018). Development and psychometric testing of the Workplace Civility Index: A reliable tool to assess workplace civility. *Journal of Continuing Education in Nursing, 49*(9), 400–406.

Craft, J., Schivinski, E. L., & Wright, A. (2020). The grim reality of nursing incivility. *Journal for Nurses in Professional Development, 36*(1), 41–43.

Cypher, R. L. (2021). Whistleblowing in healthcare: Allegations to actions. *Journal of Perinatal & Neonatal Nursing, 35*(1), 12–15.

Grant, S., Davidson, J., Manges, K., Dermenchyan, A., Wilson, E., & Dowdell, E. (2020). Creating healthful work environments to deliver on the Quadruple Aim: A call to action. *The Journal of Nursing Administration, 50*(6), 314–321.

Greene, M. T., Gilmartin, H. M., & Saint, S. (2020). Psychological safety and infection prevention practices: Results from a national survey. *American Journal of Infection Control, 48*(1), 2–6.

Hancock, B., & Meadows, M. T. (2020). The nurse manager and professional governance: Catalysts for leadership development. *Nurse Leader, 18*(3), 265–268.

Hashish, E. (2020). Nurses' perception of organizational justice and its relationship to their workplace deviance. *Nursing Ethics, 27*(1), 273–288.

Institute of Medicine (US) Committee on the Work Environment for Nurses and Patient Safety. (2004). In A. Page (Ed.), *Keeping patients safe: Transforming the work environment of nurses.* Washington (DC): National Academies Press (US).

Institute of Medicine (IOM). (2000). *To err is human: Building a safer health system.* Washington, DC: National Academies Press.

Lake, E. T., Sanders, J., Duan, R., Riman, K. A., Schoenauer, K. M., & Chen, Y. (2019). A meta-analysis of the associations between the nurse work environment in hospitals and 4 sets of outcomes. *Medical Care, 57*(5), 353–361.

Lasater, K. B., Germack, H. D., Small, D. S., & McHugh, M. D. (2019). Hospitals known for nursing excellence perform better on value based purchasing measures. *JONA: The Journal of Nursing Administration, 49*(10S), S40–S49.

McCright, M., Blair, M., Applegate, B., Griggs, P., Backus, M., & Pabico, C. (2019). Addressing workplace violence with the Pathway to Excellence® framework. *Nursing Management, 50*(8), 10–13.

Medeiros, M. (2019). Improving outcomes, sharing innovations, celebrating excellence. *Nursing Management, 50*(1), 10–11.

Mengstie, M. (2020). Perceived organizational justice and turnover intention among hospital healthcare workers. *BMC Psychology, 8*(19). https://doi.org/10.1186/s40359-020-0387-8.

Mento, C., Silvestri, M. C., Bruno, A., Muscatello, M. R. A., Cedro, C., Pandolfo, G., & Zoccali, R. A. (2020). Workplace violence against healthcare professionals: A systematic review. *Aggression & Violent Behavior, 51.* 3–8.

Minarik, P., & Catramabone, C. (1998). Collective participation in workforce decision-making. In D. Mason, D. Talbot, & J. Leavitt (Eds.), *Policy and politics for nurses: Action and change in the workplace, government, organizations and community* (3rd ed.). Philadelphia: Saunders.

Munro, C. L. (2020). Healthy Work Environment: Resolutions for 2020. *American Journal of Critical Care, 29*(1), 4–6.

Olender, L., Capitulo, K., & Nelson, J. (2020). The impact of interprofessional shared governance and a caring professional practice model on staff's self-report of caring, workplace engagement, and workplace empowerment over time. *Journal of Nursing Administration, 50*(1), 52–58.

O'Rourke, M. W. (2021). Work Engagement: Passion–Role Clarity Connection in a Turbulent Time. *Nurse Leader, 19*(2), 204–209.

Oss, J. A., Schad, E. A., Drenth, A. R., Johnson, L. M., Olson, J. M., & Bursiek, A. A. (2021). Driving nurse satisfaction through shared governance. *Nurse Leader, 19*(1), 47–52.

Patient Safety Network (PSNET). (2019). *High Reliability.* Retrieved from https://psnet.ahrq.gov/primer/high-reliability.

Porter-O'Grady, T. (Ed.). (2009). *Interdisciplinary shared governance: Integrating practice, transforming health care* (2nd ed.). Sudbury, MA: Jones and Bartlett Publishers.

Porter-O'Grady, T. (2019). Principles for sustaining shared/professional governance in nursing. *Nursing Management, 50*(1), 36–41.

Porter-O'Grady, T., & Clavelle, J. T. (2020). The structural framework for nursing professional governance: Foundation for empowerment. *Nurse Leader, 18*(2), 181–189.

Press Ganey. (2016). *2016 nursing special report: The role of workplace safety and surveillance capacity in driving nurse and patient outcomes [White Paper].*

Rehder, K., Adair, K., Hadley, A., McKittrick, K., Frankel, A., Leonard, M., Christensen Frankel, T., & Sexton, J. (2020). Associations between a new disruptive behaviors scale and teamwork, patient safety, work-life balance, burnout, and depression. *The Joint Commission Journal on Quality and Patient Safety, 46*(1), 18–26.

Richey, K., & Waite, S. (2019). Leadership development for frontline nurse managers promotes innovation and engagement. *Nurse Leader, 17*(1), 37–42.

Rodríguez-García, M. C., Márquez-Hernández, V. V., Belmonte-García, T., Gutiérrez-Puertas, L., & Granados-Gámez, G. (2020). How Magnet hospital status affects nurses, patients, and organizations: A systematic review: Findings support the pursuit of Magnet recognition. *American Journal of Nursing, 120*(7), 28–38.

Saunders, J., Sridaromont, K., & Gallegos, B. (2021). Steps to establish a healthy work environment in an academic nursing setting. *Nurse Educator, 46*(1), 2–4. https://doi.org/10.1097/NNE.0000000000000829.

Sherman, R. O. (2019). *Nurse leader coach: Become the boss no one wants to leave.* (Self-published).

Sherman, R. O., & Cohn, T. M. (2019). Promoting professional accountability and ownership: Nursing leaders set the tone for a culture of professional responsibility. *American Nurse Today, 14*(2), 24–26.

The Joint Commission. (2018). *Sentinel Event Alert 59: Physical and verbal violence against health care workers.* Retrieved from https://www.jointcommission.org/resources/patient-safety-topics/sentinel-event/sentinel-event-alert-newsletters/sentinel-event-alert-59-physical-and-verbal-violence-against-health-care-workers/#.Yi5yenrMLnY.

The Joint Commission Center for Transforming Healthcare. (2021). *High reliability in health care is possible.* Retrieved from https://www.centerfortransforminghealthcare.org/high-reliability-in-health-care/.

Ulrich, B., Barden, C., Cassidy, L., & Varn-Davis, N. (2019). Critical care nurse work environments 2018: Findings and implications. *Critical Care Nurse, 39*(2), 67–84.

Veazie, S., Peterson, K., & Bourne, D. (2019). *Evidence Brief: Implementation of High Reliability Organization Principles.* Washington, DC: Evidence Synthesis Program, Health Services Research and Development Service, Office of Research and Development, Department of Veterans Affairs. VA ESP Project #09-199. Retrieved from https://www.hsrd.research.va.gov/publications/esp/high-reliability-org.cfm.

Vessey, J. A., & Williams, L. (2021). Addressing bullying and lateral violence in the workplace: A quality improvement initiative. *Journal of Nursing Care Quality, 36*(1), 20–24.

Wilson, R. C., & Galuska, L. (2020). Professional governance implementation: Successes, failures, and lessons learned. *Nurse Leader, 18*(5), 467–470.

13

Solving Problems and Influencing Positive Outcomes

Sylvain Trepanier and Jeannette T. Crenshaw

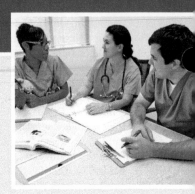

ANTICIPATED LEARNING OUTCOMES

- Apply a decision-making model to identify the best options to solve a problem.
- Analyze the decision-making style of a nurse leader or manager.
- Value the concept of influence as it relates to leadership and management in nursing.

- Implement strategies that have a positive influence in work settings, professional organizations, and health policy.

KEY TERMS

coalition

decision-making

influence

negotiating

problem-solving

THE CHALLENGE

Healthcare managers are faced with numerous and complex issues in providing quality services for patients within a resource-scarce environment. Stress levels among staff can escalate when problems are not resolved, leading to decreased morale, productivity, and quality service. This was the situation I encountered in my previous job as an administrator for California Children Services (CCS). When I began my tenure as the new CCS administrator, staff expressed frustration and dissatisfaction with staffing, workload, and team communication. This led to high staff turnover, lack of teamwork, customer complaints, unmet deadlines for referral and enrollment cycle times, and poor documentation. In addition, the team was in crisis, characterized by infighting, blaming, lack of respectful communication, and lack of commitment to program goals and objectives. Because I had not worked as a case manager in this program, it was hard for me to determine how to address the staff's problems. I wanted to be fair but thought that I did not have enough information to make immediate changes. My challenge was to lead this team to greater compliance with state-mandated performance measures.

What would you do if you were this nurse?

Vickie Lemmon, RN, MSN
Director of Clinical Strategies, Operations WellPoint, Inc.,
Ventura, California

INTRODUCTION

Solving problems and influencing positive outcomes are essential skills for effective nursing practice as you lead, manage, or follow. The challenges we face often are complex and have critical consequences. These challenges require thoughtful consideration. How we address these challenges reflects on us, regardless of our role. The ability to effectively make decisions and influence positive outcomes is necessary to manage and deliver care and is essential for planned change. Technological, social, political, and economic changes and the COVID-19 worldwide pandemic have dramatically affected healthcare and nursing practice. Increased patient acuity; shorter hospital stays; shortage of healthcare providers; advanced technology; greater emphasis on quality and patient safety; value-based purchasing; "pay for performance"; and the continuing shift from inpatient to home health, ambulatory, and community-based healthcare are just some of the changes that require nurses to make effective decisions and identify solutions to inevitable problems caused by change.

Moreover, increased diversity in patient populations, professional healthcare roles, and employment settings require effective problem-solving skills. More emphasis is placed on person- and family-centered care plus the recognition of patients as full partners in decision-making. Continuing emphasis also is placed on problem-solving in collaboration with interprofessional teams as the foundation for evidence-based results. The term *VUCA* (volatility, uncertainty, complexity, and ambiguity) creates the current context for solving problems in healthcare—and in many other fields. Nurses must possess the knowledge, skills, and attitudes required for effective problem-solving, decision-making, and influencing. These competencies are essential for all nurses, especially nurses with leadership and management responsibilities regardless of their practice setting.

PROBLEM-SOLVING

Attributed to Einstein is this wisdom: "If I were given an hour to solve a problem upon which my life depended, I would spend 40 minutes analyzing the problem, 15 minutes planning the solution, and 5 minutes executing the solution." Thus, the effective leader anticipates problems and develops methods for dealing with them. The leader who defines a problem has the potential to create a cogent solution.

Problem-Solving Process

Several approaches to problem-solving and decision-making exist. First, examine the problem-solving and decision-making model illustrated in Fig. 13.1. Then, review the Decision-Making Format in Box 13.1, which includes a series of questions to help the nurse leader or manager to define a problem, identify and rank possible solutions, and implement and evaluate a plan to solve a problem.

Initial Evaluation

Before attempting to solve a problem, a nurse needs to ask several questions:
1. Is it important?

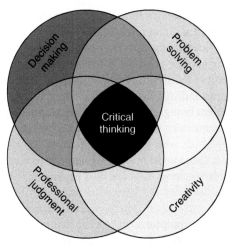

Fig. 13.1 Problem-solving and decision-making model.

BOX 13.1 Decision-Making Format

Objective: _____

Options	Advantages	Disadvantages	Ranking

Add more rows as necessary. Rank the priority of options, with "1" being most preferred. Select the best option.

Implementation plan: _____

_____

Evaluation plan: _____

_____

2. Do I "own" the problem? (i.e., is it mine to resolve to someone else's?)
3. Do I want to do something about it? (e.g., is it a priority?)
4. Am I qualified to handle it?
5. Do I have the authority to address the problem?
6. Do I want to do something about it? (e.g., do I have the knowledge, interest, time, and resources to address the problem?)
7. Can I delegate it to someone else?
8. What benefits will be gained from solving it?

If the answers to questions 1 through 6 are "no," why waste time, resources, and personal energy? Now, make a conscious decision to ignore the problem, refer or delegate, or consult or collaborate to solve it. On the other hand, if the answers are "yes," the nurse accepts the problem and assumes responsibility for it.

After identifying the problem, nurses then decide whether the problem is within their control and whether it is significant enough to require intervention. Sometimes individuals believe they need to "solve" every problem brought to their attention. Some situations, such as some interpersonal conflicts, are best resolved by the individuals who own the problem. A "do nothing" approach (*purposeful inaction*) may be indicated when the problem belongs to others or is beyond one's control.

Some decisions are "givens" because they are based on firmly established criteria within an organization, built on the traditions, values, doctrines, culture, or policies. Every leader and manager has to work within mandates established by persons higher in the organizational structure.

Although managers may not have the authority to control certain situations, they may be able to influence outcomes. For example, because of losses in revenue, members of the administration team decided to eliminate the clinical educator positions in a home health agency and give the responsibility for clinical education to senior home health nurses. The manager does not have the control to reverse this decision. Nevertheless, the manager can explore nurses' concerns and fears regarding this change and facilitate the transition by preparing them for their new role and, as appropriate, share the concerns with those responsible for the decision.

These two scenarios are not examples of a *do-nothing* approach since the manager took deliberate action. Nor are these strategies examples of a *laissez-faire* (i.e., uninvolved) approach. In these examples, the manager consciously chose not to intervene.

Define the Problem, Issue, or Situation

To solve a problem, the leader must first understand it. Before accurately diagnosing an issue, leaping to a solution may appear to save time, but it often becomes a temporary "fix" and may make the problem worse. Markowitz (2020) developed a simple four-step process to help a leader or manager avoid the urge to solve problems with a "Band-Aid": "(1) Go and see, (2) frame your problem properly, (3) think backward, and (4) ask why." (Refer to the Literature Perspective).

LITERATURE PERSPECTIVE

Resource: Markovitz, D. (2020). How to avoid rushing to solutions when problem-solving. *Harvard Business Review*. Retrieved from https://hbr.org/2020/11/how-to-avoid-rushing-to-solutions-when-problem-solving.

Markowitz's (2020) simple four-step process can help nurse leaders rushing to a solution without fully understanding a problem that needs resolving. Busy leaders, who frequently are in the midst of complex and stressful situations, often feel an urge to quickly solve a problem to "check it off their list" and move on to the next issue. To avoid this urge, use Markowitz's four simple steps:

1. *Go and see.* This step reminds us that to solve a problem, we must first accurately state the problem. To

arrive at a decision takes not only the data you can observe on a spreadsheet from your office but also getting facts that can be obtained only by observing the problem and talking to those involved with the problem.

2. *Frame your problem properly.* Avoid stating the problem ambiguously or as a solution. If you state a problem as "We need more staff on the night shift," the only possible solution is to hire more staff. Were several nurses on the night shift ill and unable to work their shift? Did the unit receive more admissions this month than usual? Markowitz recommends that if you see only one solution to your problem, reconsider it.

LITERATURE PERSPECTIVE—cont'd

3. *Think backwards.* Instead of thinking forward to a quick but possibly inadequate solution, think backwards. First, map out the problem, so you know what caused it. Identify the contributing factors. An effective way to identify the causes is to use a fishbone diagram illustrating the root causes that led to the problem (the effect). See Fig. 13.2 for an example of a fishbone diagram.
4. *Ask why.* To find a root cause, ask "why" repeatedly. Each time, you will get closer to the root cause of the problem you need to solve. Once you can describe the root cause, you can identify a sustainable solution rather than a quick fix.

Implications for Practice

Although it takes more time, defining a problem well leads to effective solutions and ultimately will save the time lost implementing the wrong solution. H. L. Mencken, an American journalist in the 20th century, wrote: "For every complex problem, there's a solution that is simple, neat, and wrong." Using Markowitz's four-step strategy can lead to a clearly defined problem with a solution that is more likely to be effective.

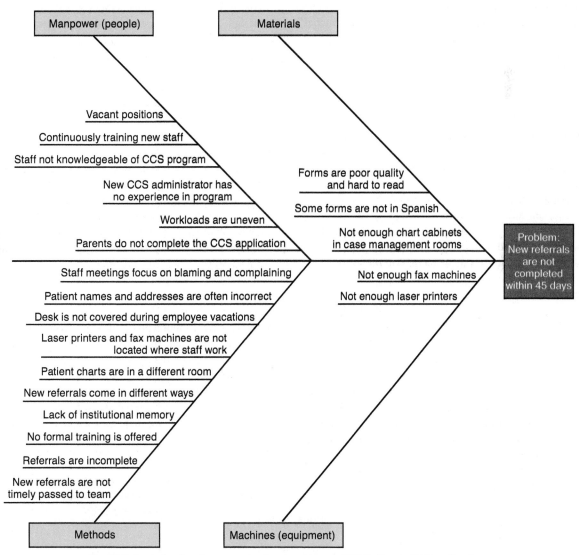

Fig. 13.2 Analysis of root causes of referral problems. *CCS,* California Children Services.

Prioritizing Problems

Nurses need to determine how to establish priorities for solving problems. For example, do you tend to work on issues chronologically, in order of complexity, or order of importance? Deciding which problem takes precedence and why and which issues can be "on the back burner" can help us avoid using valuable time addressing concerns that seem urgent and/or easy but not actually the most important. (Refer again to the Decision-Making Format in Box 13.1.)

Identifying Problems

Recognizing and identifying problems are vital steps in the problem-solving process. The most common cause for failure to resolve a problem is inaccurately identifying that problem. The quality of the outcome requires recognizing and targeting the underlying causes (*root causes*).

Problem identification is influenced by the information available; by the values, attitudes, and experiences of those involved; and by time. Allow adequate time for gathering facts about the problem. Too often, we do not allow enough time to collect and organize data about a problem, leading to unsatisfactory outcomes. Because problems in healthcare are complex and rarely have a single root cause and simple solution, nurse leaders and managers should harness the power of asking questions.

One method for harnessing the power of asking questions is to use the simple analysis technique called the *5 Whys*, developed in the 1930s by the founder of Toyota Industries, Sakichi Toyoda (MindTools, n.d.) After answering the preliminary question of why the problem has occurred, "why" should be asked again, a second, third, fourth, and even fifth time. Each answer provides greater clarity to the problem-solvers' understanding of root causes. Using the 5 Whys can keep problems from resurfacing because this technique uses *countermeasures*, not solutions. Countermeasures are actions that focus on the accurately identified root causes of a problem rather than on the symptoms of a problem (McMahon, 2020). By using the 5 Whys countermeasures technique, we can avoid treating problems simplistically and prevent them from recurring.

Differentiating between an actual problem and the symptoms of a problem is essential. For example, consider the problem of an inadequately stocked emergency cart with missing emergency medications and with equipment that fails to function. Individuals charged with resolving this problem may discover that this is symptomatic of an underlying problem, perhaps inadequate staffing, or an inadequate staffing mix. Based on correctly identifying the problem, one solution might be to assign checking and stocking the emergency cart to unlicensed personnel in the unit.

In work settings, problems often fall under specific categories or issues, described as the *Four Ms: m*anpower, *m*ethods, *m*achines, and *m*aterials. Examples of manpower issues include inadequate staffing or staffing mix and knowledge or skills deficits. Methods issues include communication problems and lack of protocols. Machine issues include lack of equipment or malfunctioning equipment. Materials issues include inadequate supplies or defective materials. A *fishbone diagram*, also known as a *cause-and-effect diagram*, is a valuable model for categorizing the possible causes of a problem. The fishbone diagram graphically displays, in increasing detail, the possible causes of a problem and its root causes. This tool helps problem solvers focus on the root causes of a problem instead of being sidetracked by personal interests, issues, or team members' agendas. A fishbone diagram creates a snapshot of the collective knowledge of a team and helps build consensus about a problem. The "effect" is generally a problem statement, such as decreased morale, and the problem is placed at the right end of the figure (the "head of the fish"). The major categories of causes are the main bones of the fish, which are supported by smaller bones representing issues that contribute to the leading causes. An example of a fishbone diagram appears in Fig. 13.2.

Gather Data

After identifying the problem, individuals or teams can focus on gathering and analyzing data to resolve an issue. Assessment through the collection of data is a continuous and dynamic process. The data collected include objective information (facts) and subjective information (intuition, beliefs). Information gathered should be valid, accurate, relevant to the issue, and timely. Moreover, individuals involved in the process need access to these data and sufficient resources to make cogent decisions.

Analyze Data

Data are analyzed to refine the problem statement further and identify possible solutions. The nurse leader or manager needs to differentiate a problem from what is merely its symptoms. For example, a nurse manager is concerned by the latest quality improvement (QI) report showing that nurses are not documenting patient education. Does this evidence mean that patient education is not being done? Is lack of documentation the problem? Perhaps lack of documentation is a symptom of the actual problem. On further analysis, the manager may discover that nurses do not know how to document patient teaching using the new computerized documentation system. By distinguishing the problem from its symptoms, the correct solution can be identified and implemented. This example is one in which asking the *5 Whys* could be effective.

Develop Solutions

Rigid "black and white" thinking hampers the quality of problem-solving and outcomes. For example, nurses who are unhappy with their work situation might think of only two options—stay or resign. This illustrates rigid thinking. "Either/or" thinking significantly limits the possibilities for solutions and the quality of outcomes.

Developing solutions requires critical thinking. Critical thinking requires the ability to use "logic and reasoning to identify the strengths and weaknesses of alternatives to clinical or practice problems" (ANCC, 2021, p. 57). Nurses and nurse managers who think critically and are flexible, open-minded, and creative enable themselves to develop a range of possible solutions. Everyone has preconceived ideas when confronted with specific situations. Putting preconceived notions on hold and considering alternatives is beneficial but challenging. Consider asking these questions to help identify options:

- Am I jumping to conclusions?
- If I were (insert name of a role model), how would I approach the issue?
- How are my beliefs and values affecting my decision?

Select a Solution

The problem solver then objectively weighs each options according to its risks, unintended consequences, and possible outcomes. Criteria for evaluation include variables such as cost-effectiveness, time, and legal and ethical considerations. The options are then ranked in the order in which they are likely to result in the desired outcome. The solution selected should be the most feasible one, with the fewest undesirable consequences and the most positive outcomes. Nurses can ask themselves whether they are choosing a solution because it is the best one or the easiest one. Making effective decisions based on a thorough assessment of a situation is the key to successfully resolving a problem and contributing to a nurse's effectiveness as a leader.

Implement the Solution

The planned solution requires a defined strategy, often implemented in phases. The phases may include revision of policies and procedures, education, and documentation. In addition, the nurse leader or manager may need a contingency plan (a *Plan B*) if the original solution does not resolve the problem or address unintended consequences if they arise.

Evaluate the Result

Considerable time and energy are allocated to identify the problem or issue, generate possible solutions, select the best solution, and implement the solution. However, time for evaluation and monitoring might be overlooked. Establishing early in the process how assessment and monitoring will occur, who will be responsible for it when it takes place, and the desired outcome can ensure that the nurse or nurse manager critically evaluates whether a problem has been resolved. The key is to learn from mistakes and use the experiences to help guide future actions. Henry Ford said, "Failure is only the opportunity to begin again, this time more intelligently" (Brainy Quote, n.d.).

Influence

Resolving a problem effectively also requires the ability to influence. Influence is the ability to impact someone's behavior and requires a strong emotional connection with self and others (Laker & Patel, 2020). For example, nurses and nurse managers influence by working with and through others. The good news is that influence is a skill that can be learned. The ability to influence others requires a trusting relationship. Laker and Patel conducted a meta-analysis to identify how influential leaders throughout history mastered the art of influence. They identified two main approaches: transactional influence and transformational influence. Transactional influence, often referred to as a *top-down* approach, focuses on tasks accomplished by a follower and includes a directive approach between a leader and a follower. This approach may be best suited for crises. Transformational influence is focused on the encouragement and support of followers by leaders. The leader using transformational influence is a role model and a motivator, offering vision and empathy. Laker and Patel remind us that "behind every great leader is an army of followers acting in support of their mission or cause."

Laker and Patel (2020) describe specific ways to develop the art of influence using a transformational approach:

1. Establish rapport and trust with those you wish to influence.
2. Be an active listener, as opposed to a transmitter of information.
3. Demonstrate commitment to your team.
4. Be a role model and express appreciation for team members.

If you are a first-time manager or new in your position, spend time getting to know your team. This will build trust, which is the magic ingredient that positively influences the members of your team. Take time to visit with the members of the group. Ask them questions. Show a genuine interest in getting to know them and let them know you care about who they are. Learn what they appreciated most about the "best boss" they ever worked for. Find out what motivates them and what disappoints or frustrates them. Team members can use this same approach to learn more about their colleagues and their manager. When we focus on learning about others, we are more effective in communicating with them, which leads to positive influence.

Theodore Roosevelt said, "Nobody cares how much you know until they know how much you care" (Andrew, 2015). Showing compassion and empathy, along with active listening, demonstrates that you care. Be sure also to use curiosity in every interaction. Prepare a list of questions to help you have engaging conversations with everyone on your team. For example, initiate a conversation by asking a follow-up question related to something you learned during a previous conversation with a colleague. If someone shared getting ready to attend a special event, ask about the event. This shows that you care enough to remember what was discussed during the last conversation—consider using reminder notes about topics you plan to discuss during a future dialogue. Robert McNamara, the former U.S. Secretary of Defense, reminded us that "Brains are like hearts. They go where they are appreciated" (Andrew, 2015).

EXERCISE 13.3 List the name of five to six people with whom you work most frequently. List at least five facts about them that are not observable attributes (e.g., wears glasses). Set a timer so that you accomplish this in less than 3 minutes.

Be sure to recognize everyone, especially those who meet or exceed expectations. However, remember that not everyone appreciates the same form of recognition. Therefore, it's essential to inquire how others like to be recognized.

Make sure to support all of the team members by demonstrating a commitment to their development and growth. This does not occur by happenstance. It requires a deliberate, active involvement on your part. As you share your vision, be sure to identify how you see others' contributions to the vision. Invite them to describe how they see their own contribution. To do that, offer all team members an opportunity to meet with you to assess their potential and to develop a meaningful plan for the future. Staying focused on a vision is extremely important. It is the work of a leader to do so.

THEORY BOX

Key Contributor	Key Ideas	Application to Practice
Cialdini, R. B. (2016). *Pre-Suasion: A Revolutionary Way to Influence and Persuade*. New York: Simon & Schuster.	Cialdini's Theory of Influence, the basis on which Pre-Suasion is built, consists of 6 key principles. 1. Reciprocity—the expectation that a favor needs to be returned 2. Consistency—living to one's promises and to make those public 3. Social proof—influence others who is "like me" 4. Liking—the idea that we tend to want to associate with people we like—and follow them 5. Scarcity—we want something that is rare or limited in quantity (product or knowledge) 6. Unity—the need to belong and feel a part of something	Nurse leaders are consistently asking staff and others to try new things—to change procedures, for example. Cialdini's theory is a great framework to assist nurse leaders in leveraging the team to do great things. Nurse leaders need to develop a strong relationship with physician colleagues, for example, so that they, in return, can assist and support a new practice in any given environment.

Influence and Empowerment

According to Kanter's structural empowerment theory (1977, 1979), the role of managers is to provide the "power tools" that will, in turn, empower employees to find meaning in their work and accomplish great things. In 1991, Mechanic described empowerment as integrating one's goals with belief in one's ability to achieve them and the confidence that efforts to achieve one's goals will influence life's outcomes. Empowerment is illustrated in the behaviors of nurse leaders and managers as they facilitate, coach, teach, mentor, and collaborate. Nurse leaders in all practice settings exercise their empowerment s they make professional judgments in their daily work. Effective nurse leaders and managers empower their followers to practice autonomy and inspire them to develop professionally. Nursing empowerment improves the profession and improves the quality of the care that nurses provide while enhancing job satisfaction (Tan & Conde, 2021). Empowered nurses also support their patients and families so that they can participate actively in their care.

Influence and Organizational Savvy

Another way to think about influence might be explained by Cialdini's work about persuasion (2001). See Theory Box. Nowhere are persuasion skills more needed than in health care organizations where so many structural silos intersect with each other in so many situations. To accomplish most of our work, we have to be able to persuade others to our way of thinking. Cialdini further expanded his work to focus on how we might make people even more receptive to our persuasive techniques by focusing on the conditions that serve, in a sense as precursors for being persuaded (Cialdini, 2016).

To use influence effectively in any organization requires an understanding of how the system functions. Developing organizational savvy includes identifying the decision-makers, those persons who have a high level of influence with the decision-makers, and informal yet influential leaders within any setting. An influential senior clinical nurse may have more decision-making power related to direct patient care than the nurse manager. A senior clinical nurse may have more clinical expertise and greater knowledge about the history of the unit and its personnel than a nurse manager with excellent management and leadership skills who is new to the unit.

Executive assistants of a chief nursing officer (CNO) are usually powerful, although not consistently recognized as such. For example, a CNO's assistant influences the flow of information provided to the CNO; makes decisions about who can meet with the CNO and when; and, in triaging incoming and outgoing mail, informs the CNO when a document needs immediate attention or places a memo under a stack of mail for review at a later time.

Collegiality and Collaboration

Nursing does not exist in a vacuum, nor do nurses work in isolation from other nurses, other professionals, or support personnel. Nurses function within a wide range of organizations, such as schools, hospitals, community health organizations, governments, insurance companies, professional associations, and universities. Nurses are noted for having divided views about the appropriate educational level for entry into practice. Nurses are also noted for their reticence to join nursing organizations that influence numerous public health areas, including public health policy.

Developing a sense of unity requires that nurses act collaboratively and collegially in the workplace and other organizations, such as professional associations. Collegiality demands that nurses value the accomplishments of nursing colleagues and express a sincere interest in their efforts. Turning to colleagues for advice and support empowers colleagues and, at the same time, expands one's power base. One does not have to be a friend to everyone who is a colleague. Collegiality demands mutual respect, not friendship. Nurses should recognize that unity of purpose does not preclude diversity of thought.

Collaboration and collegiality require that nurses work collectively to ensure that the voice of nursing is heard in the workplace and public policy arenas. Nurses need to use collaboration and collegiality to address various concerns, including abuse and safety issues that might be resolved in the workplace and might need to be addressed through legislative action.

Volunteering to serve on committees and task forces in the workplace, not just within the nursing department but also on organization-wide committees, develops opportunities to work with various people and learn new skills for influencing others. One way for nurses to stay current with issues and to create alliances is to become an active member of nursing organizations, including state nursing organizations and those organizations with a specialty focus. Since all nurses are leaders, nurses can become involved in the American Organization for Nursing Leadership (AONL), and its state and local chapters. If eligible, you can become active in nursing's professional honor society, Sigma Theta Tau International (STTI), and its local chapter. Being a part of the AONL and STTI allows opportunities to advance the influence of nursing and to improve healthcare.

If the workplace has a shared governance council, becoming involved in the council's committees, task forces, and work groups allows you to share your energy, ideas, and expertise. Many organizations have interdisciplinary committees that bring together nurses, physicians, and other healthcare professionals to improve professional collaboration and the quality of patient care. Becoming an active, productive member of these interprofessional groups creates new ways to deal with healthcare issues and problems.

Communicate in a manner that facilitates a partnership approach to quality care delivery. One of the competencies required of all healthcare professionals and outlined in the AACN Essentials is to communicate in a manner that facilitates a partnership approach to quality care delivery. This competency allows the ability to work collaboratively, using integrated professional perspectives, to provide healthcare across practice settings (Schot et al., 2020). Nurses can be the "bridge" to overcome gaps in collaborative practice due to their strategic position in providing patient care. Although work still needs to be done to ensure that nurses can practice with full autonomy, within their scope of practice, and as full partners on the healthcare team, nurses are increasingly recognized by interprofessional colleagues as essential members of the healthcare team who effectively collaborate with physicians and other healthcare professionals.

A Professional Practice Image

Recognizing the competencies that nurses bring to the care of patients allows nurses to demonstrate a positive and professional attitude about being a nurse to nursing colleagues, patients and their families, other colleagues in the workplace, and the public, including businesses, places of worship, and the public policy sector. This recognition facilitates the exercise of power among colleagues while educating others about nurses and nursing. A powerful image is an essential aspect of demonstrating this positive professional attitude. The current practice of nurses to identify themselves by the first name may only decrease their power image in the eyes of stakeholders, including physicians. Physicians are always addressed as "Doctor." When they address others only by their first names, inequality of power and status is evident. The use of first names among colleagues is not inappropriate so long as everyone is playing by the same rules. Managers may want to enhance the empowerment of their staff members by encouraging them to introduce themselves as "Dr.," "Ms.," or "Mr."

Arriving at work, appointments, or meetings on time, looking neat and appropriately attired for the work setting or other professional situation, and speaking positively about one's work are examples of how easy it is to demonstrate a positive, powerful, and professional attitude. Referring to practitioners of medicine as physicians rather than doctors helps reinforce the idea that many other practitioners, including nurses, hold doctoral degrees although they do not practice medicine.

The American Nurses Credentialing Center's (ANCC) Magnet® program recognizes organizations characterized by work environments that empower nurses (ANCC, 2020). Nurses who work in Magnet®-recognized organizations report higher job satisfaction. In addition, Magnet®-recognized organizations have higher nurse retention rates and reduced turnover.

RESEARCH PERSPECTIVE

Resource: Trépanier, S.-G., Peterson, C., Fernet, C., Austin, S., & Desrumaux, P. (2021). When workload predicts exposure to bullying behaviours in nurses: The protective role of social support and job recognition. *Journal of Advanced Nursing, 77*(7), 3093–3103.

Trépanier et al. (2021) conducted a longitudinal study to explore the impact of poor-quality work environments on bullying behaviors in the workplace and social support in the workplace and job recognition on bullying behaviors. The characteristics of poor-quality work environments included high workload, role conflict, and low autonomy and support. The researchers found that as negative work-related factors increased over time so did the bullying behaviors of nurses. However, the researchers found that when workplace social support and job recognition were high, these factors had a buffering (mediating) effect on

bullying behaviors. In addition, they found that as workload stress increased, so did nurses' exposure to bullying behaviors. However, when job recognition and social support in the workplace was high, nurses' exposure to bullying behaviors did not increase despite high levels of workload stress.

Implications for Practice
The workplace in healthcare is complex and highly stressful. A significant yet simple strategy that nurse leaders and managers can use to ameliorate the impact of a stressful workplace environment is to integrate staff support and recognition into the workplace culture. Ensuring staff support and job recognition can reduce, over time, the bullying behavior perpetrated on nurses associated with stressful workload.

Transformational leadership is foundational to the work culture in those organizations with Magnet® recognition.

Bullying

Although bullying is described elsewhere in this book, it is discussed here as an example of ineffective use of power. Furthermore, such behavior weakens our influence, which provides another reason to address this issue. The Research Perspective illustrates the impact of poor-quality work environments on bullying in nursing and potential strategies to mediate the effect.

Developing Coalitions

A coalition is a group of individuals or organizations with a common interest who agree to work together toward a common goal. The exercise of power is often directed at creating change. Although an individual can often be effective at exercising power and creating change, creating specific changes within most organizations requires collective action. Coalition building is an effective political strategy for collective action.

The goals of coalitions often focus on an effort to effect change. The networking among organizations that results in coalition building requires members of one group to reach out to other groups. This often occurs at the leadership level and may come through formal mechanisms such as letters that identify an issue or problem—a shared interest—around which a coalition could be built. For example, a state nurses association may invite the leaders of organizations interested in child health (e.g., organizations of pediatric nurses,

public health nurses, and physicians; plus elementary school teachers, school nurses, and daycare providers) and consumers (e.g., parents) to discuss collaborative support for a legislative initiative to improve access, including equity of immunization programs in urban areas, rural areas, and underserved communities. Such coalitions of professionals and consumers are powerful in influencing public policy related to healthcare.

Collaboration among groups and individuals with shared interests and goals often results in greater success in effecting change and exercising power in the workplace and within other organizations, including legislative bodies. A group of diverse nursing organizations may come together as a coalition to support a modification of the state nursing practice act. Expanding networks in the workplace, as suggested earlier in this chapter, facilitates creating a coalition by developing a pool of candidates for coalition building before they are needed. Examples of effective strategies to develop a coalition include:

- Inviting people with common goals to lunch or coffee to begin building a coalition around an issue. Discuss shared interests and gain the commitment of the individuals.
- Meeting informally with members of a committee or task force that is working on the same issue. Attend the open meetings of professional groups that share the same interests as the organization to which you belong.
- Seeking representation from the diverse members of the community where you are focused.
- Sharing ideas on how to create the desired change most effectively while building coalitions.

Coalition building is an essential skill for involvement in public policy. Nursing organizations often use coalition building when dealing with state legislatures and Congress. For example, changes in nurse practice acts to expand opportunities for advanced nursing practice have been accomplished in many states through coalition building. State medical societies or the state agencies that license physicians often oppose such changes. Efforts by a single nursing organization (e.g., a state nurses association or a state nurse practitioners organization), representing a limited nursing constituency, often lack the clout to overcome opposition by the unified voice of the state's physicians. However, the unified effort of a coalition of nursing organizations, other healthcare organizations, and consumer groups can be powerful in effecting change through public policy.

Negotiating

Although we do not typically think of negotiating, or bargaining, as a formal decision-making process, it is an essential skill for personal, organizational, and political power. Negotiation is a process of making trade-offs. Children are natural negotiators. Often, they will initially ask their parents for more than what they are willing to accept in privileges, toys, or activities. The logic is simple to children: ask for more than is reasonable and negotiate down to what you want!

Negotiating often works the same way within organizations. People will sometimes ask for more than they want and be willing to accept less. In other situations, both sides will enter negotiations asking for radically different things. Still, both may be willing to settle for a position that differs markedly from their respective original positions. In the simplest forms of bargaining, each participant has something that the other party values: goods, services, or information. At the "bargaining table," each party presents an opening position. Then, the process moves on until they reach a mutually agreeable result, or until negotiations fail, and one or both parties walk away from the bargaining table.

Bargaining may take many forms. For example, individuals may negotiate with a supervisor for a more desirable work schedule or with a peer for a schedule change to attend an out-of-town conference. A nurse manager may sit at the bargaining table with the department director during budget planning to negotiate to expand funded education hours for the nursing unit's budget for the coming year. Representatives of a coalition of nursing organizations meeting with a legislator may negotiate with the legislator over sections of a proposed healthcare-related bill to eliminate or modify sections that are not in the best interests of nurses, patients, or the healthcare system. Nurses may bargain with nursing and hospital administration over wages, staffing levels, or the working conditions and policies that govern clinical practice. Another type of negotiation is *collective bargaining*, regulated by state and federal labor laws, which usually involves representation by a state nurses association or a nursing or nonnursing labor union (see Collective Action in Chapter 14).

Successful negotiators are well informed about not only their positions but also those of the opposing side. Negotiators must be able to discuss the pros and cons of both positions. They can assist the other party in recognizing the costs versus the benefits of each position. These skills are also essential to exercising power effectively within the arenas of professional and legislative politics. For example, when lobbying a member of the legislature to support a bill desired by nurses, one must understand the position of those opposed to the bill so that they can effectively advocate for their position and answer questions that the legislator may ask.

Taking Political Action to Influence Policy

In the 1990s, Carolyn McCarthy was a licensed practical nurse from New York when a tragedy turned her life upside-down. Her husband was killed, and her son injured, by a shooter on the Long Island Railroad. She sought the support of her elected member of Congress on gun control legislation because of her tragedy. He refused to support such legislation. She took extraordinary action, changing her party affiliation and then running against the incumbent for his seat in Congress. She served in the U.S. Congress until 2014. There are, of course, other nurses in local politics, state houses, and the U.S. Congress. However, their numbers are few. As a result, the distinct perspective of nursing may not be as visible as it could be if more nurses were elected officials.

Running for office at any level of government is essential to be sure that the nursing perspective is part of the policy discussion. However, it is not the only action a nurse might take to participate in policy development. Gaining political skills, like any other skill set, is a developmental process. Some suggested strategies for developing political skills are presented in Box 13.2. Learning one's strengths and areas for improvement requires self-study. The Political Astuteness Inventory (adapted) (Goldwater & Zusy, 1990) is a helpful tool in

---

BOX 13.2   Developing Political Skills

- Build a working relationship with a legislator, such as your state senator or representative or member of the U.S. Congress and the legislative staff members.
- Join and be an active member of your state nurses' association affiliated with the American Nurses Association.
- Join a specialty nursing organization related to your clinical specialty (e.g., critical care, pediatrics) or specialty role in nursing (nurse practitioner, manager).
- Invite a legislator to a professional organization meeting.
- Invite a legislator or staff person from the legislator's office to spend a day with you at work.
- Register to vote and vote in every election.
- Join your state nurses' association's government relations or legislative committee and political action committee (PAC); join the ANA's PAC.
- Be in touch with your federal and state legislators on nursing and healthcare issues, especially related to specific bills, by writing letters, making telephone calls, or sending emails.
- Participate in Nurse Lobby Day and meet with your state legislators.
- Work on a federal or state legislative campaign.
- Visit your U.S. senators and member of Congress if visiting in the Washington, DC area to discuss federal legislation related to nursing and healthcare or visit their local offices.
- Get involved in the local group of your political party.
- Run for office at the local, county, state, or congressional level.
- Enhance the image of nursing in all your policy efforts.
- Communicate your message effectively and clearly.
- Develop your expertise in shaping policy.
- Seek appointive positions or elective offices to shape policy more effectively.

From Kelly, K. (2015). Power, politics, and influence. In P. Yoder-Wise (Ed.), *Leading and managing in nursing* (6th ed.). St. Louis: Mosby.

---

determining how well prepared you are to influence legislative politics and public policy, especially public policy related to healthcare (Box 13.3).

EXERCISE 13.4 Complete the Political Astuteness Inventory. Based on your responses and score, identify the number of items needed to elevate your score to the next level (e.g., from 10–19 to 20–29). Describe how you can implement a personal plan to address each of the items you selected to change. [As an example, you might have scored 18 and know you need to select 2 items to elevate your score to the next category (20–29). You choose items 15 and 34 because you didn't know that information. Your plan is to use your state government directory and determine who is your state senator and then to review the state board of nursing web site to determine how the state board of nursing is comprised.

Many social, technological, scientific, and economic trends have shaped nursing's ability to exercise power in the political arena. Although some failures have occurred in moving nurses to autonomous professionals, we also have experienced many successes. For example, in 1988, in response to a nursing shortage, the American Medical Association (AMA) proposed a new category of the healthcare worker, the registered care technologist (RCT). The proposal suggested that the RCT be trained in a hospital and be primarily responsible for carrying out physician's orders in medication administration, test orders, and discharge plans (Jonas, 2003). However, nurses believed that this recommendation, similar to the training of the hospital-based nurse, was not the answer to the nursing shortage. Nurses and nursing organizations responded powerfully. Nursing leaders came together in "summit meetings" to formulate powerful responses to the AMA and implemented a range of actions, including public education and the education of legislators. As a result of nurses' use of their power, a new category of workers was not formed.

The personal power strategies mentioned earlier in this chapter are also crucial for building one's political power. Nurses can no longer be passive observers of the political world. Political involvement is a professional responsibility, not just a privilege; political advocacy is a mandate. And, with the rise of the role of media in our lives, we need to be savvy about how we use media to further our work.

CONCLUSION

Sometimes, individuals and groups do not adopt a structured problem-solving approach because it takes too much time, the process may be tedious, stakeholders are too busy to get involved, or participants may perceive that little or no recognition for their participation is likely. Leaders should be cognizant of these potential barriers and should be prepared to prevent or minimize them.

Whether they are managers, leaders, or followers, all nurses need adequate decision-making and problem-solving skills to be effective in their roles. Regardless of the

BOX 13.3   Political Astuteness Inventory

Place a checkmark next to those items for which your answer is "yes." Then, give yourself 1 point for each "yes." After completing the inventory, compare your total score with the scoring criteria at the end of the inventory.

1. I am registered to vote.
2. I know where my voting precinct is located.
3. I voted in the last general election.
4. I voted in the last two elections.
5. I recognized the names of the majority of the candidates on the ballot and was acquainted with the majority of issues in the last election.
6. I stay abreast of current health issues.
7. I belong to the state professional or student nurse organization.
8. I participate (e.g., as a committee member, officer) in this organization.
9. I attended the most recent meeting of my local nurses' association.
10. I attended the last state or national convention held by my organization.
11. I am aware of at least two issues discussed and the stands taken at this meeting.
12. I read literature published by my state nurses' association, a professional journal/magazine/newsletter, or other literature on a regular basis to stay abreast of current health issues.
13. I know the names of my senators in Washington, DC.
14. I know the name of my representative in Washington, DC.
15. I know the name of the state senator from my district.
16. I know the name of the state representative from my district.
17. I am acquainted with the voting record of at least one of the previously mentioned state or federal representatives in relation to a specific health issue.
18. I am aware of the stand taken by at least one of the previously mentioned state or federal representatives in relation to a specific health issue.
19. I know whom to contact for information about health-related issues at the state or federal level.
20. I know whether my professional organization employs lobbyists at the state or federal level.
21. I know how to contact these lobbyists.
22. I contribute financially to my state and national professional organization's political action committee (PAC).
23. I give information about effectiveness of elected officials to assist the PAC's endorsement process.
24. I actively supported a senator or representative during the last election.
25. I have written to one of my state or national representatives in the last year regarding a health issue.
26. I am personally acquainted with a senator or representative, or member of his or her staff.
27. I serve as a resource person for one of my representatives or his or her staff.
28. I know the process by which a bill is introduced in my state legislature.
29. I know which senators or representatives are supportive of nursing.
30. I know which house and senate committees usually deal with health-related issues.
31. I know the committees of which my representatives are members.
32. I know of at least two health issues related to my profession that are currently under discussion.
33. I know of at least two health-related issues that are currently under discussion at the state or national level.
34. I am aware of the composition of the state board that regulates my profession.
35. I know the process whereby one becomes a member of the state board that regulates my profession.
36. I know what DHHS stands for.
37. I have at least a vague notion of the purpose of the DHHS.
38. I am a member of a health board or advisory group to a health organization or agency.
39. I attend public hearings related to health issues.
40. I find myself more interested in political issues now than in the past.

Scoring:
0–9: Totally unaware politically/apathetic
10–19: Slightly more aware of the implications of the politics of nursing/buy-in
20–29: Beginning political astuteness/self-interest to political sophistication
30–40: Politically astute, an asset to nursing/leading the way

Adapted from Goldwater, M., & Zusy, M. J. L. (1990). *Prescription for nurses: Effective political action*. St. Louis: Mosby; with permission by M. Goldwater.

problem-solving approach, using a systematic approach will help address issues in an organized and focused manner.

Influence is played out every day in every setting. Politics are played out and in every setting. Effective use of influence and politics can improve healthcare delivery and patient outcomes. Nursing leaders can be influential and politically savvy in positive, practical ways.

THE SOLUTION

In a previous job, I had used interprofessional process improvement teams that consisted of key stakeholders to initiate process improvement. I chose to try this concept again. Our team consisted of the public health nurse (PHN) case managers, the California Children Services (CCS) caseworkers, the billing and claims staff, the CCS medical director, clerical, and support staff, and me. I believed that a group approach to these problems would yield the most information and gain the greatest support for any changes that would be made. The team met weekly for an hour. We began by identifying our customers and key stakeholders and their expectations. This was extensive and took a few months to complete. Key stakeholders included the patients (children) and their parents; the providers (physicians and hospitals); pharmacists; vendors; representatives from schools, insurance plans, and other agencies; taxpayers (state and county); and our team members. The expectations for each stakeholder were listed, discussed for clarity, and recorded. During this exercise, the team learned a great deal about each person's job duties (a few surprises) and how each stakeholder's role affected other team members' ability to do their job. As the team began understanding each person's job and issues, they focused less on blaming and more on how to change our processes.

Next, the team brainstormed (divergent thinking) a list of issues. The numerous issues were then grouped according to similarity, and duplicates were eliminated. Multi-voting was then used to determine the three highest-priority issues. Our number one problem is related to cycle time. When a client is referred to CCS, determining eligibility, opening (or denying) the case, and authorizing care are vital cycles. Patient care is often coordinated based on the client's eligibility, and service delays can result when the process is not completed on time. The reasons for our failure to meet these deadlines seemed overwhelming and beyond our ability to resolve. We needed a method to find the root causes to improve our performance. We chose to use a fishbone diagram, also known as a *cause-and-effect diagram*. Our problem was, "New referrals are not completed within 45 days." We categorized our known barriers on the four bones of the fish: manpower, methods, machines, and materials. Once we had identified the factors contributing to our problem, we prioritized them and generated action plans for each major factor. These action plans were extensive and involved implementing training and education programs, redesigning workspace for greater efficiency, purchasing more equipment, revising job descriptions, increasing provider outreach activities, and more. Performance data did not improve during the initial year of our process improvement initiative, and I chose not to share it with staff to avoid demoralizing them. My management team and I were taking a leap of faith that our process would eventually result in the desired outcome of meeting the performance metrics.

It took 18 months for CCS to "turn the corner," but once improvement started, it was exponential. The cycle time measure for "referral to case open" was initially 57 days. Two years later, it was 30 days. The cycle time "referral to deny" began at 97 days, and two years later was down to 39 days. Most important, the cycle time "referral to first authorization" decreased from an initial 189 days to just 49 days! It was at this time that I shared the outcome data with the team. They were ecstatic! I asked the team to list the problems they believed we had solved through our process improvement team's efforts. They listed (1) improved staffing, (2) increased staff morale and decreased turnover (all the positions were now filled), (3) better understanding of the job expectations and the rationale behind those expectations, (4) improved teamwork, and (5) more efficient and effective workspace. They have maintained enthusiastic support of the Performance Improvement Team (PIT), and participation remains high. The team is still highly focused on problem-solving. I have learned that when assuming leadership of a department in which one has no experience, a structured team approach to information gathering, assessment of data, identification of problems, and implementation of action plans can be highly effective in the resolution of priority problems.

Would this be a suitable approach for you? Why?

Vickie Lemmon

REFLECTIONS

Consider a recurring problem you face. What have you done to try to resolve the issue? What else could you do? Who is a trusted ally who could offer a fresh view of the problem? What are you willing to risk to use a new approach?

BEST PRACTICES

Critical thinking enables a nurse to make effective decisions, influence positive healthcare outcomes, and develop political savvy. Critical thinking allows the nurse leader and manager to implement change from the current state to the desired state. Building this competence requires scheduled time for reflection. "Unplugging" and unwiring lead to effective reflection and decisions that improve outcomes for patients/clients, their families, and those who care for them.

TIPS FOR SOLVING PROBLEMS AND INFLUENCING POSITIVE OUTCOMES

Political savvy is "the ability to maximize and leverage relationships in order to achieve organizational, team, and individual goals" (Center for Creative Leadership, Leading Effectively Staff, 2020). Leaders and managers with political savvy are viewed as authentic and honest (Table 13.1). Leaders and managers who are not politically savvy may be seen as self-serving or controlling. Fortunately, we can develop political savvy. The Leading Effectively Staff from the Center for Creative Leadership suggest six behaviors to improve your political savvy:

1. *Hone your powers of perception.* This includes developing the ability to sense what motivates people and to "read" nonverbal behaviors.
2. *Practice **influence.*** At the core of practicing **influence** is establishing rapport and communicating well.
3. *Learn to network effectively.* Networking includes building friendships and strong working relationships. Not only does networking involve helping you to achieve your goals but it also involves "returning the favor"—reciprocating.
4. *Think before you speak.* Leaders and managers must develop the art of knowing when to speak up immediately, when postponing a discussion might lead to better outcomes, or when something is better left unsaid.
5. *Manage up—to a point.* Managing up means developing effective relationships with those you report to, but not at the expense of establishing effective relationships with team members and those throughout an organization or agency.
6. *Be sincere.* Leaders and managers with political savvy are authentic. They inspire trust; leaders and managers can use these simple strategies to develop their "political savvy quotient":
   - Learn to read others (emotional intelligence).
   - Be willing to risk a different view and be equally willing to stop trying to **influence** people who don't want to be influenced—unless they are required to make a change.
   - Know who your boss's boss is.
   - Don't say no to an opportunity—it might open a different door.

TABLE 13.1   Authentic Leadership Characteristics and Behaviors Related to Power and Influence

Characteristics	Description of Behavior
Self-aware and genuine	Self-actualized, aware of strengths, limitations, and emotions. Recognizes that self-actualization is forever ongoing. Behavior is consistent in private and public. Open about mistakes. Does not fear looking weak.
Mission-driven and focused on results	Puts the organization ahead of self-interest. Pursues organizational results, not power, money, or ego.
Leads with the heart and the mind	Not afraid to show emotions, vulnerability. Connects with employees—communicates problems in a direct manner; directness without being cruel.
Focuses on the long term	Concerned about what happens to the organization over the long term. Nurtures individuals and the organization with patience.

Modified from Kruse, K. (2013). *Authentic Leadership.* https://www.forbes.com/sites/kevinkruse/2013/05/12/what-is-authentic-leadership/#2b8d8019def7.

- Show up.
- Listen to what people say and find a common concern/value.
- Know what you value in life and be true to those values.
- Know the staff of a legislator even better than you know the legislator.
- Participate at the state level in any policy day activities sponsored by nursing.
- Modify any form email before sending it to your legislator/city council representative or others.
- Be sure to include a local perspective to help the recipient understand or recall the emotion of the facts.
- Establish a relationship before it is needed.
- Act as if you belong—you do.
- Keep a record of key people you meet so you can help them recall who you are the next time you know you will see them.
- Watch what you post on social media—you never know where it goes after it leaves your device.
- Learn people's names—and something about them.
- Seek additional information from other sources, even if they do not support the preferred action.
- Learn how other people approach decision-making and problem-solving.
- Talk with colleagues and supervisors who you believe are effective problem solvers and decision makers.
- Observe positive role models in action, such as clinical nurse specialists, clinical nurse leaders, educators, and managers.
- Review journal articles and relevant sections of textbooks on strategies to enhance your ability to problem solve and exert influence.
- Use new approaches to problem resolution (after calculating potential risks to self and others.
- Become an active member of selected nursing organizations, especially your state nurses' association, and a specialty organization.
- Develop a powerful personal and professional self-image.
- Invest in your nursing career by continuing your education.
- Make nursing your career, not just a job.
- Develop networking skills.
- Be visible and competent in the organizations in which you work and network.
- Be politically savvy.

REFERENCES

American Nurses Credentialing Center (ANCC). (2021). *The essentials: Core competencies for professional nursing education*. Retrieved from https://www.aacnnursing.org/Portals/42/AcademicNursing/pdf/Essentials-2021.pdf.

American Nurses Credentialing Center (ANCC). (2020). About Magnet. In *New 2020 Magnet and mission statement*. Retrieved from https://www.nursingworld.org/organizational-programs/magnet/about-magnet/.

Andrew, M. F. (2015). *People don't care how much you know until they know how much you care*. Linked in. Retrieved from. https://www.linkedin.com/pulse/show-how-much-you-care-michael-f-andrew.

Brainy Quote. (n.d.). Henry Ford. Retrieved from https://www.brainyquote.com/quotes/henry_ford_121339.

Center for Creative Leadership, Leading Effectively Staff. (2020). *6 Aspects of Political Skill*. Retrieved from https://www.ccl.org/articles/leading-effectively-articles/6-aspects-of-political-skill/.

Cialdini, R. B. (2001). *Influence: Science and practice* (4th ed.). Allyn and Bacon.

Cialdini, R. B. (2016). *Pre-Suasion: A Revolutionary Way to Influence and Persuade*. London: Random House Books.

Goldwater, M., & Zusy, M. J. L. (1990). *Prescription for nurses: Effective political action*. St. Louis: Mosby.

Jonas, S. (2003). *An introduction to the U.S. health care system* (5th ed.). New York: Springer.

Kanter, R. M. (1977). *Men and Women in the Corporation*. New York, NY: Basic Books.

Kanter, R. M. (1979). Power failure in management circuits. *Harvard Business Review, 57*(4), 65–75.

Kruse, K. (2013) What is authentic leadership? Forbes. https://www.forbes.com/sites/kevinkruse/2013/05/12/what-is-authentic-leadership/.

Laker, B., & Patel, C. (2020). Strengthen your ability to influence people. *Harvard Business Review*. Retrieved from https://hbr.org/2020/08/strengthen-your-ability-to-influence-people.

Markovitz, D. (2020). How to avoid rushing to solutions when problem-solving. Harvard Business Review. Retrieved from https://hbr.org/2020/11/how-to-avoid-rushing-to-solutions-when-problem-solving.

McMahon, T. (2020). Focus on counter measures, not solutions. *A Lean Journey.com*. Retrieved from http://www.aleanjourney.com/2020/07/focus-on-countermeasures-not-solutions.html.

Mechanic, D. (1991). Adolescents at risk: New directions paper presented at the seventh annual conference on health policy. Cornell University Medical College.

MindTools. (n.d.). 5 Whys: Getting to the root of a problem quickly. Retrieved on April 9 2022 from https://www.mindtools.com/pages/article/newTMC_5W.htm.

Schot, E., Tummers, L., & Noordegraaf, M. (2020). Working on working together. A systematic review on how healthcare professionals contribute to interprofessional collaboration. *Journal of Interprofessional Care, 34*(3), 332–342.

Tan, H. D. T., & Conde, A. R. (2021). Nurse empowerment—Linking demographics, qualities, and performances of empowered Filipino nurses. *Journal of Nursing Management 29*(5), 1302–1310.

Trépanier, S.-G., Peterson, C., Fernet, C., Austin, S., & Desrumaux, P. (2021). When workload predicts exposure to bullying behaviours in nurses: The protective role of social support and job recognition. *Journal of Advanced Nursing, 77*(7), 3093–3103.

CASE STUDY 13.1 Next-Generation Nclex® Case Study

Question 1
NGN Item Type: Multiple Response

A direct care nurse brings a concern to her unit's nurse manager. She is worried about the outcome of an interdisciplinary team meeting for one of her clients, an older adult man who is being discharged from the hospital after a bout of pneumonia. The interprofessional treatment team is recommending that the client be placed in a long-term care facility because of his declining mental acuity and the fact that he lives alone. Most of the client's children agree with the team's recommendations. However, after the most recent team meeting, the client's youngest daughter told the nurse she was willing to move in with her father to provide the necessary support. The daughter indicated that her father preferred this alternative, although the rest of family is skeptical that this is a good idea. The direct care nurse is asking for help from the nurse manager to "change the treatment team's decision."

The nurse manager must decide how to proceed to solve this problem. What questions should the nurse manager ask himself to determine his response to this request?

Select all that apply.
a. "Am I qualified to handle this issue?"
b. "Do I have the knowledge, interest, time, and resources to deal with this?"
c. "Do I have the authority to do anything?"
d. "What negatives could occur from addressing this issue?"
e. "Will taking action enhance my position as a nurse manager?"
f. "Has the nurse making the request used good judgment in the past?"

Question 2
NGN Item Type: Multiple Response

The nurse manager agrees to talk to the social worker who is the team leader responsible for this client's discharge plan to gather more information. The social worker indicated that the client was evaluated by a neurologist during his hospitalization. The neurologist's report noted that although the client can take care of his personal activities of daily living, he seems unable to make decisions that would allow him to cook, clean, or drive. The social worker noted that the adult children have had trouble agreeing on a plan to care for their father. The majority of the children were skeptical of the youngest daughter's ability to care for their father because of her past behaviors.

Based on this information, the team unanimously believed that the client would be better served by being transferred to a long-term care facility. The social worker tells the nurse manager that the direct care nurse on this interprofessional team had been very quiet during all team conferences, saying little about the nursing aspects of the client's care. She reported that at the end of the last team meeting, she asked each of the team members to contact her if they had information about the client that might have an impact on the team's final recommendation. The nurse manager must determine what his role should be in helping the direct care nurse deal with this situation.

Select all that apply.
a. The direct care nurse might be intimidated by the roles and credentials of those participating in the interprofessional team.
b. Members of the interdisciplinary team were aggressive in recommending a transfer to a long-term care facility.
c. The team leader did not encourage diversity of thought among the interprofessional team.
d. "Someone" in power at the hospital has a financial interest in the long-term care facility being recommended.
e. The direct care nurse may not have the skills to communicate with this group.
f. The client's youngest daughter may have a history of irresponsibility, saying she will do something and then not following through.

CASE STUDY 13.1 Next-Generation Nclex® Case Study—cont'd

Question 3

NGN Item Type: Multiple Response Select N

The nurse manager recognizes that he must help the direct care nurse work effectively with the treatment team to make recommendations for this client. Choose the most likely hypotheses by dragging possible hypotheses in Column A to Column B.

Which three (3) possible solutions seem to be most appropriate for this situation?

a. Ask the direct care nurse to have a meeting with the social worker regarding her conversation with the client's youngest daughter.

b. Ask the nurse to practice how she will present her conversation with the client's youngest daughter and her recommendations to the interprofessional team.

c. Indicate to the nurse that her job performance evaluation will be affected by her future performance in the treatment time.

d. In a one-to-one conference, ask the nurse to evaluate her contributions to the interprofessional team and what, if anything, she would do differently,

e. Ask the nurse if her shyness has hampered her performance in other situations.

Question 4

NGN Item Type: Matrix Multiple Response

The nurse manager must identify the actions he should take to help the direct care nurse in her role in the interdisciplinary team. **Mark as indicated or contraindicated the following actions that the nurse manager could take to help the nurse improve her competency in advocating for the patient in interprofessional team meetings.**

Potential Interventions	Indicated	Contraindicated
a. Ask the direct care nurse to set up an appointment with the nurse manager.		
b. Ask the direct care nurse to evaluate her own performance in the interprofessional treatment team, compare her self-evaluation to others' performance, and provide ways in which she might change her performance.		
c. Counsel the direct care nurse regarding the expectations of the organization for nurses participating in interprofessional team conferences.		
d. Role play with the direct care nurse as a presentation to the interprofessional team ways she might present information regarding her conversation with the client's youngest daughter.		
e. Suggest that the direct care nurse ask the social worker to schedule another meeting of the interprofessional team.		
f. Indicate to the direct care nurse that her failure to advocate for the patient in the team conference will be noted on her annual performance evaluation.		

Question 5

NGN Item Type: Multiple Response Select N

The direct care nurse may have responded in a variety of ways to the nurse manager's interventions to improve her competency in advocating for the patient during interprofessional team meetings.

Choose three (3) of the following potential responses from the direct care nurse to the interventions that demonstrate a positive professional growth for the direct care provider.

a. Procrastinates making an appointment with the nurse manager.

b. Makes excuses for her lack of advocacy for the patient in past team meetings, blaming others for her reticence.

c. Admits to her fear that other members of the interprofessional team might judge her if she spoke up in the meetings.

d. Effectively role plays communication with the interprofessional team that advocates for the patient.

e. Evaluates her lack of advocacy for the patient in past team meetings, identifying ways she might improve in the future.

f. Resists providing the social worker a report of her discussion with the client's youngest daughter.

14

Delegating: Authority, Accountability, and Responsibility in Delegation Decisions

Maureen Murphy-Ruocco

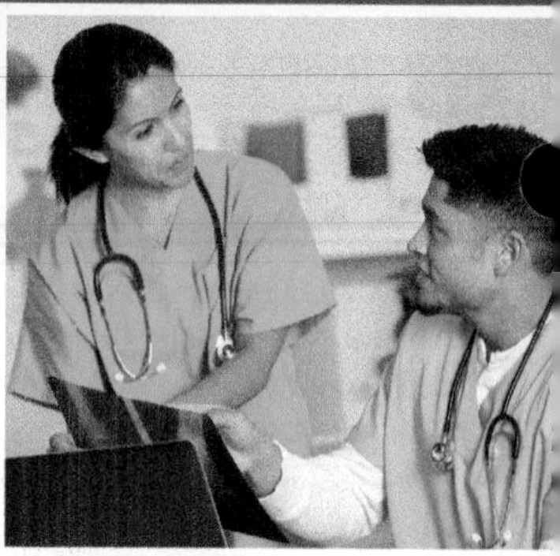

Copyright © SDI Productions/iStock/Thinkstock.

ANTICIPATED LEARNING OUTCOMES

- Examine the role of the employer/nurse leader, licensed nurse, and delegatee in the delegation process.
- Distinguish between authority, accountability, and responsibility in the delegation process.
- Explain how a nurse delegates successfully to a delegatee in the delegation process.
- Create strategies to overcome underdelegation, overdelegation, and improper delegation.
- Comprehend the legal authority of the registered nurse in delegation.

KEY TERMS

accountability
assignment
authority
delegatee
delegated responsibility
delegation
delegator
individual accountability
legal authority
nurse practice acts (NPAs)
organizational accountability
responsibility
supervision
unlicensed nursing personnel/assistive personnel (UNP/AP)

THE CHALLENGE

During the spring of 2021, much of the country was reopening as the numbers of critically ill individuals infected with SARS-CoV-2 (COVID-19) were decreasing. Many communities had been in quarantine for approximately one year. In the United States, the government mandated the wearing of masks in public places. The U.S. Food and Drug Administration's emergency authorization of COVID-19 vaccines was primarily responsible for the relaxation of these quarantine restrictions. These constraints created many hardships for individuals, families, and communities. One major hardship was the large number of healthcare workers who became fatigued, physically and emotionally. Some even left their healthcare positions permanently because of enormous amounts of stress and the impact of coping with the large number of deaths. This created a serious shortage of highly skilled, experienced professionals for hospitals. As a result, hospitals restricted the availability of scheduled elective procedures to provide resources for severely ill COVID patients. Many individuals postponed preventive care and other treatments due to the potential exposure to this highly contagious virus. When hospitals began to

THE CHALLENGE—cont'd

reinstate these procedures, they found they needed additional staff. Many nursing schools graduated students earlier than expected to provide care for the large number of individuals coming into hospitals for those procedures and the delayed surgeries.

The registered nurse in charge of the surgical unit was informed by the Admissions Department that two new patients would arrive within the next half hour. Once the patients arrived, they would be due in the operating room within the hour. As the registered nurse, I was assigned these two new patients. I had been working in the hospital for eight years and on the surgical unit for two years. Their nursing admission assessment had to be completed prior to going to surgery. I was working with a UNP/AP who had worked on the unit as a senior nursing student. The first patient arrived on the unit and I informed the

UNP/AP that I was going to do the first patient admission. The second patient arrived within seconds of the first patient and I instructed the UNP/AP to take care of the second patient. After completing the first patient admission and managing an urgent issue on the unit, I was approached by the UNP/AP who stated she had taken care of the second patient admission and provided me the nursing admission assessment. As the registered nurse, I realized that the UNP/AP made nursing assessments and judgments that were not within her scope and function.

What would you do if you were this nurse?

Kathryn King-Dyker, RN, MSN
Former Clinical Nurse II, Hackensack University Medical Center,
Hackensack, New Jersey

INTRODUCTION

Delegation, an art and skill of professional nursing, is a complex decision-making strategy implemented to accomplish nursing's goals of providing safe, efficient, and high-quality person-centered care. Effective delegation occurs when nurses know and understand their state's nurse practice act (NPA), rules and regulations, and policies in their jurisdictions (National Council of State Boards of Nursing [NCSBN] & American Nurses Association [ANA], 2019). The delegation process requires understanding the concepts of authority, accountability, and responsibility. The process must include determining each patient's condition, assessing the level of education, training, and competence of the delegatee, and examining the level of supervision required related to the delegated responsibility. Effective delegation, learning how to distribute delegated responsibilities, builds confidence in the delegatee, allowing them to provide care for patients safely and effectively. Conversely, ineffective delegation creates apprehension in the delegatee about providing patient care safely and effectively. Delegation strategies often improve as the nurse gains more knowledge and clinical experience and transitions from a novice through other levels of nursing development, known as advanced beginner, competent, proficient, and expert (Benner, 1984). Delegation is the most effective professional leadership and management strategy that nurses implement in clinical practice to improve the safety and quality of person-centered care.

DEFINITIONS

Delegation, a multifaceted decision-making process, is learned and is an essential nursing competency. The principles of effective delegation are derived from the corresponding states' NPAs and through an understanding of the concepts of responsibility and accountability. Delegation is "allowing a delegatee to perform a specific nursing activity, skill or procedure, that is beyond the delegatee's traditional role and not routinely performed" (NCSBN & ANA, 2019, p. 2). Delegated responsibility refers to a nursing activity, skill, or procedure that is transferred from a licensed nurse to a delegatee (NCSBN & ANA, 2019, p. 2). Accountability is "to be answerable to oneself and others for one's own choices, decisions, and actions as measured against a standard" (ANA, 2015, p. 41).

Delegation always involves at least two individuals, delegator and delegatee, who engage in open communication to achieve a goal. The terms *delegator* and *delegatee* represent two key roles enacted in the process of delegation. The delegator is the individual who delegates a nursing responsibility. The NCSBN and ANA (2019) define a licensed nurse as an advanced practice registered nurse (APRN), registered nurse (RN), or licensed practical nurse/licensed vocational nurse (LPN/LVN). The National Guidelines for Nursing Delegation (NCSBN & ANA, 2019) state that an APRN can delegate to RNs, LPNs/LVNs, and assistive personnel (AP), referred to in this chapter as unlicensed nursing personnel/assistive personnel (UNP/AP). RNs can delegate to LPNs/LVNs and/or UNP/AP; in some NPAs and states/jurisdictions, LPNs/LVNs may be permitted to delegate to UNP/AP. However, the National Guidelines for Nursing Delegation reinforce that these guidelines do not apply to the transfer of responsibility for care of a patient between healthcare providers, such as from an RN to another RN or an LPN/LVN to another LPN/LVN, because this transfer of care for the patient is considered a "handoff."

A delegatee is an individual who is delegated a nursing responsibility by a licensed nurse (APRN, RN, or LPN/LVN (if a jurisdiction NPA allows). The delegatee must be competent to perform the delegated responsibility and must verbally accept the responsibility (NCBSN & ANA, 2019). Many nonlicensed delegatees function in a supportive role to the RN or LPN/LVN and may have other titles, across states, such as patient care technicians (PCTs), certified nursing assistants or aides (CNAs), certified medication assistants (CMAs), and home healthcare aides. Licensed nurses do not supervise all assistive personnel. For example, physical therapy technicians work under the authority of the physical therapist, as they are trained to perform selected physical therapy activities. Regardless of who supervises the UNP/AP, licensed nurses exchange appropriate information and collaborate with all disciplines to create productive interprofessional teams for the best delivery of high-quality healthcare.

ASSIGNMENT VERSUS DELEGATION

In the workplace, nurses must differentiate between assignment and delegation. An assignment is defined as performing a fundamental skill on the job, such as "routine care, activities and procedures that are within the authorized scope of practice of the RN or LPN/VN or part of the routine functions" of the UNP/AP (NCSBN & ANA, 2019, p. 2). Assignments are the distribution of work that each qualified individual is responsible for during the work period. Once the nurse knows that the routine care, activities, and procedures are part of the individual's basic educational training, the nurse can make appropriate assignments. However, the nurse must validate that the assignment was completed and performed correctly. Once an assignment requires a specific type of knowledge or skill, the nurse must consider this delegation and must validate the competency of the delegatee.

Delegation occurs when delegatees are requested to perform a specific nursing activity, skill, or procedure outside their traditional role that is not routinely performed. The delegatee must have completed additional education and training, and successfully validated competency to perform the care related to the delegated responsibility (NCSBN & ANA, 2019). Competency validation relates to how safely individuals can perform the delegated responsibility and their role and function in the healthcare facility. The licensed nurse, who delegates responsibility, maintains overall accountability for the patient. However, the delegatee still maintains responsibility for the activity, skill, or procedure. The licensed nurse can never delegate nursing judgment or critical decision-making, both of which are authorized in the state's NPA. However, specific nursing responsibilities can be delegated because they have the legal authority to delegate under the NPA. When delegating to a licensed nurse, the delegated responsibility must be within the parameters of the delegatee's authorized scope of practice under the NPA (NCSBN & ANA, 2019).

Therefore, the decision of whether to delegate is based on the licensed nurse's clinical judgment, which considers the condition of the patient, the competence of all members of the nursing team, and the degree of supervision required. The licensed nurse should delegate only when confident that the delegatee's competency has been validated.

HISTORICAL PERSPECTIVE

In the 1970s and 1980s, RNs entered the profession with relatively limited content knowledge and/or clinical experience about delegation and how, what, and when to delegate. During that time, most healthcare occurred in acute care hospitals, staffed by RNs, LPNs/LVNs, and nurse's aides, now referred to as UNP/AP. Concepts such as "team nursing" permitted LPNs/LVNs and UNP/AP to function as part of a nursing team, limiting the number of RNs employed on the unit. This allowed for a portion of direct patient care to be provided by LPNs/LVNs and UNP/AP. Direct patient care included providing physical comforts and basic treatments to patients. As the complexities of patient care delivery increased, the work demand and expectation of RNs became more challenging, creating the need to employ more UNP/AP to support patient care. Even though in the mid-1990s a shift occurred to a primary nursing model (all professional nurses), it shifted back to a multilevel nursing model (RNs mixed with LPNs/LVNs and UNP/AP). At that time, fiscal constraints and new complexities in healthcare created an urgent need for nurses to learn more about how to use delegation skills to deliver safe and effective nursing care. As the healthcare industry began to emphasize community-based care, the need for delegation and supervision of others became even more evident.

During the early part of the 21st century, the ANA and the NCSBN became increasingly concerned about the quality of delegation. In 2005, both the ANA and NCSBN adopted position papers on delegation with slightly different definitions; however, both agreed that delegation is an essential nursing skill. In 2015, the NCSBN convened two expert panels from education, research, and practice to discuss the literature on and issues related to delegation, and to evaluate the research completed by the NCSBN's Center for Regulatory Excellence Grant Program. Their goal was to develop National Guidelines for Nursing Delegation that provided clear direction and standardization of the delegation process, from an organizational and patient care perspective for safe delegation. In 2016, the NCSBN and ANA published the National Guidelines for Nursing Delegation. In 2019, the National Guidelines for Nursing Delegation were revised and updated, replacing older NCSBN and ANA Joint Statements on Delegation. These guidelines apply to all levels of nursing licensure—APRNs, RNs, and LPNs/LVNs—where the NPAs are silent (NCSBN & ANA, 2019). However, the National Guidelines for Nursing Delegation emphasize that they do not apply to the transfer of responsibility for care of a patient between licensed healthcare professionals. Nurses are educated to conduct assessments, plan, evaluate, and apply nursing judgment. Nurses need to understand that the pervasive function of "clinical reasoning, nursing judgment, or critical decision making cannot be delegated" (NCSBN & ANA, 2019, p. 3).

With ongoing changes in the healthcare environment, including high patient acuity rates, complexity of patients' chronic conditions, technological advances, and extreme challenges, such as COVID-19, for the healthcare delivery system, nurses must become expert delegators. A comprehensive knowledge base in delegation, diagnostic reasoning, and clinical decision-making skills is required since nurses are delegating more patient care responsibility while continuing to provide expert nursing care. Because of limited nursing resources in different regions and in certain facilities, it may be necessary to delegate responsibilities beyond the traditional role of healthcare providers. Thus, delegators must understand the delegation process, their state NPA, and the roles and responsibilities of other healthcare providers, including APRNs, RNs, LPNs/LVNs, and UNP/AP. The overarching goal of effective delegation decisions is the protection of the public.

NATIONAL GUIDELINES FOR NURSING DELEGATION

The National Guidelines for Nursing Delegation (NCSBN & ANA, 2019) identify the roles and responsibilities of the employer/nurse leader, licensed nurse, and delegatee in the delegation process (Fig. 14.1). The delegation process commences with members at the administrative level of the organization deciding what nursing responsibilities can be delegated and to whom and under what circumstances, developing policies and procedures on delegation based on these decisions, evaluating the delegation process on a periodic basis, and creating a positive culture and work environment (NCSBN & ANA, 2019). The National Guidelines for Nursing Delegation provides an exceptional graphic that describes the role, function, and collaborative work relationships among those in the role of the employer/nurse leader, licensed nurse, and delegatee. (See Fig. 14.1.)

The responsibilities of the employer/nurse leader include the ability to identify a nurse who can provide oversight of a delegated responsibility through an assessment process, and is ultimately accountable for a safe healthcare environment. That designated nurse leader must develop and support a delegation committee—ideally composed of nurse leaders—who determine what nursing responsibilities can be delegated, to whom, under what circumstances, and periodically review delegation policies and procedures. This will ensure consistency with nursing practice trends, the state/jurisdiction's NPAs, and patient safety. The employer/nurse leader must communicate the responsibilities related to delegation to licensed nurses and educate them about what can be delegated. This communication should include the competencies that are required of the delegatee to perform a specific nursing responsibility safely. On an ongoing basis, the employer/nurse leader must provide individuals access to training and education for delegated responsibilities.

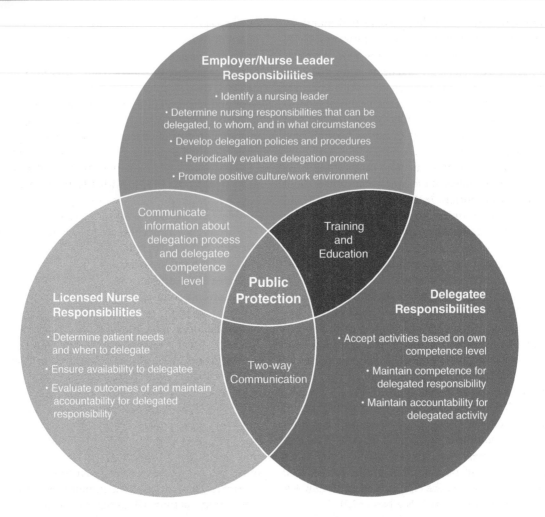

Employer/Nurse Leader Responsibilities
- Identify a nursing leader
- Determine nursing responsibilities that can be delegated, to whom, and in what circumstances
- Develop delegation policies and procedures
- Periodically evaluate delegation process
- Promote positive culture/work environment

Communicate information about delegation process and delegatee competence level

Training and Education

Public Protection

Licensed Nurse Responsibilities
- Determine patient needs and when to delegate
- Ensure availability to delegatee
- Evaluate outcomes of and maintain accountability for delegated responsibility

Two-way Communication

Delegatee Responsibilities
- Accept activities based on own competence level
- Maintain competence for delegated responsibility
- Maintain accountability for delegated activity

NCSBN's position papers on delegation and working with others:

Fig. 14.1 The National Council of State Boards of Nursing (NCSBN) Model and position paper on delegation describes the responsibilities of the employer or nurse leader, licensed nurse, and delegate. (From National Council of State Boards of Nursing & American Nurses Association. [2019]. *National Guidelines for Nursing Delegation.* https://www.ncsbn.org/NGND-PosPaper_06.pdf).

Additionally, they must provide documented evidence of periodic competency validation, a procedure to validate the delegatee's knowledge and competence related to the delegated responsibility. All competency validations should be measured at the appropriate level of the APRN, RN, LPN/LVN, or UNP/AP.

The delegation process must be periodically evaluated and documented, and include resolutions for the issues identified to ensure patient safety. For effective delegation, the employer/nurse leader must promote a positive culture and work environment that supports person-centered care. The licensed nurse's responsibilities include knowledge and understanding of when and what to delegate, the ability to determine patients' needs and conditions, the state's or jurisdiction's provisions for delegation, employer policies and procedures regarding delegating a specific responsibility, and what can and cannot be delegated based on the practice setting.

The licensed nurse must be available to the delegatee to provide guidance as well as to respond to any questions related to the delegated responsibility. The nurse's communication needs to be clear and concise and the delegatee needs to know how to communicate immediately with the nurse if a change in the status of the patient occurs. If the patient's condition or other circumstances warrant, the nurse should assist or complete the delegated responsibility. After completion of the delegated responsibility, the nurse should follow up with the delegatee as well as the patient. The nurse must provide feedback about the delegation process, evaluate the delegatee's competency, and report any issues to the nurse leader, including whether the delegatee needs any additional training or support. The nurse must evaluate outcomes of, and maintain accountability for, the delegated responsibility.

The delegatee's responsibilities include the ability to accept the delegated responsibility based on one's level of education, competence, and comfort given the patient's condition or circumstances in the practice setting. The delegatee should confirm acceptance of the delegated responsibility or nonacceptance of the delegated responsibility if uncomfortable. It is essential to maintain ongoing competence for delegated activities, skills and procedures as well as attend additional training when appropriate. To ensure continuity of care, delegatees must maintain two-way communication with the licensed nurse in charge of the patient and maintain responsibility for completing the delegated activity, skill, or procedure. According to the facility policy, delegatees must provide timely and accurate documentation regarding their delegated responsibility (NCSBN & ANA, 2019).

The employer/nurse leader must communicate information with the licensed nurse and UNP/AP about the delegation process, provide education and training of employees, and communicate the level of competence of the delegatee. Successful delegation is influenced by several factors: effective communication, level of competence, role clarification, and collaborative work relationships (NCSBN & ANA, 2019). The overall goal of delegation is to achieve quality person-centered care and provide exemplary public protection.

EXERCISE 14.1 Interview a nurse leader about the leader's role and what support the employer provides in the delegation process. Discuss these findings with a small group of colleagues. What can you conclude?

EFFECTIVE COMMUNICATION: AN ESSENTIAL COMPETENCY FOR SUCCESSFUL DELEGATION

Effective communication involves a two-way exchange between the delegator and delegatee. The nurse must provide communication that is clear, concise, timely, and reliable to produce safe and efficient person-centered care. Maintaining two-way communication, requesting information from the delegatee, and teaching how, when, and what to report are essential. A clear understanding between the delegator and delegatee about the delegated responsibility creates a greater chance of producing optimum outcomes for person-centered care.

A delay in communicating information can interfere with clinical decision-making and have a negative impact on person-centered care. For example, when a person's health status rapidly changes (e.g., one or more of the patient's vital signs rapidly changes), specific information can lose its value or become irrelevant to the patient's condition when not reported in a timely manner. When the reported information is incomplete, it leads to poor clinical judgments that may have adverse effects on person-centered care. A two-way communication and follow-through system established between the delegator and delegatee allows person-centered care to be altered, if necessary, in a timely manner.

Improving lines of communication can occur by appreciating and valuing each other. Healthy work relationships among all personnel, including licensed nurses and UNP/AP, promote a "synergy between team members," enabling them to work together more effectively. Understanding another individual and developing a trusting relationship are critical components to successful delegation. Trust is developed through the knowledge of one another's capabilities and encouragement of others. Delegating with confidence requires considerable trust between two or more individuals to create an effective team. For example, a delegatee who does not concur with the philosophy of the facility (e.g., the goals of hospice care) might have a negative impact on person-centered care. Building on the communication strength and understanding the communication challenges of the team prove to be an effective strategy for maintaining effective communication. Strategies for communication related to delegation appear in Box 14.1. The nurse needs to be an advocate for and effectively

---

BOX 14.1   Strategies for Communication Related to Delegation

Giving information. This role applies to both the delegator and delegatee. The delegator must provide sufficient information about the patient, situation, delegated responsibility, monitoring process, and desired outcomes. In turn, the delegatee must report back to the delegator to indicate deviations from any of those elements.

Giving direction. This role applies to the delegator. If a delegatee has not performed a delegated responsibility previously or is new to the unit, considerable direction (and additional guidance) may be expected. The delegator is expected to be as specific as possible in what the delegated responsibility entails, how often reports to the delegator are needed, and what constitutes an immediate concern. With experienced delegatees, the direction may be more generalized (e.g., please check the patient's blood pressure every 2 hours, assist the patient out of bed to the chair, and check the blood pressure as soon as the patient is sitting in a chair). More detailed direction may be necessary for a delegatee

depending on the complexity level of the delegated responsibility.

Seeking clarity. This role applies to both the delegator and delegatee. The delegator determines whether the delegatee understands what is expected in relation to the delegated responsibility and reporting requirement. The delegatee must understand the delegator's general standards for general statements such as, "immediately report any change in the patient or something unusual." A repeat-back communication method can be used by both delegator and delegatee to ensure that they understand each other.

Seeking advice. This role applies mostly to the delegatee but may be used by the delegator. Examples include finding other ways to solicit information from patients or ways to perform a delegated responsibility when a patient's physical condition prevents a typical approach. To a lesser extent, this technique can be used by the delegator to determine how to support the delegatee in performing a delegated responsibility.

---

communicate the needs of the patient to the appropriate members of the healthcare team. The interprofessional team members should be aware of the goals of care, treatments, and interventions. This level of communication decreases misunderstandings and conflicts, eliminates fragmentation of care, prevents errors, and enhances patient safety (ANA, 2020).Documentation, a form of communication, must be accurate, complete, and provided in a timely manner. Nurses have a legal and ethical responsibility to communicate and document the person-centered care provided.

DELEGATION AND THE DECISION-MAKING PROCESS IN NURSING

To be an effective delegator, the nurse should consider a series of questions and reflect on the answers before delegating; examine the questions in Box 14.2. Once a decision to delegate is made, the nurse confers with the delegatee to communicate critical details (Fig. 14.2). Each of the questions in Box 14.2 can guide nurses in deciding whether a particular delegation can be achieved while ensuring patient safety. Organizations often have roles

---

BOX 14.2   Key Questions to Consider in Delegation

- Does the Nurse Practice Act laws, rules, or regulations restrict delegation in the given situation?
- Do organizational policies support delegation in the given situation?
- Does the delegator have the authority, within the delegator's scope of practice, to delegate a nursing responsibility in the given situation?
- Does the delegator know to whom and under what circumstance to delegate a nursing responsibility?
- Does the delegator know that nursing responsibilities that require nursing judgment or critical decision-making can never be delegated?

- Does the patient's acuity level limit or prevent the delegation decision-making process?
- Does the delegatee have the level of education or training, degree of competence, and comfort to carry out the delegated responsibility safely?
- Does the delegatee know how to alert the delegator about specific signs and symptoms for a specific patient in a specific situation?
- Will supervision be readily available?

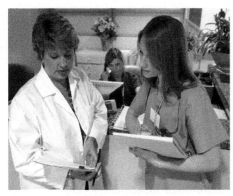

Fig. 14.2 The nurse must confer with the UNP/AP related to any situation involving delegation.

for UNP/AP that are facility dependent. Just because a particular task could be delegated in a home healthcare environment does not necessarily mean that task can be delegated in an acute care or long-term care facility. Furthermore, just as nurses specialize, so do UNP/AP. The UNP/AP may receive delegations that would not be appropriate on another unit or in another setting.

In the provision of nursing care, delegation is built on a foundation that emphasizes professional nursing practice. Delegation, a critical leadership skill, must be learned and implemented effectively to accomplish a nursing goal. During the delegation process, the nurse must perform a critical assessment, make a judgment, and decide whether to delegate. This process can be especially challenging for nurse managers. One strategy for learning how to be an effective delegator is to use some of the concepts learned in the nursing process. Begin with assessment and planning and then proceed with implementation and evaluation.

Assessment and Planning

Assessment begins with selecting a designated nurse leader who has the ability to make a thorough assessment about the facility and who implements appropriate staffing models for delegation while maintaining accountability for safe person-centered care. Appropriate nurse staffing is a critical requisite for delivering safe, quality healthcare at every level of practice and in every setting (AMN Healthcare, 2018). To optimize health system performance, the Institute for Healthcare Improvement (IHI) Quintuple Aim initiative focuses on improving the patient's experience of care, including quality of care and satisfaction, improving health

of populations, reducing per capita cost of healthcare, improving the work life of healthcare providers and advancing health equity (IHI, 2022).

During assessment, the nurse considers critical questions and evaluates the answers to differentiate what is and is not appropriate to delegate (see Box 14.2). The nurse must ensure that the laws, rules and regulations, and policies support delegation and that it is within the nurse's role. The authority to delegate differs across states; thus, all nurses must verify their jurisdiction's statutes and regulations. Once an assessment of the patient's needs is completed, a nurse manager or charge nurse should determine whether the delegating nurse is competent to make delegation decisions. This determination is usually based on educational level, validated competency, or additional continuing education. Once the delegating nurse is considered competent, the selection of a delegatee occurs. This step is extremely important because the delegatee's work affects the success of the healthcare team. However, the nurse may or may not have the opportunity to select a particular delegatee for the team.

Before delegating, the nurse must determine whether the activity, skill, or procedure is appropriate to delegate to a delegatee. The nurse must determine whether the delegatee has the knowledge, skill, and ability to accept the delegation and whether the delegatee's ability matches the care needs of the patient. If the nurse believes that it is not an appropriate match, delegation should not occur. The nurse must convey a consistent message to the delegatee that performing the activity, skill, or procedure is one component of person-centered care. Although the performance of a psychomotor task is essential for providing person-centered care, it is the second component—the nursing process, performed by the nurse—that determines factors for nursing action. The direct care nurse also assesses the situation to determine whether the facility has policies, procedures, and protocols for the delegated responsibilities. If the policies, procedures, and protocols are not documented, they must be instituted as soon as possible. In addition, appropriate supervision must be available to the delegatee. Box 14.3 reviews elements to consider during assessment and planning in the delegation process. During the COVID-19 pandemic many protocols were adjusted, allowing for as much flexibility as possible due to limited staff with specific expertise in clinical areas, and limited equipment and supplies, provide the best person-centered care outcomes.

BOX 14.3   Assessment and Planning in the Delegation Process

Assessment

The delegator should:

- Ensure that state laws and institutional policies support delegation
- Determine whether the delegated responsibility is within the scope of the delegating nurse practice and whether the delegator is competent to delegate
- Assess the client's needs, stability, health condition, and predictability of the risks and responses
- Assess whether the task is appropriate to delegate to a delegatee
- Determine whether a specific delegatee has the experience and educational background to complete the task safely and effectively
- Consider the type of healthcare facility related to the delegated responsibility
- Determine whether the institution's policies and procedures allow for this type of delegation to a delegatee
- Assess whether the nurse can provide appropriate guidance, support, and supervision of the delegated responsibility

Planning

The delegator should:

- Identify the delegated responsibility, how it should be accomplished and the expected outcomes
- Determine the delegatee's understanding of the delegated responsibility and expectations
- Alert the delegatee to any specific patient conditions, characteristics or concerns
- Reinforce a willingness to guide and support the delegatee
- Convey expected observations to be reported and recorded
- Specify reporting time frames and/or dates expected
- Specify any concerns or emergency situations that warrant prompt reporting
- Validate the delegatee's willingness to accept the delegated responsibility
- Emphasize the importance of timely, accurate, and complete documentation
- Determine any specific patient requirements, characteristics or concerns to be addressed

The delegatee should:

- Comprehend the delegated responsibility
- Ask questions and seek clarification regarding the delegated responsibility if needed
- Specify any performance limitations regarding the delegated responsibility (e.g., never completed the delegated responsibility before or completed it only once or infrequently)
- Request additional training or supervision if needed
- Affirm an understanding of expectations related to delegated responsibility
- Review the emergency action/communication plan
- Inform the delegator that you cannot accept the delegated responsibility because of a knowledge deficit related to education, training or comfort level

Implementation and Evaluation

Implementation

During implementation, the delegator allocates work to delegatees and gives them the responsibility to perform the work. When delegating work, the nurse is merely sharing a set of functions to ensure quality outcomes. In essence, sharing work does not negate the nurse's accountability for total person-centered care. The definition of *delegation* emphasizes that patient care itself is not delegated; only a group of activities, skills, or procedures is delegated. Thus, the final accountability remains with the delegator. For example, requesting an individual to perform a delegated responsibility within a defined set of functions or asking the person to perform the same delegated responsibility as the previous day can be expected. For delegation to be effective, the nurse must understand that sharing activities is essential to benefit person-centered care and the professional aspects of care may never be delegated. The role of the nurse in providing safe, effective, person-centered care is critical, whether person-centered care is performed by an individual nurse or by another member of the team through the process of delegation. Individual actions and collaboration with other healthcare team members achieve optimal care (ANA, 2020).Critical thinking, diagnostic reasoning, and the ability to synthesize information from various sources are what characterize the nurse, a licensed professional, who implements safe and effective nursing care.

The nurse has the ultimate responsibility for person-centered care and the ability to supervise the delegatee's performance of the delegated responsibility and to ensure compliance with standards of practice, policies, and procedures. Supervision is the nurse's ability to provide direction, guidance, support, feedback, and evaluation to the delegatee for the accomplishment of a delegated responsibility. Delegatees must be provided the appropriate information, materials, resources, and technology as well as guidance and support to perform the delegated responsibility successfully. The level of supervision should correlate with the experience of the delegatee and the level of complexity of the delegated responsibility. For example, when new skills are being acquired by the UNP/AP, the nurse should provide more support, guidance, and oversight of a delegated responsibility.

During supervision, the nurse should ask the delegatee a series of questions such as, "Has the delegated responsibility been completed?" "What changes were observed with the patient?" and "How did the patient respond?" Open-ended questions allow the nurse to gain pertinent information from the delegatee about the delegated responsibility. This also allows for the experienced nurse to identify delegatee's verbal or nonverbal clues about how comfortable they are with performing the delegated responsibility. For example,

a delegatee who has functioned in a physician's office for a long time and are not used to working under the direction of a nurse may appear concerned about being supervised by a nurse. Initiating a conversation about the nurse's role and function in the facility and why supervision is necessary can eliminate or diminish any negative feelings about being supervised. Similarly, delegatees should feel free to ask questions about the delegated responsibilities, how best to perform them, the patient's condition, and how and when to report relevant information. The nurse must validate that the delegatee knows to ask questions and offer observations about anything that will enhance patient safety. Effective teams communicate specific time frames for meetings to ensure that delegated responsibilities occur within the agreed upon time frame. Specific time frames may include before and after breaks and meals, and any time delegatees have any questions or concerns. It is important to recognize the contributions of delegatees toward person-centered care. "Recognition is one thing that simply cannot be overdone" (Tye, 2020, p. 71). Recognition of all members of the healthcare team enhances collegiality and collaboration. Box 14.4 reviews elements to consider during implementation.

BOX 14.4 Implementation and Evaluation During Delegation

Implementation

The nurse must:

- Review the delegated responsibility, how it should be accomplished, and expected outcomes as implementation begins
- Reinforce any specific patient requirements, characteristics or concerns
- Provide available resources necessary to complete the delegated responsibility
- Intervene based on the patient's needs and/or complexity of the delegated responsibility on a timely basis
- Supervise the delegatee's ability to complete the delegated responsibility based on education and experience
- Provide appropriate feedback on a timely basis

The delegatee should:

- Complete the delegated responsibility according to established standards
- Ask questions or seek clarification when necessary

- Adhere to specified and agreed upon reporting times
- Report any specific concerns or emergency situations immediately

Evaluation

The nurse reviews if the:

- Delegated responsibility was successfully performed
- Expected person-centered care outcome(s) were successfully achieved
- Communication was timely and effective
- Strengths/challenges were identified
- Strengths/challenges created a platform for a quality improvement plan
- Quality improvement plan allowed for addressing concerns/issues and provided constructive feedback for the nurse and delegatee
- Quality improvement plan allowed for appropriate training and education
- Team was acknowledged for contributions to safe and effective person-centered care

Supervision can also vary in different types of health-care facilities, potentially resulting in role confusion among RNs and LPN/LVNs. For example, in long-term care facilities, an LPN/LVN may be responsible for a nursing unit with a registered nurse supervising patient care. In long-term care facilities, the role of RNs and LPNs/LVNs may not be well delineated. This creates an environment in which LPNs/LVNs may be responsible for delegation that exceeds their scope of practice. Variation in NPAs and administrative codes leads to role confusion among LPNs/LVNs regarding their scope of practice, especially as it relates to delegation and supervision of others. This can create a negative impact on the relationship between the RN and LPN/LVN.

Evaluation

Evaluation, often overlooked in the delegation process, should be completed because it allows time to reflect on delegation decisions. It provides the nurse time to determine whether the delegation was successful and to identify the strengths and challenges related to the delegation decision. Evaluation and constructive reflection allow us to build on the strengths, learn from the challenges, and implement quality measures to improve delegation decisions.

When delegators decrease the amount of direct person-centered care they perform, they automatically increase their supervision of others. Giving clear directions, asking for and receiving quality feedback regarding delegated responsibilities and having an agreed upon schedule for checkpoints are essential for a well-executed plan. An evaluation plan is influenced by factors such as knowledge of and experience with the delegatee, the number of delegatees and patients for whom the delegator is accountable, the geographic design of the location, the stability of the patients, and the resources available. Evaluating how the delegatee and patients are doing throughout the work period is critical to work performance and the outcomes of person-centered care.

The delegator should provide constructive feedback to a delegatee regarding their work-related performance. To convey satisfaction with a delegatee's performance that is less than satisfactory diminishes the credibility of the nurse. A verbal attack on a delegatee does not produce effective change and potentially undermines any long-term working relationship. For example, a verbal attack such as "What is wrong with you today?" is not effective to elicit feedback. The detrimental impact of incivility, in nursing education and practice, has been documented in the literature (Olsen et al., 2020, p. 319). It is also common in the workplace. The best strategy is to provide open, honest, and constructive feedback such as "Let me demonstrate a more effective way to perform the task." Honest feedback about work-related performance and specific strategies for change provide the delegatee a quality improvement plan.

Another concern regarding delegation is when individuals lack the competence to hold their current position. One strategy for managing this issue is to temporarily lower expectations and provide additional support. This strategy allows individuals to build on their strengths, minimize weaknesses, and gain confidence. However, the delegator and leaders must examine the effect that lowering expectations for an individual has on other team members. Many questions need to be considered in the decision: Why is one employee held to the standard and another is not? Who becomes responsible for the work that one individual cannot accomplish? Is it fair to compensate an individual for work that does not meet performance expectations? What are the potential liabilities of altering the standards of performance? Since making delegation decisions is a complex process, nurses must understand that delegating to individuals who are not capable of performing safely and effectively and then not intervening creates a high risk for legal liability. Work should not be delegated if the delegator knows that the delegatee is not competent to perform the delegated responsibility. In addition to the legal ramifications of poor delegation decisions, ethical considerations should also influence the nurse's decisions. Box 14.4 reviews elements to consider for evaluating delegation decisions.

Nurses always have accountability for assessment, diagnosis, planning, nursing judgment, and evaluation of person-centered care. Evaluation and constructive feedback are essential components for continuous quality improvement and effective nursing management. RNs are accountable for evaluation and the overall patient outcomes (Barrow & Sharma, 2020). The ability to make effective delegation decisions and to be accountable for providing safe, competent, and effective person-centered care is a critical competency for nurses in the 21st century.

EXERCISE 14.2 Interview three licensed nurses. Ask them what they believe their responsibilities are in the delegation process. Discuss these responsibilities with a small group of colleagues.

ORGANIZATIONAL AND INDIVIDUAL ACCOUNTABILITY

Organizational accountability, the ability to secure the necessary resources for the healthcare team to provide safe and effective person-centered care, is a crucial component of delegation. Highly productive organizations often use a relationship-based leadership model that fosters interprofessional communication and collaboration among all members of the healthcare team. Building positive relationships with patients, professionals, and other healthcare team members "is an imperative for nurse executives striving to create and sustain caring practice environments" (Prestia & Dyess, 2020, p. 330). This promotes a positive culture and work environment that supports person-centered care, necessary for effective delegation. Successful organizations close the gap between the "values posted on the lobby wall and the attitudes and behaviors that are actually reflected in workplace culture" (Tye, 2020, p. 67).

A shared governance model, a framework for organizing nursing care, is often used when hospitals seek Magnet® recognition. A shared governance model, an accountability-based leadership model, fosters structural empowerment, transformational leadership, development of new knowledge, and evidence-based practice improvements and innovations. Successful organizations that achieve Magnet® status, through an extensive evaluation process, usually have supportive work environments and support healthcare teams to function effectively. Making appropriate decisions depends on how well the organization provides adequate resources, including an appropriate ratio of RNs to LPNs/LVNs and UNP/AP. Chief nursing officers (CNOs) are accountable for establishing systems to assess, monitor, verify, communicate, and evaluate competency requirements related to delegation.

Individual accountability is another component of delegation. This term refers to individuals' abilities to explain their actions and results. Accountability is to be "answerable to oneself and others for one's choices, decisions and actions as measured against standards..." (ANA, 2015, p. 41). Individual or personal accountability is a "culture of ownership" in which individuals hold themselves to higher standards to be " held accountable" (Tye, 2020, p. 67). The *Code of Ethics for Nurses with Interpretive Statements* (2015a) is composed of nine provisions and describes the ethical obligations of all nurses. The Code's Provision 4 focuses on the nurse's authority, accountability, and responsibility for nursing practice and how decisions and actions must be consistent with promoting health and providing high-quality healthcare. Provision 4 also has four interpretive statements related to responsibility and obligations to the patient. The first interpretive statement emphasizes the importance of the role of "authority, accountability, and responsibility" in nursing practice. The second interpretive statement reviews "accountability for nursing judgment, decision making, and actions" and emphasizes that technology is viewed as only as an aid to care and cannot be substituted for nursing actions, judgment, and accountability. The third interpretive statement addresses the nurses' responsibilities related to "accountability for nursing judgment, decision making, and actions" and requires nurse executives to empower nurses to actively engage, participate, and contribute to organizational committees and institutional review boards. The fourth interpretive statement addresses the "assignment and delegation of nursing activities or tasks." This statement indicates that nurses cannot delegate nursing assessment and evaluation and emphasizes that employer policies do not release nurses of this responsibility in the delegation process. Legally, nurses have authority, accountability, and responsibility for the quality of person-centered care provided in accordance with the scope and standards of nursing practice, nurse practice acts, and rules and regulations.

LEGAL AUTHORITY TO DELEGATE

Legal authority, by virtue of the professional nursing license, is the ability to delegate a nursing responsibility to a competent individual. However, the nurse retains accountability for ensuring that the delegated responsibility is completed by the right person and that the person is supervised appropriately.

A critical component of delegation is authority, and the delegated responsibility must comply with the law, such as the state's NPA, and comply with the educational preparation and certification of the delegatee. Nurses must be able to articulate their scope of practice and responsibility of nursing care congruent with standards of practice and state nurse practice act. Most state NPAs address the concept of delegation, including some rules and regulations governing when and what can be delegated. State boards of nursing are vested in protecting the public; therefore, they regulate the educational preparation and practice of professional nursing. Nurses must be engaged in nursing at the individual, organizational, and legislative level because "nursing practice drives value, and nurses have a direct and intimate influence on the quality, safety and costs of patient centered care" (ANA, 2020, p. 4)

Legally, delegation is a complex process. First, the delegator is personally responsible for prudent action. If the delegated responsibility is not performed within acceptable standards, a potential for nursing malpractice emerges. Failure to delegate and supervise within acceptable standards may extend to direct corporate liability for the facility. Whenever care is provided by another individual rather than a nurse, the accountability for care remains with the delegator even though others provide various aspects of care. This view of professional liability is consistent with the concept that licensure conveys both privilege and expectation. Specific knowledge about nursing and delegation is necessary to make appropriate nursing judgments. The Literature Perspective is an exemplar of wrongful delegation of patient care. Nurses are legally accountable and liable for their actions and those of their delegatees. Since the role of the nurse evolves over time, nurses must maintain current and accurate knowledge about the scope of nursing liability.

LITERATURE PERSPECTIVE

Resource: Reiner, G. (2020). Nurse legal case study: Wrongful delegation of patient care. Georgia Nursing, 80(2), 12.

A registered nurse (RN) employed by a home healthcare agency received a call from a certified nursing assistant (CNA) who was at a patient's home and informed the RN that the patient's gastrointestinal (GI) tube fell out during the night. The RN informed the CNA that the patient would have to go to the emergency room (ER) to have the GI tube reinserted and it would be several hours before she could visit the patient. However, the family did not want to bring the patient to the ER and decided to wait for the RN to visit the patient. The CNA informed the RN that she felt comfortable reinserting the GI tubes because she had experience doing it from working in a nursing home. The RN agreed to allow her to reinsert the GI tube but informed her not to restart any tube feedings. After 45 minutes, the CNA confirmed with the RN that the GI tube was reinserted, without difficulty, and she had checked the GI tube for proper placement. Several hours later, the RN arrived at the patient's home and observed the patient receiving a tube feeding. The daughter denied being told by the CNA to stop the tube feedings until the RN arrived. The patient was complaining of nausea and abdominal pain. The physical assessment revealed abdominal distention and pain on palpation. The RN called 911 to access emergency medical assistance and the patient was transported to the hospital. The patient was diagnosed with peritonitis due to improper placement of the GI tube.

The family filed a lawsuit against the RN and the home healthcare agency. The allegations against the RN included failure to contact provider for an order to reinsert the GI tube; wrongful delegation of patient care to assistive personnel; failure to follow agency's policies and procedures on delegation, GI tube insertion, and supervision of assistive personnel; and failure to ensure that patient and family received communication to withhold GI tube feedings. As mandated by state law, the nurse was reported to the National Practitioner Data Bank (NPDB). The case was settled before trial, and the cost was estimated at more than $255,000 to defend and settle the case on behalf of the insured nurse.

Implications for Practice

The RN delegator nurse needs to know and understand the employer's policies and procedures for safe clinical practice and delegated responsibilities for safe patient care. Verifying the delegatee's knowledge, skills, abilities, education, training, experience, competency, and diversity awareness, as well as determining the complexity of patient, are necessary before delegating responsibility to a delegatee. The nurse must also monitor and evaluate the patient care outcomes and patients' responses to care. Providing feedback to delegatees regarding their performance of delegated responsibility is essential. Informing the executive nursing leadership and risk management about issues related to delegating to a delegatee is essential to improve the quality of patient care. Nurses must understand that not being knowledgeable about the scope and standards of nursing practice and the policies and protocols of an organization is not a legal defense, especially if a nurse has received education on such policies and protocols. Nurses must never delegate clinical reasoning, nursing judgment, or critical decision-making related to the delivery of person-centered care.

LEARNING HOW TO DELEGATE: DIFFERENT STRATEGIES FOR SUCCESS

The Five Rights of Delegation

The five rights of delegation, Table 14.1, is a valuable tool to assist nurses in making effective delegation decisions. The first column of Table 14.1 contains the five delegation rights, the second column provides specific questions to ask yourself before delegating, and the third column indicates that if the response to all of the questions regarding the five rights is "yes," then it is appropriate to delegate. The five rights include how to delegate the right task, under the right circumstances, to the right person, with the right direction and communication, and under the right supervision. The direct care nurse's communication style influences how the delegatee responds to delegated responsibilities and influences teamwork and relationships. The fourth right of delegation—the "right directions and

TABLE 14.1   The Five Rights of Delegation

Delegation Rights	The Right Questions (Answer all Questions)	The Right Response (If all of the answers are yes, it's the...)
Task	Is the delegated responsibility appropriate to delegate based on the individuals' job description and facility policies and procedures? Is the delegated responsibility legally appropriate to delegate?	Right task
Circumstance	Is the delegation process appropriate to the situation? Is the environment conducive to completing the delegated responsibility safely? Are the equipment and resources available to complete the delegated responsibility? Do staffing ratios demand the use of high-level delegation strategies? Does the delegatee have appropriate supervision to complete the delegated responsibility?	Right circumstances
Person	Is the prospective delegatee a willing and able employee? Does the delegatee have the knowledge and experience to perform the specific delegated responsibility safely? Does the delegatee have the expertise to complete the delegated responsibility safely and effectively in relation to the acuity of the patient?	Right person
Direction/ communication	Do the delegator and delegatee understand a common work-related language? (Do terms such as *time frame*, *patient needs*, and *critical* mean the same to each of them?) Does the delegator provide clear and concise directions for the delegated responsibility? Does the delegatee understand the assignment, directions, limitations, and expected results as they relate to the delegated responsibility? Do the delegator and delegatee know how to maintain open lines of communication for the purpose of questions and feedback? Does the delegatee understand how, what, and when to report to the delegator?	Right direction/ communication
Supervision	Is it clear that the delegatee will provide feedback related to the delegated responsibility when appropriate? Is the delegator able to monitor and evaluate the patient appropriately?	Right supervision

Adapted from National Council of State Boards of Nursing & American Nurses Association. (2019). *National Guidelines for Nursing Delegation*. https://www.ncsbn.org/NGND-PosPaper_06.pdf (Copyright © 2022 M. Murphy-Ruocco).

communication"—is the foundation of delegation. Mindful communication, a two-way process, is necessary for effective delegation. Mindful communication involves active participants giving and receiving information, allowing for questions and clarifications. The nurse communicates information about the delegated responsibility, ensures that the delegatee understands the delegated responsibility, provides necessary clarification, and determines whether the delegatee feels comfortable accepting the delegated responsibility. High quality information presented by the direct care nurse in a timely, meaningful, and effective manner and in the right context can significantly shape the quality and safety of patient care.

Assessing Ability and Willingness for Delegation: Situational Leadership® Model

The Situational Leadership® Model, originally designed by Paul Hersey, is based on the relationship between leaders and followers. It provides a framework to examine and analyze situations based on the Performance Readiness® Level that a follower exhibits in performing a specific task, function, or objective. Once leaders diagnose the individual's Performance Readiness® Level, they adapt their behavior (amount of task behavior and amount of relationship behavior), communicate so that followers understand and accept how they will be supported, and continue to support their ongoing and advanced development. The Situational Leadership® Model transcends cultural and generational differences and equips leaders with the skills to drive behavior to enhance productivity (The Center for Leadership Studies, 2017).

The Situational Leadership® Model can be used to determine the Performance Readiness® Level of the delegatee and the type of relationship needed to make nursing delegation successful. Multiple factors influence the effectiveness of the leader, including an assessment of personality characteristics, the readiness level of the individual as it relates to the type of task and goals to be attained, and specific environmental conditions.

The Situational Leadership® Model describes two factors that need to be assessed to determine the followers' Performance Readiness® Level: ability and willingness. How these factors interact with each other must also be considered. Ability relates to knowledge and skills in a specific situation. Willingness relates to the individual's attitude, confidence, and commitment toward the

specific situation. Ability usually does not change from one moment to another, whereas willingness can fluctuate from one moment to another. If a delegatee indicates reluctance to perform some type of work, the delegator must evaluate the situation to determine whether the issue is a knowledge deficit or a psychomotor deficit that interferes with performing the work, or whether the delegatee is bored, anxious, upset, or just unwilling to meet the expectation. If the delegatee is less able or unwilling to perform in a specific situation, the delegator must remain actively engaged in the situation. Thus, the greater the ability and willingness of the delegatee, the more likely the delegator can implement delegation strategies while interacting with an individual in a specific situation.

The Situational Leadership® Model describes the leadership style required of an effective leader and its relationship between the amount of guidance and direction (task behavior) and amount of socioemotional support (relationship behavior) needed in the given situation. This determines the best approach a leader can use based on the Performance Readiness® Level of the delegatee. If the delegatee has limited knowledge and ability to perform a task, the delegator needs to provide more guidance. However, if the relationship is limited (when two or more individuals are unlikely to work together again), the delegator simply "tells" the individual what to do and how to perform. The Situational Leadership® Model describes the leader's behavior as guiding or "telling." If a situation involves a new task and the relationship is ongoing (two individuals who will usually continue to work together), the delegator explains what to do and how to do it. The Situational Leadership® Model describes the leader's behavior as explaining, or "selling." Logically, if producing outcomes in a given situation is the driving force, the delegator is much less likely to spend the time and effort investing in limited relationships than in established relationships. If the delegatee has the ability and willingness, but the relationship between the delegator and delegatee is relatively new, they need to establish mutual expectations and conditions of performance. The Situational Leadership® Model describes the leader's behavior as involving or "participating." If the delegatee has the ability, and willingness, expertise to accomplish the work, and an established relationship, the Situational Leadership® Model describes the leader's behavior as entrusting or "delegating."

Applying the Situational Leadership® Model can be useful in real work-related situations. For example, when a new team begins to work together to build a trusting relationship, the delegator must evaluate the ability and willingness of the delegatee. If the ability and willingness is low, the delegator uses the leadership style of telling or selling. If the nature of the relationship is limited, such as when someone is going to work for only half a day on the unit, the leadership style should be "telling," because it provides a fair amount of guidance but limits the time spent on the interactions. If the relationship is developing or ongoing, the delegator needs to understand the delegatee's motivation related to the situation. In that case, the leader's style should be "selling," which takes more time but leads to a supportive relationship. If the relationship is new or developing, more support is needed—the delegator and delegatee need to interact in a participatory manner. When a delegatee has a high degree of ability and willingness and is familiar with the expected task, little guidance is required. Thus, the greater the ability and willingness of the delegatee, the more likely the delegator can implement delegation strategies while interacting with that individual in a specific situation. In other words, both the amount of guidance (task behavior) and the amount of support (relationship behavior) would be relatively low, which works well for established work relationships. However, delegation can be viewed as a spectrum of behaviors based on the context and needs in a specific situation. To achieve effective outcomes, knowing how to interact with a given delegatee is one of the key challenges for the delegator. The Theory Box illustrates how the Situational Leadership® Model applies to nursing. Table 14.2 presents the delegatee's condition, relevance to the delegator, terminology, and a clinical exemplar on how to structure communication with the delegatee to achieve a goal. (For a visual representation of this information, enter the words *situational leadership Hersey* in a search engine and use the image feature to find the original model.)

Challenges of Delegating to Unlicensed Nursing Personnel/Assistive Personnel

Delegation to unlicensed nursing personnel/assistive personnel (UNP/AP) may be challenging because their educational preparation and job descriptions are not consistent across states or within organizations and need greater public accountability. Some facilities have UNP/AP with different designation levels, a higher-level designation indicating the ability to perform more delegated responsibilities. The education of UNP/AP, coupled with facility policies, define how they may or may not function. Healthcare facilities have descriptors of what tasks, activities, or procedures they may perform in a particular position. Their job description defines the authority for the specific position.

With advances in healthcare, more tasks, activities, and procedures may need to be delegated to assist nurses in the delivery of quality person-centered care. The increases in patients' complexity and fiscal constraints have "cultivated an environment in which delegation is necessary" (Barrow & Sharma, 2020, p. 3). Even when policies

THEORY BOX

Situational Leadership® Model

Theory	Key Ideas	Application to Practice
Situational Leadership (Hersey 2006)	The Situational Leadership® Model contends that leaders need to examine and analyze the Performance Readiness® Level of the follower and adapt their behavior (amount of task behavior and relationship behavior) needed to be successful in a given situation.	Nurses must analyze an individual's Performance Readiness® Level: ability and willingness related to the delegated responsibility to determine whether delegation is appropriate. Nurses make decisions based on this analysis. Before delegating, the nurse must assess the amount of guidance/direction (task behavior) and the amount of socioemotional support (relationship behavior) a leader must provide to the delegatee for a delegated responsibility. Delegatees may need different levels of guidance and support for different delegated responsibilities.

TABLE 14.2 Communicating with a Delegatee

Delegatee Condition	Delegator Relevance	Terminology	Clinical Exemplar
Has limited knowledge and ability to perform the task	Requires more guidance	Tell (if the relationship is not going to be ongoing)	"It is important that you take his blood pressure every 15 minutes."
Has ongoing relationship, but a new task is delegated	Requires explanation	Sell	"This is what you need to accomplish; in fact, let me show you what is necessary."
Has willingness and ability, but the relationship is new	Requires that both individuals create mutual expectations and conditions for performance	Participate	"Please tell me how you go about performing this procedure, and I will share with you my expectations about how frequently and under what conditions we need to communicate/report to each other."
Has established relationship and expertise	Little guidance is needed	Delegate	"I know you know what you are doing and when to report. Just remember that I am available to you at any time if an issue or concern arises. Thank you for being part of the team."

and protocols within a facility indicate that an individual may perform a delegated responsibility on behalf of a nurse, the delegatee must be competent to perform the delegated responsibility. To assist with the challenges of delegating, nurses can use four elements to determine the abilities of the UNP/AP to perform the task or activity. These four elements are safety, critical thinking, stability, and time. One of the elements may play a more important role than another in different patient care situations. For example, when critical-thinking skills are of utmost importance for person-centered care, other elements may be relatively less important in the delegation decision. Therefore, making decisions about to whom to delegate, what to delegate, and when to delegate is a complex process. Safety is a basic physiologic need; when a patient is unsafe for any reason, delegation may not be appropriate. Exceptions to this rule are usually related to monitoring behaviors of patients (e.g., when patients are placed on suicide precautions). Critical thinking, the intensity and complexity of nurses' decision-making processes, is vital to patient care decisions. For example, simple (straightforward) patient teaching, such as hand washing, can be performed by UNP/AP. Complex (multifaceted) patient teaching, such as diabetic teaching, cannot be delegated.

Stability, the patient's level of strength or steadiness, is also a major factor in making person-centered care decisions. The greater the stability of a patient, the more likely the UNP/AP can provide safe patient care. Time, the intensity and length of the interaction with the patient, is also a significant factor to consider in planning person-centered care. For example, emergency facilities may employ fewer UNP/AP because patients are less stable compared with extended-care and long-term care facilities, where patients are more stable. Tasks, activities, or procedures can be delegated when the delegatee has the appropriate work and performance abilities. Tasks, activities, and procedures can still be delegated when a delegatee has limited work and performance abilities, but the delegator must educate, monitor, and evaluate care very closely to ensure quality person-centered care. Due to a dramatic amount of resignations during 2020, considerable restructuring and redesigning of how care is delivered was reconceptualized. LPN/LVNs, who were once not hired in many hospitals, were reintroduced into demanding roles. The role of UNP/AP was also reexamined in light of the COVID-19 pandemic. Many changes began to occur due to the demands the pandemic placed on healthcare system.

With the shortage of nurses and a growing population of patients living at home with chronic conditions and disabilities, nurses must examine their attitudes regarding delegation and eliminate any unnecessary challenges when delegating responsibilities to competent delegatees. With our increasingly complicated healthcare system and the various healthcare providers who care for patients, nurses need to delegate appropriately. At first, this situation may seem overwhelming; however, if patients are in stable condition and the nursing care is somewhat predictable, care may be manageable. When delegatees are well-prepared providers of routine care and the care environment is limited to a designated area, responsibilities are less challenging. If these factors are not consistent, the responsibility for an increased number of patients may become overwhelming. When delegatees render a portion of the care, these factors need to be assessed to determine the appropriateness of the patient care workload and whether it can be managed safely and effectively in each clinical situation. Educating delegatees on how to implement a delegated responsibility is crucial for positive outcomes. The Research Perspective provides an exemplar of an innovative educational approach to elevate the knowledge, skills, and attitudes of delegatees.

RESEARCH PERSPECTIVE

Resource: More, L., & Parson, L. (2020) Using innovative education to elevate unlicensed assistive personnel practice. *Nursing Economics, 38*(2), 86–93.

A study was conducted in a large pediatric care organization with primary and specialty outpatient services in which differences in clinical practice and communication techniques of medical assistants (MAs) contributed to error and inconsistencies in patient care practices. The executive leadership team identified stakeholders who would guide the standardization and implementation of the educational program and others who could participate in the development of and strategic plan for completion of a 6-month MA program. A survey, direct observation, and feedback from leaders, providers, peers, and RNs about the current practices of MAs were completed. Survey data indicated that MAs "did not feel valued while working and communicating in teams" and observations indicated "inconsistencies and inaccuracies with skill performance and communicating with families."

Additional gaps included lack of consistency in their formal MA educational programs, level of experience, training, skills validation, and certification. These inconsistencies may lead to negative patient care outcomes. The Logic Model, a theoretical framework, has a visual depiction connecting resources (inputs), activities, or processes that were implemented (outputs) and outcomes/measures for the program. A small group of educators, managers, RNs, MAs, and the MA Educational Coordinator met to plan the program. The goal was to focus on concepts of professionalism and its alignment with skill performance. Enhancement of communication skills, standardization of clinical skills and development of "soft skills" to enhance patient/family experience was the focus of the program. Evidenced-based frameworks, theories, and program evaluations were used to assist MAs in improving the safety of patient care and improving patient care outcomes.

Implications for Practice

Evidence-based frameworks and theories provided a solid foundation for the development of comprehensive educational programs. Using the Logic Model, an educational blueprint provided key strategies and steps to achieve desired behavior change in practice. Using adult learning theory allowed educators to understand how individuals learn, retain knowledge, and become competent. Using evidence-based teaching strategies, for example, combining "chunks of information" into meaningful groups stimulated the brain to learn. Using all 3 learning domains, cognitive, affective, and psychomotor in the teaching/learning process created the best learning outcomes. Formative evaluations, questions, quizzes, observations, homework, and reflections assisted student understanding, and allowed for a change in teaching strategy to improve student learning. A curriculum incorporating adult learning theories, evidence-based teaching strategies, including formative and summative evaluations, facilitated the development of knowledge, skills, and attitudes (KSA) and behavioral change in individuals to enhance the delivery of safe patient care.

Additionally, consumers, nurses, and delegatees must work collaboratively to improve the quality of community living for patients and individuals with disabilities within a broad regulatory framework. Thus, nurses must acquire competency skills in critical thinking, clinical practice, organization, leadership, communication, and time management to meet the challenges of delegation decisions.

Challenges Delegating to Diverse Team Members

Delegation, a complex decision-making process, is successful when effective delegation strategies are learned and implemented by nurses. The nurse's crucial challenge is to fully understand the specific skill set and capabilities of each delegatee on the team.

Delegation can be further influenced by other factors, such as age, sex/gender, and race, and ethnicity. Each generation of nurses have made significant impacts on the nursing profession; however, we need to be mindful not to make generalizations about any one age, sex/gender, race, or ethnic group. That said, millennial nurses have different nursing expectations than previous generations of nurses because they have been significantly impacted by the Internet, social media, mobile communication, and significant societal changes (AMN Healthcare, 2018). They bring new perspectives and expectations related to leadership, work culture, advanced nursing education, and career advancement. Millennial nurses seek to have a meaningful impact on decision-making at the organizational level and on the delivery of person-centered care. They seek a value-based organizational culture that allows for more collaboration, greater autonomy, and even greater authority. "Millennial nurses are more attracted to leadership opportunities than their generational counterparts" (Faller & Gogek, 2019, p. 135). They seek leaders who are very effective, whom they can trust, and who care about them and their careers. (Faller & Gogek, 2019).

An individual's sex/gender also plays a role in learning delegation skills. "The perceptions of men about subtle discrimination, biases, feelings of isolation, 'feminized' curriculum and instructional approaches" have been reported in small studies for over two decades (Hoffart et al., 2019, p. 99). However, in a study of accelerated second-degree nursing students, male students expressed more confidence in leadership competences than female students (Hoffart et al., 2019). More research is needed to better understand the complexities of how sex and gender influence the delegation process.

Ethnicity also plays a role in the process of delegation because individuals from diverse cultures perceive information and their ability to direct others to perform tasks differently. Cultural background can influence how the delegator is heard or viewed in the delegation process. Different cultures communicate differently. "Reframing through cultural respect contributes to promising practices that are connected to social interaction and professional learning that are historically and sociopolitically contextualized" (Botelho & Lima, 2020, p. 317). Diverse cultural, educational, and experiential backgrounds also shape the quality, meaning, and clarity of the information communicated between the delegator and the delegatee. Nurses must be culturally competent and understand that healthcare outcomes improve when the workforce "reflects the diversity of the population served" (Weston et al., 2020, p. 72).

Selecting a delegatee who has the specific skill set for the particular delegated responsibility is a more productive strategy than just selecting a competent individual. A new nurse in a workplace may find delegation decisions difficult, not yet knowing the capabilities of delegatees. Working with a delegatee as a team to deliver person-centered care allows the nurse to assess the delegatee's ability, and willingness. Other challenges with teams, especially diverse teams, include the nurse's ability to provide clear and concise directions and expectations, create open and honest lines of communication, provide appropriate resources, and ensure that the delegatee knows how to function and understands the time frame. Clear expectations about task accomplishments and making sure that the expectations are understood provide a structure for ongoing supervision and evaluation of a delegatee.

If a nurse observes a problem or issue related to delegation but does not have authority specific to the situation and no safety issues, urgency to intervene, or potential negative patient outcomes exist, the nurse can assist other nurses with their delegation decisions by using three strategies: *asking, offering,* and *doing.* The first strategy, asking, begins with questions related to the problem or issue regarding person-centered care. Often, asking questions provides an opportunity to open lines of communication and may allow the delegator to examine the situation differently and reassess the situation. The second strategy, offering, involves making a suggestion that can facilitate the achievement of a desirable person-centered care outcome. The third strategy, doing, occurs by demonstrating the specific task or behavior to improve person-centered care.

> **EXERCISE 14.4** Review a delegation decision made by a nurse related to a clinical experience in your practice setting. After reviewing the nurse practice act and professional standards, provide answers with an evidence-based rationale to the following questions:
> - Did the nurse make clear what was delegated? Why or why not?
> - Were the delegation decisions logical? Why or why not?
> - Were the delegation decisions made within legal and ethical parameters?

Barriers to Effective Delegation

Barriers to effective delegation impede the success of the healthcare team and include underdelegation, overdelegation, and improper delegation. Underdelegation occurs when nurses do not have the confidence to make an effective delegation decision, lack the time to delegate, choose to complete the responsibility themselves, lack the confidence in the delegatee's abilities to complete the task, or fear a loss of control. Nurses with limited delegation experience can misuse valuable resources, whereas others believe delegation is too time-consuming or requires more energy than doing it themselves. Other nurses may have difficulty trusting others and/or are unable to delegate appropriately because they fear the loss of control. The nurse's fear is often perceived as a lack of trust, which can create a toxicity in the workplace and impair innovation. Toxicity occurs when "teams stop collaborating, communication breakdown occurs, unreasonable goals are set, or excessive internal competition is encouraged" (Weberg & Fuller, 2019, p. 22). In the ever-changing healthcare setting, knowing and valuing how to be a successful delegator achieves optimum person-centered care outcomes.

Once the delegatee understands the delegated responsibility and is competent to perform the task or activity, any unnecessary interference or micromanaging by the delegator, unless for a safety or ethical concern, can cause the delegatee to lose confidence or become frustrated and erode the trust relationship. Teams that feel "under threat or undervalued can create pockets of toxicity that metastasize over time" (Weberg & Fuller, 2019, p. 23). Once nurses know that delegatees have been trained, educated, and evaluated on a particular task or activity, they usually become more comfortable assigning a delegated responsibility to a delegatee. Developing and maintaining working relationships is complicated and challenging. Once delegatees develop a trusting relationship with the nurse and understand that the ultimate goal of nursing delegation is to maximize person-centered care outcomes, delegatees become more receptive to constructive feedback. This delegation process creates a collaborative and productive work environment. The nurse who trusts, respects, and allows ownership to delegatees regarding the delegated responsibility makes delegatees feel valued, competent, and an integral part of the healthcare team. How leaders interact with the team will "greatly influence how your team makes decisions, interprets information, and engages in a culture of ownership" (Weberg & Fuller, 2019, p. 22). Effective delegation decisions do not release power of control; rather, they enhance the productivity, accomplishment, and success of the healthcare team.

Overdelegation occurs when the nurse overburdens a delegatee with too many delegated responsibilities. This occurs when the delegator has difficulty organizing work, has poor time management skills, and is overwhelmed. A delegatee who is overburdened and overworked becomes overwhelmed, experiences employee burnout, and decreases the productivity of the healthcare team. Nurses must develop exemplary organization skills, including time management skills, and foster open communication with the delegatee so that, when necessary, the delegatee can respectfully refuse a delegated responsibility. Nurses who maintain clinical practice, mentor delegatees, and are responsive to the delegatees' needs increase the productivity of the healthcare team.

Improper delegation is delegating responsibilities beyond the delegatee's training or education or assigning a delegated responsibility without providing adequate information or data to successfully complete the delegated responsibility. Nurses must determine whether delegatees are capable of performing the delegated responsibility according to their job description or whether it requires specialized knowledge and skills that would not be appropriate for their role and function in the facility. Improper delegation can lead to inadequate care for the patient, failure to meet the standards of care and can cause potential harm to patients. This creates a potential for liability for the nurse and the healthcare facility.

EXERCISE 14.5   Interview a nurse and a delegatee about their perspective related to barriers to delegation. Compare and contrast the similarities and differences in the two perspectives and roles.

Building Effective Nurse Delegators and Interprofessional Teams

In a nurse's career, high-quality clinical delegation experiences and engagement with a nursing mentor foster professional self-confidence. These experiences advance the nurse's ability to become a successful delegator. Nurses must keep current in delegation decisions by enrolling in continuing education programs to reinforce what, when, and how to effectively delegate. These programs create opportunities for all healthcare professionals to keep current in their fields and adapt to the ever-changing healthcare environment.

Building a cohesive interprofessional healthcare team begins with understanding the individual members of the team, their roles and functions, and their disciplines. Learning with and understanding the role and responsibilities of other healthcare professionals creates a respect for the contributions that all healthcare providers make to patient care. Teams feel valuable when their input and ideas are included in leadership decision-making (Weber & Fuller, 2019). Interprofessional collaboration reflects shared decision-making and prevents fragmentation in person-centered care while increasing the effectiveness of the healthcare team. Building collaborative staff relationships, based on trust and respect, is necessary for effective delegation and interprofessional teamwork.

Successful nurse executives demonstrate the value of caring, often referred to as the caring essentials, through "clinical presence, facilitating dialog, affirming relationships, balancing limited resources and having the strength to persist" (Prestia & Dyess, 2020, p. 329). The Quintuple Aim's fourth tenet provides nurse executives guidance on how to improve healthcare quality but does not provide guidance on the science of caring or teaching the core business skill, caring for people (Prestia & Dyess, 2020). Nurse executives who acquire both skills can have a greater impact on the organizational success. Nurse executives who do not engage in valuing their healthcare team can negatively impact organizational effectiveness and the quality of healthcare provided.

Creating positive, collaborative partnerships among nurse leaders at healthcare facilities and faculty at colleges of nursing can increase experiences in interprofessional practice. Nurse leaders, licensed nurses, and faculty should collaborate on evidenced-based research studies and projects and disseminate the outcomes to enhance person-centered care. These partnerships can be twofold: they may provide nurse leaders, and licensed nurses, adjunct faculty positions at colleges and universities and offer faculty opportunities to remain clinically competent. Curricula that offer structured nursing leadership experiences, with faculty mentoring students in small group seminars, foster leadership skills and enhance professional nursing socialization. Intentional teaching strategies are "designed and incorporated throughout the curriculum in multiple contexts and with increasing complexity to provide students multiple opportunities for learning and demonstrating competencies" (American Association of Colleges of Nursing, 2021, p. 18). Nursing internships that provide delegation and supervisory experience of delegatees can enhance an individual's clinical experience and confidence, allowing the individual to learn how to delegate safely and effectively.

To continue to attract and retain high-quality nurses, healthcare organizations, nurse executives, nursing deans, and faculty need to meet the current expectations of the nursing workforce. These expectations include supportive leadership, positive culture, transparency, quality care, and continuing professional development. Emerging from the COVID-19 pandemic offered many healthcare delivery lessons and ample opportunities to reframe and restructure how we deliver the best-quality healthcare. An organizational culture that supports collaborative interdisciplinary practice and ability to identify and document challenges, including barriers, to healthcare delivery produces the best patient outcomes as well as professional nursing outcomes (Martin & Zoinierek, 2020).

CONCLUSION

Delegation, a multifaceted decision-making process, is a learned skill related to how to make appropriate nursing judgments, achieve nursing goals, and improve person-centered care. Effective delegation skills are essential competencies to practice as a nurse in the 21st century. Multiple factors play a role in the ability of the nurse to delegate effectively. These factors include, but are not limited to, the nurse's educational preparation, demographic area, state nurse practice acts, leadership style, employment area, clinical experience, and self-confidence. The nurse must understand the delegation process, develop critical judgment skills, and

effectively use delegation skills to maximize productivity while providing safe, high-quality, cost-effective person-centered care.

THE SOLUTION

As the registered nurse, when I received the UNP/AP nursing admission assessment for the second patient, I became aware of my error, miscommunication. I realized I did not follow four of the five rights of delegation. I did not delegate the right task, under the right circumstances, to the right person, with the right directions and communication.

Upon reflection, I remembered saying "take care of" the second patient, rather than communicating specifically what I wanted the UNP/AP to do. This communication was vague and nonspecific. In addition, the UNP/AP failed to clarify or ask questions concerning what I meant by "take care of" the second patient. The UNP/AP thought she could

complete the nursing admission assessment on the second patient because she had completed nursing admission assessments before as a senior nursing student. However, at that time, she was supervised by nursing faculty.

I came to realize how important it is to follow the five rights of delegation and ensure my communication is clear, concise, timely and reliable to produce safe and efficient patient care. Clarifying the delegaee's role with him/her, and reinforcing my ability to answer questions would have prevented any miscommunications.

Would this be a suitable solution for you? Why?

Kathryn King-Dyker

REFLECTION

Since delegation is such a multifaceted decision-making process, we must learn to become reflective practitioners. What aspect of delegation do you consider most challenging? What type of education or training would

assist you in managing the challenges of delegation? How comfortable are you with the delegation process? What element of the delegation process will you do well? What element will you likely seek support for initially?

BEST PRACTICES

Delegation, a complex decision-making process, is successful when effective delegation strategies are learned and implemented by nurses. A nursing internship or residency can enhance an individual's clinical experience and confidence to delegate safely and effectively. As nurses

continue to adapt to the rapidly changing healthcare environment, nurse managers must continue to support nurses with clinical experiences and continued professional education that enhance their leadership skills, allowing them to effectively delegate and supervise others.

TIPS FOR DELEGATION

- Develop and maintain policies and procedures that describe to whom and what can be delegated.
- Maintain documentation of periodic competency validations for all employees, measured at the appropriate level of the APRN, RN, LPN/LVN, or UNP/AP.
- Promote a positive work culture and environment.
- Understand the organizational structure, policies, and culture of the facility to make effective delegation decisions.
- Comprehend the job description of individuals before delegating responsibilities.

- Assess the knowledge, skills, willingness, and readiness of the individual before delegating responsibilities.
- Use the state NPA and scope and standards of nursing practice to determine how to appropriately delegate responsibilities.
- Use assessment, planning, implementation, and evaluation to determine whether a delegated responsibility can be and/or was successfully delegated.
- Provide clear and concise directions regarding the delegated responsibility.

- Ensure that the delegatee understands that it is essential to immediately notify the nurse if the status of the patient changes.
- Evaluate the effectiveness of delegating responsibilities to others on a regular basis.

- Confirm acceptance or denial of the delegated responsibility by the UNP/AP based on their own level of competence and comfort.
- Maintain accountability for delegated responsibilities.

REFERENCES

American Association of Colleges of Nursing (AACN). (2021). *The essentials: Core competencies for professional nursing education.*

American Nurses Association (ANA). (2015). *Code of ethics for nurses with interpretive statements.* Silver Spring, MD: Author.

American Nurses Association (ANA). (2020). *ANA's principles for nurse staffing* (3rd ed.). Silver Spring, MD: Author.

AMN Healthcare. (2018). *Survey of millennial nurses: A dynamic influence on the profession.* Retrieved from https://www.amnhealthcare.com/industry-research/survey-of-millennial-nurses-2018.

Barrow, J. M., & Sharma, S. (2020). *Five rights of nursing delegation.* Treasure Island, FL: StatPearls Publishing.

Benner, P. (1984). *From novice to expert: Excellence and power in clinical nursing practice.* Menlo Park, CA: Addison-Wesley Publishing Company.

Botelho, M. J., & Lima, C. A. (2020). From cultural competence to cultural respect: A critical review of six models. *Journal of Nursing Education, 59*(6), 311–318. https://doi.org/10.3928/01484834-20200520-03.

The Center for Leadership Studies. (2017). *Situational leadership: Relevant then, relevant now.* Cary, NC: Leadership Studies, Inc.

Faller, M., & Gogek, J. (2019). Break from the past: Survey suggests modern leadership styles need for Millennial nurses. *Nurse Leader, 17*(2), 135–140. https://doi.org/10.1016/j.mnl.2018.12.003.

Hoffart, N., McCoy, T. P., Lewallen, L. O., & Thorpe, S. (2019). Differences in gender-related profile characteristics, perceptions, and outcomes of accelerated second degree nursing students. *Journal of Professional Nursing, 35*(2), 93–100. https://doi.org/10.1016/j.profnurs.2018.10.003.

Institute for Healthcare Improvement (IHI). (2022). *Triple aim for populations.* http://www.ihi.org/Topics/TripleAim.

Martin, E., & Zoinierek, C. (2020). Beyond the nurse practice: Making a difference through advocacy. *Online Journal of Issues in Nursing, 25*(1). Retrieved from https://doi.org/10.3912/OJIN.Vol25No01Man02.

National Council of State Boards of Nursing & American Nurses Association. (2019). *National guidelines for nursing delegation.* Retrieved from https://www.ncsbn.org/NGND-PosPaper_06.pdf.

Olsen, J. M., Aschenbrenner, A., Merkel, R., Pehler, S. R., Sargent, L., & Sperstad, R. (2020). A mixed-methods systematic review of interventions to address incivility in nursing. *Journal of Nursing Education, 59*(6), 319–326. https://doi.org/10.3928/01484834-20200520-04.

Prestia, A. S., & Dyess, S. M. (2020). Losing sight: The importance of nurse leaders' maintaining patient and staff advocacy. *Nurse Leader, 18*(4), 329–332. https://doi.org/10.1016/j.mnl.2020.04.005.

Tye, J. (2020). Living your values. *Nurse Leader, 18*(1), 67–72. https://doi.org/10.1016/j.mnl.2019.11.012.

Weberg, D., & Fuller, R. M. (2019). Toxic leadership: Three lessons from complexity science to identify and stop toxic teams. *Nurse Leader, 17*(1), 22–26. https://doi.org/10.1016/j.mnl.2018.09.006.

Weston, C., Wise-Mathews, D., Pittman, A., & Montalvo-Liendo, N. (2020). One in diversity: Obtaining nursing excellence in diversity and opportunities for improvement. *Journal of Cultural Diversity, 27*(3), 69–73.

CASE STUDY 14.1   NEXT-GENERATION NCLEX® CASE STUDY

Next-Generation NCLEX® case studies are included in select chapters to familiarize you with these new testing items for the NGN exam.

Learning Outcome:
Apply regulations to the process of delegation.

Cognitive Skill:
Take Action

A registered nurse working on the 7p-to-7a shift in an acute care facility is responsible for making assignments for the following 7a-to-7p shift. Three staff available to be assigned include an experienced RN, a novice LPN/LVN, and an experienced unlicensed nursing personnel/assistive personnel (UNP/AP). Although there are twenty patients on this unit, six patients' conditions require, by regulation, a certain level of preparation and competence by the staff, including:
- A 79 y/o patient with an indwelling catheter that requires removal during the 7a-to-7p shift.
- A 50 y/o patient newly diagnosed with type 2 diabetes mellitus who needs teaching regarding the diagnosis.
- An 85 y/o patient with a diagnosis of urinary tract infection (UTI) who requires collection of a daily urine specimen.
- A 75 y/o patient with dementia who requires care of an ileostomy and scheduled tube feedings.
- A 63 y/o patient who is expected to be discharged home with IV antibiotic therapy.
- A 56 y/o patient, newly admitted, with a diagnosis of R/O bladder cancer.

For each patient below, click to specify the available staff that, *by regulation*, might be assigned to meet their care needs. Note: Some of the patients may be assigned to more than one of the choices.

Patient	RN	LPN/LVN	UNP/AP
A 79 y/o patient with an indwelling catheter that requires removal during the 7a-to-7p shift.			
A 50 y/o patient newly diagnosed with type 2 diabetes mellitus who needs teaching regarding the diagnosis.			
An 85 y/o patient with a diagnosis of urinary tract infection (UTI) who requires collection of a daily urine specimen.			
A 75 y/o patient with dementia who requires care of an ileostomy and scheduled tube feedings.			
A 63 y/o patient who is expected to be discharged home with IV antibiotic therapy.			
A 56 y/o patient, newly admitted, with a diagnosis of R/O bladder cancer.			

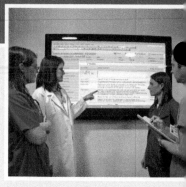

15

Effecting Change, Large and Small

Mary Ellen Clyne

ANTICIPATED LEARNING OUTCOMES

- Examine the steps in the strategic planning process.
- Examine the use of select functions, principles, and strategies for initiating and managing change.
- Explore the various methods for sustaining change.

KEY TERMS

barriers

change agents

change leaders

change process

complexity theory

facilitators

learning organization

planned change

strategic plan

strategic planning process

SWOT analysis

unplanned change

THE CHALLENGE

Clara Maass Medical Center established a vision to be best in class for Excellence in Patient Safety and Quality. To make such a planned change, the organization developed a strategic plan and goals to make this vision a reality. The organization began the journey to become a High Reliability Organization (HRO), with the ultimate goal of causing no harm to patients and staff. I knew our vision could only become a reality by effecting change, big and small. This would have to be accomplished by having a fully engaged healthcare team. I wanted to ensure that all staff felt as if they were a part of this journey and a change agent.

I did not want the staff to ever feel fearful to speak up for safety due to a power distance (meaning that if a staff member perceives that another person could have more power or influence than they do, the staff member is not comfortable in speaking up for safety because of the potential consequences). To that end, if a team member does not speak up for safety, it can result in an error or harm to those who are entrusted with their care. One example is our initiative for all staff and medical personnel requiring

hand washing upon entering and leaving a patient's room. Let's say, a staff member observes that a physician did not wash their hands before entering a patient's room and the staff member did not say anything and allows this to happen; there is a potential to cause harm.

In my role, I want to empower the staff to be change agents and an active participant with setting the course for our organizational vision, understanding our strategic plan, positively impacting our goals, and ultimately ensuring the safety of those who we care for as well as for each other. How could I transform the culture for frontline nurses to speak up for safety without resistance? How could I best support the staff to be empowered to speak up for safety? How would the staff adjust to the change? *What would you do if you were this nurse?*

Teresa Di Elmo, MSN, RN
Chief Nursing Officer, Clara Maass Medical Center, Belleville, New Jersey

INTRODUCTION

From an organizational perspective, as we think about affecting change, big and small, there is a strategic plan (a written plan of action that anticipates the future so that an organization can adapt and survive in a changing and competitive environment) that drives both planned change and unplanned change. The strategic planning process allows for an organization to conduct a realistic examination of its current state, where it needs to be, how to get to where it needs to be, and how people determine how well they are doing (Rasouli et al., 2020).

In an effort to effect change, big and small, nurses throughout a healthcare organization need to be involved in the strategic planning process and consider how the overall plan influences the work throughout the organization. Although an organization is guided by its strategic plan, the reality is that the strategic plan is made up of goals and tactical plans that must be executed. The organization has to be ready for change when executing the strategic plan because change is inevitable. Nurse leaders, nurse managers, and frontline nurses must know that they can influence the strategic plan and affect change. In an effort to assist nurses in this endeavor, remember that the only thing constant is change. To that end, all of us nurses should participate in our organization's strategic plan and strategic planning process because of the instrumental role we can play with affecting change and to support the vision of the organization you are aligned with.

Take a moment and ask yourself the following: how comfortable am I with change; how comfortable am I at accepting change; and am I willing to embrace change? To be effective, nurses must understand the nature of change and how to effectively navigate the change process. Nurses working in any setting (at the bedside, in clinics, in ambulatory centers, and in patients' homes) not only support patients in changing their behavior and making healthy choices but also must now foster innovation and promote change in the workplace to adopt best practices, advance patient safety, and improve patient outcomes.

Nurses have the ability to excel as change leaders, no matter the role. As the change process transpires, nurse leaders are focused on ensuring the delivery of safe and effective care. Specifically, the nurse leader is assessing for any potential disruption and chaos of

TABLE 15.1 Attributes Characterizing Change Agents

Attribute	Key Points
Commitment to a better way	Excited about designing a better future
Courage to challenge power bases and norms	Closest to the work
Go beyond role, take initiative, think outside the box	Assurance of change happening
Persona	Self-motivated, generate enthusiasm
Caring	Commitment to patients and their welfare
Humility	About the change, not about "me"
Sense of humor	Self-support through challenges

Data from Katzenbach, J. R., Beckett, F., Dichter, S., Feigen, M., Gagnon, C., Hope, Q., & Ling, T. (1996). *Real change leaders.* New York: Random House.

change to be transparent to the patients served as well as ongoing monitoring for sustainabilty. All nurses are change agents (Table 15.1) because of their ability to prepare for, implement, and sustain change (Gunty et al., 2019).

STRATEGIC PLANNING

The focus of the strategic planning process is designed to encompass the organization's mission, vision, and values; environmental factors (internal and external); strategies; goals; and tactical plans, which are continuously being monitored, evaluated, and changed as needed (Fig. 15.1). Five phases comprise the strategic planning process:

- Phase 1—Conduct an environmental scan, SWOT analysis (strength and weaknesses are assessed from an internal perspective; opportunities and threats are assessed from an external perspective, outside of the organization).
- Phase 2—Strategic vision and mission are established and revised as appropriate.

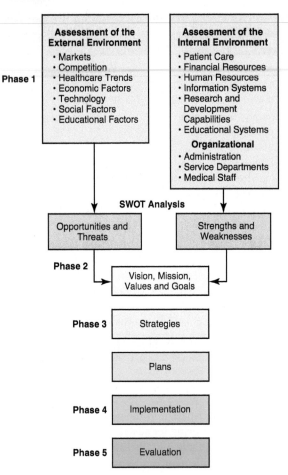

Phase 1

Assessment of the External Environment	Assessment of the Internal Environment
• Markets	• Patient Care
• Competition	• Financial Resources
• Healthcare Trends	• Human Resources
• Economic Factors	• Information Systems
• Technology	• Research and Development Capabilities
• Social Factors	• Educational Systems
• Educational Factors	

Organizational
• Administration
• Service Departments
• Medical Staff

SWOT Analysis

Opportunities and Threats

Strengths and Weaknesses

Phase 2 — Vision, Mission, Values and Goals

Phase 3 — Strategies

Plans

Phase 4 — Implementation

Phase 5 — Evaluation

Fig. 15.1 Key steps in the strategic planning process.

EXERCISE 15.1 A chief nursing officer (CNO) is embarking on the Magnet® journey and is working with the nursing leadership team, various professional practice councils, and the frontline nursing staff to create a strategic plan for nursing. The CNO would like to complete an internal environmental assessment regarding the current status of nursing excellence. The nurse leaders and frontline nurses are assigned to examine the strengths and weaknesses of the nursing department, examine the quality patient care outcomes indicators, and examine the patient experience scores of a Magnet®-designated organization and review their outcomes on the website *www.hospitalcompare.gov*.

Select a hospital. Evaluate it and determine its strengths and weaknesses. Do the quality scores demonstrate excellence?

REASONS FOR STRATEGIC PLANNING

The complexity of the healthcare environment means that it is ever changing. The strategic plan is fluid, agile, and adaptable (Posch & Garaus, 2020). It is the organizational vision for the future (Fig. 15.2). The strategic planning process leads to goal achievement, gives meaning to work life, and provides direction and improvement for operational activities of the organization (George, Walker, & Monster, 2019).

The strategic plan cannot happen in a silo—nurses can be instrumental in this process. Nurses can develop

- Phase 3—Strategic development whereby strategies are developed and a plan is written to address the SWOT analysis.
- Phase 4—Implement the strategy by selecting the best strategic options for the organization that balance its potential with the challenges of changing conditions, taking into account the values of its management and its social responsibilities; prepare the strategy and tactical plan to support the strategy; and execute the plan.
- Phase 5—Monitor the progress by evaluating the strategy to determine success. This phase is ongoing and can be changed as needed (unplanned change) and revised as appropriate.

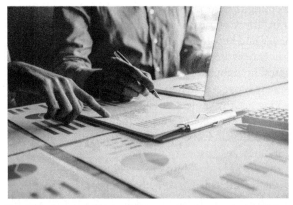

Fig. 15.2 A strong and dynamic strategic plan results in efficient and effective use of resources. (Copyright © Sarinyapinngam/iStock/Thinkstock.)

a nursing strategic plan that supports the goals and objectives of the organization (Lal, 2020). Nurses are the driving force that can implement and monitor the strategic plan to ensure success by demonstrating improvements in patient safety, quality, patient experience, and reducing the cost of care delivery (Lal, 2020).The fact is, without change (planned or unplanned) and without nurses as change agents, a healthcare organization is unlikely to actualize its vision and effectively execute its strategic plan (Lal, 2020).

THE NATURE OF CHANGE

The nature of change is constant and can be resisted by some. Yet, it is inevitable that change will occur either on a personal or organizational level. To that end, change can be initiated by the individual, the system, or imposed by either. Lewin (1951) opines that change can be planned and unplanned. Planned change is considered to be deliberate, organized, and has the goal of improvement. Unplanned change is considered to be disconcerting, unanticipated, and adaptive (Gunty et al., 2019).

All change, no matter how it is perceived, either positively or negatively, big or small, can be scary and generate fear because of the potential uncertainty and unknown. Some individuals embrace change more readily while others may be resistant to change (Miake-Lye et al., 2020). Nurses and nurse leaders can be successful change agents by understanding and being equipped to navigate and manage the change process (Posch & Garaus, 2020). Certainly, the American Association of Colleges of Nursing (AACN) (2022) competence to improve quality and ensure safety (6.2) implies the ability to plan for and respond to planned or unplanned change.

THE CHANGE PROCESS

When implementing change, one must have a working knowledge of the change process in order to effectively navigate change (Nilsen et al., 2020). One must also be mindful of systems theory and how it can impact change—if one part of the system is changed, then it affects the overall system. Additionally, if a vulnerabilty or weakness is present/identified, the system will be able to adapt and remain stable. Of note,

open systems are also influenced by both the internal and external environment. Here is an example that illuminates how both the internal and external environment of open systems can influence the change process: If one thinks about a healthcare system and the frontline nurses who work within, nurses are affected by internal factors such as the availability and quality of resources, the levels of staffing, and the processes used to manage patient care. External factors such as disease, social determinants of health, lifestyle patterns in the community population, healthcare regulation and reimbursement, and the supply of healthcare workers also affect the system.

Planned Change

Lewin (1947), one of the first theorists to study the process of planned change, determined that change has three stages. The first stage/preparation stage begins when assisting a person, group, or organization to move from the current behavior or process (unfreezing). The second stage begins when there is a move toward the new desired future state/reality (moving). The third stage begins when the new change is hardwired and sustained (refreezing). During the first stage (unfreezing), one must be cognizant that this stage involves helping others to overcome inertia—the desire to keep things the same. For example, unfreezing is when a nurse encounters a patient who realizes the need to adopt a diabetic diet after being diagnosed with type 2 diabetes or an organization acknowledges the need to change its delivery care model to achieve the goal of lowering the cost of care. Thus, unfreezing is the step during which individuals and organizations come to the realization that the need to change exists and then begin to implement that change.

During the stage of unfreezing, evaluation regarding the benefits and the costs of implementing the change must be considered. This decision could affect the motivation level generated to make the change. This evaluation is known as the *force field analysis*, which is described as the forces or influences that affect whether change occurs (Lewin, 1951). There are two forces in this evaluation. One force favors change—facilitators—in which case change will be more likely to occur. The other force is against change—barriers—in which case change will be less likely to occur. By understanding the force field analysis, nurses will have the perspective and insight as to what it will take to make and sustain a change. Specifically, it is key for change agents to assess and determine whether individuals see the need to unfreeze by listening to all participants involved in the change and answering the question, "Do they have a shared vision for the change?"

From an organizational perspective, change is accomplished through individual change. Thus, one must understand the power of maintaining the status quo. Unless individuals perceive that change will make things better, those demonstrating resistance and putting up barriers will limit the success of the change. As in the Challenge, the needed changes in getting the staff to speak up for safety and feel comfortable enough in asking a clarifying question to those who did not wash their hands upon entering a patient's room is about unfreezing. During this stage of change, the change agent understands what people fear and how to best address those fears. Our normal tendency has focused on what needs to change and how we will make that change. What people want to know, however, is why change is needed. Change is a lot of work.

The second stage of change (moving) is when planned interventions and strategies are executed to support the implementation of the necessary change by utilizing methods such as education about the need for the change, vision building to conceptualize and bring life to the change, involving individuals/key stakeholders in the process of planning and making the change, and implementing small steps toward the change. Information gleaned during the analysis of the forces (facilitators and barriers) can be utilized to guide the change agent in making a plan and developing strategies to ensure effective implementation of the change goal.

The final stage (refreezing) focuses on sustaining the change. During this time, the change agent works to reinforce the new, desired behaviors and processes by way of positive reinforcement, reward and recognition, and providing feedback. The nurse manager must be the leader of change, taking ownership by continuing to monitor and reassess the successfulness of the change and compliance to required changed behaviors or processes, measuring the impact of the changes, and updating the frontline nurses on the progress being made.

EXERCISE 15.2 Think about Lewin's force field analysis, which identifies facilitators and barriers, and apply it to the following situation. Use a scale of 1 to 5 to rate the potential strength of each in favoring or hindering attainment of the change. Use +5 for the highest positive strength toward change occurring and +1 for the weakest. Use −5 for the greatest negative strength against the change and −1 for the weakest.

Leaders at the Center of Excellence for Latino Health were concerned about the results from the Community Health Needs Assessment (CHNA) for the Latino/Hispanic population they serve. The assessment revealed that diabetes, hypertension, and obesity were negatively impacting their health. The nurses provided health education in the community following religious services. The nurses were culturally competent and culturally sensitive, able to develop a true trusting relationship with the participants, and able to communicate in their language. The frontline nurses provided education on the impact of diabetes, hypertension, and obesity and promoted various healthy choices to achieve their health goals. The participants learned how to take their own blood pressure with return demonstration as well as to recognize when the results were considered high, normal, and low. The house of worship was provided with blood pressure equipment for self monitoring and several participants agreed to be the blood pressure champion for ongoing support. Historically, programs held after their religious services offered soda, high-fat and high-calorie food options, and the food portions were large. The participants live in what is considered a food desert. Issues of food insecurity and very limited access to fresh produce were common. Many of the participants expressed their love of salt added to their food. Therefore, the frontline nurses created a dinner meeting and held a cooking demonstration, introducing participants to the use of a salt substitute. Some of the participants were willing to make the switch. When the frontline nurses instructed them on the particulars of portion size, the participants said they never realized what one portion size was. Some even verbalized that they were unknowingly overeating by two to three portions during a meal. Although some of the participants were enlightened and open to the potential of making healthy choices, others were less than enthusiastic about using the salt substitute. Last, but not least, another request for change was to switch out the soda for water and do away with the high-fat/high-calorie foods. One proposal was that if someone wanted soda, the person would have to pay for it.

THEORY BOX
Planned Change

Key Contributors	Key Idea	Application to Practice
Seven Phases of Planned Change Lippitt et al. (1958)	1. The client system becomes aware of the need for change. 2. The relationship is developed between the client system and change agent. The leader of a change must be committed to the change. 3. The change problem is defined. Creating a change team enhances the diversity of thinking about a potential progam. 4. The change goals are set and options for achievement are explored. 5. The plan for change is implemented. 6. The change is accepted and stabilized. 7. The change entities redefine their relationships. A group may disband or identify another issue.	Change can be planned, implemented, and evaluated in seven sequential phases. Ongoing sensitivity to forces in the change process is essential. Nurses are accountable for quality care and changes often lead to enhanced safety and quality. Goals can drive change at any level of an organization. Action must occur among the people involved in the problem. Major goal attainment needs to be celebrated and reinforeced for the change to be retained.

Adapted from Lippitt, R., Watson, J., & Westley, B. (1958). *The dynamics of planned change.* New York: Harcourt Brace.

Lewin's work has been the foundation for many change theorists. Other theorists, such as Lippitt et al. (1958) have been able to further evolve Lewin's theory of change to include three human factors that come into play during the second stage of change (see the Theory Box). The three human factors that set the stage to foster and embrace change are (1) asking probing questions to clarify the problem requiring the change; (2) examining the various ways to address the problem, developing commitment and buy-in to one of those plans; and (3) moving individuals/stakeholders to actually make the change—going from intending to change to actually making the change in behaviors and processes (Lippitt et al., 1958). The influence of the change agent cannot be underestimated. Lippitt et al. (1958) revealed that the effectiveness of the change agent due to the relationship the change agent had with the group made a significant difference in successfully accomplishing the change. The Literature Perspective illustrates a complex planned change.

Unplanned Change

Although simplistic, Lewin's theory described unplanned change. In evaluating the various theories that align with unplanned change, complexity theory aligns the best because it provides the framework to better understand how to navigate unpredictable events that we may encounter. Complexity theory describes change as the following: emergent, that is, it may appear chaotic but there is a balance between order and disorder; it is not consid-ered to be episodic, rather, it is agile and adaptive because the system adjusts and realigns, recreating itself continuously; it is influenced by all individuals/stakeholders and subsystems in an organization; and a paradigm shift occurs. The change experience operates from a top-down model whereby leaders design the future state and impose it on the current system (command and control) to make it one in which change is organic and systemic, emerging throughout the system, across departments and professions, as an adaptive response fostered by decentralized decision-making and collaboration.

The second Literature Perspective provides thoughts about how frontline nurses can be innovators and change agents. An illustration of this is the Magnet Recognition Program® in the United States. The American Nurses Credentialing Center (ANCC) awards this status to hospitals that meet or exceed a set of standards designed to measure the quality and effectiveness of nursing in their organizations (ANCC, 2019).

As a nurse leader, you need to be the champion of change, even if the chances of failure are great. A review of the literature demonstrates that close to 70% of all change strategies fail, whether change is planned or unplanned (Nilsen et al., 2020). Organization and individual stakeholders can articulate the vision and develop exceptional plans to execute change but still not be successful because they may have underestimated the impact of the human factor and how this change will affect people (Nilsen et al., 2020).

LITERATURE PERSPECTIVE

Resource: Nether, K., Thomas, E., Khan, A., Ottosen, M., & Yager, L. (2022). Implementing a robust process improvement program in the neonatal intensive care unit to reduce harm. *Journal for Healthcare Quality, 44*(1), 23–30.

This article provides an example of how nurses can be successful change agents. It focuses on the way in which neonatal intensive care nurses successfully reduced preventable harm to critically ill neonates and how they could hardwire their processes for sustained improvements to ensure patient safety. The nursing leadership team, staff nurses, medical staff, and parents/guardians of the critically ill neonates were engaged in implementing change that focused on three measurable outcomes for improvement: prevention of central line bloodstream infections (CLBSIs), improving the nutritional status for low-birthweight neonates, and avoidance of unplanned extubations.

The neonatal intensive care team members were on a journey toward high reliability and were committed to ensuring zero harm events for the neonates. The overall goal was to intentionally change the culture of safety in the neonatal intensive care unit and sustain those changes. It was paramount for the team members to improve their confidence and knowledge in safety concepts and safety tools. This was accomplished by online training and in-person classes on the management of the safety concepts and tools, mentoring, and change management.

This was completed in two phases: the improvement phase (first phase) and control phase (second phase).

The results of this planned change by the nurses and the multidisciplinary team demonstrated not only significant improvement but sustained improvements. Specifically, post-implementation, there was a 67.1% reduction in CLBSIs, which was sustained for 17 months in the first phase of the change, followed by a 77.9% improvement in the second phase of the change. The nutritional status of the neonates improved by 63% in phase one and 35% in phase two with sustainability not yet determined. The amount of unplanned extubations was reduced by 22.7% in phase one and 54.3% in phase two and sustained for 20 months. Overall, the confidence and knowledge of the team demonstrated a positive impact and suggested that this improvement led to achievement in sustainability results and changing the culture of safety. The team followed the rules of engagement for planned change, which was also beneficial and led to achieving their three goals.

Implications for Practice
Specific strategies can foster efforts for frontline nurses to be successful change agents. The lived experience of frontline nurses prepares them to identify opportunities that can positively impact the care of those they serve and to contribute to the overall goals for the nursing strategic plan.

LITERATURE PERSPECTIVE

Resource: Cusson, R., Meehan, C., Bourgault, A., & Kelley, T. (2020). Educating the next generation of nurses to be innovators and change agents. *Journal of Professional Nursing, 36*(2), 13–19.

The purpose of this article was to identify how nurses can be innovators and change agents. Introducing this concept into the nursing education curriculum is important. The article discusses the significance of nurses understanding the benefits of thinking creatively and becoming inspired to be engaged in change. Additionally,

it allows for nurses to have a voice and be empowered to make change.

Implications for Practice
The strategy of providing education for nurses based on the principles of being an innovator and a change agent can lead to an empowered nursing workforce making a difference in the outcomes of their patients. When nurses are willing to think out of the box and be open to change, it may lead to new possibilities.

The nurse manager has an awesome responsibility to function as a change leader in the healthcare system. This requires developing a critical change management acumen that includes the ability to examine personal resistance against the change, assess for poor motivation to adopt new technologies, and be confident in gathering and communicating evidence-based practice strategies. Additionally, the change agent needs to be cognizant of the degree to which the change does not conflict with personal values, the context through how change advances in the organization, and the overall impact that the amount of substantive changes individuals must make in their behavior all influence change outcomes.

PEOPLE AND CHANGE

Change, whether planned or unplanned, has an impact on people. Change can be initiated, mandated, or directed by either internal or external sources. Change agents need to understand that the potential response/reaction to the change process by individuals/groups may vary across the continuum from full rejection to complete acceptance (Nilsen et al., 2020). This holds true when considering a person's participation level in the change process; participation can vary across the continuum from total disengagement to full engagement (Miake-Lye et al., 2020).

Some initial responses to change may come across as reluctance and resistance, which may surface if people feel that it threatens their personal security (Nilsen et al., 2020). For example, when an organization is considering a restructure, the reality is that there is a potential for various changes of positions that will affect the staff. For example, a frontline nurse position might be eliminated from one department and the nurse offered another less desirable position. This could result in that frontline nurse feeling disgruntled, disheartened, and could even lead to survivor's guilt if the frontline nurse retained a position over a colleague who lost a job/role.

The Institute for Healthcare Improvement (IHI) encourages organizations to consider making change that focuses on rapid, small tests of change which are often at the point of care (http://www.ihi.org/resources/Pages/HowtoImprove/ScienceofImprovementImplementingChanges.aspx). This method allows for a nursing unit to experience unit-based decision-making to change processes and policies that revolve around staff members who have firsthand knowledge about working on the unit and depends highly on their ongoing adaptation to evolving realities.

All nurses have the capacity to be change agents because they proactively assist in helping others to transform by advocating for openness and improvement. Nurses who act as change agents fully understand the change process and are committed to the opportunity for growth. Additional characteristics of a change agent is being an optimist, having influence with colleagues, knowing how to build networks, and being able to facilitate communication. Nurses who function as positive change agents within the healthcare system are willing to try new things, stay abreast of new evidence about best practices, are open to change, are respected, and are role models. See Table 15.2 for an example of a self-assessment related to receptivity to change. Assessment of organizational culture and the readiness of staff and others to engage in making or participating in a change,

TABLE 15.2 Self-Assessment: How Receptive Are You to Change and Innovation?

Read the following items. Circle the answer that most closely matches your attitude toward creating and accepting new or different ways.

1. I enjoy learning about new ideas and approaches.	Yes	Depends	No
2. Once I learn about a new idea or approach, I begin to try it right away.	Yes	Depends	No
3. I like to discuss different ways of accomplishing a goal or end result.	Yes	Depends	No
4. I continually seek better ways to improve what I do.	Yes	Depends	No
5. I commonly recognize improved ways of doing things.	Yes	Depends	No
6. I talk over my ideas for change with my peers.	Yes	Depends	No
7. I communicate my ideas for change with my manager.	Yes	Depends	No
8. I discuss my ideas for change with my family.	Yes	Depends	No
9. I volunteer to be at meetings when changes are being discussed.	Yes	Depends	No
10. I encourage others to try new ideas and approaches.	Yes	Depends	No

If you answered "yes" to 8 to 10 of the items, you are probably receptive to creating and experiencing new and different ways of doing things. If you answered "depends" to 5 to 10 of the items, you are probably receptive to change conditionally based on the fit of the change with your preferred ways of doing things. If you answered "no" to 4 to 10 of the items, you are probably not receptive, at least initially, to new ways of doing things. If you answered "yes," "no," and "depends" an approximately equal number of times, you are probably mixed in your receptivity to change based on individual situations.

whether minor or extensive, sets the stage for the selection and use of change strategies (Miake-Lye et al., 2020).

An example of the readiness of staff is found in Exercise 15.3. The willingness of the two nurses in this exercise to learn new skills and the combined talents of the nursing, clinical education, and administrative managerial staff to work together successfully helped achieve the very different nursing and organizational skills required by the new infusion center.

EXERCISE 15.3 Responsibilities for promoting change can vary depending on the role a nurse plays in an organization. View this short case study from the perspectives of a manager and a clinical nurse educator. Discuss the responsibilities each nurse would have in transitioning two frontline nurses to work in a new infusion center and identify the appropriate functions.

Both frontline nurses were long-term employees; one was from the medical-surgical float pool and the other was the logistics coordinator (responsible for determining all patient placement and bed assignments) whose position was eliminated because of budget reductions. The chief nursing officer developed the overall vision for this planned change and provided the following: (1) goals for the new infusion program, (2) activities essential for implementation goals, and (3) a timeline to accomplish the planned change. The nurse manager and the clinical nurse educator agreed to check in with each other daily and meet weekly for a more formal review of the team's progress. Part of this plan includes the option to adjust it based on the potential for any unexpected changes. The two frontline nurses would begin their new position in 4 weeks and the plan would be executed.

What would be the nurse manager's responsibility in implementing this change? What would be the clinical nurse educator's responsibility in implementing this change? What are some unexpected issues that may occur requiring the nurse manager and clinical nurse educator to modify the goal, activities, or time frame of the project (dynamic quality of process)? What feedback from the nurse manager, clinical nurse educator, and the two frontline nurses transitioning would be important in guiding the overall process?

EXERCISE 15.4 Answer the self-assessment questions in Table 15.2 to determine how receptive you are to change.

We know that the more rapidly change can be incorporated, the more effective the organization is at remaining relevant. Connecting early adopters, such as the unit-based champions/change agents, to new ideas and to innovations, such as national peers of an IHI Web-based learning community, keeps them at the cutting edge. When these two groups are supported, an early majority can be recruited to support the change initiative. If as a frontline nurse you realize you are usually a laggard, look to be sure that rejection of new ideas is about some concern with the idea, not with just resisting change. Insight can be gained by using Exercise 15.5.

EXERCISE 15.5 Reflect on a time when a particular individual tried to get you or a group to do something in a work or personal situation. Share what rationale supported the decision of whether to go along with it. Looking back on it, do you believe that the idea was worthwhile? Was the person making the suggestion known, understood, and trusted? Would you say that the person making the request was aware of the real situation or had that person not received official sanctioning to influence activities? Does it resonate with you that change agents need specific qualities and abilities to be trusted by others?

CONTEXT AND CHANGE

Although the people who make up an organization have a great impact on change processes, so, too, does the culture of the organization. Understanding the impact of organizational culture is key when it comes to change. When an organization is open and has its finger on the pulse of the realities facing the communities served and the larger industry and regulatory context, they are more viable, fluid, and responsive to change (Lal, 2019). From a nursing perspective, organizations that support the efforts to strive for Magnet® status or are designated as a Magnet® facility are an excellent illustration of learning organizations because they promote a shared governance philosophy grounded in the openness and empowerment of the nurse in shared decision-making power. Thus, the frontline nurses are engaged, their voices are heard, they have a seat at the table, and they know best what changes need to be made that will positively impact patient outcomes. To that end, when an organization fully supports nurses on the Magnet® journey, it not only benefits nursing but also transcends the entire organization. Since 2007, the Institute of Medicine (now the National Academy of Medicine) has encouraged organizational change that improves the quality of care and reduces costs by creating learning healthcare systems in America (Institute of Medicine, 2012). Nurses are instrumental in driving these results. Although implementing change can be complex, nurse leaders can use strategies to assist with the successful adoption of change. Box 15.1 provides an overview of six change support strategies that leaders can adopt.

Managing and inspiring change is a major task for all nurse leaders in healthcare (Nghe et al., 2020). The nurse leader must develop a positive working relationship with the nurses and staff based on reciprocal trust. Once this relationship is established, the nurse leader is more likely to be present in the moment and to truly listen and understand what matters to frontline nurses. This provides the nurse leader the opportunity to serve as a facilitator, promoting the sharing of ideas, fears, and honest reactions to the change proposal. Although nurse leaders can certainly inspire people to change, ultimately the individual must decide that the change matters (Austin et al., 2020). When nurses are inspired, the nurse leader can build on that and mentor frontline nurses as the change agents who are engaged in the change process (Nghe et al., 2020).

Today's dynamic environment means that nurse leaders will have less time to plan and that plans must be constantly updated and amended (Fig. 15.3). Classic elements of effective change implementation can be found in Box 15.2. Past leadership theories place the leader at the helm, in command of the ship. Today's leader must work to solve process problems with the team and empower them to be part of the solution. Nurse leaders will be the ones who keep patient care at the center of

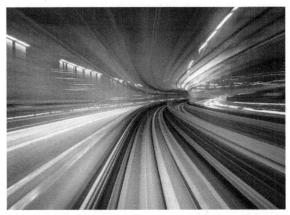

Fig. 15.3 Change happens quickly in healthcare. (Copyright © Ikunl/iStock/Thinkstock.)

BOX 15.2 Classic Principles Characterizing Effective Change Implementation

- Change agents within healthcare organizations use personal, professional, and managerial knowledge and skills to lead change.
- The recipients of change believe they own the change.
- Administrators and other key personnel support the proposed change.
- The recipients of change anticipate benefit from the change.
- The recipients of change participate in identifying the problem warranting a change.
- The change holds interest for the change recipients and other participants.
- Agreement exists within the work group about the benefit of the change.
- The change agents and recipients of change perceive a compatibility of values.
- Trust and empathy exist among the participants of the change process.
- Revision of the change goal and process is negotiable.
- The change process is designed to provide regular feedback to its participants.

Adapted from Harper, C. L. (2007). *Exploring social change* (5th ed.). Englewood Cliffs, NJ: Prentice Hall.

BOX 15.1 Change Support Strategies

- Promote acceptance of the change by viewing the change as a positive experience.
- Develop skills essential for supporting the change.
- Reduce negative influences and behaviors in the group experiencing the change.
- Mobilize positive peer support for the change.
- Create financial incentives that reward change agents.
- Make structure and process modifications to support the change initiative.

Adapted from Patterson, K., Grenny, J., Maxfield, D., McMillan, R., & Switzler, A. (2011). *Change anything*. New York: Hatchette Book Group.

every decision, who will advance the ethos of nursing and who will connect change to what matters to frontline nurses (Nghe et al., 2020).

CONCLUSION

Nurse leaders have business skill competencies that empower them to facilitate the strategic planning process, giving them the credibility to be strategic leaders and change leaders. Nurses in direct care need to be engaged in the strategic planning and change process to be effective in implementing the plan and goals of the organization. A strategic plan is deemed successful when demonstrated intentional improvement in outcomes is evident.

Whether delivering direct care, serving as a nurse leader, or providing clinical education, embracing change is the new imperative for nurses. Contemporary nursing requires that we celebrate more innovation and risk taking, decide to "break the rules" whenever possible to promote improvement, and embrace a spirit of curiosity as we explore the benefits of change.

THE SOLUTION

The frontline nurses received didactic education on the guiding priniciples of a High Reliability Organization (HRO). The concept of power distance was introduced. The frontline nurses shared examples of their lived experience of various power distance situations they encountered and discussed retrospectively the impact of that situation. The frontline nurses were instructed on the methodologies utilized in an HRO. To best address the power distance concerns, the team did role-playing exercises. I wanted the frontline staff to know that I was here to support them and they did not have to be fearful when having a questioning attitude even when the power distance presented itself to the situation. The bottom line was, if there is a concern for safety, the frontline nurse is empowered to ask a clarifying question because that is how we can ensure the safety of our patients and entire staff. We also created a safety hero award, which has been well received. The nurse leaders were also part of the education and training. The leadership in the organization also conducted leadership rounds to reinforce the HRO practices and rounded with intent to validate, celebrate, reward and recognize the frontline nurses for great catches and utilization of the tool to keep everyone safe. Seeing the enthusiasm, I was able to tap into the frontline nurses to be safety coaches. This allowed for another level of engagement and commitment from the frontline nurses, who are just incredible change agents. The culture has embraced this new paradigm and the entire team and the physicians are on this journey. The power distance concern was eradicated and the cross checks/clarifying questions have become the new norm.

Would this be a suitable approach for you? Why?

Teresa Di Elmo

REFLECTIONS

Think back on your experiences thus far. In what way have you been involved with strategic planning? What can you do to convey to others the importance of nurses being engaged in the strategic planning process? What are you willing to commit to in terms of involvement in the future?

Throughout your career, you will face many changes and challenges as you work to become highly competent in a given role or field. How can the content in this chapter help you prepare for those changes? What change support strategies are you going to use? How can you approach this as a planned change to promote your success?

BEST PRACTICES

As busy as we are in our practice areas, we all need to connect with the strategic planning process and the resultant plan. The process allows us to shape the direction of the organization from our perspective and the plan itself serves as the roadmap to the future. Being able to adapt quickly to unplanned change is increasingly an important skill in any nursing position because change continues to happen quickly.

▮ TIPS FOR LEADING CHANGE

- As the nurse leader, be clear about the vision for change.
- As the nurse manager, when managing change, ensure that you are connected to frontline nurses and that you are present in the moment for them by listening to their thoughts, ideas, and concerns about the change.
- As the nurse leader, recognize and mentor their change agents.

- As frontline nurses, be aware of their potential to resist change and be supportive when they are attempting to embrace it.
- As frontline nurses, recognize that your lived experience prepares you to share your views when a planned or unplanned change occurs. Your expertise can assist in the successful execution of the change.

REFERENCES

American Association of Colleges of Nursing (AACN). (2022). Quality and Safety Education for Nurses (QSEN). Retrieved from http://www.aacn.org/Quality-Safety-Education.

American Nurse Credentialing Center (ANCC). (2019). *Magnet Recognition Program® overview.* Washington, DC: The National Academies Press. Retrieved from https://www.nursingworld.org/organizational-programs/magnet/.

Austin, T., Chreim, S., & Grudniewicz, A. (2020). Examining health care providers' and middle-level managers' readiness for change: a qualitative study. *BMC Health Services Research, 20,* 47. https://doi.org/10.1186/s12913-020-4897-0.

Cusson, R., Meehan, C., Bourgault, A., & Kelley, T. (2020). Educating the next generation of nurses to be innovators and change agents. *Journal of Professional Nursing, 36*(2), 13–19.

George, B., Walker, R. M., & Monster, J. (2019). Does strategic planning improve organizational performance? A meta-analysis. *Public Administration Review, 79*(6), 810–819.

Gunty, A., Van Ness, J., & Nye-Lengerman, K. (2019). Be a change agent: tools and techniques to support organizational and individual transformation. *Journal of Vocational Rehabilitation, 50*(3), 325–329.

Harper, C. L. (2007). *Exploring social change* (5th ed.). Englewood Cliffs, NJ: Prentice Hall.

Institute of Medicine (IOM). (2012). *Best care at lower cost: The path to continuously learning health care in America.* Retrieved from http://www.nationalacademies.org/hmd/Reports/2012/Best-Care-at-Lower-Cost-The-Path-to-Continuously-Learning-Health-Care-in-America.aspx.

Katzenbach, J. R., Beckett, F., Dichter, S., Feigen, M., Gagnon, C., Hope, Q., & Ling, T. (1996). *Real change leaders.* New York: Random House.

Lal, M. (2020). Why you need a nursing strategic plan. *The Journal of Nursing Administration, 59*(4), 183–184.

Lal, M. (2019). Leading effectively through change. *The Journal of Nursing Administration, 49*(12), 575–576.

Lewin, K. (1947). Frontiers in group dynamics: Concept, method, and reality in social science, social equilibria and social change. *Human Relations, 1*(1), 5–41.

Lewin, K. (1951). *Field theory in social science.* New York: Harper Torchbooks.

Lippitt, R., Watson, J., & Westley, B. (1958). *The dynamics of planned change.* New York: Harcourt Brace.

Miake-Lye, I., Delevan, D., Ganz, D., Mittman, B., & Finley, E. (2020). Unpacking organizational readiness for change: An updated systematic review and content analysis of assessments. *BMC Health Services Research, 20,* 106. https://doi.org/10.1186/s12913-020-4926-z.

Nether, K., Thomas, E., Khan, A., Ottosen, M., & Yager, L. (2022). Implementing a robust process improvement program in the neonatal intensive care unit to reduce harm. *Journal for Healthcare Quality, 44*(1), 23–30.

Nghe, M., Hart, J., Ferry, S., Hutchins, L., & Lebet, R. (2020). Developing leadership competencies in midlevel nurse leaders. *The Journal of Nursing Administration, 50*(9), 481–488.

Nilsen, P., Seing, I., Ericsson, C., Birken, S., & Schildmeijer, K. (2020). Characteristics of successful changes in health care organizations: An interview study with physicians, registered nurses and assistant nurses. *BMC Health Services Research, 20,* 147. https://doi.org/10.1186/s12913-020-4999-8.

Patterson, K., Grenny, J., Maxfield, D., McMillan, R., & Switzler, A. (2011). *Change anything.* New York: Hatchette Book Group.

Posch, A., & Garaus, C. (2020). Boon or curse? A contingent view on the relationship between strategic planning and organizational ambidexterity. *Long Range Planning, 53*(6), 101878.

Rasouli, A., Ketabchi Khoonsari, M. H., Ashja' ardalan, S., Saraee, F., & Ahmadi, F. Z. (2020). The importance of strategic planning and management in health: A systematic review. *Journal of Health Management and Informatics, 7*(1), 1–9.

Next-Generation NCLEX® case studies are included in select chapters to familiarize you with these new testing items for the NGN exam.

Learning Outcome:
Analyze results of an initial assessment to determine which findings supports a potential action or hinder the action; or when additional information is needed.

Cognitive Skill:
Evaluating Outcome

A direct-care nurse who is actively involved in the governance of their assigned surgical unit has been asked by their nurse manager to participate in a strategic planning committee to explore the addition of a bariatric surgical service at the hospital. The nurse is excited and delves into the strategic planning literature to be prepared for this opportunity. She realizes that she must be able to participate in developing strategies that reflect the environmental scan recently competed. The Strategic Planning Committee is to review the Environmental Scan done by the Administration. The findings were as follows:
- Determining the need for more bariatric surgeries in the area has been difficult.
- The hospital has a positive cash flow, limited debt, and sufficient reserves for expansion.
- A competing hospital across town has a robust bariatric service, led by a well-regarded chief of service.
- A new surgeon has moved to town and would like to increase his bariatric practice.
- Members of the medical staff of the hospital have strong negative feelings regarding starting such a service.
- The operating room (OR) facilities are currently providing services at peak capacity Monday through Friday.
- Additional space could be converted into more OR rooms.
- The Director of Surgical Services is an experienced nurse who is responsible for the preoperative areas, the operating rooms, and the postanesthesia recovery room. She plans to retire in 6 months.
- The nurse managers of the preoperative areas, the OR, and postanesthesia recovery unit all have 5 years or less experience and have been at the hospital for less than a year.
- The hospital is experiencing a shortage of nurses overall, particularly on the medical-surgical units.

For each of the findings of the environmental analysis, indicate whether the finding supports moving forward with the planning process, reduces the likelihood that the bariatric service would be successful, or more information is needed.

Findings	Supports moving forward	Reduces likelihood of success	Needs more information
Determining the need for more bariatric surgeries in the area has been difficult.			
The hospital has a positive cash flow, limited debt, and sufficient reserves for expansion.			
A competing hospital across town has a robust bariatric service, led by a well-regarded chief of service.			
A new surgeon has moved to town and would like to increase his bariatric practice in this area.			
Members of the medical staff of the hospital have strong negative feelings regarding starting such a service.			
The OR facilities are providing services at peak capacity Monday through Friday.			
Additional space could be converted into more OR rooms.			
The Director of Surgical Services is an experienced nurse who is responsible for the preoperative areas, the operating rooms, and the postanesthesia recovery room. She plans to retire in 6 months.			
The nurse managers of the preoperative areas, the OR, and postanesthesia recovery room all have 5 years or less experience and have been at the hospital for less than a year.			
The hospital is experiencing a shortage of nurses overall, particularly on the medical-surgical units.			

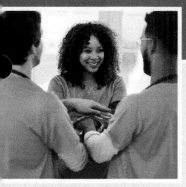

16

Copyright © Dean Mitchell/iStock/Thinkstock.

Building Effective Teams

Karren Kowalski

ANTICIPATED LEARNING OUTCOMES

- Evaluate the differences between a group and a team.
- Value four key concepts of teams.
- Describe the process of debriefing team functioning.
- Apply the guidelines for acknowledgment to a situation in your clinical setting.
- Compare a setting that uses agreements with your current clinical setting.
- Develop an example of a team that functions synergistically, including the results that such a team would produce.
- Discuss the importance of a team to patient safety and quality.

KEY TERMS

acknowledgment	debriefing	interprofessional teams
active listening	dualism	synergy
commitment	group	team

THE CHALLENGE

An extensive "team" of people works together to care for a neonate in a neonatal intensive care unit (NICU). The team includes registered nurses, physicians, respiratory therapists, physical therapists, social workers, neonatal nurse practitioners, and ancillary staff. Occasionally, specialists are consulted for specific cardiac, neurologic, or gastrointestinal problems. These are intermittent "team" members who play a crucial role in the baby's care.

Recently, a new group of specialists joined our team. They were identified as a top-notch group who would, by virtue of their expertise and reputation, increase the census and revenues for the hospital. Our team was excited to have this opportunity to grow in an area in which we had infrequent experience. However, integration of these new team members did not go smoothly. Clinical disagreements, communication breakdowns, and interpersonal conflicts occurred. The experience evolved into mutual distrust and control issues.

As disagreements, insults, and complaints escalated on both sides, the situation came to a defining moment when the director of the specialty group said, "I'm never bringing any of our patients here. I'm sending them to the PICU [pediatric intensive care unit]." The response from the NICU team was, "Fine with us—we don't need you, your patients, or the hassle." It seemed reasonable to not work together because, in fact, functionally we were already not working together. This response was in direct conflict with our belief that we could provide a valuable service and make a difference for both the patients and their families. This posed a dilemma for the staff, but everyone felt the situation was hopeless.

(Continued)

INTRODUCTION

As we experience crises such as the impact of the COVID-19 pandemic, as well as cost-cutting and quality and safety issues in healthcare, teamwork becomes crit-ical. The adage "If we do not all hang together, we will all hang separately" was never more true than now as we move through an era in which nursing is accountable for quality patient outcomes that affect reimbursement for care and the institutional financial bottom line. On top of all that, we don't have a sufficient amount of nurses to provide care for the high demands placed on most orga-nizations. To create finely tuned teams, communication skills (see Chapter 8) must improve. All team members must focus on improving their own skills, as well as supporting other team members, to grow in effectively building their team. These skills will be increasingly im-portant as teams negotiate a crisis-focused healthcare system that includes rapidly changing inpatient unit configurations, learning new isolation techniques, and ever changing personal protective equipment (PPE) in addition to state and federal payment systems and regulations. Between 2020 and 2021, we saw how read-ily nurses rose to these challenges associated with the pandemic and how effective the members were within the team and with patients and families. We also saw the toll that this intense effort took on the members of the team—not only nurses—to maintain that level of commitment.

In our society, because of the emphasis placed on the individual and individual achievement, teamwork is the quintessential contradiction. In other words, with all of the focus on individuals, we still need individu-als to work together in groups to accomplish goals and keep patients safe. In today's world, a nursing unit or team might have representatives from four or five dif-ferent generations: The Veteran Generation (less than 2%), Baby Boomers, Generation X, Millennials, and Generation Z or iGen (Tanner, 2020). The differences in these generations can be staggering, which is challeng-ing for functioning as a team if we fail to seek mutual interests. Fortunately, recent efforts have been in the di-rection of lessening the views of differences and more in the direction of increasing the views of commonalities in teams in the workplace. This effort has the potential to allow for recognition of differences, race, gender, age, sex, and so forth, while focusing on our commonali-ties—we are here because we all are smart, we care, we are experts in certain aspects of the profession of nurs-ing, and so forth.

GROUPS AND TEAMS

One definition of group is a number of individuals as-sembled together or having some unifying relationship. In groups, performance and outcomes are a result of the work of individual group members. Groups could be all of the parents in an elementary school, all of the mem-bers of a specific church, or all of the students in a school of nursing, because the members of these various groups are related in some way to one another by definition of their involvement in a certain endeavor.

A group of people does not constitute a team. Surbhi (2018) describes the differences between groups and teams and delineates a team as a collection of people collaborating in specific work or activity that focuses on a specific goal or outcome (see Table 16.1).

A team is an assemblage of people with a high degree of interdependence geared toward the achievement of a goal or task. Often, we can recognize intuitively when the designated team is not functioning effectively. We say things such as "We need to be more like a team" or "I'd like to see more team players around here." Consequently, in the process of defining *team*, effective versus ineffective teams must be considered. Teams are a collective of people who have defined objectives; ongo-ing positive relationships; effective, respectful commu-nication; and a supportive environment. In healthcare, teams are focused on accomplishing specific tasks and are essential in providing cost-effective, high-quality healthcare. As healthcare crises occur, resources are

TABLE 16.1 Comparison of Groups and Teams

Basis for Comparison	Group	Team
Definition	A collection of individuals who work on completing a task	An assemblage of people having a collective identify, joined together to accomplish a goal
Leadership	Only one leader	More than one leader and may change according to skill set
Members	Independent	Interdependent
Process	Discuss, decide, and delegate	Discuss, decide, and *do*
Work products	Individual	Collective
Focus on	Accomplishing individual goals	Accomplishing team goals
Accountability	Individually	Either indvidually or mutually

expended more prudently or prove scarce. In response, patient care teams must develop clearly defined goals, use creative problem solving, and demonstrate mutual respect and support. Facilities with ineffective teams may not survive the current changes in healthcare.

EXERCISE 16.1 Think of the last team or group in which you participated. Think about what went on in that team or group. Specifically, think about what worked for you and what did not work. Use the "Team Assessment Exercise" in Box16.1 to assess specific aspects of your team. Address each of the identified areas and discover how well your team or group functioned. Think about roles, activities, relationships, and general environment. Consider examples of shared decision-making, shared leadership, shared accountability, and shared problem solving. These are the concepts that can be used to evaluate the functioning of almost any team of which you are a member.

In a smoothly functioning team, each nurse is responsible for care provided to the patient and for the care provided by the whole team. In thinking about the whole team in a hospital setting, consider such activities as bedside shift handoffs when the teams from both

BOX 16.1 Team Assessment Exercise: Are We a Team?

Directions: Select a team with which you work. Place a checkmark beside each item that is true of your team. If the statement is not true, place no mark beside the item.

1. The language we use focuses on "we" rather than "you" or "I."
2. When one of us is busy, others try to help.
3. I know I can ask for help from others.
4. Most of us on the team could say what we are trying to accomplish.
5. What we are trying to accomplish on any given work day relates to the mission and vision of nursing and the organization.
6. We treat each other fairly, not necessarily the same.
7. We capitalize on people's strengths to meet the goals of our work.
8. The process for changing policies, procedures, equipment is clear.
9. Meetings are focused on the goals we are trying to achieve.
10. Our outcomes reflect our attention to goals and efforts.
11. Acknowledgment is individual and goal-oriented.
12. Innovation is supported by the team and management.
13. The group makes commitments to each other to ensure goal attainment.
14. Promises are kept.
15. Kindness in communication is evident, especially when bad news is delivered.
16. Individuals can describe their role in the overall work of the group.
17. Other members of the team are seen as trustworthy and valued.
18. The group is cost-effective and time-effective in attaining goals.
19. No member is excluded from the process of decision making.
20. Individuals can speak highly of their team members.

Tally the number of checkmarks and multiply that number by 5. The resultant number is an assessment of how well your team is functioning. The higher the score, the better the functioning.

shifts are present and collaborating with one another. Think also of interprofessional rounding when nurses, physicians, pharmacists, physical therapists, case managers, and social workers, to name a few, are present to assess and plan with the patient for the care that is needed. Think about how each of these professional groups communicate respectfully with one another. Huddles also allow nursing staff to focus on how they may best collaborate to provide care for the patient. This interactivity of the team promotes the best possible care for the patient and family while demonstrating the value of nursing (Albert et al., 2021).

When a team functions effectively, a significant difference is evident in the entire work atmosphere—the way in which discussions progress, the level of understanding of the team-specific goals and tasks, the willingness of members to listen, the manner in which disagreements are handled, the use of consensus, and the way in which feedback is given and received. The classic work done by McGregor (1960) and the more recent work by Farnsworth, Clark, Becton, Wysocki, and Kepne (2022) shed light on some of these significant differences, which are summarized in Table 16.2 (Eventus Training & Events, 2013).

Ineffective teams are often dominated by a few members, leaving others bored, resentful, or uninvolved. Leadership tends to be autocratic and rigid, and the team's communication style may be overly stiff and formal. Members tend to be uncomfortable with conflict or disagreement, avoiding and suppressing it rather than using it as a catalyst for change. When criticism is offered, it may be destructive, personal, and hurtful rather than constructive and problem centered. Team members may begin to hide their feelings of resentment or disagreement, sensing that these feelings are "dangerous." This creates the potential for later eruptions and discord. Similarly, the team avoids examining its own inner workings, or members may wait until after meetings to voice their thoughts and feelings about what went wrong and why.

In contrast, the effective team is characterized by its clarity of purpose, informality and congeniality, commitment, and a high level of participation. The members' ability to listen respectfully to each other and communicate openly helps them handle disagreements in a civilized manner and work through them rather than suppress them. Through ample discussion of issues, they reach decisions by consensus. Roles and work assignments are clear, and members share the leadership role, recognizing that each person brings unique strengths to the group effort. This diversity of styles helps the team adapt to changes and challenges, as does the team's ability and willingness to assess its own strengths and weaknesses and respond to them appropriately. Because of the importance of effective teams, we have seen the movement from the Triple aim to the Quntiple Aim with the fourth aim addresses, which incorporates the climate in which care is delivered, reflecting the tenets of the Magnet® program.

TABLE 16.2   Attributes of Effective and Ineffective Teams

Attribute	Effective Team	Ineffective Team
Goals	Task or objective is understood and supported by team members.	Team interaction fails to clarify the task or objective of group.
Contributions	All team members participate in discussion and comments are pertinent.	A few members dominate the discussion and minimize others' contributions.
Environment	Informal, comfortable, relaxed.	Indifferent, bored, tense.
Leadership	Shared and shifts according to expertise.	Autocratic and remains with the chairperson.
Assignments	Clearly stated, assigned, and accepted.	Unclear and lacks clarity regarding who is doing specific tasks.
Listening	Listen attentively to each member; every idea is heard.	Members do not listen; ideas are ignored, judged, and overridden.
Conflict	Members are comfortable with disagreement, with no conflict avoidance.	Disagreements are ignored or suppressed; voting results and minority are disconnected.
Decision-making	General agreement reached by consensus.	Actions or voting occurs before examination or resolution of real issues.
Self-evaluation	Conscious of its own process; ongoing evaluation; assesses interferences with team function.	Group avoids any discussion of effectiveness or operation.

Adapted from Eventus Training & Events. (2013). [Effective vs ineffective teams.] www.eventus.co.uk/effective-vs-ineffective-teams/.

The challenges encountered in today's healthcare systems are prodigious. Patient safety issues are at the forefront. Ongoing rounds of downsizing, budget cuts, declining patient days, reduced payments, staff layoffs, and use of travel nurses to meet crises abound. The latest analysis of patient outcome data indicates a decline in patient safety performance, as evidenced by the rise in nurse-sensitive indicators such as falls, central line–associated bloodstream infection (CLABSI) and catheter-associated urinary tract infection (CAUTI) rates, which is a reversal of prepandemic trends (Business Wire, 2021). Effective teams participate in effective problem solving, increased creativity, and improved healthcare. The effects of smoothly functioning teams on patient safety and the creation of a just culture are critically important. It is challenging to be a smoothly functioning team if the members are constantly changing.

CREATING EFFECTIVE TEAMS

When thinking about teams, consider the power of teamwork and what can be accomplished by a group of people working synergistically—people who are able to work together in a complementary way. The historical basis of theory related to teams is most commonly attributed to Tuckman, who proposed the 5 stages of group development in 1965. As the Theory Box shows, these five stages were seen as sequential and evolving. In the classic work of LaFasto and Larson (2001), in which they studied 600 teams and 6000 team members, the two key factors that emerged in the effectiveness of team functioning were great relationships between team members and excellent communication skills. Both of these concepts are complex and worth exploring in

more detail. For example, building relationships has two major aspects: behaviors, or what people do with each other; and characteristics, or who they are as human beings.

Building Relationships

Being in a relationship is about being connected or related and having mutual dealings, connections, or feelings between two parties. Specific learned behaviors, demonstrated by team members, can accelerate building extraordinary relationships among team members. Occasionally, a team member can shoulder the responsibility for criticism or for what did not work on behalf of the team. Taking the criticism, especially if you are not emotionally attached and can remain objective, demonstrates a willingness to go out of the way to support a team member. Thus, another team member can have the space to de-escalate and gain control of one's emotions. Such support can go a long way toward developing relationships. Another aspect of building relationships is the ability for you to "step in" to help without being asked. A subtle difference exists between someone who volunteers help before being asked and someone who agrees to help only after being asked. A true builder of relationships pays close attention to the well-being of others and is proactive. This is also a demonstration of caring and serendipitously builds stronger relationships.

In building relationships, you can anticipate the "question under the question." Often, team members will ask a more superficial question than the one they really want to ask. A colleague asking about an issue raised in the last meeting may actually be seeking a deeper understanding and appreciation of that colleague's contribution to the team. For example, asking questions to

THEORY BOX

Key Contributor	Key Ideas	Application to Practice
Tuckman, B. (1965). Developmental sequence in small groups. *Psychological Bulletin, 63*, 384–399.	Composed of 5 stages 1. Forming: Personal relations focused on safe behaviors, learning the group. 2. Storming: Competition and conflict; defining rules and roles. 3. Norming: Cohesion, active recognition of contributions, asking questions, shared leadership, group belonging. 4. Performing*: Interdependence, dynamic adjustments, problem solving, productivity. 5. Adjourning: Disengagement.	Building in time for groups to work through the stages of development in addition to the tasks themselves.

*Note: Not all groups will achieve the performing stage.

obtain more clarity following such interactions with a grateful acknowledgment of team members' curiosity can increase the quality of the relationship.

You must be willing to demonstrate thoughtfulness of others by giving unexpected praise or acknowledgment. Take time each day to do something nice for a teammate just because you can. This approach can be coupled with a desire to help, not because you need something from someone, but because you can support or help someone else. Approach relationship building from the perspective of the other person, not from your perspective or your needs. In other words, give more than you receive. Valuing every member of the team can have major positive outcomes. Find something positive about all team members and their contributions. Every human being is important, as is every job. Recognition is critical to retention of team members—while that recognition needs to come from the leader, it is also valued from peers.

Communicating Effectively

The connection existing between relationship building and effectively communicating feelings and concerns is significant to the creation of effective teams. Likewise, communication in the work environment is not only important to creating a healthy work environment that retains nurses but also essential to reduction of medical errors (American Association of Critical Care Nurses (AACN, 2016). The AACN conducted some of the first original research on communication in the intensive care unit (ICU), reporting these critical findings in the book entitled *Silence Kills* done by the AACN, AORN, and VitalSMarts (Maxfield, Grenny, McMillan, Patterson, & Switzler, 2005). This seminal work reported that communication breakdown was detrimental to patients and could even cause death. This work led to the creation of the guidelines for a healthy work environment with an emphasis on effective communication. The second edition of these guidelines (AACN, 2016) were widely adopted across facilities to increase the quality of the work environment. These skills are crucial to smoothly functioning teams. An example of a commonly used tool for effective communication is SBAR (Situation, Background, Assessment, Recommendation), which is discussed in the communications chapter.

During the COVID-19 pandemic, we discovered that a key way we communicated was with technology, primarily through email and text messaging, as we had to reach many people quickly. Because we are seeing only words when using technology rather than experiencing the full spectrum of communication, it is difficult to determine the other aspects of communication such as body language, facial expression, and tonality. Thus, strategies to increase the effectiveness of email communication would be important, as the Literature Perspective describes.

LITERATURE PERSPECTIVE

Resource: Medland, J. (2020). Leveraging email to build healthy effective teams. *Nurse Leader, 19*(2), 40–46.

The author identifies email as occupying nearly 25% of a leader's workday—and this was *prior* to the virtual work environment necessitated by the COVID-19 pandemic (Medland, 2020). This work emphasizes the importance of communicating clearly and in a meaningful way both as leaders and clinical nurses. Email must be able to connect team members, including feelings of social well-being and a sense of being related. This approach stresses the importance of the care and attention devoted to email communication. Analysis of thousands of email messages over a 12-month period revealed the importance of the following. (1) The sender should tailor the message so that it is meaningful to the recipients (other team members), creating a connection between sender and receivers, supporting receivers in feeling capable/successful in their work, and feeling engaged with the sender. (2) The sender must also invest in what matters to the other team members and, over time, the cumulative communication pattern should make a deep and lasting impact on the receiver. (3) The emails need to be positive in tone and conversational, including hope, curiosity, and affirmation, or a "thumbs up" to the receiver. (4) The messages can attend to team members by building their emotional well-being, addressing their concerns, and exchanging feedback. (5) Emails can be connecting when they serve as a vehicle to help others be successful in their jobs, especially when they are feeling uncertain or insecure about how to proceed.

Implications for Practice
By using a few basic rules, team leaders and team members can use emails to further develop and enrich the functioning of the team. Practicing being thoughtful and caring rather than being in a hurry or viewing emails in a negative light or as a chore can make this strategy effective. Employing simple but powerful strategies can enhance the functioning of the team, connecting the members while promoting individual team member autonomy.

For purposes of establishing effective teams, consider some additional aspects of communication. These skills are essential to clinical practice, to building teams, and to leadership. Because communication consists of both verbal and nonverbal signals, humans are continuously communicating thoughts, ideas, opinions, feelings, and emotions. Once the message is sent, the first impression of the communication usually is lasting. However, it is often an unconscious response or reaction. To become more aware of communication in teams, consider the following model.

Positive Communication Model

Whenever human beings are in distress, unengaged, disengaged, or have an emotional reaction to a situation or the actions of another, a conditioned response is to move into one or all of the following: blame, judgment, or demand. These are depicted in the awareness model found in Fig. 16.1. With effort and practice, it is possible to create a communication interaction that produces a significantly improved outcome.

When individuals react at the feeling level, they tend to move unconsciously to blame. By taking accountability for these feelings, they can move out of blame and

own feelings by stating, "I feel ...." Likewise, when individuals are trapped in distress or reaction at the thinking level, they most often turn to judgment. By thinking compassionately, we can dismantle the judgment and state what we think in a compassionate way: "I think ...." Finally, when in distress, individuals may make demands that are often unreasonable. By calming ourselves, we can find respect for the other human being and make a request for what we want for ourselves in a given situation: "I want...." Wanting the other person to change is pointless because it is unlikely to happen and we don't control the other person.

Most broken relationships are stuck in blame, judgment, and demand. Being accountable, compassionate, and respectful helps clarify what goes on inside each of us.

All individuals need to feel that their skills, tools, and contributions are needed and valued and that each of us is respected for what personal contributions are offered to the workplace, team, or group. Everyone has weaknesses—emphasizing these or spending time in ongoing correction is not productive. Rather, focus should be placed on people's strengths, specifically acknowledging and emphasizing what people do well.

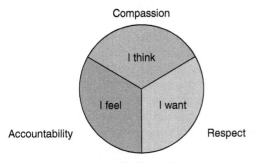

Fig. 16.1 Awareness model: Differentiating between unconscious and conscious responses.

> **EXERCISE 16.2** Think of an example or a recent incident when you were very upset or felt stuck in blame, judgment, and/or demand. You might even write down what you were feeling in that moment, what it was about for you, and what you wanted for yourself. Share the issue or problem situation with someone and practice talking using "I feel," "I think," and "I want" instead of blame, judgment and/or demand.

Characteristics of Leaders

When we think about leading a team, most of us have had positive and challenging experiences with teams. It is possible to think about qualities or characteristics of effective team leaders. The good news is each of these characteristics is possible to learn, practice, and continuously improve. We have selected five time-tested characteristics as examples (Kowalski & Yoder-Wise, 2003).

Character

Team leaders and effective team members demonstrate a strong, positive character. So, what is character? It is who we are at our center—what motivates us—what drives us to accomplish goals and tasks. It is who we are and what we do when no one else knows or sees us. It is the internal matter that makes us who we are. For effective team leaders, this is the core element. Other elements that comprise characteristics of leaders include commitment, compassion, confidence, and connectedness. We develop character, both positively and negatively, each day with every decision we make.

Commitment

Commitment is a state of being emotionally impelled and is demonstrated when a sense of passion and dedication to a project or event—a mission— exists. Often, this passion looks a little outrageous as people go the extra mile because of their commitment. They do whatever it takes to accomplish the goals or see the project through to completion. The work on peak performance by Charles Garfield (2021) during the 1960s provides an example of commitment in his description of the team that created the lunar landing module for the first man to walk on the moon. Team members demonstrated behaviors that looked odd, including working extended hours and shifts, calling in to see how the project was progressing, and sleeping at their workstations to not be separated from the project—all because they knew that they were part of something that was much larger than themselves. They were a part of sending a man to the moon, something that human beings had been dreaming about for thousands of years. It was a historic moment, and people were intensely committed to making it happen.

Many people go through their entire lives hating every single day of work. Obviously, most people who hate their work are not committed. Because we spend an extensive amount of time in the work setting, we must enjoy what we do for both physical and mental well-being. If this is not the case for you, then try to find a different job or profession—one you might love. Life is too short to do something that you hate doing every day. While you are moving into whatever you decide you love doing, commit yourself to doing your best at whatever you are currently doing. Be 100% present wherever you are. Do the best work you are capable of doing. This honors you as a human being, and it honors your coworkers and patients.

> **EXERCISE 16.3** Review the eight questions about exploring commitment in Box 16.2. Spend at least 20 minutes in a quiet place thinking about and writing answers to these eight questions. Pay particular attention to Question 7.

BOX 16.2   Exploring Commitment

The key to finding your compelling mission or passion that will lead you to success and peak performance is to ask yourself the right questions. Your answers to these questions will help you understand what you need to know about yourself. Read each question, then think carefully for a few minutes, and answer each question honestly. Do not censor or edit out anything, even if it seems impossible or unrealistic—allow yourself to be surprised. Let your imagination soar.

1. Am I deriving any satisfaction out of the work I am now doing?
2. If they did not reward (praise or pay) me to do what I now do, would I still do it?
3. What is it that I really love to do?
4. What do I want to pursue with my time and energy that is worthwhile?
5. What motivates me to reach out and do my best to excel?
6. What is it that only I can say to the world? What needs to be done that can best be done only by me?
7. If I won $40 million in the lottery tomorrow, how would I live? What would I do each day and for the rest of my life?
8. If I were to write my own obituary right now, what would be my most significant accomplishment? Is that enough?

Repeating this exercise often will give you additional insights and information about what you really want and love to do. If taken seriously, the exercise should help you have an understanding of why you selected this profession and whether you have the stamina to do whatever it takes to make a contribution and to make a difference in the practice of nursing.

Compassion

When we think of compassion or sympathetic consciousness toward others' distress with a desire to alleviate this distress and taking action to do so, it is clear that this demonstrates caring. These sentiments are likely to lessen suffering and decrease the time required for recovery. When these emotions are demonstrated by the team leader, it increases the probability that emotional healing will begin and increases the attachment of the team members to their peers and the organization. Team members may adopt the behavior demonstrated by the leader and understand that under similar circumstances, they would also be treated with compassion and caring. If this behavior increases the cohesiveness of the team, it is easy to see how it can also affect the perception of the organization and its ability to maintain exemplary care during difficult times, such as the COVID-19 pandemic. Such behavior can also foster the capacity to adapt, heal, and achieve organizational goals. In Magnet® organizations, where leaders have demonstrated compassion and caring, the clinical nurses identify these behaviors as the reason for their choice to remain in the facility.

Confidence

To effectively demonstrate compassion, connectedness with team members, and the commitment to activate these behaviors, leaders must be confident in their own abilities and trust themselves, which can create a boldness and self-assurance that evolves their leadership style and capacity to lead. Such capacity enables the leader to grow personally and professionally and to exhibit the inner drive to build on the achievements of the previous day and move the team forward in accomplishing the goals of the team. With this kind of attitude and approach, the leader can confront ongoing challenges. The most obvious challenge that can deter the effectiveness of the leader is fear—fear of failure, of looking bad, or of being judged by team members or supervisors. Fear is augmented by directing negative talk to oneself, such as "that was a stupid thing to do" or "I never should have said that." With a concerted effort, we can substitute these messages with a positive perspective that focuses on what is learned from an incident that didn't evolve the way we had hoped. This positive approach actually negates the need to be perfect and addresses the ability to handle the challenges of daily life. When the leader demonstrates confidence and positivity, team members are encouraged to adopt the same approach.

Behaviors of Great Team Members

Teams function with varying levels of effectiveness. The interesting part of these variations is that effectiveness can be created systematically. Truly effective teams are ones in which people work together to produce extraordinary results that could not have been achieved by any one individual. This phenomenon is described as synergy. In the physical sciences, synergy is found in metal alloys. Bronze, the first alloy, was a combination of copper and tin and was found to be much harder and stronger than either copper or tin separately. Because the tensile strength of bronze cannot be predicted by merely adding the tensile strength of tin and copper, it is far greater than simple addition. Working cooperatively, an effective team produces extraordinary results that no one team member could have achieved alone. To create synergy consistently, certain basic rules must be followed: establish a clear purpose, use active listening, tell the truth, be compassionate, be flexible, commit to resolution, and capitalize on what individuals bring to the team.

Establish a Clear Purpose

Creating a smoothly functioning team requires a clear purpose. Just as a clear purpose is everything to an organization, purpose is everything for a team. A clear purpose articulates why the team exists and what problems the team is to solve (O'Brien et al., 2019). All members of the team must understand the reason for the creation of the team, determine what they wish to accomplish (as delineated by defined goals and objectives), and express their beliefs regarding the value and feasibility of the goals and tasks. Teams function best when the members can not only tell others about their purpose but also define and operationalize succinctly the meaning and value of this purpose. Being aware of what each can contribute and expect allows all other members to capitalize on individual talent and support each other in goal attainment.

Use Active Listening

Active listening means that you are completely focused on the individual who is speaking. It means listening without judgment. It means listening to the essence of the conversation so that you can actually repeat to the speaker most of the speaker's intended meaning. It means being 100% present in the communication. This requires the skill of active listening. Examples of how to validate that active listening is occurring appear in Table 16.3.

Developing a defensive response or argument in your head while the other person is still speaking is not active listening. To listen actively, a person must be absorbing words, posture, tone of voice, and all of the queues accompanying the message so that the intent of the communication can be received.

Tell the Truth

To *tell the truth* means to speak clearly to personal points and perspectives while acknowledging that they are merely personal perspectives. If an observation is made about the tone or behavior of a speaker that affects the ability of others to hear the message, feedback can be provided in a way that does not make the speaker

TABLE 16.3   Active Listening

Use of Active Listening	Examples
To convey interest in what the other person is saying	I see! I get it. I hear what you're saying.
To encourage individuals to expand further on their thinking	Yes, go on. Tell me more.
To help individuals clarify the problem through their own thinking	Then the problem as you see it is …
To get individuals hear what they have said in the way it sounded to others	This is your decision, then, and the reasons are … If I understand you correctly, you are saying that we should …
To pull out the key ideas from a long statement or discussion	Your major point is … You believe that we should …
To respond to people's feelings more than to their words	You feel strongly that … You do not believe that …
To summarize specific points of agreement and disagreement as a basis for further discussion	We seem to agree on the following points … But we seem to need further clarification on these points …
To express a consensus of group feeling	As a result of this discussion, we as a group seem to feel that …

wrong. This is accomplished in an objective rather than subjective manner using neither a cynical nor a critical tone of voice or by asking a question for clarification. To be effective, one must own, or be responsible for, personal opinions and attitudes.

Be Compassionate

To *be compassionate* means to have a sympathetic consciousness of another's distress and a desire to alleviate the distress. Consequently, focusing time and energy on making the other person wrong, especially when your perspective differs from that person's, is inappropriate. The goal is to listen from a caring perspective—one that is focused on understanding the viewpoint of the other person rather than insisting on the "rightness" of one's own point of view.

Be Flexible

Flexibility and openness to another person's viewpoint are critical for a team to work well together. No single person has all the right answers. Therefore, acknowledging that each person has something to contribute and must be heard is important. Flexibility reflects a willingness to hear another team member's point of view rather than being committed to the "rightness" of a personal point of view.

Commit to Resolution

To *commit to resolution* means that one can agree to disagree with someone even when that perspective is different. Rather than assuming the person is wrong, this is a commitment to hear that person's perspective, listen to the real message, identify differences, and creatively seek solutions to resolve the areas of differences. In this way, a common understanding and shared commitment to the issue can be reached. Both parties then need to agree that they feel heard and agree to the resolution. This differs greatly from compromise and majority vote seen in the democratic process. When compromise exists, acquiescence or relinquishing of a significant portion of what was desired likely occurred. This generally leaves both parties feeling negative about themselves or the agreement. Consequently, most compromises must be reworked at some future date. Working on conflict and its resolution (Box 16.3) is time-consuming and essential to effectively functioning teams (Civico, 2019). Commitment to resolution is integral to the needs of the team. One team member may disagree with another team member, but the successful work of the team is at stake in this conflict. Without commitment to resolution for the sake of the team, individuals often have less impetus to seek a common ground or to agree to disagree.

The team is not successful when one team member becomes a self-proclaimed expert who has the "right" answer. Nor is it successful when people fail to speak. Each team member has good ideas, which need to be shared. They may not be shared, however, when someone feels uncomfortable in the team. It is difficult to speak up and appear wrong or inadequate. The challenge each person faces is to push through discomfort and become a full participant in problem identification and resolution for the overall benefit of the team.

BOX 16.3   Aspects of Conflict

Destructive

- Diverts energy from more important activities and issues
- Destroys the morale of people or reinforces poor self-concepts
- Polarizes groups so they increase internal cohesiveness and reduce intergroup cooperation
- Deepens differences in values
- Produces irresponsible and regrettable behavior, such as name-calling and fighting

Constructive

- Opens up issues of importance, resulting in their clarification
- Results in the solution of problems
- Increases the involvement of individuals in issues of importance to them
- Causes authentic communication to occur
- Serves as a release for pent-up emotion, anxiety, and stress
- Helps build cohesiveness among people sharing the conflict, celebrating in its settlement, and learning more about each other
- Helps individuals grow personally and apply what they learn to future situations

Acknowledge

Part of focusing on people's strengths is being willing to acknowledge peers, leaders, and the other significant people in one's life (Fontes, 2020). It is important to understand that acknowledgment means validating others and the importance of their contribution. This recognition gives team members a feeling of fulfilment and purpose in their work. For leaders, acknowledgment of team members needs to evolve into an intrinsic attribute or part of their growth and development rather than a tool to motivate team members. Because we all want to be validated for our contributions, acknowledgment needs to be a priority for team leaders.

In contrast, some leaders focus on correction. Consequently, many of us spend a large portion of our time correcting others rather than appreciating them for all of the attributes they demonstrate. Focusing on strengths rather than on weaknesses is far more productive and leads to excellence. According to the classic work of Gallup about people's strengths as reported by Rath (2007), weaknesses will never be improved to more than average or mediocre. If the focus is on improving our strengths, it is much easier to excel and then to be acknowledged for what we do well. Focusing on weaknesses tends to decrease the appreciation and, thus, the acknowledgments. Furthermore, we seem to believe that a finite number of acknowledgments exist. This attitude of scarcity of acknowledgments leads to stinginess in acknowledging people. Of course, this approach is a bit ridiculous. Acknowledgments are infinite. The more we sincerely give to others and to ourselves, the smoother the team functions. On the other hand, we do not always give acknowledgments in a way they can be received and valued. Box 16.4 can serve as a guide for giving acknowledgments.

BOX 16.4   Guidelines for Acknowledgment

1. Acknowledgments must be specific. The specific behavior or action that is appreciated must be identified in the acknowledgment; for example, "Thank you for taking notes for me when I had to go to the dentist. You identified three key points that needed to be reported."
2. Acknowledgments must be "eye to eye," or personal. Look people in the eye when you thank them. Do not run down the hall and say "Thanks" over your shoulder. Written appreciation also qualifies as "eye to eye."
3. Acknowledgments must be sincere, that is, from the heart. Each of us recognizes insincerity. If you do not truly appreciate a behavior or action, do not say anything. Insincerity often makes people angry or upset, thus, defeating the goal. Further, it discredits the person who is insincere.
4. Acknowledgments are more powerful when they are given in public. Most people receive pleasure from public acknowledgment and remember these occasions for a long time. For people who are shy and may prefer no public acknowledgment, this is an opportunity to work on a personal growth issue with them. Public acknowledgment is an opportunity to communicate what is valued.
5. Acknowledgments need to be timely. The less time that elapses between the event and the acknowledgment, the more powerful and effective it is and the more the acknowledgment is appreciated by the recipient.

EXERCISE 16.4 Within the next 3 days, find three opportunities to acknowledge a peer or acquaintance using the five guidelines for acknowledgment shown in Box 16.4. Use these same guidelines to acknowledge yourself for something you have done well.

Debriefing

The general definition of debriefing is to carefully review upon completion or to question someone about a completed undertaking. The most common use of debriefing in nursing is with the use of simulation. The International Nursing Association for Clinical Simulation and Learning Healthcare Simulation Standards of Best Practice: The Debriefing Process (2021) describes debriefing as a reflection or a conscious consideration of the meaning and implication of an action, which includes the assimilation and understanding of knowledge, skills, and attitudes. Reflection can lead to new interpretations or understanding by participants who can reframe the situation or scenario cognitively as an essential part of learning. The skills of the debriefer are important to ensure the best possible learning outcomes. Debriefing is one example of the process of reflection. Likewise, the exercises in this chapter are an opportunity to practice debriefing and to determine what was learned in the exercise.

KEY CONCEPTS OF TEAMS

In rare instances, a team may produce teamwork spontaneously, like kids in a schoolyard at recess. However, most management teams learn about teamwork because they need and want to work together. This kind of working together requires that they observe how they are together in a group and that they unlearn ingrained self-limiting assumptions about the glory of individual effort and authority that are contrary to cooperation and teamwork. Team dynamics, when valued by all members of the team, facilitate the team's work. Keys to the concept of team include the following:

- Conflict management
- Singleness of mission
- Willingness to cooperate
- Commitment

Conflict Management

Realizing that conflict is fundamental to the human experience can be helpful. Conflict is an integral part of all human interaction. Therefore, the challenge is to recognize the breakdown in the communication process and to deal appropriately with it (Albert et al., 2021). Conflicts are usually based on a person's attempts to protect self-esteem or to alter perceived inequities in power because most human beings believe that other people have greater power. Thus, those who feel this way believe that they are unlikely to achieve their objectives. For example, the following steps can be helpful in resolving conflict between two nursing assistants on one's team:

- Identify the triggering event.
- Discover the historical context for each person.
- Assess how interdependent they are on each other.
- Identify the issues, goals, and resources involved in the situation.
- Assess the impact on the current work.
- Uncover any previously considered solution.
- Determine how the individuals can move forward.

Assessing the level of working relationship between the conflicted parties is essential, particularly if they work together on a regular basis.

The word *team* is usually reserved for a special type of working together. This working together requires communication in which the members understand how to conduct interpersonal relationships with their peers in thoughtful, supportive, and meaningful ways. Working together requires that team members are able to resolve conflicts among themselves in ways that enhance rather than inhibit their working relationship. In addition, team members must be able to trust that they will receive what they need while being able to count on one another to complete tasks related to team functioning and outcomes. To communicate effectively, people must be willing to confront issues and to express openly their ideas and feelings—to use interactive skills to accomplish tasks. In nursing, constructive confrontation has not been a well-used skill. Consequently, if communication patterns are to improve, the onus is on each of us as individuals to change communication patterns. In essence, for things to change, each of us must change.

Singleness of Mission

Every team must have a purpose—that is, a plan, aim, or intention. However, the most successful teams have a mission—some special work or service to which the team is 100% committed. The sense of mission and purpose must be clearly understood and agreed to by all (Ready Training On-Line, 2021). The more powerful and visionary the mission is, the more energizing it will be to the team. The more energy and excitement engendered, the more motivated all members will be to do the necessary work. The mutuality of the work to be accomplished can help bring the members of a team, even one with great diversity, together to accomplish a goal.

Willingness to Cooperate

Just because a group of people has a regular reporting relationship within an organizational chart does not mean that the members are a team. Boxes and arrows are not in any way related to the technical and interpersonal coordination or the emotional investment required of a true team. In effective teams, members are required to work together in a respectful, civil manner. Most of us have been involved in organizations in which some people could accomplish assigned tasks but were not successful in their interpersonal relationships. In essence, these employees received a salary for not getting along with people. Some of these employees have not worked cooperatively for years! Organizations can no longer afford to pay employees to not work together. Personal friendship or socialization is not required, but cooperation is a necessity. Traditionally, these interpersonal skills were considered "soft" skills and were difficult to identify or to hold team members accountable for them. Currently, in most organizations, employees can be terminated for a lack of willingness to work cooperatively with team members.

EXERCISE 16.5 Think about the last event in which you were either involved in or observed major conflict. Identify what triggered the event; reflect on what the context was for each person; assess the relationship and identify the issues, goals, and resources for each; think about the impact on the current work environment; discover any possible solutions both currently and previously; and discover possible ways the individuals can move forward in working together.

ISSUES THAT AFFECT TEAM FUNCTIONING

When individuals come together purposefully to form a team, they spend considerable time in group process or social dynamics, which allows them to advance toward becoming a team and completing a goal. Each person within the emerging team struggles with key issues about cooperation, power, appreciation, agreements, emotions, trust, differences, and feedback that must continually be reevaluated and renegotiated.

"In" Groups and "Out" Groups

Most of us want to be valued and recognized by others as a part of the group, one who "knows" or understands. Most people want to be at the core of decision-making, power, and influence. In other words, they want to be part of the "in" group. Researchers have demonstrated that those who feel "in" cooperate more, work harder and more effectively, and bring enthusiasm to the group. The more we feel we are not a part of the key group, the more "out" we feel—the more we withdraw, work alone, daydream, and engage in self-defeating behaviors. Often, intergroup conflict results when individuals who feel they are "out" and want to be "in" create a schism or a division that prohibits the team from accomplishing its goals. The concept of "in" group is conveyed in the term *belonging*. When we consider efforts related to diversity, equity, inclusion, and belonging, we understand how valuable the sense of being in the "in group" is to having a sense of belonging. People don't want to feel as if they are merely an employee of some organization—they want to feel connected to others at work. Most of us want to belong to a group.

Dualism

Our society tends to be dualistic in nature. Dualism means that most situations are viewed as right or wrong, black or white. Answers to questions are often reduced to "yes" or "no." As a result, we sometimes forget that a broad spectrum of possibilities actually exists. Exercising creativity and exploring numerous possibilities are important. This allows the team to operate at its optimal level.

An extension of this idea of dualism is a person who is a self-proclaimed expert, to whom it is critically important to be right and acknowledged as right and who becomes judgmental of others whose perspectives and opinions differ. Consequently, being able to tell the truth to a team member and to encourage team members to stretch and look at different ways of functioning is vital. This requires strong negotiation and conflict resolution skills, something for which few of us have been trained. If self-proclaimed experts think we are judging them, they will not hear the questions, observations, or the "truth" because the message will appear to be proving them wrong. Going beyond dualism is critical to the team.

Power and Control

Everybody wants at least some power, and everybody wants to feel in control. When faced with changes that we cannot influence, we feel impotent and experience a loss of self-esteem. Consequently, we want to feel that we are in control of our immediate environment and that we have enough power and influence to get our needs met. When a situation or an event arises that we cannot handle, we attempt to compensate for it in some way; most of these ways are not productive to smoothly functioning teams. You may have been "right," but the sense of a loss of control or power is very uncomfortable, sometimes resulting in stress and fear. Mature behavior is required to maintain a positive, problem-solving approach.

EXERCISE 16.6 Think about a time when you and a small group wanted to change something—such as a scheduled time (a class or meeting), an assignment, or an outcome measure (grading curve of a test or a performance evaluation criterion)—and the person "in charge" adamantly refused. How did you feel? What was the response? Did you engage in gossip to make others appear wrong?

Use, Develop, and Be Appreciated for My Skills and Resources

Each member of the team has unique skills and resources to bring to the team's goals and tasks. The Gallup (2020) research makes it quite clear that one of the most powerful indicators of a successful, supportive work environment can be predicted by the scores from the following question: "At work, do you have the opportunity to do what you do best every day?" When the score is low in this area, team members clearly do not believe their skills are recognized, well used, or appreciated. To accomplish the goal of having all team members believe that their skills are recognized, encouraged, and used and their growth encouraged requires a strong, knowledgeable *team leader*. Fewer than 20% of employees feel their strengths are used every day (Gallup, 2020). When nurses do not believe their skills are used, they are more prone to be in the "out group." This leads to being unengaged and even disengaged in the workplace. This is not supportive of a positive, creative work environment or of developing effective teams.

Group Agreements

One of the most helpful tools available is to have team members enter into an agreement about their relationships with one another. This can take place in various ways. Multiple types of guidelines can even be used to set the context for how people relate. Many hospitals and facilities have service agreements that new employees accept when they are first hired. These are often in the employee handbook and are used to hold people accountable for behaviors. One example of a set of agreements comes from the Colorado Center for Nursing Excellence, the nursing workforce center for the state (Box 16.5). These are called the "Commitment to My Team Members." They have gone through multiple transitions and redesigns, but the basic tenets are essentially the same. People

---

BOX 16.5   Commitment to My Team Members

- I accept responsibility for establishing and maintaining healthy interpersonal relationships with every member of this team. I recognize that the words, actions, and attitudes of each of us individually reflect on the whole of the Colorado Center for Nursing Excellence.
- I will respectfully speak promptly with any team member with whom I am having a problem. The only time I will discuss it with another person is when I need assistance in reaching a satisfactory resolution. The goal of a conversation with a trusted colleague is not to complain or triangulate but to gain insight into resolution. I will always remember to "take the mail to the correct address."

- I will establish and maintain a relationship of trust with every member of this team. My relationships with each of you will be equally respectful, regardless of job title, level of educational preparation, or any other differences that may exist.
- I will accept each team member as they are today, forgiving past problems and asking each person to do the same with me.
- I will remember that no one is perfect and that our errors will be accepted as opportunities for forgiveness, growth, and learning.
- Because all members of our team are leaders and followers, we are committed to finding solutions to

BOX 16.5   Commitment to My Team Members—cont'd

problems and embracing accountability for the success of the whole organization.

- My words, actions, and attitudes make my team members feel appreciated, included, and valued. I will have fun and keep a sense of humor at work.
- As leaders we practice what The Center teaches.

I expect and accept if at any time I do not comply with the above statements my team members will have a confidential conversation with me directly in order to raise awareness and accountability to the above commitments.

I agree to hold myself accountable to the above commitments in an effort to promote a healthy learning environment.

Editorial Comments

The staff at the Colorado Center for Nursing Excellence adapted these agreements in 2010 from similar agreements used previously in other facilities by Dr. Kowalski. The staff included both professional and support personnel. These agreements are reviewed at each monthly "all staff meeting." This review serves as a reminder of how the team works together, and each person considers these agreements integral to the smooth functioning of the team.

Different projects have different team members as the leader, and the remainder are followers. Sometimes, the leader of a specific project is a support person and the followers, both professional staff and support staff, take direction from that person.

The Center delivers educational offerings on leadership, teaching, quality, and safe patient care and presentations. The common threads exemplified in the above agreements are taught, and each member of the team is expected to demonstrate the behaviors we teach to participants.

From Colorado Center for Nursing Excellence. (n.d.). Commitment to my team members. https://www.coloradonursingcenter.org/documents/misc/team_commitment.pdf.

---

must agree on the goals and mission with which they are involved. They have to reach some understanding of how they will exist together. Tenets or agreements such as "I will respectfully speak promptly with any team member with whom I have a problem" go a long way to avoid gossiping, backbiting, bickering, and misinterpreting others. These team agreements are reviewed regularly (e.g., monthly or quarterly), because this process helps members of the team be accountable for upholding the agreements and receive/give feedback when the agreements have been violated or need to be changed. Without agreement, people have implicit permission to behave in any manner they choose toward one another, including angry, hostile, hurtful, and acting-out behavior. What is different about these agreements from the statements found in employee handbooks is that they are fluid. Team agreements require review and input from the team members and adjustments are made in the words, not necessarily the standards. This mutual agreement among the members of the team, including the leader, allows for everyone to hold everyone else accountable.

> **EXERCISE 16.7** Think about a group meeting you attended that did not go well. Identify three examples of a group agreement that might have improved the tone and outcomes of the meeting.

Managing Emotions

Probably one of the greatest fears in team building is that people will become emotional, that they will lose control of themselves or the environment, or that they will appear weakened or vulnerable. Management and leadership are usually more willing to deal with the "thinking" side than the "feeling" side of individuals within the team. Today, considerably more patience is exhibited with the stress in the workplace and the emotional responses it evokes. Positive emotions can create excitement, positive energy, and creativity. At the same time, extreme emotions of a more negative nature can block effective communication and positive problem solving.

If you feel yourself begin to escalate emotionally, it may be helpful to strive to keep your composure through slowing your breathing and consciously relaxing the tense areas of your body. You might also attempt to identfy the threat to yourself, especially the thoughts that had you respond emotionally. Do your best to maintain direct eye contact. If you disagree, do so promptly without emotion. In spite of your best intentions, you may sometimes respond in a negative way. If this response occurs, attempt to understand your emotional response and understand that anger often covers other emotions, such as fear or emotional pain.

If you are dealing with an angry team member, try to identify the "real" feeling the individual is experiencing.

Let your emotional team member vent; listen to what the individual has to say. Another strategy could be to encourage the team member to move or sit down. If possible, affirm the individual's emotions/feelings without necessarily agreeing with the point being made. Don't dismiss or negate the team member's feelings. Use the individual's name several times to affirm individuality and importance.

Ask for more details. Attempt to determine what is threatening to the team member, such as loss of approval or control or fear of failure. Does the individual feel taken advantage of? If possible, encourage the person to identify optional solutions. Discourage interruptions when you are speaking and even suggest a brief break (possibly time to take deep breaths). If the team member is completely out of control, let the person know that you take this situation very seriously and that the current emotional upset is not acceptable. Remind the person of team agreements.

Whether you are a team member or the team leader, specific behaviors such as meditation, physical activity, or yoga can help support you in maintaining an even emotional approach in these difficult situations. Remember that the team members know these same strategies and likely will be irritated by repetitive implementation of them. Acknowledge the upset and ask that the team member put the concern in writing so that the leader and/or the team can give further consideration to the issue.

Trust

Trust is the basis by which leaders and managers facilitate the activities and progress of the team. Trust is critical to effective interactions and is defined as a firm belief in the reliability, ability, and truth of another person or a thing. Canadian philosopher Paul Thagard (2019) describes trust as a set of behaviors that depend on another, a probability that a person will behave in specific ways. Furthermore, he believes that trust is an abstract mental attitude that views someone as dependable, for example, it is confidence and a feeling of security that a partner truly cares. Warrell (2020) believes that the most significant aspect of trust is the trust we have in ourselves, that within us are the resources we need to handle whatever unfolds in our lives. Furthermore, the author believes that trust is not only the core of relationships but also the currency of influence in both the specific workplace and the entire organization, which is described as the three core domains of trust: competence, reliability, and sincerity. Competence refers to a specific skill set. For

example, you might trust me to teach you about leadership and administration, but you would not want me to attempt to take care of you in the critical care unit if that is not my area of expertise (and you shouldn't, as my clinical background is obstetrics).

Reliability relates to counting on a person to manage and honor commitments. A team member may be trusted as competent at a specific task but may have a track record of tardiness or sloppy work, which prevents you from complete trust. It comes down to this: Can your word be trusted?

Sincerity is related to the assessment of someone's integrity, to the fundamental nature of their character. It is the most pivotal in the decision to trust someone and it is the most important aspect of leadership. It is why allegations of impropriety or infidelity in leaders is so devastating. For example, in a marriage, infidelity has a devastating effect, whereas forgetting an anniversary is much less damaging. Likewise, when colleagues talk about you behind your back, it is much more significant than if they are chronically late to meetings. Sincerity also relates to how much someone cares about what you care about, such as a sick or dying relative. In the case of a severe family illness, do your colleagues even acknowledge they know about the situation and do they check on you? If the answer is no, trust is eroded. We are supposed to care about those who are part of our workplace relationships. When trust erodes, influence, intimacy, and relationships also erode. If this continues in a downward spiral, organizations fail from lack of collaboration, understanding, and effective problem solving, those things which are most closely related to success.

Trust is also a major issue among newly formed teams and their members. One of the first questions to come up when joining a team is whom can you trust or not trust. Team members model trust through behaviors such as facilitating the establishment of ground rules and agreements by which the team will function and hold team members accountable. Trust is probably the most delicate aspect within relationships and is influenced far more by actions than by words. Therefore, what people do is more powerful than what they say. Trust is a fragile thread that can be severed by one act. Once destroyed, trust is more difficult to reestablish than it was to create initially.

Accepting and Celebrating Differences

Every human being is different, with different backgrounds, different races and ethnicities, different skill sets, different strengths, and different approaches. Yet, it is not unusual for us to assume that team members are like us. Other team members must understand us and can even see or appreciate our "point of view." If we go into the situation with the awareness that not everyone is like us, we can reach out to other team members. We can always build from one connection to other connections. Appreciating differences may help us capitalize on talents we do not possess or value a behavior or situation from a different perspective. We should celebrate the fact that we may complement each other.

Giving and Receiving Feedback

Feedback is like plant food; it allows human beings to learn and to grow. Feedback may not always feel great, but it can be very good for you. Many of us are more anxious about receiving feedback than about giving feedback. It is very helpful to attempt to listen to feedback with an openness and to clarify anything that might be unclear. Assume the best of intentions. Work not to be defensive but rather to search for the pearl—the grain of truth that can support your learning and growing. Any information received can be accepted and incorporated or rejected. It just might be information about a "blind spot" that you may have never seen. When giving feedback, focus on how you would like to receive it. Remember to ask questions and to focus on growth. Tonality and how something is said is of premier importance.

EXERCISE 16.8 Think about the last team project in which you participated. What worked about the team? What did not work about the team? Were there members who did not carry their share of the work? Was there a team member who was a "know it all"? How did you handle the situation? Was there a person on the team who took the lead? How many of the qualities of a good team player do you possess? Be honest. What are areas in which you could improve? What are your strengths, that is, where do you shine?

INTERPROFESSIONAL TEAMS

Interprofessional teams are essential to providing quality person-centered care, as the Research Perspective illustrates (Dwiel, Weilnau, Hunt, Phillips, & Sullivan, 2019). Nurses, physicians, dietitians, social workers, case managers, pharmacists, and physical therapists, to name a few, must work together to achieve

cost-effective care while providing the highest quality of care in the healthcare setting. Nurses who are committed to quality care delivery in a true partnership approach have an effective communication style that conveys this team spirit. This means that efforts must be made to understand the various roles and backgrounds of each profession and to convey competently what nurses' roles and responsibilities are. At the same time, nurses are frequently leading teams comprising licensed practical/licensed vocational nurses and technicians or assistants of various kinds. Here, again, it is critical to understand everyone's role and job description as well as each person's background and identity. In addition, the collaboration needed in interprofessional teams cannot be created without mutual trust and respect among the members (Baird et al., 2019).

Core competencies for interprofessional collaborative practice were developed in 2016 by an expert panel of the Interprofessional Education Collaborative, consisting of the following groups: the American Association of Colleges of Nursing, American Association of Colleges of Osteopathic Medicine, American Association of Colleges of Pharmacy, American Dental Education Association, Association of American Medical Colleges, and the Association of Schools of Public Health.

The identified competency domains include the following: Values/Ethics for Interprofessional Practice, Roles/Responsibilities, Interprofessional Communication, and Teams and Teamwork (Interprofessional Education Collaborative [IPEC], 2016).

The Teams and Teamwork competency includes the following aspects of team functioning (IPEC, 2016):

- Describe the process of team development and the roles and practices of effective teams.
- Engage other health professionals—appropriate to the specific care situation—in shared patient-centered problem solving.
- Integrate the knowledge and experience of other professions to inform care decisions.
- Apply leadership practices that support collaborative practice and team effectiveness.
- Engage self and others to constructively manage disagreements about values, roles, goals, and actions among healthcare professionals and with patients and families.
- Share accountability with other professions, patients, and communities for outcomes.
- Reflect on individual and team performance for individual as well as team performance improvement.

RESEARCH PERSPECTIVE

Resource: Dwiel, K., Weilnau, T., Hunt, L., Phillips, R., & Sullivan, E. (2019). Building improvement capacity to create strong, effective primary care teams in community health centers. *The Joint Commission Journal on Quality and Patient Safety, 45*(12), 838–840,

The authors describe a multidisciplinary project funded by the Health Resources and Services Administration (HRSA) that taught team-based approaches focused on improving patient and provider experiences. These efforts were focused on 18 community health centers (CHCs) and partnered with the Massachusetts League of Community Health Centers to expand the knowledge of providers and clinic personnel to improve the quality of team-based ambulatory care using the patient-centered medical home (PCMH) model. The purpose of the project was to employ Advancing Teams in Community Health programs (ATPs), equipping these CHC teams with quality improvement (QI) tools and effective teaming skills using the Agency for Healthcare Research and Quality (AHRQ) TeamSTEPPS program. This was a 10-month program creating strong and effective interprofessional teams that would execute improvements aligned with the needs of the CHCs. These teams comprised CHC staff and students and included a three-day in-person learning session, eight webinars, and two coaching site visits with the practice improvement coaches who specialized in QI for primary care practice transformation. Optional coaching was available via phone and email. The curriculum established a shared understanding of the evidence for team-based care, principles of effective team structures and management, communication strategies, and QI processes.

The project leaders used the Patient-Centered Medical Home Assessment (PCMH-A) tool to measure the teams' improvement over the 10-month period. The assessments were completed at the beginning and end of the project. The tool asked teams to rate their performance on 33 areas associated with the eight change concepts: care coordination, enhanced access, patient-centered interactions, organized evidence-based care, continuous and team-based healing relationships, empanelment, quality improvement strategy, and engaged leadership. Even a relatively short program focused on forming multidisciplinary teams with strong QI skills can demonstrate positive perceptions of team improvement in these eight concepts. The outcomes suggest sustainable skill building at the individual level and improvement in the care that patients received from the team.

Implications for Practice

This project demonstrated improvements in the team relationships, goals, and interactions with patients. Ambulatory care has been ignored for decades—it is powerful to see team building and quality care for patients improve with these interventions. Interprofessional teams may function a bit differently in ambulatory settings but can still be pivotal in increasing the quality of patient care.

- Use process improvement strategies to increase the effectiveness of interprofessional teamwork and team-based care.
- Use available evidence to inform effective teamwork and team-based practices.

This work begins with education and transitions to practice and is the wave of the future, even though some practitioners are resistant to adapting traditional roles and responsibilities.

Several additional aspects of interprofessional work are crucial to creating and maintaining these teams. O'Conner (2019) identifies five benefits to this collaboration, which begins with improved patient care and outcomes. When the team works together, each member brings unique perspectives and valuable insights about the patient. Due to these different perspectives, each specialty can notice different symptoms and consider different possibilities and, when amalgamated, create a more comprehensive, holistic view of the patient. These perspectives are shared in collaborative patient rounds or in "team" meetings. Second, this collaboration can reduce medical errors. As discussed previously, communication breakdowns can have costly consequences that range from missed symptoms to misdiagnoses and medication errors or even death. Collaborative team care can catch such errors and avoid complications. Third, treatment can be expedited by collaboration that decreases the healthcare waiting game, such as physicians waiting for specialist consultations or laboratory results. The Joint Commission has identified improved staff communication and acquisition of important test results as a National Patient Safety Goal. Fourth, collaboration can reduce inefficiencies and healthcare costs by improving the patient experience (and, thus, the Hospital Consumer Assessment of Healthcare Providers and Systems) and by delivering improved patient outcomes such as reduction in falls, decreased length of stay, and increased discharges prior to noon (to facilitate admissions). Last, staff relationships and job satisfaction can be improved through leveling the "playing field" and acknowledging each profession's vital role on the care team, providing a sense of team camaraderie. This can increase staff retention, as many nurses stay at facilities where they are liked and respected as important team members.

EXERCISE 16.9 Identify a problem that you have heard discussed in a healthcare setting—for example, awkward timing of admissions and discharges, running out of supplies, or conflicts in scheduling procedures. Make a list of all of the different professions and support staff who might be involved with that issue in some way and who would need a voice during efforts to improve the situation.

THE VALUE OF TEAM BUILDING

When things are not going well in an organization and problems need to be resolved, the first intervention people think of is "team building." Naturally, for teams (a collection of people relying on each other) to be effective, they must function smoothly and communicate effectively to create the best possible work environment. The problem is that when organizations are facing difficulties, they generally do not have teams whose members function well together. Team building and consultants can help; however, to sustain smoothly functioning teams, leadership is critical.

Regardless of the problem, appropriate assessment of the team is essential (see Exercise 16.1). The success of the team depends on its members and its leadership. Providing feedback in a manner in which it can be heard and growing the team creates value in the team.

A resurgence in team building has occurred. Corporations are once again focused on the importance of teams. Mojica (2019) believes that team building activities are particularly vital to the success of small businesses, and most nursing units or clinics are essentially a small business. Vogt (2017) demonstrates that team-building exercises can build trust, ease conflicts, increase collaboration, and increase the effectiveness of communication. She further believes that increasing mutual trust through team-building activities can increase the codependence on one another in the team, thus, increasing the efficiency and the productivity. Team building can ease conflicts by supporting team members to know each other better on a personal level, to bond with one another, and to become more comfortable with each other's personalities. Team-building activities can increase collaboration among the team members and increase their awareness of interdependency.

Lencioni (2020) builds a strong case for dealing constructively with building an underlying foundation for teams. He believes that three major components of smoothly functioning teams must be created:
- Mutual trust among the members
- A strong sense of team identity (that the team is unique and worthwhile)
- A sense of team efficacy (that the team performs well and its members are synergistic in their manner of working together)

At the heart of these components are the emotions we often work so hard to keep out of the workplace. However, as human beings, we function the same way in both our work and personal lives. Mutual trust can be developed only when each team member tells the truth about feelings, thoughts, and wants and listens and supports other members of the team to do likewise. We all yearn to be a part of something bigger than ourselves—to do something important that makes a difference. Well-functioning teams allow this to happen (Fig. 16.2). Developing such teams can increase nursing job satisfaction and group cohesiveness, decrease nurse turnover rates, and promote patient safety and quality outcomes.

Understandable anxiety exists concerning the safety of being vulnerable and exposed if personal issues are revealed. That is why it is helpful for a team-building facilitator to make a thorough assessment of major issues and the willingness on the part of members to work on issues. One approach is to interview members of the team individually to discover the critical issues. The types of questions that might be asked, found in Box 16.6, provide some sense of the major issues within the team so that the facilitator has a better understanding of how to work with its members.

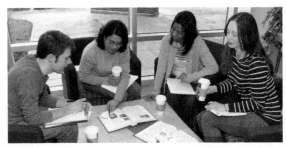

Fig. 16.2 Teams can form strong relationships external to the work environment.

BOX 16.6   **Interview Questions for Team Building**

1. What do you see as the problems currently facing your team?
2. What are the current strengths of your institution or work group? What are you currently doing well?
3. Does your boss do anything that prevents you from being as effective as you would like to be?
4. Does anybody else in this group do anything that prevents you from being as effective as you would like to be?
5. What would you like to accomplish at your upcoming team-building session? What changes would you be willing to make that would facilitate a smoother-functioning team and accomplishment of the team goals?

Because people spend such a large percentage of their time in the work setting, it would be unrealistic to believe that they are continually in an unemotional and controlled state. Human beings simply do not function that way. What is observed are people's aspirations, their achievements, their hopes, and their social consciousness. They are observed falling in love; falling in hate and anger; winning and losing; and being excited, sad, fearful, anxious, and jealous. Consequently, these feelings are important components of organizational life and can undermine work effectiveness. Most of us know of situations in which, because of an emotional disagreement, two individuals have avoided each other for years. Because of the power of emotions and the inevitability of their presence, their effect on interpersonal relationships and their influence on productivity, quality of work, and safety of patients, emotions should be a high priority when examining the functioning of the team. Fortunately, research addresses the importance of emphasizing the "emotional intelligence" of individuals when working in teams in the classic work by Goleman (2011). Those teams that address these issues are much more successful and create a more positive work environment than those that do not.

Suppressing emotions at work is neither healthy nor constructive for team members. When emotions are handled appropriately within the team, several positive outcomes are possible for the work setting. One creates a sense of internal comfort with the workings of the team and the organization. When stress is lowered and kept at lower levels, on average, problems are much more easily resolved. This phenomenon is similar to releasing steam slowly with a steam valve rather than having the gasket blow. Interpersonal relationships on the team are more stable, and people have a sense of closer ties and collegiality when emotions are addressed. Fewer negative relationships or interactions develop, which results in more effective and pleasant working relationships all around.

Work group effectiveness improves when the team is functioning smoothly and emotions and feelings are being addressed on a routine basis rather than waiting for a volcanic eruption. The daily routines of frustration and boredom and retreat from the group are likely to undo a team. People who are engaged and have leaders who help them achieve goals are more effective. The skills and tools previously discussed (e.g., speaking supportively) are the basic tools one needs to handle the emotional aspects of the team. Coping with emotional upset must be a conscious choice, one that requires practice to improve the skill.

THE ROLE OF LEADERSHIP

Teams usually have a leader. In addition, teams function within large organizations that have leaders. Team building, which can be a costly endeavor in terms of consultation fees as well as work time and team resources, is difficult to undertake and of questionable effectiveness without the approval and support of the leader. Although very strong teams may be able to educate themselves regarding some issues, such as establishing goals and priorities or clarifying their own team process, addressing any kind of relationship issue among team members without a more objective outside party or skilled leader facilitating the process is exceedingly difficult.

Because leadership is such a pivotal part of smoothly functioning teams, it is illuminating to examine leaders more carefully. Truly progressive leaders understand that leadership and followership are not necessarily a set of skills or role-playing; rather, these are qualities of character. Leadership and followership is as much about character and development as it is about education. Leaders realize their capacity for influence, risk taking, and decision-making more fully. Team building is a natural outgrowth. This type of leader understands that the best in a person is tied intimately to the individual's deepest sense of self—to one's spirit (Yoder-Wise et al., 2020). The efforts of leaders must touch the spiritual aspect in themselves and others. The same could be said for skillful followers. Warren Bennis (2009) once said that leaders simply care about more people. Consequently, this caring manifests itself in doing whatever it takes to improve team functioning. This may imply involving oneself in team building with the team. The risk in such an endeavor is that the team leader is open to being vulnerable, to being judged by others, and to being wrong. However, if the leader has been a role model for the team agreement and has held people accountable to these statements, the team-building exercise will not degenerate into judging and placing blame.

If true leadership is about character development as much as anything, then character development is also beneficial for followers—that is, members of the team. The areas of character development often addressed include communication, particularly those aspects of speaking supportively that enhance understanding the other person's message while avoiding placing blame and justifying. Box 16.7 highlights an example of character development from personal experience, the concept of self-confidence.

BOX 16.7   The "Can Do" Brigade: An Army Nurse's Study in Character Development

As life events are reviewed, important or pivotal learning can be identified. One life event that significantly affected me was the year I spent as an Army Nurse Corps officer in South Vietnam. This was the first time I remember an awareness and understanding of confidence in the face of incredible obstacles. I had spent the first 10 months of my nursing career in labor and delivery at Indiana University before volunteering for a guaranteed assignment to Vietnam. I went to Fort Sam Houston for 6 weeks of basic training, where they taught me really important things like how to salute, how to march, and how many men are in a battalion. No one ever asked me if I could start an IV or draw a tube of blood. This was important because Indiana University had the largest medical school class in the United States at that time and nurses did nothing that interfered with medical education. Therefore I had never started an IV or drawn blood. When I arrived in Saigon, they put me in a sedan with another nurse and sent me up to the Third Surgical Hospital, one not unlike the one in *M*A*S*H*. We even had a Major Burns—that was not his name but it was his function. Surgical hospitals receive only battle casualties; their purpose is to stabilize and to transport.

The Third Surgical Hospital was located in the middle of the 173rd Airborne Brigade, whose job it was to defend the Bien Hoa Air Base, where all the sorties in the south were flown during the war. We were stopped at the gate by an MP who stepped up and saluted very snappily. He knew that a staff car must contain either a very-high-ranking officer or, if it was his lucky day, females.

When I was in Vietnam, 500 American women and 500,000 American men were there. The MP looked in the window, saluted snappily, and said "Afternoon, ma'am!" He wanted to know where we were going; he talked to us for a few minutes and assured us that if there was anything he could do for us, we should just give him a call. He saluted us and said, "can do." I didn't understand because I did not know that there are units with very high esprit de corps who attach snappy little sayings at the end of things like salutes, phone conversations, memos, and so forth. The 173rd was the "can do" brigade.

When we got to the hospital and met the chief nurse, she took us down to the mess hall and introduced us to all the doctors and nurses. We were sitting and having coffee when the field phone rang in the kitchen and the mess sergeant yelled out, "Incoming wounded." Everybody got up and started to leave for the preop area. I just sat there until the chief nurse said, "Come on." I said, "You don't understand, I deliver babies." She was not impressed! She took me by the arm and led me to preop.

When we got there, we discovered there were not just a few incoming wounded, there were more than 30, and some were very seriously injured. She immediately told the sergeant to call headquarters battalion of the 173rd Airborne and tell them that the Third Surg needed blood. She turned to me and said, "Lieutenant, you are responsible for drawing 50 units of fresh whole blood." I was shocked! I had never drawn a tube of blood, but I found in the back section of preop a Specialist 4th class who was already setting up "saw horses" and stretchers, putting up IV poles, and hanging plastic blood sets. I started to help, and soon I heard trucks out back. I opened the door and looked outside. There were two huge Army trucks, and kids—17, 18, 19, and 20 years old—were jumping out. They were covered with red mud from the bottom of their boots to the tops of their helmets. I looked at them, and I looked at the clean cement floor, and in an instant, my mother came to me. I put my hand on my hip and said, "Where have you boys been?" One PFC stepped forward and saluted me very snappily and said, "Ma'am, we just came in this afternoon from 30 days in the field, we have been out in the rice paddies chasing the Viet Cong, we have not had a hot meal, and we've not had a shower, but Sergeant Major said the Third Surg needs blood!" He saluted smartly and said, "can do!" They were very clear. After 30 days of chasing and being chased by the Viet Cong, giving a unit of blood was easy. "Can do!" They were confident. They were kids who had looked into the face of death. At that moment, I knew if they *can do*, I Can Do! Life requires confidence. With confidence, you can make your dreams come true!

Confidence, which loosely translates as faith or belief that one will act in a correct and effective way, is a key aspect of character. Thus, it follows that confidence in oneself can be closely tied to self-esteem, which is satisfaction with oneself. The greatest deterrent to self-esteem and self-confidence is fear. Fear is described by some as "false evidence appearing real." Working on self-confidence requires an attitude of belief, of confidence, of I "*can do*" whatever is required.

```
False
Evidence
Appearing
Real
```

Leading the team is clearly not the easiest thing to do, but neither is being an active, fully participating member of the team. Both require taking risks, including being in a relationship. Being in a team-building experience and hearing those things that have not worked for people in their interactions with peers and the leader can be scary but worthwhile. It requires a focus on personal and professional growth. It requires building character.

CONCLUSION

Whether a nurse is a leader, manager, or member of the team, effective performance requires commitment to the group. Forging new relationships and strengthening old ones are typically facilitated by deliberate actions ranging from creating clarity of purpose through holding each other accountable.

THE SOLUTION

The first question that needed to be asked was, "Were we committed to providing the most optimal care for the neonate?" In other words, why would teamwork be important in this situation? What's the vision or mission? After achieving agreement among the NICU team, we strategized on how to create a "team" with the specialists. Making our intent clear was very important. A meeting with the director of the specialty team, the NICU medical director, and nursing leadership was arranged. We discovered that we shared a common goal: to provide the best care possible for the baby. Keeping that goal as the focus, we then identified areas of mutual respect. From there, both sides were willing to listen to each other's concerns. Care guidelines could be identified, as well as areas of responsibility. Ideas on how to improve the communication process were also discussed. A plan based on patient needs, complete with agreements, was implemented.

Were we a team yet? The answer is "no." There was still a little skepticism and reserve. Everyone seemed to have a "wait-and-see" attitude. The first big chance was identified when the specialty group insisted that a patient of theirs be admitted to the NICU because they believed it was the best place for the baby to be. Another measurable outcome was having the agreements honored. This reinforced to everyone that his or her concerns had been heard and respected. Mutual trust was building, and a collegial relationship began. A year later, it is hard to imagine that this situation ever occurred. There is enthusiasm for this specialty's physicians and their patients. It is certainly a change in attitude.

There are many components to team building, but the most important component is to be clear about your mission and intentions and to be clear in communication when working with potential team members. The intention to provide the best care possible assisted each one of us to be more open, creative, and trusting. These are all necessary components of team building. Remember, teams are made up of individuals. Ask yourself if you are willing to accept responsibility for your response and actions. Be the change that you want to see.

Would this be a suitable approach for you? Why?

Diane Gallagher

▮ REFLECTIONS

Consider the following questions, then write a one-paragraph summary. When could you have been more effective as a team member or group leader recently?

What personal behavior could you improve in your next group or team experience?

BEST PRACTICES

For teams to function at their best, they need to communicate effectively and to build valued relatlionships. They must care about each other and the team's purpose or mission. They are considerate of each other and fulfill their commitments to each other and the team. They tell the truth and acknowledge good work and innovative ideas. They support each other through successes and challenges.

TIPS FOR TEAM BUILDING

- Commit to the purpose of the team.
- Develop team relationships of mutual respect.
- Communicate effectively, and listen actively.
- Create and adhere to team agreements concerning function and process.
- Build trust.

REFERENCES

Albert, N., Pappas, S., Porter-O'Grady, T., & Malloch, K. (2021). *Quantum leadership: Creating sustainable value in healthcare.* Burlington, MA: Jones and Bartlett Learning.

American Association of Critical Care Nurses (ACCN). (2016). *AACN standards for establishing and fostering healthy work environments.* Retrieved from https://www.aacn.org/nursing-excellence/standards/aacn-standards-for-establishing-and-sustaining-healthy-work-environments.

Baird, J., Ashland, M., & Rosenbluth, G. (2019). Interprofessional teams: Current trends and future directions. *Pediatric Clinics of North America, 66*(4), 739–750.

Bennis, W. (2009). *On becoming a leader.* Reading, MA: Addison-Wesley.

Business Wire. (2021). New Press Ganey findings show healthcare safety scores fell amid the pandemic. Retrieved from https://www.businesswire.com/news/home/20211021005658/en/New-Press-Ganey-Findings-Show-Healthcare-Safety-Scores-Fell-Amid-the-Pandemic#.YXKXVH8aZRE.linkedin.

Civico A. (2019) How to manage conflict in the workplace. *Psychology Today.* Retrieved from https://www.psychology-today.com/us/blog/turning-point/201902/how-manage-conflict-in-the-workplace.

Dwiel, K., Weilnau, T., Hunt, L., Phillips, R., & Sullivan, E. (2019). Building improvement capacity to create strong, effective primary care teams in community health centers. *The Joint Commission Journal on Quality and Patient Safety, 45*(12), 838–840.

Eventus Training & Events. (2013). [Effective vs ineffective teams.] Retrieved from www.eventus.co.uk/effective-vs-ineffective-teams/.

Farnsworth, J., Clark, L., Becton, C., Wysocki, A., & Kepne, K. (2022). Building teamwork and the importance of trust in a business environment. https://edis.ifas.ufl.edu/pdf%5CHR%5CHR01800.pdf. Retrieved June 6, 2022.

Fontes, A. (2020). *The power of acknowledgement.* Retrieved from https://www.pmi.com/our-transformation/voices-of-change/power-of-acknowledgement/.

Gallup. (2020). *What is employee engagement and how do you improve it?* Retrieved from www.Gallup.com/workplace/285674/improve-employee-engagement-workplace.aspx.

Garfield, C. (2021). Peak performance and organizational transformation: An interview with Charles Garfield. www.education.edu/ir/library/html/erm/erm9958.html. Retrieved on 9 June, 2022.

Goleman, D. (2011). *The brain and emotional intelligence: New insights.* Northampton, MA: More Than Sound.

International Nursing Association for Clinical Simulation and Learning (INACSL) Standards Committee, Decker, S., Alinier, G., Crawford, S. B., Gordon, R. M., Jenkins, D., & Wilson, C. (2021). Healthcare Simulation Standards of Best Practice™: The Debriefing Process. *Clinical Simulation in Nursing, 58*(2021), 27–32.

Interprofessional Education Collaborative Expert Panel (IPEC). (2016). *Core competencies for interprofessional collaborative practice: 2016 update.* Washington, DC: Interprofessional Education Collaborative.

Kowalski, K., & Yoder-Wise, P. S. (2003). Five Cs of leadership. *Nurse Leader, 1*(5), 26–31.

LaFasto, F., & Larson, C. (2001). *When Teams Work Best: 6000 Team members and leaders tell what it takes to succeed.* Thousand Oaks, CA: Sage Publishing.

Lencioni, P. (2020). *Motive: Why so many leaders abdicate the most important responsibility.* Hoboken, NJ: John Wiley & Sons, Inc.

Maxfield, D., Grenny, J., McMillan, R., Patterson, K., & Switzler, A. (2005). Silence kills: The seven crucial conversations for healthcare. https://psnet.ahrq.gov/issue/silence-kills-seven-crucial-conversations-healthcare. Retrieved on 7 June, 2022.

McGregor, D. (1960). *The human side of enterprise*. New York: McGraw-Hill.

Medland, J. (2020). Leveraging email to build healthy effective teams. *Nurse Leader*, *19*(2), 40–46.

Mojica, M. (2019). *Why team building is important for your business*. Retrieved from https://complianceandethics.org/why-team-building-is-important-for-your-business/.

O'Brien, D., Main, A., Kounkel, S., & Stephen, A. (2019). *Purpose is everything: How brands that authentically lead with purpose are changing the nature of business today*. https://www2.deloitte.com/us/en/insights/topics/marketing-and-sales-operations/global-marketing-trends/2020/purpose-driven-companies.html.

O'Conner, W. (2019). *5 Benefits of interprofessional collaboration in healthcare*. Retrieved from https://tigerconnect.com/blog/5-benefits-of-interprofessional-collaboration-in-healthcare/.

Rath, T. (2007). *Strengths finder 2.0*. New York: Gallup Press.

Ready Training On-Line. (2021). *Mission possible*. Retrieved from https://readytrainingonline.com/articles/team-mission/.

Surbhi, S. (2018). *Difference between group and team*. Retrieved from https://keydifferences.com/difference-between-group-and-team.html.

Tanner, R. (2020). *Understanding and Managing the 4 Generations in the Workplace*. Retrieved from https://managementisajourney.com/understanding-and-managing-the-4-generations-in-the-workplace.

Thagard, P. (2019). *Treatise on Mind and Society*. Oxford, UK: Oxford University Press.

Tuckman, B. (1965). Developmental sequence in small groups. *Psychological Bulletin*, *63*, 384–399.

Vogt, C. (2017). Importance of team-building activities. www.linked-in.com/pulse/importance-team-building-activities-crystal-vogt-ranaivomanana. Retrieved on 8 June, 2022.

Warrell, M. (2020). *The life-changing power of trusting yourself*. Melbourne, Australia: John Wiley & Sons.

Yoder-Wise, P., Kowalski, K., & Sportsman, S. (2020). *The leadership trajectory: Developing legacy leaders-ship*. St. Louis, MO: Elsevier.

CASE STUDY 16.1   NEXT-GENERATION NCLEX® CASE STUDY

Next-Generation NCLEX® case studies are included in select chapters to familiarize you with these new testing items for the NGN exam.

Question 1

Learning Outcomes:

Develop actions to address conflict among staff, evaluating the results of these interventions.

Cognitive Skills:

Recognize cues, analyze cues, generate solutions, take action, and evaluate outcomes.

Two unlicensed assistive personnel (UAP) are working on a unit. One of the UAPs has been working in the facility for 10 years but has just transferred to the unit. The transfer was the result of several negative annual personnel evaluations addressing the UAP's difficulty in establishing a good relationship with colleagues. The second UAP has recently moved to the area but has experience as a UAP in a hospital in another city.

The two UAPs have been assigned to the same shift in the unit for the last two months. They initially worked well together but seemed to develop an animosity to each other after both were caring for an extremely ill patient who developed a preference for the second UAP. In recent weeks, they have had several confrontations about who is responsible for various tasks on the unit or which approach toward clients was most appropriate. On three occasions, they have been seen having an intense argument in public spaces.

The nurse manager of the unit knows she must do something to address this conflict. Complete the diagram below by specifying which condition is most likely present in the unit, two actions the nurse manager should take to address that condition, and two parameters the nurse manager should monitor to determine the effectiveness of her interventions.

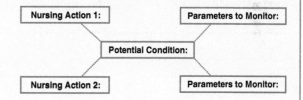

Nursing Action	Potential Condition	Parameters to Monitor
a. Assess the interdependence of both UAPs having the conflict.	a. Jealousy of UAP 2 by UAP 1.	a. Evaluate the UAP's response to nurse manager's assessment of the conflict.
b. Reprimand both UAPs.	b. Arrogant behavior by UAP 2.	b. Assessing the perceptions of members of the team about the UAP's behavior.
c. Fire the UAP who is most at fault for causing the conflict.	c. Dissatisfaction of many of the unit staff.	c. Assessment of the behavior of both UAPs one month after the nurse manager's conference with both UAPs.
d. Discuss expectations with each UAP in individual conferences with the Nurse Manager.	d. Conflict between the UAPs on one of the staff teams.	d. Reviewing each UAP's behavior during their annual evaluation one year from now.
e. Teach conflict resolution to staff on the unit.		e. Remove one of the UAPs from the unit.

(Continued)

CASE STUDY 16.1   NEXT-GENERATION NCLEX® CASE STUDY—CONT'D

Question 2

Learning Outcomes:

Using the Interdisciplinary Team Core Competencies for Collaborative Practice, evaluate the effectiveness of the various team interactions.

Cognitive Skill:

Evaluate Outcomes

A nurse leader is responsible for evaluating the effectiveness of the interprofessional teams in her organization, using the Interdisciplinary Team Core Competencies for Collaborative Practice. Which of the following situations reflect such practice?

Select all that apply.

a. The psychiatrist, nurse, social worker, and a representative of other therapies in a behavioral healthcare facility meet weekly to discuss a patient's care.

b. The nurse manager of an oncology unit indicating that because of staff shortages, unit nurses will no longer participate in team meetings until further notice.

c. Following a negative outcome of a client in a long-term care (LTC) facility, the team implemented a review of the client's record.

d. A member of a team in an acute care setting brings several research articles supporting a novel approach to caring for clients typically on the unit. The senior members of the team reject the recommendation for a resulting change without discussion.

e. Following a disagreement regarding care, the team leader said, "Let us take a breath—then adjourn and see if we can find evidence to support the various positions. We can then reconvene to discuss."

f. After ongoing arguments about the process of team functioning, the leader of the team disbands it, indicating that he will appoint new members of the team.

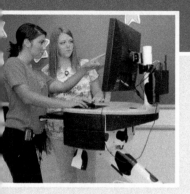

17

The Impact of Technology

Joan Benson, Kathryn Hansen, and Jenny Horn

ANTICIPATED LEARNING OUTCOMES

- Examine various technologies and how they can play a role in impacting patient safety.
- Provide definitions for the core components of informatics: data, information, and knowledge.
- Compare and contrast the different types of technology for capturing data at the point of care.

- Apply how decision support systems have impacted patient care in your lived experience.
- Explore the issues of patient safety, ethics, and information security and privacy within information technology.

KEY TERMS

bar-code technology
big data
biomedical technology
clinical decision support
clinical decision support systems
communication technology
computerized provider order
    entry (CPOE)
dashboard
data

data analytics
database
electronic health record (EHR)
electronic medical record (EMR)
informatics
information
information technology
innovation
knowledge technology
knowledge worker

Point of care or bedside
    technology
Quality and Safety Education for
    Nurses (QSEN)
real-time
smart card
smart technology
speech recognition (SR)
telehealth
wearable technology

THE CHALLENGE

In 2008, clinical and information systems teams collaborated to implement a "big bang" electronic health record (EHR) project that impacted workflows and documentation for pharmacy, laboratory, allied health, medicine, and nursing. Over the years, data elements have been added to the EHR to meet regulatory, accrediting, and other requirements, contributing to increased nursing documentation burden and decreased satisfaction. Questions to consider when EHR documentation updates are needed for us to support healthcare and

(Continued)

371

INTRODUCTION

Technology continues to be an integral part of patient care delivery in the hospital, ambulatory, and home environments. Intravenous pumps, biomedical monitoring, phones, and wearables are just some of the ways technology has become smarter, with the ability to monitor patients in critical, noncritical, and remote settings. New nurses entering the profession may be part of the generation that hasn't been exposed to anything before the Internet, cell phones, social media, clinical information systems (IS), applications, and technologies. Healthcare is a technology and an information-intensive business. Therefore, the success of nurses using biomedical technology, information technology (IT), and knowledge technology contributes to patient care delivery, outcomes, and clinician experience and efficiencies.

Competency in informatics and healthcare technology is required for nurses in today's healthcare environment. The new American Association of Colleges of Nursing (AACN) Baccalaureate *Essentials* (2021) has devoted an entire competency domain to this topic. The *Essentials* describe competence in informatics and healthcare technology as the "use of information and communication technologies and informatics processes to provide care, gather data, form information to drive decision making, and support professionals as they expand knowledge and wisdom for practice. Informatics processes and technologies are used to manage and improve the delivery of safe, high-quality, and efficient healthcare services in accordance with best practice and professional and regulatory standards" (AACN, 2021).

Quality and Safety Education for Nurses (QSEN) has also identified informatics competency as a necessary component of the knowledge, skills, and attitudes necessary to continuously improve the quality and safety of health care (QSEN, 2021). Nurses use data and information daily from technology for decision-making, communication, and delivery of care that is outcomes driven. Focusing on the use of technology for patient care is essential as nurses, IT team members, and leadership collaborate to ensure that nurses have the right technology to support the right care at the right time for the right patient outcomes.

The TIGER Initiative, an acronym for *T*echnology *I*nformatics *G*uiding *E*ducation *R*eform, was formed in 2004 as an effort to bring together nursing stakeholders to develop a shared vision, strategies, and specific actions for improving nursing practice, education, and the delivery of patient care using health information technology. The TIGER Informatics Competencies Collaborative (TICC) team developed informatics recommendations for all practicing nurses and graduating nursing students that are embedded within the AACN Baccalaureate Essentials and the QSEN informatics competencies. The TIGER Nursing Informatics Competencies Model includes the following three parts:

1. Basic computer competencies
2. Information literacy
3. Information management (American Nurses Association [ANA], 2015)

Nurses are knowledge workers who need data and information to provide effective, efficient, safe patient care. According to the ANA *Nursing Informatics: Practice Scope and Standards of Practice,* "knowledge is information that is synthesized so that relationships are identified and formalized" (2015, p. 2). Data and information must be accurate, reliable, and presented in an actionable form. Technology can facilitate and extend nurses' decision-making abilities and support nurses in numerous ways, including creating a clinical data pool for the conduct of research.

TYPES OF TECHNOLOGIES

As nurses, we use, manage, and rely on technology to care for patients. When properly developed and applied, technology can enhance the healthcare team's ability to collect, manage, share data and information to achieve desired outcomes (ANA, 2015). The report by the Institute of Medicine (IOM, now the National Academy of Medicine), *Health IT and Patient Safety: Building Safer Systems for Better Care* (IOM, 2012) suggests that health information technology (HIT) can promote safe and quality care that is delivered effectively and efficiently with improved communication and decreased costs. With the ongoing healthcare landscape changes and complexities, technology will continue to evolve, advance, and revolutionize patient care delivery and outcomes.

Nurses interact with many different types of technology at the bedside and beyond. Point of care or bedside technology includes biomedical technologies with computer terminal access to patient data and biometric measures from physiologic monitoring and testing. Smart technology enables linking of the right data and information at the right time from various systems and interfaces. Wearable technology promotes chronic condition monitoring and tracking within the patient's home and nonclinical environments. Information technology and knowledge technology make up the infrastructure to acquire, review, integrate, and use data and information from applications and devices for knowledge to make patient care decisions.

Point of Care and Smart Technology

Biomedical technology at the bedside is used for (1) physiologic monitoring, (2) diagnostic testing, (3) intravenous fluid and medication dispensing and administration, and (4) therapeutic treatments. Physiologic monitoring systems measure heart rate, blood pressure, and other vital signs. They also monitor cardiac rhythm; measure and record central venous, pulmonary wedge, intracranial, and intraabdominal pressures; and analyze oxygen and carbon dioxide levels in the blood. Analysis of adverse events in hospitalized patients have indicated that many physiologic abnormalities are not detected early enough to prevent the event, even when some of the abnormalities are present for hours before the event occurs (Munroe et al., 2020). As bedside devices and monitoring systems have become smarter, data can be pushed to the care team via alerts within the EHR.

Patient surveillance systems are designed to provide early warning of a possible impending adverse event. One example is a system that provides wireless monitoring of heart rate, respiratory rate, and attempts by a patient "at risk for falling" to get out of bed unassisted. Smart beds can initiate alarms based on patient movement to help minimize patient falls. They can minimize other complications as well; for example, pressure sores can be prevented with a bed that has the ability to turn patients.

Innovative technology permits physiologic monitoring and patient surveillance by expert clinicians who may be distant from the patient. The remote or virtual intensive care unit (vICU) is staffed by a dedicated team of experienced critical care nurses, physicians, and pharmacists who use state-of-the-art technology to leverage their expertise and knowledge over a large group of patients in multiple intensive care units (Williams et al., 2019).

Diagnostic Testing

Dysrhythmia monitoring systems can also be used for diagnostic testing. The computer, after processing and analyzing the ECG, generates a report that is confirmed by a trained professional. ECG tracings can be transmitted from remote sites, such as the patient's home, to the physician's office or clinic. Patients with implantable pacemakers can have their cardiac activity monitored without leaving home.

Other systems for diagnostic testing include blood gas analyzers, pulmonary function systems, and ICP monitors. Laboratory medicine is virtually all automated with information systems that receive, schedule, and track specimen tests and collections. In addition, point-of-care testing devices extend the laboratory's testing capabilities to the patient's bedside or care area. Test result values can display result values, ranges, and trends. An alert to the appropriate clinician can be pushed when values are critical or outside the normal range for the patient. Point-of-care blood glucose monitors can download results of bedside testing into an automated laboratory results system and the patient's electronic record. Results can be communicated quickly and trends can be analyzed throughout patients' hospital stays and ongoing at ambulatory or home care visits. The necessary insulin doses based on evidence for tight blood glucose control can be calculated and evoke electronic orders for administration. Data collection from patients with chronic conditions such as diabetes may be used within disease registries to help track clinical care and outcomes by promoting the integration of diagnostic test results with the appropriate orders-based intervention.

Intravenous Fluid and Medication Administration

Intravenous (IV) fluid and medication distribution and dispensing via automated dispensing cabinets (ADCs) have been a hospital staple since the 1980s when they were first introduced to enable medication storage and dispensing near the point of care. ADCs have contributed to decreased time for medication availability and administration, greater protection and tracking of medications (especially controlled substances), and improved accuracy of drug charge capture. Real-time ADC communication with the EHR allows the nurse to see patient information at the point of care to help reduce the risk of medication errors. The Institute for Safe Medication Practices (ISMP) developed guidelines and core practices for safe medication administration and ADC use that are available on the ISMP website (*www.ismp.org/resources/guidelines-safe-use-automated-dispensing-cabinets*) (ISMP, 2020).

Bar code scanning of the medication ordered by the physician, verified by the pharmacist, and obtained from the ADC helps the nurse ensure that the right medication is given to the right patient at the right time. This closed-loop medication process ensures that all members of the care team are using one single patient file and source of truth. Alerts and real-time messages may be sent electronically across systems at any point of the medication process via smart technology functionality to enhance care team communication, efficiencies, and delivery of safe patient care.

Smart technology relies on interfaces so that information can be gathered and shared across systems to support patient care. Smart IV pumps can deliver fluids, blood and blood products, and medications either continuously or intermittently at rates between 0.01 and 999 mL per hour. IV smart pumps promote safety, accuracy, advanced pressure monitoring, ease of use, and versatility. Many smart pumps can interface with the EHR as the nurse verifies the IV medication order, dose, and rate on the pump to reduce the risk of manual programming errors. The EHR can then receive smart pump data to help the nurse manage the infusion, patient's physiologic status, and interventions.

Therapeutic Treatments

Treatments may be administered via implantable infusion pumps that administer medications at a prescribed rate and can be programmed to provide boluses or change doses at set points in time. These pumps are commonly used for hormone regulation, hypertension, chronic intractable pain, diabetes, venous thrombosis, and cancer chemotherapy. Therapeutic treatment systems may be used to regulate intake and output, regulate breathing, and assist with patient care. Intake and output systems are linked to infusion pumps that control arterial pressure, drug therapy, fluid resuscitation, and serum glucose levels. These systems calculate and regulate the IV drip rate.

Increasingly sophisticated mechanical ventilators are used to deliver a prescribed percentage of oxygen and volume of air to the patient's lungs and to provide a set flow rate, inspiratory-to-expiratory time ratio, and various other complex functions with less trauma to lung tissue than was previously possible. Computer-assisted ventilators are electromechanically controlled by a closed-loop feedback system to analyze and control lung volumes and alveolar gases. Ventilators also provide sophisticated, sensitive alarm systems for patient safety.

In the newborn and intensive care nursery, computers monitor the heart and respiratory rates of babies. In addition, newborn nursery systems can regulate the temperature of the infant's environment by sensing the infant's temperature and the air of the surrounding environment. Alarms can be set to notify nurses when preset physiologic parameters are exceeded. Computerized systems monitor fetal activity before delivery, linking the ECGs of the mother and baby and the pulse oximetry, blood pressure, and respirations of the mother.

Biomedical technology affects nursing as nurses provide direct care to patients treated with new technologies: monitoring data from mobile devices, administering therapy with updated evidence-based techniques, and evaluating patients' responses to care and treatment.

Nurses must be aware of the latest technologies for monitoring patients' physiologic status, diagnostic testing, drug administration, and therapeutic treatments. Nurses need to identify the data to be collected, the information that might be gained, and the many ways that the data can be used to provide new knowledge (Fig. 17.1). More importantly, nurses must remember that biomedical technology supplements, but does not replace, the skilled observation, assessment, and evaluation of the patient.

Biomedical technology is designed to help keep patients safe and to alert staff of changes in the patient's condition. As early as 2013, a Sentinel Event Alert from The Joint Commission (TJC, 2015) brought attention

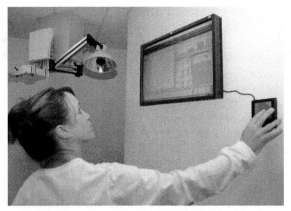

Fig. 17.1 Patient data displayed with computerized systems to provide meaningful information and trends.

to alarm fatigue or alarm desensitization from biomedical technology. The overuse of alarms from infusion pumps, feeding devices, monitors, and ventilators can cause sensory strain. Staff who are overwhelmed by the sheer number of alarms can miss or delay responding, leading to sentinel events or even patient death. Desensitization and alert fatigue have become a national problem (Phillips et al., 2020). Nursing leaders must be aware of how these technologies fit into the delivery of patient care and the strategic plan of the organization in which they work. They must have a vision for the future and be ready to suggest innovative solutions that will assist nurses across specialties and settings to improve patient care safety and quality.

EXERCISE 17.1 List the types of biomedical technology available for patient care in your organization. List ways that you currently use the data and information gathered by these systems. How do these help you care for patients? Can you think of other ways to use the technology and/or the data or information? For example, data from biomedical devices might be sent directly to the EHR, negating the need for transcription of a result into the patient's chart. Nurses spend many hours learning to use biomedical devices and to interpret the data gained from them. Have we come to rely too heavily on technology rather than on our own judgment? You might consider using your computer skills to draw a concept map to illustrate the relationships between the types of biomedical, diagnostic, therapeutic, and information technologies available in healthcare organizations you have worked in.

Wearable Technology

Continuous dysrhythmia monitors and electrocardiograms (ECGs) provide visual representation of electrical activity in the heart. They can be used for surveillance and detection of dysrhythmias and for interpretation and diagnosis of the abnormal rhythm within the hospital, ambulatory, and home settings. As these systems have grown increasingly sophisticated, integration with wireless communication technology permits new approaches to triaging alerts to nurses about cardiac rhythm abnormalities. Voice technology and integrated telemetry and nurse paging systems have enhanced our accuracy and timelines in intervening in critical patient situations. Patient access to health information and communications via a portal further promotes communication and sharing of vital data and information from in-home monitoring devices and applications. Biomedical devices for physiologic monitoring can be interfaced with clinical information system technology. Monitored vital signs and invasive pressure readings can be downloaded directly into the patient's electronic medical record, where the nurse confirms their accuracy and affirms the data entry.

Continuous glucose monitoring (CGM) can be used to monitor blood glucose levels in diabetics and provide data throughout the day rather than intermittently checking glucose measurements three to four times per day with finger sticks. CGM aids in providing trend information and helps to identify and prevent unwanted periods of hypo- and hyperglycemia. Blood glucose levels can be downloaded and reviewed with the patient and provider or Certified Diabetes Educator (CDE) to enhance diabetes education, compliance, and care. This type of monitoring can also be done inside and outside of a hospital setting to ensure that data is available to the right clinician at the right time for the right interventions and outcomes.

Information Technology

Health care is an information-intensive and knowledge-intensive enterprise. Information technology can help healthcare providers acquire, manage, analyze, and disseminate both information and knowledge. Healthcare in the 21st century should be safe, effective, patient-centered, timely, efficient, and equitable (IOM, 2001). To achieve that, we need a comprehensive view. This objective isn't new—as a result of information technology, however, it is manageable.

Computers offer the advantage of storing, organizing, retrieving, and communicating digital data with accuracy and speed. Patient care data can be entered once, stored in a database, and then quickly and accurately retrieved many times and in many combinations by healthcare providers and others. A database is a collection of data elements organized and stored together. Data processing is the structuring, organizing, and presenting of data for interpretation as information. For example, vital signs for one patient can be entered into the computer and communicated on a graph; many patients' blood pressure measurements can be compared with the number of doses of antihypertension medication. Vital signs for male patients between the ages of 40 and 50 years can be correlated and used to show relationships with age, ethnicity, weight, presence of comorbid conditions, and so on.

Humans process data continuously, but in an analog form. Computers process data in a digital form. Data processed by computers is done faster and more accurately than humans and provides a method of storage for data retrieval as needed. The Theory Box provides key concepts of information processing. Box 17.1 describes the development of information management skills from novice to expert.

BOX 17.1 Development of Information Management Skills: Novice to Expert Practice

Novice nurses focus on learning what data to collect, the process of collecting and documenting the data, and how to use this information. They learn what clinical applications are available for use and how to use them. Computer and informatics skills focus on applying concrete concepts.

As nurses grow in expertise, they look for patterns in the data and information. They aggregate data across patient populations to look for similarities and differences in response to interventions. Expert nurses integrate theoretical knowledge with practical knowledge gained from experience.

Expert nurses know the value of personal professional reflection on knowledge and synthesize and evaluate information for discovery and decision-making.

KNOWLEDGE TECHNOLOGY

Knowledge technology consists of systems that generate or process knowledge and provide clinical decision support (CDS). Defined broadly, CDS is a clinical

THEORY BOX

Information Theory

Key Contributor	Key Ideas	Application to Practice
Locsin (2005)	The realities of continuously advancing technologies in healthcare necessitate that contemporary nursing practice incorporate both the concepts of technology and caring. Nurses practice in environments requiring technological expertise. Technology has transformed the practice of nursing with the coexistence of caring and technology. Competency with technology is demonstrated by registered nurses in skillful, intentional, deliberate, and authentic activities that engage technology in caring for patients and families. Nurses can build a strong connection with patients and families through the competent use of technology.	Nurses at all stages of professional development need to acquire the skills to use technology competently. When nurses are adept in the use of technology, they engage it to care for patients. For example, the best online resources for patient/family education can be linked to clinical information systems and accessed when the ideal teaching moment is identified. Nurses can influence patients and families to engage in their own care. Providing patients an electronic copy of their record or making patients aware of a patient portal, enrolling them in a portal account, and teaching them how to use it are steps toward strengthening patient access to their health information and engagement in their own healthcare.

Modified from Locsin, R. C. (2005). *Technological competency as caring in nursing: A model for practice.* Indianapolis, IN: Sigma Theta Tau International.

computer system, computer application, or process that helps health professionals make clinical decisions to enhance patient care. The clinical knowledge embedded in computer applications or work processes can range from simple facts and relationships to best practices for managing patients with specific disease states, new medical knowledge from clinical research, and other types of information. Among the most common forms of CDS are drug-dosing calculators—computer-based programs that calculate appropriate doses of medications after a clinician inputs key data (e.g., patient weight or the level of serum creatinine). These calculators are especially useful in managing the administration of medications with a narrow therapeutic index. Allergy alerts, dose range checking, drug–drug interaction, and duplicate order checking are other common applications of CDS.

Clinical decision (or diagnostic) support systems (CDSSs) are interactive computer programs designed to assist health professionals with decision-making tasks by mimicking the inductive or deductive reasoning of a human expert. The basic components of a CDSS include a knowledge base and an *inferencing mechanism* (usually a set of rules derived from the experts and evidence-based practice). The knowledge base contains the knowledge that an expert nurse would apply to data entered about a patient and information to solve a problem. The inference engine controls the application of the knowledge by providing the logic and rules for its use with data from a specific patient. The advent of Watson has helped determine interventions while collecting more data for making decisions. Watson, named after the founder of IBM, is the company's artificial intelligence (AI) platform. AI applications use computer language to learn, adapt, and predict. Extracting data from the EHR and has the potential to improve patient care by supporting clinical decision-making. AI proved useful during the COVID-19 pandemic for detection and diagnosis, monitoring the effectiveness of treatment, contact tracing, and treatments and vaccine development (Clipper, 2020). The Literature Perspective discusses the need for rapid adoption of technology during the COVID-19 pandemic.

Box 17.2 illustrates the use of an expert system for determining the maximum dose of pain medication that can be given to a patient safely after an invasive procedure. The knowledge base contains eight items that are to be considered when giving the maximum dose. The inference engine controls the use of the knowledge base by applying logic that an expert nurse would use in making the decision to give the maximum dose. This decision frame states that if pain is severe (A) or a painful procedure is planned (B), and there is an order for pain medication (C) and the time since surgery is less than 48 hours (H) and the time since the last dose is greater than 3 hours (G), and there are no contraindications to the medication (D) or history of allergy (E) or contraindication to the maximum dose (F), then the "decision" would be to give the dose of pain medication. The rules are those that expert nurses would apply in making the decision to give pain medication.

LITERATURE PERSPECTIVE

Resource: Golinelli, D., Boetto, E., Carullo, G., Nuzzolese, A. G., Landini, M. P., & Fantini, M. P. (2020). Adoption of digital technologies in health care during the COVID-19 pandemic: Systematic review of early scientific literature. *Journal of Medical Internet Research, 22*(11), 1–23.

The COVID-19 pandemic forced the use of technology in healthcare. Prior to the pandemic, some viewed the use of new technologies as a nuisance and were resistant to adopt digital solutions. Diagnosis, prevention, adherence, treatment, lifestyle, and patient surveillance were identified as patient needs that could be addressed by digital technologies. AI was used in diagnosis and screening of COVID-19 using results from chest computed tomography (CT) images; there was also use of a low-cost app for uploading test results. Apps for contact-tracing were used by many people and surveillance of Internet searches and social media usage were monitored. Telehealth allowed patients to increase their access to mental health care during the pandemic.

A systematic review discussed the need to track a large population of patients and the need for rapid diagnostic tests and screening for COVID-19 favors the adoption of digital technologies in healthcare. The review found that implementation of digital solutions was needed expeditiously and viewed the crisis as an opportunity to take advantage of ideas and solutions that may become best practice for the future.

Implications for Practice

This review highlights the importance of digital technologies not only during a pandemic but also in all healthcare situations.

BOX 17.2 **Expert Decision Frame for "Give Maximum Dose of Pain Medication"**

The Knowledge Base

A. Pain score
B. Invasive procedure scheduled
C. Opiate analgesic ordered
D. Contraindications to the medication
E. History of allergic reaction to opiate analgesics
F. Contraindication to maximum dose of opiate analgesic
G. Time since last dose of opiate analgesic administered
H. Time since surgical procedure

The Inference Engine

Give the maximum dose of pain medication if (A or B) and (C and H < 48 hours and G > 3 hours) and not (D or E or F)
OR
(C and H < 48 hours and G > 4 hours) and not (D or E or F)

EXERCISE 17.2 Mr. Jones's heart rate is 54 beats per minute. Tony is about to give Mr. Jones his scheduled atenolol dose. When Tony scans Mr. Jones's armband and the medication bar codes, the computer warns him that atenolol should not be given to a patient with a heart rate less than 60 beats per minute. What should Tony do?

One of the benefits of CDSSs is that they permit the novice nurse to take advantage of decision-making expertise and judgment of an expert. Nursing leaders must be aware of the usefulness of decision support systems for nursing because the development of CDS applicable to nursing practices continues to grow (Cato et al., 2020). Clinical experts are needed to develop both the knowledge in the database and the logic used to develop the rules for its application to a particular patient in a particular circumstance. Advanced critical thinking skills are needed to develop logic and rules. When these are in place, patient care quality can be standardized and improved.

Medication management has a number of high-risk and high-volume processes. New applications provide support for all aspects of the process, thereby improving safety and efficiency (Box 17.3).

INFORMATION SYSTEMS

A clinical information system can be manual or computerized—in fact, we have collected and recorded information about patients and clinical care since the dawn of healthcare. Computer information systems manage large volumes of data, examine data patterns and trends, solve problems, and answer questions. In other words, computers can help translate data into information. Ideally, data are recorded at the point in the care process where they are gathered and are available to healthcare providers when and where they are needed. This is accomplished, in part, by networking computers both within and among organizations to form larger systems. These networked systems might link inpatient care units and other departments, hospitals, clinics, hospice centers, home health agencies, and/or physician practices. Data from all patient encounters with the healthcare system are stored in a central data repository, where they are accessible to authorized users located anywhere in the world. These provide the potential for automated patient records, which contain health data from birth to death.

Adopting the technology necessary to computerize clinical information systems is complex and must be accomplished in stages. The Healthcare Information and Management Systems Society (HIMSS) has described seven stages of electronic medical record (EMR) adoption for hospitals and health systems across the globe. The seventh stage marks achievement of a fully electronic healthcare record. Stage 3 is an important stage, as it is the halfway point to complete adoption and 42% of hospitals have achieved Stage 3 or higher. (Everson et al., 2020). The HIMSS Electronic Medical Record Adoption Model (EMRAM) stages are listed and described in Table 17.1.

Nurses care for patients in acute care, ambulatory, and community settings, as well as in patients' homes. In all settings, nurses focus not only on managing acute illnesses but also on health promotion, maintenance, and education; care coordination and continuity; and monitoring chronic conditions. Ideally, clinical information systems support the work of nurses in all settings.

Communication networks are used to transmit data entered at one computer to be received by others in the network. These networks can reduce the clerical functions of nursing. They can provide patient demographic and census data, results from tests, and lists of medications. Nursing policies and procedures can be

BOX 17.3   Information Technology: Trends in the Medication Management Process

Various information technology (IT) devices and software applications are designed to support the medication management process. Each has unique functionality and targets a specific phase of the medication process.

Computerized Provider Order Entry (CPOE)
- Decision support and clinical warnings (e.g., alerts the provider of allergies, pertinent laboratory data, drug–drug and drug–food interactions)
- Automatic dose calculation
- Link to up-to-date drug reference material
- Automatic order notification
- Standardized formulary-compliant order sets
- Legible, accurate, and complete medication orders
- Decreased variations in practice
- Less time clarifying orders
- Fewer verbal orders
- No manual transcription errors

Electronic Medication Administration Record (e-MAR)
- Integration with clinical documentation (in the electronic record)
- Link to up-to-date drug reference material
- Automatic reminders and alarms for approaching or missed medication administration times
- Prompts for associated tasks or additional documentation requirements
- Alert when cumulative dosing exceeds maximum
- Legible record
- Accessible to multiple users
- Improved accuracy of pharmacokinetic monitoring (administration times are reliable)
- Record matches the pharmacy profile
- Generated reports to track medication errors with visibility of near misses
- Perpetual interface with pharmacy inventory system
- Increase the accuracy of charge capture (at the time of administration vs. when drug is dispensed)

Bar Coding and Radio-Frequency Identification (RFID) Scanning
- Medication documentation captured electronically at the time of administration (populates the e-MAR)
- Medication rights verified

- Positive patient identification
- Clinician alerted to discrepancies (e.g., wrong drug, wrong dose, wrong time, wrong patient, expired drug)
- Automatic tracking of medication errors and provides visibility to near misses

"Smart" Infusion Pumps (Medication Infusion Delivery System)
- Reduced need for manual dose/rate calculation
- Institution-defined standardized drug library (drugs, concentrations, dosing parameters)
- Software filter prevention of programming errors/programming within preestablished minimum and maximum limits before infusion can begin
- Device infusion parameter limits based on patient type or care area
- Interface with the patient's pharmacy profile with capabilities to program the pump electronically
- User alerts to pump setting errors, wrong channel selection, and mechanical failures
- Electronic notification to pharmacy when fluids or medications need to be dispensed
- Interface with the patient's e-MAR (accurate documentation of administration times and volumes infused)
- Memory functions for settings and alarms, with a retrievable log
- Electronic recording of reprogramming and limited override activity

Automated Dispensing Unit or Cabinet
- Secured drug storage
- Controlled user access—biometric identification
- Interface with the pharmacy profile—access restricted until order reviewed
- Quick access once medication order reviewed by pharmacist
- Ability to monitor controlled substance waste and utilization patterns
- Perpetual interface with pharmacy inventory

Pharmacy Automation and Robotics
- Increased accuracy and speed of dispensing

From Bell, M. J. (2005). Nursing information of tomorrow. *Healthcare Informatics, 22*(2), 74–78; Larrabee, S., & Brown, M. M. (2003). Recognizing the institutional benefits of bar-code point-of-care technology. *Joint Commission Journal on Quality and Safety, 29*(7), 345–353.

TABLE 17.1   U.S. Electronic Medical Record Adoption Model

Stage	Cumulative Capabilities
7	Complete EMR, data analytics to improve care, HIE, disaster recovery, privacy and security
6	Use of technology with medication, blood products and human milk administration, and full CDS
5	Physician documentation (templates) and protection from intrusion
4	CPOE with CDS, clinical documentation excluding ED is 90%
3	Clinical documentation is 50% and EMAR
2	CDR, controlled medical vocabulary, CDS, basic security
1	Ancillaries—laboratory, rad, pharmacy – all installed, full R-PACS
0	All three ancillaries not installed

CDR, Clinical data repository; *CDS,* clinical decision support; *CDSS,* clinical documentation support systems; *CPOE,* computerized provider order entry; *ED,* emergency department; *EMR,* electronic medical record; *EMAR,* electronic medication administration record; *HIE,* health information exchange; *R-PACS,* radiology picture archiving and communication system. From HIMSS Analytics, Healthcare Information and Management Systems Society. (2021), EMRAM: A strategic roadmap for effective EMR adoption and maturity. https://www.himssanalytics.org/emram.

linked to the network and accessed, when needed, at the point of care. Links can be provided between the patient's home, hospital, and/or physician office with computers, handheld technologies, and point-of-care devices. Day-to-day events can be recorded and downloaded into the patient record remotely in community nursing settings or at the point of care in the hospital or clinic.

As an example, assume that abdominal magnetic resonance imaging (MRI) with contrast has been ordered. In a paper-based system, handwritten requisitions are sent to nutrition services, the pharmacy, and the radiology department. With a computerized system, the MRI is ordered and the requests for dietary changes, bowel preparation medications, and the diagnostic study itself are automatically sent to the appropriate departments. Radiology compares its schedule openings with the patient's schedule and automatically places the date and time for the MRI on the patient's automated plan of care.

The images and results of the diagnostic procedure are immediately available online and within the patient's EHR.

> **EXERCISE 17.3** Select a healthcare setting with which you are familiar. What information systems are used? Make a list of the names of these systems and the information they provide. How do they help you in caring for patients or in making management decisions? Think about the communication of data and information among departments. Who can readily access the system? Do the systems communicate with each other? If you do not have computerized systems, think about how data and information are communicated. How might a computer system help you be more efficient?

Home Health and Hospice Systems

Nurses caring for patients in home healthcare and hospice must complete documentation necessary to meet government and insurance requirements. Computers assist with direct entry of all required data in the correct format. Portable computers are used to download files of the patients to be seen during the day from a main database. During each visit, the computer prompts the nurse for vital signs, assessments, diagnosis, interventions, long-term and short-term goals, and medications based on previous entries in the medical record. Nurses enter any new data, modifications, or nursing information directly. Entries can be transmitted via a home or cell phone to a main office computer or downloaded from a device at the end of the day. This action automatically updates the patient record and any verbal order entry records, home visit reports, federally mandated treatment plans, productivity and quality improvement reports, and other documents for review and signature. Laptop computers have made recording patient care information more efficient and have improved personnel productivity and compliance with necessary documentation. Additionally, the potential for errors and lack of coordination is reduced.

Placing computers or handheld devices "patient-side" permits nurses to enter data once, at the point of care (Fig. 17.2). Documentation of patient assessments and care provided at the point of care saves time, gives others more timely access to the data, and decreases the likelihood of forgetting to document vital information. Bedside technology at the point of care can support the nurse's decision-making processes (Garcia-Dia, 2020)

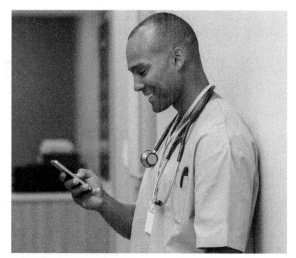

Fig. 17.2 Smartphone technology is a platform for widely used mobile clinical applications. Copyright © Ridofranz/iStock/Thinkstock.

and help reduce medication administration errors with bar code scanning and documentation at the bedside (Graham et al., 2018).

EXERCISE 17.4 Think about the data you gather as you care for a patient through the day. How do you communicate information and knowledge about your patient to others? Does the information system support the way you need this information organized, stored, retrieved, and presented to other healthcare providers? For example, if a patient's pain medication order is about to expire and you want to assess the patient's use and response to the pain medication during the past 24 hours, can the information system generate a graph that compares the time, dose, and pain score for this period? If your assessment is that the medication order needs to be renewed, how do you communicate that message to the prescriber?

Meaningful Use

The potential of EHRs to benefit caregivers, patients, and their families depends on how they are used. The Health Information Technology for Economic and Clinical Health (HITECH) Act was enacted as part of the American Reinvestment & Recovery Act in 2009 to promote meaningful use and transform how patient care is documented with the push for implementation and adoption of EHRs (U.S. Department of Health

and Human Services [DHHS], 2017). Meaningful use (MU) was a set of standards defined by the Centers for Medicare and Medicaid (CMS) incentive programs to govern the use of EHRs and allow eligible providers and hospitals to earn incentive payments by meeting specific criteria. The goal of MU was to promote the implementation and effective use of EHRs to improve healthcare in the United States (Colicchio et al., 2019). To achieve MU, eligible providers and hospitals adopted an EHR with the technical capabilities to ensure that the systems perform the defined required functions. Thereafter, providers and hospitals must use the technology to achieve specific objectives. Benefits of meaningful use of EHRs include the following:

- Complete and accurate information. With EHRs, care providers have the information they need to provide the best possible care.
- Better access to information. EHRs facilitate greater access to the information needed to diagnose and treat health problems earlier and improve health outcomes for patients. EHRs allow information to be shared among offices, hospitals, and across health systems, which facilitates care coordination.
- Patient empowerment. EHRs can empower patients and families to take a more active role in their health. They can receive electronic copies of their healthcare records and share their health information securely over the Internet with their families and care providers.

The MU objectives and measures evolved over 5 years. Stage 1 was the capturing and sharing of data via EHRs. Stage 2 was advancement of clinical processes with EHRs. Stage 3 required that physicians and hospitals use EHRs to demonstrate improved patient outcomes (Table 17.2). In 2018, the CMS renamed EHR incentive programs to Promoting Interoperability Programs, which moved EHR measurements beyond MU requirements to a focus on interoperability and improved patient access to health information (Centers for Disease Control and Prevention [CDC], 2020). According to the CDC (2020), data interoperability benefits for eligible professionals, critical care access hospitals, and eligible hospitals include:

- Bidirectional communication between state public health departments and clinical care providers
- Standardized data elements for data exchange
- Improved efficiency across the healthcare and public health system

TABLE 17.2 Stages of Meaningful Use		
Stage 1 Criteria Focus	**Stage 2 Criteria Focus**	**Stage 3 Criteria Focus**
Capturing health information electronically in a standardized format	More rigorous health information exchange (HIE)	Improving quality, safety, and efficiency, leading to improved health outcomes
Using that information to track key clinical conditions	Increased requirements for e-prescribing and incorporating laboratory results	Decision support for national high-priority conditions
Communicating that information for care coordination processes	Electronic transmission of patient care summaries across multiple settings	Patient access to self-management tools
Initiating the reporting of clinical quality measures and public health information	More patient-controlled data	Access to comprehensive patient data through patient-centered HIE
Using information to engage patients and their families in their care		Improving population health

Source: HealthIT.gov. (2019). *Meaningful use: Meaningful use and the shift to the merit-based incentive payment system.* https://www.healthit.gov/topic/federal-incentive-programs/meaningful-use. Nursing leaders can learn more about MU at https://www.healthit.gov/.

Information Systems Quality and Accreditation

Quality management and measuring patient care efficiency, effectiveness, and outcomes are necessary for accreditation and licensing of healthcare organizations. This is demonstrated by documentation of patient care processes and outcomes. The plan of care outlines what patient care needs to occur, orders are entered to prescribe needed care, and documentation confirms that the care was provided. Computers can then capture and aggregate data to demonstrate both the processes of care and the patient outcomes achieved.

The Joint Commission (TJC), an independent, not-for-profit organization, evaluates and provides accreditation and certification to more than 22,000 healthcare organizations and programs in the United States (TJC, 2020). Accreditation and certification by TJC are recognized nationwide as symbols of an organization's commitment to meeting performance standards focused on improving the quality and safety of patient care. The TJC *Comprehensive Accreditation Manual for Hospitals* and the manuals for other healthcare programs include a chapter of standards for information management. Planning for information management is the initial focus of the chapter because a well-planned system meets the internal and external information needs of an organization with efficiency and accuracy. The goals of effective information management are to obtain, manage, and use information to improve patient care processes and patient outcomes, as well as to improve other organizational processes. Planning is also necessary to provide care continuity should an organization's information systems be disrupted or fail. Adequate planning is essential to ensure privacy, security, confidentiality, and integrity of data and information.

The chapter in the TJC accreditation manual entitled "The Record of Care, Treatment and Services" (TJC, 2021) provided standards and recommendations for the components of a complete medical record. It details documentation requirements that include accuracy, authentication, and thorough, timely documentation. Other standards address the requirements for auditing and retaining records (TJC, 2021). All nurses, including nurse leaders, share responsibility to ensure that cost-effective, high-quality patient care is provided. Nursing administrative databases, containing both clinical and management data, support decision-making for these purposes. Administrative databases assist in the development of the organization's information infrastructure, which ultimately allows for links between management decisions, costs, and clinical outcomes. For example, a database can analyze patient acuity information to suggest safe nurse–patient ratios and help guide staffing decisions.

Selection of clinical information systems, software, applications, and technologies that impact patient care delivery workflows are important decisions that need to

---

BOX 17.4   Elements of the Ideal Hospital Information System

- Data are standardized and use structured terminology.
- The system is reliable—minimal scheduled or unscheduled downtime.
- Applications are integrated across the system.
- Data are collected at the point of care.
- The database is complete, accurate, and easy to query.
- The infrastructure is interconnected and supports accessibility.
- Data are gathered by instrumentation whenever possible so that only minimal data entry is necessary.
- The system has a rapid response time.
- The system is intuitive and reflective of patient care delivery models.
- The location facilitates functionality, security, and support.
- Screen displays can be configured by user preference.
- The system supports outcomes and an evidence-based approach to care delivery.

---

include the chief nursing officer and the nursing leadership team. Nurse leaders and direct care nurses must be members of the selection team, participate actively, and have a voice in the selection decision. Remember that nurses are workers who require data, information, and knowledge to deliver effective patient care. The information system must make sense to the people who use it and fit effectively with the processes for providing patient care. Box 17.4 identifies key elements of an ideal clinical information system that can guide the decision-making necessary for selecting or developing health information software. Before making a selection decision, consider visiting other organizations already using the software to obtain practical and strategic information. Discussions at site visits should include both the utility and performance of the software and the customer service and responsiveness of the vendor.

Information Systems Hardware

Placing the power of computers for both entering and retrieving data at the point of patient care is a major thrust in the move toward increased adoption of clinical information systems. Many hospitals and clinics are using several computing devices in the clinical setting—desktop, laptop, tablet computers, and smartphones—as we learn about both the possibilities and limitations of different hardware solutions. Theoretically, nurses may work best with robust mobile technology. Installing computers on mobile carts, also known as workstations on wheels or WOWs, may increase work efficiency and save time. However, if the cart is cumbersome to move around or if concern about infection risk is associated with moving the cart from one room to another, some organizations favor keeping one cart stationed in each patient care room or installing hardwired bedside computers.

Wireless Communication

Wireless (WL) communication is an extension of an existing wired network environment that transmits data signals through the air without any physical connections. Telemetry is a clinical use of WL communication. Nurses can communicate with other healthcare team members, departments, and offices and with patients using pagers, smartphones, and wireless computers. Nurses can send and receive email, clinical data, and other text messages. Internal and external policies, procedures, and evidence-based care resources can be accessed on these devices via an intranet or the Internet.

Emergency medical personnel use WL technology to request authorization for the treatments or drugs needed in emergency situations. Laboratories use WL technology to transmit laboratory results to physicians, patients awaiting organ transplants are provided with WL pagers so that they can be notified if a donor is found, and parents of critically ill children carry WL pagers when they are away from a phone. Visiting nurses using a home-monitoring system employ WL technology to enter vital signs and other patient-related information. Inpatient nurses can send messages to the admissions department when a patient is being transferred to another unit without having to wait for someone to answer the telephone. Hospitals and health systems use WL technology house-wide to deploy their information systems to the point of patient care.

New hardware for clinical information systems has both advantages and disadvantages. Portable devices, such as smartphones and tablet computers, are less expensive than placing a stationary computer in each patient room. In addition, each caregiver on a shift can be equipped with a device. Portable, handheld devices allow access to information at the point of care, both for retrieval of information and entry of patient data. Nurses may no longer need their "tool belt" when they have a smartphone device that can be used for communication, clinical documentation, and bar-code scanning, as it replaces the need to carry a phone, pager, scanner, and tablet. Disadvantages stem from smartphone or tablet size and portability. They have a small display screen, limiting the amount of data that can be viewed on the screen and the size of the font. Portable devices can also be put down and forgotten, dropped and broken, and targeted for theft. Small devices require a convenient and adequate place to store them when they are not in use and to charge their batteries. Finally, WL technology may need to be assessed and/or updated to ensure that it operates with the speed necessary to advantage busy healthcare workers in fast-paced environments, especially as an increasing number of technologies are being used by healthcare organizations.

Management of the hardware designed to take advantage of clinical information system software is important. Nursing leaders must make knowledgeable decisions about the type of hardware to use, the education needed to use it effectively, and the proper care and maintenance of the equipment. Important questions to ask include the following: What data and information do we need to gather? When and where should it be gathered? How difficult is the equipment to use? Has the hardware been tested sufficiently to ensure purchase of a dependable product? Is the wireless infrastructure stable and capable of handling new or updated technologies?

Communication Technology

Communication technology is an extension of WL technology that enables communication among mobile hospital workers. Hospital staff members wear a pendant-like badge around their neck; by simply pressing a button on the badge, they can be connected to the person with whom they wish to speak by stating the name or function of the person. This type of communication technology has become especially helpful for staff duress functionality that leverages Real Time Location Services (RTLS) to immediately locate and help a nurse who may need assistance with an aggressive patient or family member. Smartphones for voice and text communications, medication and device scanning, and review of clinical information are commonly shared devices that nurses and other healthcare team members use to enhance communication within the hospital.

Voice technology will continue to evolve and may enhance the use of computer systems in the future for nurses. Speech recognition (SR) is also known as *computer speech recognition*. The term *voice recognition* may also be used to refer to speech recognition but is less accurate. SR converts spoken words to machine-readable input. SR applications in everyday life include voice dialing (e.g., "Call home"), call routing (e.g., "I would like to make a call"), and simple data entry (e.g., stating a credit card or account number). In health care, preparation of structured documents, such as a radiology report, is possible with SR. In all of these examples, the computer gathers, processes, interprets, and executes audible signals by comparing the spoken words with a template in the system. If the patterns match, recognition occurs, and a command is executed by the computer. This allows untrained personnel or those whose hands are busy to enter data in an SR environment without touching the computer. Voice technology will also allow physically challenged individuals to function more efficiently when using the computer. SR systems recognize many words but are still immature. The speaker must use staccato-like speech, pausing between each clearly spoken word, and these systems must be programmed for each user so that the system recognizes the user's voice patterns.

Automating the healthcare delivery process is not an easy task. Patient care processes are often not standardized across settings, and most software vendors cannot customize software for each organization. Some current versions of the electronic patient record have merely automated the existing schema of the chart rather than considering how computers could permit data to be viewed or used differently from manual methods. The complexity of decision-making about health information systems software and hardware has given rise to the science of informatics.

NURSING INFORMATICS

Nursing informatics is a "specialty that integrates nursing science with multiple information and analytical sciences to identify, define, manage, and communicate data, information, knowledge, and wisdom in nursing practice" (ANA, 2015). The term *nursing informatics* was probably first used and defined by Scholes and Barber in 1980 in their address to the International Medical Informatics Association (IMIA) at the conference that year in Tokyo. They defined *nursing informatics* as "the application of computer technology to all fields of nursing—nursing services, nurse education, and nursing research" (Staggers & Thompson, 2002, p. 73).

Nursing informatics has become a thriving subspecialty of nursing that combines nursing knowledge and skills with computer expertise. Like any knowledge-intensive profession, nursing is greatly affected by the explosive growth of both scientific advances and technology. Nurse informatics specialists manage and communicate nursing data and information to improve decision-making by consumers, patients, nurses, and other healthcare providers. Nurse informatics specialists formed the American Nursing Informatics Association (ANIA) in the early 1990s to provide networking, education, and information resources that enrich and strengthen the roles of nurses in the field of informatics, including the domains of clinical information, education, and administration decision support. In addition, nursing informatics is represented in the American Medical Informatics Association (AMIA) and the IMIA by working groups that promote the advancement of nursing informatics within the larger interdisciplinary context of health informatics.

The Nursing Informatics Working Group of the AMIA defined their practice specialty as "the science and practice (that) integrate nursing, its information and knowledge, with management of information and communication technologies to promote the health of people, families, and communities worldwide" (American Medical Informatics Association, 2021). Many undergraduate and graduate nursing education programs recognize that it is essential to prepare nurses to practice in a technology-rich environment (National League for Nursing [NLN], 2015). Noting the federal initiatives pushing the adoption of EHRs throughout all healthcare institutions, the NLN recognizes the role of nurse educators in preparing the nursing workforce "to enhance patient care outcomes in a shifting health care environment" (NLN, 2015, p. 4). Certification as a nurse informatics specialist by the American Nurses Credentialing Center (ANCC) requires specific coursework and specific experience and/or continuing education.

Informatics is interdisciplinary; although specific bodies of knowledge exist for each healthcare profession (e.g., nursing, dentistry, dietetics, pharmacy, medicine), they interface at the patient. Working with integrated clinical information systems and emerging technologies demands interdisciplinary collaboration at a high level.

PATIENT SAFETY

The patient care environment is complex and prone to errors. Nurses have a major role in the quality and safety of healthcare (Phillips, Malliaris, & Bakerjian, 2021). In addition to physical challenges, resource challenges, and interruptions characteristic of nursing work, nurses are challenged by inconsistencies and breakdowns in care communication. Communication and information difficulties are among the most common nursing workplace challenges and are frustrating and potentially dangerous for patients. Effectively designed and implemented information technology has the potential to improve patient safety in the healthcare setting (Sittig et al., 2018).

Nurses, other health professionals, patients, and families rely increasingly on information technology to communicate, manage information, mitigate error potential, and make informed decisions (Sittig et al., 2018). Health information technology has the potential to improve—or obstruct—work performance, communication, and documentation (Sittig et al., 2018). Because nurses play a central role in patient care, the extent to which information technology supports or detracts from nurses' work performance may affect patient care delivery and nurse-sensitive outcomes (Moore et al., 2020). Documentation to meet organizational, accreditation, insurance, state, and federal requirements, as well as to provide information needed by other healthcare providers, imposes a heavy demand on nurses' time. Burden of documentation requirements for nurses may lead to feelings of less time for direct contact with patients and families. Patient safety needs to remain at the forefront as nursing partners with IS teams to implement, adopt, and optimize information systems, structures, and technologies.

Impact of Clinical Information Systems

Clinical information systems that provide access to patient information and clinical decision support can reduce errors and improve communication (Cline, 2020). Patient information in an electronic clinical information system enables organization and legibility of data and information that is used to make patient care decisions. Nurses see all the medications prescribed for a patient in one location, doses are written clearly, and drug names are spelled correctly. The patient problem list shows acute and chronic health conditions and complete allergy information. Abnormal findings are highlighted and can be graphed and compared with interventions. Alerts signal to nurses that critical information has been entered in the electronic record. For example, critical test results signal the need for provider notification and intervention. An alert that a patient is at risk for falling signals the need for additional monitoring and interventions to ensure safety. Nursing reminders to perform care can reduce the incidence of hospital-acquired conditions such as pressure ulcers.

When standards for care are not being followed, clinical information systems can generate reminders or propose suggestions. Rules remind care providers to perform required care. For example, when documentation is not recorded for medication administration, IV tubing change, or wound care, the information system can generate a reminder based on rules that have been agreed to by providers. Evidence-based practices are integrated in the process of care as providers are guided to select the most appropriate course of action.

Errors can be prevented by eliminating problems stemming from illegible handwriting. Computerized order entry also eliminates the nursing time required for clarification of illegible and incomplete orders. Transcription is no longer required, orders are sent directly to the performing department, and patient care needs are communicated more clearly and quickly to all clinicians. Medication dosing, drug allergy, and drug–drug interaction checking all have a significant impact on patient safety (Tolley et al., 2018).

Impact on Communication

Integrated information systems allow all members of the interdisciplinary patient care team to see pertinent patient information. The patient plan of care is based on real-time data for what is currently happening with the ability to be proactive in anticipation of what should occur in the future. The entire care team has visibility for who is responsible for the patient and who needs to communicate about the patient's care. Clinical information systems provide multiple users with simultaneous, real-time access to patient records. Patient care handoffs are safer when information is readily available and not lost in the process. Patient care processes are facilitated and treatment delays are decreased. The patient and family experience is also improved by decreasing redundant data collection by multiple members of the care team.

Impact on Patient Care Documentation

Nurses spend increasing amounts of time documenting patient care activities. Clinical documentation in an electronic information system can improve communication and coordination among providers. Ongoing education and monitoring can help clinicians increase documentation efficiency and productivity (Geier & Smith, 2019). Nurses have identified that the benefits of electronic documentation include safer medication administration and ease of access to clinical information (Schenk et al., 2021). Patients can access their own health information via secure online patient portals. The use of a portal allows the patient 24-hour access to recent visits, discharge summaries, and medications. Also, portals allow patients to communicate with their providers and nurses, request prescription refills, schedule appointments, and complete pre-visit forms, contributing to documentation within their electronic health record.

Impact on Medication Administration Processes

The *Quantros MEDMARX* database includes annual records of medication errors. Historically, approximately 25% of errors involved some aspect of computer technology as at least one cause of the error. Most of the errors related to technology involved mislabeled bar codes on medications, mistakes at order entry because of confusing computer screens, or other problems with information management (TJC, 2015). Errors also were related to dispensing devices and human factors, such as failure to scan bar codes or overrides of bar-code warnings. Computerized provider order entry (CPOE) has become an effective mechanism for improving patient safety by reducing medication errors and wrong-time administration errors (York et al., 2019). Safeguards built into clinical information systems can avert an error, but awareness of the potential for new issues is vital. Bar-code technology ensures that the right patient gets the right medication, in the correct dose, by the appropriate route, and at the right time. However, this technology must not impede nurses' care of patients. Faced with urgent or emergent situations with patients, technical difficulties, or poor work redesign, unorthodox and potentially unsafe workarounds are sometimes invented when the medication administration system is not usable and obstructs patient care (van der Veen et al., 2018). Closed-loop electronic prescribing, dispensing, and bar-code patient identification systems reduce prescribing errors and medication adverse

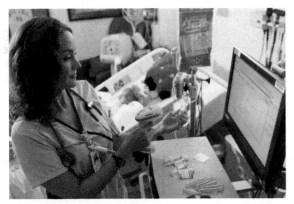

Fig. 17.3 Bar-code medication administration "closes the loop" on medication safety by providing a double-check of the "rights" of medication administration at the point nurses actually give patients their medications.

events and increase confirmation of patient identity before administration (Fig. 17.3). Human errors in prescribing cannot be eliminated as people, process, and technology are always components of any new or updated information system that impacts care delivery (Thompson et al., 2018).

SAFELY IMPLEMENTING HEALTH INFORMATION TECHNOLOGY

Opportunities for nurses to embrace technology that improves patient safety abound by reducing hospital-acquired infections, promoting antimicrobial

stewardship, implementing automated dispensing systems, and more (Astier et al., 2020). Despite the promise of positive outcomes from clinical information systems, success is not a guarantee. Nurses need to work with their IS counterparts to remain alert to potential limitations as increasing use of technologies and automation may create opportunities for new types of errors and less transparency (Astier et al., 2020). As McBride eloquently stated in the early 2000s, still applicable today, "Information technology is not a panacea, and will not fulfill its promise unless it is harnessed in support of foundational values" (McBride, 2005). Nurses must stay connected with the ongoing information technology advances and take active roles in ensuring that IT supports nursing practice and patient care outcomes.

According to TJC, as new and updated health information technology is adopted, users must be mindful of the safety risks and preventable adverse events that implementation can create (TJC, 2015). Any form of technology has the potential to adversely affect patient care safety and quality if designed or implemented improperly. TJC suggests 13 actions, which are presented in Table 17.3. Clinical information systems, structures, and technologies need to align with the organizational strategy and culture, the information needs of its users, and clinical processes and practices. The successful implementation of technology requires a shared responsibility and multifaceted approach, looking at the people, processes, environment, and technology involved (Sittig et al., 2018).

TABLE 17.3 The Joint Commission Recommendations for Safely Implementing Health Information Technology
Suggested Action
1. Examine work processes and procedures for risks and inefficiencies. Resolve problems identified before technology implementation. Involve representatives of all disciplines—clinical, clerical, and technical—in the examination and resolution of issues.
2. Involve clinicians and staff who will use or be affected by the technology, along with information technology (IT) staff with strong clinical backgrounds, in the planning, selection, design, reassessment, and ongoing quality improvement of technology. Involve pharmacists in planning and implementing any technology that involves medication.
3. Assess your organization's technology needs. Require IT staff to interact with users outside their own facility to learn about real-world capabilities of potential systems from various vendors; conduct field trips; look at integrated systems to minimize the need for interfaces.

(Continued)

TABLE 17.3   The Joint Commission Recommendations for Safely Implementing Health Information Technology—cont'd

Suggested Action

4. Continuously monitor for problems during the introduction of new technology and address issues as quickly as possible to avoid workarounds and errors. Consider an emergent issues desk staffed with project experts and champions to help rapidly resolve problems. Use interdisciplinary problem solving to improve system quality and provide vendor feedback.

5. Establish training programs for all clinical and operations staff, designed appropriately for each group and focused on how the technology will benefit staff and patients. Do not allow long delays between training and implementation. Provide frequent refresher courses or updates.

6. Develop and communicate policies delineating staff authorized and responsible for technology implementation, use, oversight, and safety review.

7. Ensure that all order sets and guidelines are developed, tested, and approved by the Pharmacy and Therapeutics Committee (or equivalent) before implementation.

8. Develop a graduated system of safety alerts in the new technology to help clinicians determine urgency and relevancy. Review skipped or rejected alerts. Decide which alerts need to be hard stops in the technology and provide supporting documentation.

9. Develop systems to mitigate potential computerized provider order entry (CPOE) drug errors or adverse events by requiring department and pharmacy review and sign off. Use the Pharmacy and Therapeutics Committee (or equivalent) for oversight and approval of electronic order sets and clinical decision support (CDS) alerts. Ensure proper nomenclature and printed label design, eliminate dangerous abbreviations and dose designations, and ensure electronic medication administration record (e-MAR) acceptance by nurses.

10. Provide environments that protect staff doing data entry from undue distractions when using the technology.

11. Maximize the potential of the technology to maximize safety. Continually reassess and enhance safety effectiveness and error detection. Use error-tracking tools, and evaluate events and near-miss events.

12. Monitor and report errors and near-miss events. Pursue potential system errors or use problems with root cause analysis or other forms of failure-mode analysis. Consider reporting significant issues to external reporting systems.

13. Reevaluate the applicability of security and confidentiality protocols. Reassess Health Insurance Portability and Accountability Act (HIPAA) compliance periodically to ensure that the addition of technology and the growing responsibilities of IT staff have not introduced new security or compliance risks.

Relying too heavily on health information technology for communication can reduce teamwork and may negatively affect patient safety and care quality (Astier et al., 2020). Although improved access and better-organized information can eliminate nurses' need to locate information for other care providers, information technology should not eliminate the need for personal communication and teamwork. Successful development and implementation of nursing information technology depend on nurses working in partnership with organizational leadership, information systems vendors, and systems analysts to create tools that truly benefit nurses.

When nurses have the systems and tools needed to provide patient care effectively and efficiently, safety and care quality will follow. Direct-care nurses must work with informatics nurses and information system developers and programmers in system development, implementation, and ongoing improvement. By combining computer and information science with nursing science, the goals of supporting nursing practice and the delivery of high-quality nursing care can be achieved (Ruppel & Funk, 2018). The Research Perspective identifies some recommendations related to health information technology successes and failures.

RESEARCH PERSPECTIVE

Resource: Moore, E. C., Tolley, C. L., Bates, D. W., & Slight, S. P. (2020). A systematic review of the impact of health information technology on nurses' time. *Journal of the American Medical Informatics Association, 27*(5), 798–807.

The potential to use health information technology as a tool to manage effective use of nursing resources is emerging and being tested by leaders in nursing informatics. Leaders must balance nursing staffing and care quality against financial constraints in an era of cost containment.

Little agreement exists about the best approach to achieve nurse–patient ratios that support safe, high-quality nursing care for all patients. A strict ratio may ignore individual patient care needs, whereas attempts to capture details about care needs or derive a formula that

precisely predicts care needs and forecasts required staff requirements are very difficult and have not been broadly agreed on.

A systematic review of the relationship between health information technology and nurses' time was conducted to better understand areas for cost savings. The review found that health information technology systems increased nursing documentation time yet also allowed nurses to spend more time performing direct patient care.

Implications for Practice

Health information technology can result in value-added activities for care providers. As staffing concerns continue to be addressed, consideration of documentation of nurses' time and value needs to be included.

IMPLICATIONS FOR PRACTICE

Administering medications, monitoring patients after a procedure, and admitting a new patient for an inpatient stay are a few examples of the need for electronic measurement. Numerous other examples show value in nursing care. Imagine that a patient you are caring for complains of light-headedness and nausea. When documenting vital signs, you note that the blood pressure measurement is lower than it was the day before. Graphing the values across several days illustrates a steady decline in the readings. Reviewing the medication list, you note the patient is receiving hydralazine (Apresoline). Processing the data that you have collected, you implement "falls precautions," send a communication order to monitor blood pressure and other symptoms frequently, and notify the physician if the situation has not changed.

> **EXERCISE 17.5** Think about the data that you gather and document every day: vital signs, intake and output, laboratory and test results, and the patient's responses to care. What data did you automatically combine or reorganize to help you decide aspects of patient care? How did you use this information to improve your patient's outcome? How and with whom did you communicate the data and information? How did technology combine or organize data?

FUTURE TRENDS AND PROFESSIONAL ISSUES

Biomedical and Wearable Technology

Devices are becoming smarter every day, and the technology now exists to integrate pump data into the EHR. The nurse validates input from the smart pumps. Integration allows providers to see titration and changes in physiologic parameters, allows the pharmacy to know when a continuous infusion is running low, and is a time saver for nurses who no longer must manually input each data point (Fig. 17.4). Continuous monitoring of patients with chronic conditions such as diabetes and cardiovascular diseases can be done from their home environment. Continuous glucose monitoring devices can monitor blood glucose levels in diabetics and provide data throughout the day with data sent to the clinical team to enhance communication, compliance, and care. Implantable cardiac arrhythmia devices enable patients and the care team to monitor electrical activity in the heart wherever the patient is with alerts and notifications sent and received for real-time surveillance and interventions. Smartphones can track exercise, sleep, behavior, and mood status to promote physical and emotional wellness with data that can be sent via an app to the patient's care team.

Information Technology

Healthcare in the United States is expensive and of variable quality. Recognizing that informatics can play an

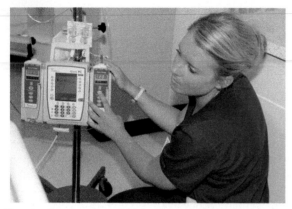

Fig. 17.4 Smart pumps offer integration between the pump and the electronic health record, including auto-pump programming.

important role in controlling costs and improving quality, the federal government's economic stimulus plan in 2009 earmarked $20 billion for health information technology. Hospitals and physician practices were incentivized to use the money wisely and follow meaningful use guidelines to ensure safe, quality care and outcomes. This effort has also encouraged the health information technology industry to move toward strong mandated data standards. Data standards are at the foundation of integrated, interoperable information systems that facilitate transfer of data from an emergency department or operating room to inpatient hospital units and enable electronic patient health information exchange between hospitals and physician offices in different parent organizations.

Use of information technology for COVID-19 testing, vaccination administration and recording, and contact tracing became prevalent with the 2020 pandemic. Contact tracing leverages data and information to help prevent the spread of infectious diseases by identifying at-risk individuals and/or populations exposed to the infection. Health departments, schools, businesses, healthcare providers, and healthcare organizations rely on access to infectious disease and vaccine data and information to monitor and communicate risks for future outbreaks.

Electronic Patient Care Records

Multiple terms have been used to define electronic patient care records, with overlapping definitions. Both electronic health records (EHRs) and electronic medical records (EMRs) have gained widespread use, with some health informatics users assigning the term *EHR* to a global concept and *EMR* to a discrete localized record. An EHR refers to an individual patient's medical record in digital format. The EHR is a longitudinal electronic record of patient health information generated across encounters in any care delivery setting. EHR systems coordinate the storage and retrieval of individual records with the aid of computers. The EHR is most often accessed on a computer, often over a network, and may include EMRs from many locations and/or sources. Among the many forms of data often included are patient demographics, health history, progress and procedure notes, health problems, medication and allergy lists (including immunization status), laboratory test results, radiology images and reports, billing records, and advance directives.

Credit card–like devices called smart cards store a limited number of pages of data on a computer chip. The implementation of computer-based health information systems has led to computer networks that store health records across local, state, national, and international boundaries. The smart card serves as a bridge between the clinician terminal and the central repository, making patient information available to the caregiver quickly and cheaply at the point of service because the patients bring it with them. This will help coordinate care; improve quality-of-care decisions; and reduce risk, waste, and duplication of effort. Patients are mobile and consult many practitioners, thereby causing their records to be fragmented. With the electronic smart card, patients, providers, and notes can be brought together in any combination at any place. Box 17.5 provides examples of the types of data that are recorded on smart cards.

Data Privacy and Security

Data protection, systems' security, and patient privacy are concerns with electronic health records. However,

---

BOX 17.5   Contents of Smart Cards

1. Patient demographics and photo identification
2. ICE—in case of emergency—contact and other key information
3. Patient medical history: for example, allergies, medications, immunizations, laboratory results
4. Past care encounter summaries, including surgical procedures
5. Patient record locations and electronic address information
6. Ability to upload or download patient information

patients' rights to privacy of their data must be maintained whether recorded in a manual or automated system. The Health Insurance Portability and Accountability Act (HIPAA) of 1996 developed federal regulations to protect the privacy and security of health information. The privacy rule protects who can access electronic, written, oral patient health information while the security rule requires electronic health security (U.S. Department of Health and Human Services, 2020). With computerized data, any person with the proper permission may access the information anywhere in the world, and multiple people can do so simultaneously.

Information security and privacy are important concerns as development of electronic health information systems and technologies continue to advance. A firewall protects the information in the central data repository from access by unauthorized users. It is a network security measure that keeps electronic intruders from accessing an organization's data on its private network while allowing members of the organization to reach the Internet. Encryption of data is a must when shared via the Internet.

The 21st Century Cures Act in 2016 was a driver for electronic access, exchange, and use of health information. The Office of the National Coordinator for Health Information Technology (ONC) finalized the Cures Act to include interoperability provisions that promote patient control of their health information (ONC, 2020). Cybersecurity and information blocking have become center stage as organizations work to comply with information privacy, security, and access regulations. Dedicated teams are often in place to focus on monitoring for information system threats or disruptions and implementation of protective measures. Access limitations, user authentication, and audit trails are mechanisms that may be in place to help protect confidential information within the EHR and mobile devices that may be managed by the organization. Clinical and IS collaboration are necessary to ensure compliance of organizational policies on the use, security, and accuracy of electronic health information.

TELEHEALTH

Telehealth is the use of modern telecommunications and information technologies for the provision of healthcare to individuals at a distance and the transmission of information to provide that care. This is accomplished by using two-way interactive videoconferencing and high-speed telephone lines, fiber-optic cable, and satellite transmissions. Patients sitting in front of the teleconferencing camera can be diagnosed, treated, monitored, and educated by nurses and physicians. In response to the COVID-19 crisis, an emergency declaration allowed the CMS to expand Medicare's telehealth benefits. This expanded reimbursement and access to telehealth benefited all Americans with healthcare covered by the CMS, and private insurers quickly followed. The regulatory guidelines relaxed and reimbursement expanded. Temporary changes in licensure requirements allowed providers to practice across state lines and changes in reimbursement encouraged hospitals to begin or increase their telehealth services. Telehealth visits protected health professionals and patients from COVID-19 exposure, increased access to healthcare, conserved supplies and hospital beds, and supported specialty care (Clipper, 2020). ECGs and radiographs can be viewed and transmitted. Sophisticated electronic stethoscopes and dermascopes allow nurses and physicians to hear heart, lung, and bowel sounds and to look closely at wounds, eyes, ears, and skin. Ready access to expert advice and patient information is available no matter where the patient or information is located. Patients in rural areas and prisons especially benefit from this technology.

The cardiac high-acuity monitoring program (CHAMP) is an in-home monitoring system for patients with single-ventricle (SV) cardiac disease. Home monitoring is completed using a tablet to input data; the data are stored in a cloud-based secure system and transferred to the EMR daily. This secure portal can alert the caregiver team to changes in the patient's condition and allow for quick adjustments to the plan of care. This monitoring program has decreased interstage mortality by greater than 40% (Rudd et al., 2020).

The COVID-19 pandemic highlighted the use of telecommunication in supporting distance learning, which has been possible for some years, with enhanced opportunities to engage learners in online classrooms. With online—or "virtual"—classrooms, learners from anywhere in the world with computer access can log into a university or other group online learning system via the Internet.

Informatics

In 2011, the HIMSS identified that just over 90% of American hospitals had implemented some component of an EMR. The specialty of nursing informatics has been recognized by ANA since 2001 and today more than 8000 nurses are practicing in informatics. Many more are needed to achieve widespread development and adoption of effective health information systems (Sensmeier, 2020).

Many opportunities exist to improve the safety, efficiency, and effectiveness of nursing care. The goal of informatics nurses and nursing leaders is to use information technology to ensure that critical information is available to caregivers at the point of care to make healthcare safer and more effective while improving efficiency. This requires interconnected and integrated healthcare technology across hospitals, healthcare systems, and geographic regions. Standards for data systems that operate efficiently with one another (termed *interoperability*) and attention to data security and patient privacy are necessary.

Nurses are working as leaders in several national initiatives to lay the groundwork and guide progress toward the goal of a nationwide health information network. Every nurse can embrace technology to improve nursing practice. The informatics role uses the informatics skills of consultation, systems analysis and design, policy development, and use of IT to enable quality improvement, research, and evaluation (Sensmeier, 2020).

Knowledge Technology

Technology has the potential to shorten the many years that currently exist between the development of new knowledge for patient care and the application of that knowledge in real-time practice with patients. Increasingly, patient conditions that are directly influenced by nursing care are part of the CMS pay-for-performance program and TJC "Never Events" initiative. Having the best knowledge available regarding clinical phenomena is increasingly important. The focus of nursing care includes medication management, activity intolerance, immobility, risk for falls and actual falls, risk for skin impairment and pressure ulcer, anxiety, dementia, sleep, prevention of infection, nutrition, incontinence, dehydration, smoking cessation, pain management, patient and family education, and self-care.

Technology can also present some challenges. First, the challenge of synthesizing the knowledge available

in a manner that is useful to clinicians is critical. Then, computerized information systems are needed to provide clinical decision support at the point of care. Finally, the computer system must collect good clinical data to promote ongoing knowledge development for nursing care of patients and families. Several "intelligent" clinical information systems are in development. These systems translate nursing knowledge into reference materials that can be accessed at the point of care.

PROFESSIONAL, ETHICAL NURSING PRACTICE AND NEW TECHNOLOGIES

Technology has and will continue to transform the healthcare environment and the practice of nursing. Nurses are professionally obligated to maintain competency with a vast array of technological devices and systems. Baseline informatics competency is a necessity for nurses to practice, communicate, and deliver care.

Because of the increasing ability to preserve human life with biomedical technology, questions about living and dying have become conceptually and ethically complex. Conceptually, it becomes more difficult to define what is extraordinary treatment in extending human life because technology has changed our concepts of living and dying. A source of ethical dilemmas is the use of invasive technological treatment to provide patients with extraordinary means and to prolong life for patients with limited or no decision-making capabilities. Nurses are concerned with individual patient welfare and the effects of technological intervention on the immediate and long-term quality of life for patients and their families. Patient advocacy remains an important function of the professional nurse.

Safeguarding patients' welfare, privacy, and confidentiality is another obligation of nurses. Security measures are available with computerized information systems. However, it is the integrity and ethical principles of system end-users that provide the final safeguard for patient privacy. System users must never share the passwords that allow them access to information in computerized clinical information systems. Each password uniquely identifies a user to the system by name and title, gives approval to carry out certain functions, and provides access to data appropriate to the user. When a nurse signs on to a computer, all data and information that are entered or reviewed can be traced to that password. Every nurse is accountable for all actions taken using that nurse's password. All nurses must be aware of their responsibilities for the confidentiality and security of the data they gather and for the security of their passwords.

Nurse managers must ensure that policies and procedures for collecting and entering data and the use of security measures (e.g., passwords) are established to maintain confidentiality of patient data and information. They have the responsibility to manage data to effectively lead change. This can be accomplished through documentation audit tools and system compliance reports. Nurse managers must also be knowledgeable patient advocates in the use of technology for patient care by referring ethical questions to the organization's ethics committee.

> **EXERCISE 17.6** Think about the use of the Internet in healthcare. How do you use it to look up healthcare information? How would you advise a patient to select appropriate sites?

CONCLUSION

Biomedical information, communication, and knowledge technology will form a bond in the future, linking people and information together in a rapidly changing world of healthcare. With new technology comes the need for a new set of competencies. Nursing participation in designing this exciting future will ensure that the unique contributions of nurses to patient and family health and illness care are clearly and formally represented.

THE SOLUTION

A systematic review of the literature related to nursing documentation informed our team of the effect of regulatory, accrediting, and other requirements as nurses spend more and more time entering data into the EHR that is not valuable or used to drive patient care. The literature also revealed a need to define what is essential for nurses to document in the EHR. Documentation optimization was necessary for us, as our nurses longed for less time on the computer and more time for care coordination and patient and family interactions.

Our nurse leaders, direct care nurses, and clinical informatics teams collaborated to optimize and define essential data elements for our admission history intake documentation. Federal and state regulatory requirements were taken into consideration, as well as quality and safety policies, to determine essential nursing documentation data elements. We leveraged timers embedded within our EHR as practice-based evidence to expose nursing documentation time and data elements most often documented within the admission history intake database. Nursing practice and care team implications were taken into consideration to ensure our EHR documentation and system updates supported interdisciplinary workflow, communication, and patient outcomes.

Information technology has become a standard for healthcare delivery within our organization as we rely on the EHR to support clinical practice and deliver safe, efficient, quality patient care. Our efforts to optimize and define what is essential for nurses to document is ongoing to ensure the right questions are asked at the right time to coordinate the right care. By optimizing and defining essential data elements, our nurses spend nearly 30% less time for admission history intake documentation! Clinical and informatics collaboration for documentation updates using regulatory requirements, literature review, and data analysis has become standard work for continuous optimization to improve nurse, patient, and family experiences at our organization.

Would this be a suitable approach for you? Why?

Jenny Horn

REFLECTIONS

Have you used more than one information system during your academic preparation in nursing? If yes, what advantages in design and implementation could you detect in one setting or another?

Have you used the same information system in more than one setting? If so, did you detect differences in how the system was designed and implemented in different settings?

If you were to participate on the HIT selection or implementation planning teams in your role as a registered nurse, are you confident you could identify features in the system with potential to either support or threaten patient safety? What do you believe are the most critical?

▊ BEST PRACTICE

Health information technology (HIT) has the potential to reduce healthcare costs, improve efficiency, and enhance patient care safety and quality. HIT must be designed, implemented, adopted, and continuously improved to positively enable healthcare quality and safety.

Nurses and Information Systems (IS) need to partner to provide HIT that is safe and enables easy entry and retrieval of data, has simple and intuitive user interfaces, supports clinical practice, and permits seamless system interoperability.

▊ TIPS FOR MANAGING INFORMATION AND TECHNOLOGY

- Create a vision for the future.
- Match your vision to the institution's mission and strategic plan.
- Learn what you need to know to fulfill the vision.
- Join initiatives that are moving in the direction of your vision.
- Be prepared to initiate, implement, and support new technology.
- Use an automated dispensing system.
- Use biometric technology.
- Use bar-coding systems/bar-code technology.
- Never stop learning, or you will always be behind.

REFERENCES

American Association of Colleges of Nursing (AACN). (2021). *The essentials: Core competencies for professional nursing education.* Retrieved from https://www.aacnnursing.org/Portals/42/AcademicNursing/pdf/Essentials-2021.pdf.

American Medical Informatics Association (AMIA). (2021). *Nursing informatics.* Retrieved from https://amia.org/communities/nursing-informatics.

American Nurses Association (ANA). (2015). *Nursing informatics: Practice scope and standards of practice* (2nd ed.). Silver Spring, MD: Nursebooks:org.

Astier, A., Carlet, J., Hoppe-Tichy, T., Jacklin, A., Jeanes, A., McManus, S., & Fitzpatrick, R. (2020). What is the role of technology in improving patient safety? A French, German and UK healthcare professional perspective. *Journal of Patient Safety and Risk Management, 25*(6), 219–224. https://doi.org/10.1177/2516043520975661.

Bell, M. J. (2005). Nursing information of tomorrow. *Healthcare Informatics, 22*(2), 74–78.

Cato, K. D., McGrow, K., & Rossetti, S. C. (2020). Transforming clinical data into wisdom: Artificial intelligence implications for nurse leaders. *Nursing Management, 51*(11), 24–30. https://doi.org/10.1097/01.NUMA.0000719396.83518.d6.

Centers for Disease Control and Prevention. (2020). Public Health and Promoting Interoperability Programs. Retrieved from https://www.cdc.gov/ehrmeaningfuluse/introduction.html.

Cline, L. (2020). How electronic health records correlate with patient-centered care. *Nursing, 50*(1), 61–63. https://doi.org/10.1097/01.NURSE.0000615140.23834.06.

Clipper, B. (2020). The influence of the COVID-19 pandemic on technology. *Nurse Leader, 18*(5), 500–503.

Colicchio, T. K., Cimino, J. J., & Del Fiol, G. (2019). Unintended consequences of nationwide electronic health record adoption: Challenges and opportunities in the post-meaningful use era. *Journal of Medical Internet Research, 21*(6), e13313. https://doi.org/10.2196/13313.

Everson, J., Rubin, J. C., & Friedman, C. P. (2020). Reconsidering hospital EHR adoption at the dawn of HITECH: Implications of the reported 9% adoption of a "basic" EHR. *Journal of the American Medical Informatics Association, 27*(8), 1198–1205. https://doi.org/10.1093/jamia/ocaa090.

Garcia-Dia, M. J. (2020). Balancing care with technology. *Nursing Management, 51*, 56. https://doi.org/10.1097/01.NUMA.0000657280.44223.10.

Geier, A., & Smith, D. (2019). The role of electronic documentation in ambulatory surgery centers. *AORN Journal, 109*(4), 444–450.

Golinelli, D., Boetto, E., Carullo, G., Nuzzolese, A. G., Landini, M. P., & Fantini, M. P. (2020). Adoption of digital technologies in health care during the COVID-19 pandemic: Systematic review of early scientific literature. *Journal of

Medical Internet Research, 22(11), 1–23. https://www.jmir.org/2020/11/e22280.

Graham, H. L., Nussdorfer, D., & Beal, R. (2018). Nurse attitudes related to accepting electronic health records and bedside documentation. *CIN: Computers, Informatics, Nursing*, 36(11), 515–520. https://doi.org/10.1097/CIN.0000000000000491.

HealthIT.gov. (2019). *Meaningful use: Meaningful use and the shift to the merit-based incentive payment system*. Retrieved from https://www.healthit.gov/topic/federal-incentive-programs/meaningful-use.

HIMSS Analytics. (2021). *EMRAM: A strategic roadmap for effective EMR adoption and maturity*. Retrieved from https://www.himssanalytics.org/europe/electronic-medical-record-adoption-model.

Institute for Safe Medication Practices (ISMP). (2020). *ISMP Targeted Medication Safety Best Practices for Hospitals*. Retrieved from https://www.ismp.org/guidelines/best-practices-hospitals.

Institute of Medicine (IOM). (2012). *Health IT and Patient Safety: Building Safer Systems for Better Care*. Retrieved from: National Academies Press. https://www.nap.edu/catalog/13269/health-it-and-patient-safety-building-safer-systems-for-better.

Institute of Medicine (IOM). (2011). *The future of nursing: Leading change, advancing health*. Washington, DC: National Academies Press.

Institute of Medicine (IOM), Committee on Quality Health Care in America. (2001). *Crossing the quality chasm: A new health system for the 21st century*. Washington, DC: National Academies Press.

Larrabee, S., & Brown, M. M. (2003). Recognizing the institutional benefits of bar-code point-of-care technology. *Joint Commission Journal on Quality and Safety*, 29(7), 345–353.

Locsin, R. C. (2005). *Technological competency as caring in nursing: A model for practice*. Indianapolis, IN: Sigma Theta Tau International.

McBride, A. B. (2005). Nursing and the informatics revolution. *Nurs Outlook*, 53(4), 183-191; discussion 192. https://doi.org/10.1016/j.outlook.2005.02.006.

Moore, E. C., Tolley, C. L., Bates, D. W., & Slight, S. P. (2020). A systematic review of the impact of health information technology on nurses' time. *Journal of the American Medical Informatics Association*, 27(5), 798–807. https://doi.org/10.1093/jamia/ocz231.

Munroe, B., Curtis, K., Balzer, S., Roysten, K., Fetchet, W., Tucker, S., Pratt, W., Morris, R., Fry, M., & Considine, J. (2020). Translation of evidence into policy to improve clinical practice: The development of an emergency department rapid response system. *Australasian Emergency Care*. S2588-994X(20)30078-6. Epub ahead of print https://doi.org/10.1016/j.auec.2020.08.003.

National League for Nursing (NLN). (2015). *Position statement: A vision for the changing faculty role: Preparing students for the technological world of health care*. https://www.nln.org/docs/default-source/uploadedfiles/about/nln-vision-series-position-statements/nlnvision-8.pdf?sfvrsn=1219df0d_0.

Office of the National Coordinator for Health Information Technology (ONC). (2020). *ONC's Cures Act Final Rule*. Retrieved from https://www.healthit.gov/curesrule/resources/fact-sheets.

Phillips, J., Malliaris, A. P., & Bakerjian, D. (2021). Nursing and patient safety. Patient Safety Network. Retrieved from https://psnet.ahrq.gov/primer/nursing-and-patient-safety.

Phillips, J., Sowan, A., Ruppel, H., & Magness, R. (2020). Educational program for physiologic monitor use and alarm systems safety. *Clinical Nurse Specialist*, 34(2), 50–62. https://doi.org/10.1097/NUR.0000000000000507.

Quality and Safety Education for Nurses (QSEN). (2021). *QSEN competencies*. Retrieved from http://qsen.org/competencies/pre-licensure-ksas/.

Rudd, N. A., Ghanayem, N. S., Hill, G. D., Lambert, L. M., Mussatto, K. A., Nieves, J. A., Robinson, S., Shirali, G., Steltzer, M. M., Uzark, K., & Pike, N. A. (2020). Interstage home monitoring for infants with single ventricle heart disease: Education and management: A scientific statement from the American Heart Association. *Journal of the American Heart Association*, 9(16), e014548. https://doi.org/10.1161/JAHA.119.014548.

Ruppel, H., & Funk, M. (2018). Nurse–technology interactions and patient safety. *Critical Care Nursing Clinics of North America*, 30(2), 203–213. https://doi.org/10.1016/j.cnc.2018.02.003.

Schenk, E., Marks, N., Hoffman, K., & Goss, L. (2021). Four years later: Examining nurse perceptions of electronic documentation over time. *Journal of Nursing Administration*, 51, 43–48. https://doi.org/10.1097/NNA.0000000000000965.

Sensmeier, J., & Anderson, C. (2020). Tracking the impact of nursing informatics. *Nursing Management*, 51(9), 50–53. https://doi.org/10.1097/01.NUMA.0000694880.86685.c1.

Sittig, D. F., Wright, A., Coiera, E., Magrabi, F., Ratwani, R., Bates, D. W., & Singh, H. (2018). Current challenges in health information technology–related patient safety. *Health Informatics Journal*, 26(1), 181–189. https://doi.org/10.1177/1460458218814893.

Staggers, N., & Thompson, C. B. (2002). The evolution of definitions for nursing informatics: A critical analysis and revised definition. *Journal of the American Medical Informatics Association: JAMIA*, 9(3), 255–261. https://doi.org/10.1197/jamia.m0946.

The Joint Commission. (2021). The Record of Care, Treatment, and Services. *Comprehensive Accreditation Manual for Hospitals*. Retrieved from https://e-dition.jcrinc.com/MainContent.aspx.

The Joint Commission (TJC). (2020). *Facts about the Joint Commission*. Retrieved from https://www.jointcommission.org/about-us/facts-about-the-joint-commission/.

The Joint Commission (TJC). (2015). *Sentinel event alert: Safe use of health information technology.* Retrieved from https://www.jointcommission.org/-/media/tjc/documents/resources/patient-safety-topics/sentinel-event/sea_54_hit_4_26_16.pdf.

Thompson, K. M., Swanson, K. M., Cox, D. L., Kirchner, R. B., Russell, J. J., Wermers, R. A., Storlie, C. B., Johnson, M. G., & Naessens, J. M. (2018). Implementation of bar-code medication administration to reduce patient harm. *Mayo Clinic Proceedings: Innovations, Quality & Outcomes, 2*(4), 342–351. https://doi.org/10.1016/j.mayocpiqo.2018.09.001.

Tolley, C. L., Forde, N. E., Coffey, K. L., Sittig, D. F., Ash, J. S., Husband, A. K., Bates, D. W., & Slight, S. P. (2018). Factors contributing to medication errors made when using computerized order entry in pediatrics: A systematic review. *Journal of the American Medical Informatics Association, 25*(5), 575–584. https://doi.org/10.1093/jamia/ocx124.

U.S. Department of Health and Human Services (DHHS). (2017). *HITECH Act Enforcement Interim Final Rule.* Retrieved from https://www.hhs.gov/hipaa/for-professionals/special-topics/hitech-act-enforcement-interim-final-rule/index.html.

U.S. Department of Health & Human Services. (2020). *The security rule.* HHS.gov. Retrieved from https://www.hhs.gov/hipaa/for-professionals/security/index.html.

van der Veen, W., van den Bemt, P., Wouters, H., Bates, D. W., Twisk, J., de Gier, J. J., Taxis, K., BCMA Study Group, Duyvendak, M., Luttikhuis, K. O., Ros, J., Vasbinder, E. C., Atrafi, M., Brasse, B., & Mangelaars, I. (2018). Association between workarounds and medication administration errors in bar-code-assisted medication administration in hospitals. *Journal of the American Medical Informatics Association, 25*(4), 385–392. https://doi.org/10.1093/jamia/ocx077.

Williams, L. S., Johnson, E., Armaignac, D. L., Nemeth, L. S., & Magwood, G. S. (2019). A mixed methods study of tele-ICU nursing interventions to prevent failure to rescue of patients in critical care. *Telemedicine and e-Health, 25*(5), 369–379. https://doi.org/10.1089/tmj.2018.0086.

York, J. B., Cardoso, M. Z., Azuma, D. S., Beam, K. S., Binney, G. G., & Weingart, S. N. (2019). Computerized physician order entry in the neonatal intensive care unit: A narrative review. *Applied Clinical Informatics, 10*(3), 487–494. https://doi.org/10.1055/s-0039-1692475.

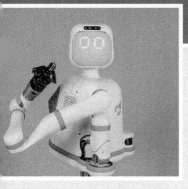

18

Artificial Intelligence

Richard Booth, Gillian Strudwick, Ryan Chan, and Edmund Walsh

ANTICIPATED LEARNING OUTCOMES

- Explore the evolving relationship between humans and emergent digital technology.
- Examine how the contemporary roles and knowledge exercised by nurses may be evolved or changed by intelligent, emergent digital technologies over the coming decades.

- Reflect on implications for nursing leadership to guide and steward aspects of the profession in digital healthcare ecosystems of the future.

KEY TERMS

artificial intelligence	data	knowledge automation
automation of inequities	electronic medical records (EMRs)	sociotechnical
barcode medication administration (BCMA)	information knowledge	task automation wisdom

THE CHALLENGE

A teaching hospital located in a large urban setting where I work as the Chief Clinical Informatics Officer implemented a barcode medication administration (BCMA) technology system to support the reduction of medication errors during the administration process. The BCMA system supported the reduction of medication errors by using barcode technology and a scanner to assist nurses with verifying the "rights" of medication administration. In order to use BCMA, nurses would first log in to the electronic health record of the client and then open a function of the electronic health record system that would allow nurses to scan the client's identifier (usually barcoded wristband) and the corresponding medication identifier (usually a barcoded package with the medication in it). If both of these identifiers correctly cross-validated with the medication order details in the administration record, the medication was confirmed by the BCMA system to be safely administered. In theory, many, if not all, of the medication errors that took place during the administration process prior to the implementation of the technology should have been eliminated with the implementation of this system. However, upon review of incident reporting data, medication errors were still occurring at the point of administration that should have been prevented by the BCMA system.

In this particular case, the Director of Clinical Informatics, the Chief Nursing Executive, project teams, and members of the quality and patient safety team and I came together to develop solutions to address these persistent medication errors discovered post-implementation of the BCMA system.

What would you do if you were this nurse?

Gillian Strudwick, RN, PhD, FAMIA
Chief Clinical Informatics Officer & Scientist
Centre for Mental Health and Addiction, Toronto, Ontario

INTRODUCTION

The profession of nursing has positioned significant elements of its tradition, values, and theory of knowledge on the need to provide interpersonal human care. As a core element of the nursing profession, the use of tools and technology to support this humanistic role has generally been viewed positively. We likely have seen the use of tools and technology as assistive either in amplifying the nursing role or evolving its presence. With the increasing use of digital health technology over the last several decades, the nursing profession has experienced shifts in various aspects of its processes and actions related to nursing care. Although the core elements that make up *nursing care* have arguably not changed, many of the processes and actions undertaken by nurses have experienced significant changes as a result of the increasing availability of artificial intelligence.

While nursing continues to play a necessary and important role within healthcare activities, the increasing presence of *intelligent* digital technologies can mimic or replicate certain aspects of human knowledge, wisdom, and actions (McGrow, 2019; Robert, 2019). More commonly referred to as *artificial intelligence*, systems containing this kind of emergent technology can be designed to mimic the various cognitive functions of humans, such as performing specific problem-solving, decision-making, and learning tasks (Booth et al., 2021). Although a certain amount of hype and over-promise remains for what these types of emergent digital technologies may offer for humans, healthcare, and the problems to be solved (Emanuel & Wachter, 2019), their increasing presence across many elements of society have become undeniable. For instance, many Internet technologies now actively utilize self-learning algorithms that can aggregate vast amounts of data about a user (and other users) to generate personalized recommendations and insights (Kumar et al., 2019). Further, the increasing presence of semi-intelligent Internet of Things (IoT) connected technologies—such as smart speakers, wearables, and home automation devices—is a further sign of the increasing embeddedness of technology in everyday activities (Kumar et al., 2019).

Although these types of emergent digital technologies may provide immense value to nursing, the profession has yet to fully grasp the impact and changes these innovations might bring. Further, the nursing profession currently lacks a critical mass of practitioners, educators, researchers, and leaders who understand the benefits, drawbacks, and future implications of these types of emergent digital technologies. We need to translate our everyday experiences into healthcare and project into the future to appreciate what lies ahead regarding the potential impact on the care we can deliver.

NURSING'S RELATIONSHIP WITH TECHNOLOGY—CURRENT DAY

Historically, nurse scholars spent considerable energy over the last several decades exploring aspects of the nursing role and its intersection with technology used in practice (Barnard & Sandelowski, 2001; Fagerhaugh et al., 1980; Henderson, 1985; Saba, 2001; Strudwick & McGillis Hall, 2015). While disagreements remain about the value and importance of technology, the view for patient care is generally positive (Barnard, 2016). Commonly, technology in the nursing profession has been conceptualized in a mechanical or industrialized sense—as being used by nurses as a mere tool or device through which nursing action can be completed, made more efficient, or improved in some way. This conceptualization of technology is logical and congruent from a humanistic lens—since technology is "not human." While this socially deterministic informed conceptualization of technology's role within healthcare is still common today, it represents a somewhat constrained interpretation of nursing's relationship with technological actors, especially moving into the future. Given the blurring and embeddedness of technology into various elements of society and everyday use, it has become increasingly difficult to separate actions conducted by humans from actions completed by nonhuman actors, such as digital technologies (Orlikowski, 2010).

Health technologies, such as electronic medical records (EMR), barcode medication administration (BCMA) systems, and other point-of-care technologies used in practice, have been found to change nursing practice and processes in both intended and unintended ways (Gephart et al., 2015). A seminal paper by Koppel et al. (2005) highlighted how a BCMA system implemented at a healthcare organization generated numerous *new* types of medication errors. These new medication errors directly resulted from the redevelopment of processes and workflow brought about by the implementation of BCMA, which replaced previous paper-based medication administration processes. Since the work of Koppel et al. (2005), an increasing recognition of *technology* can and will influence the actions of humans in both intended and unintended ways. Considerable research has been completed about unintended consequences related to health technology (Ash et al., 2007; Gephart et al., 2015; Snowden & Kolb, 2016). However, the translation of these insights into nursing practice has been slow.

Although we can conceptualize and *view* the nuanced relationship humans have with technology in many ways, we suggest a sociotechnical systems lens to better understand this relationship (Berg et al., 2003). Sociotechnical systems is a lineage of inquiry arising from post-war (World War II) coal mining research, which explored how the work practices, regulations, and design forces impacted mining activity in Britain (Trist, 1981). A more recent development of this theoretical lens generally aims to consider how humans and technical systems interrelate and apply forces on each other (Sittig & Singh, 2010) (see Theory Box). In essence, technology can influence human social systems and humans can reciprocally influence technology. Although this reciprocal human (social) and technology (technical) relationship seems straightforward, using this lens to unpack everyday actions and phenomena can result in uncovering various insights that would remain hidden if viewing reality only through either a humanistic or socially deterministic lens (Booth et al., 2016).

While traditional reflections of technology representing neutral tools or devices used by nurses in care delivery may have sufficed previously, these constrained conceptualizations will become problematic for the profession in the future due to the increasing presence of emergent digital technologies. As is true of other professions and roles in society, nursing is susceptible to technological change. Examples arising from the COVID-19 pandemic clearly demonstrated that many human tasks and behaviors once thought to be possible only through face-to-face or physically based actions have become virtualized due to necessity (Vargo et al., 2020; Webster, 2020; Wosik et al., 2020). With the effects brought about by the COVID-19 pandemic, the role and integration of technology into all facets of nursing and healthcare will become more robust in the coming decades—including the fluid relationship that humans will have with various intelligent technologies.

DATA, INFORMATION, KNOWLEDGE, AND WISDOM

Before undertaking further discussion of intelligent emergent digital technologies, we need to first understand the importance of the terms *data*, *information*, *knowledge*, and *wisdom* as related to technology used in nursing practice. According to Matney et al. (2011), the term data refers to the smallest unit of insight, commonly presented without background context, and possesses little meaning in isolation from other data. Information is described by Matney et al. (2011) as "data plus meaning" (p. 8). Therefore, information could be conceived as data that has been further contextualized to possess meaning. For instance, the number 110 and 70 are both meaningless data. If the numbers of 110 and 70 are placed within the context and alignment of representing a blood pressure reading measured in millimeters of mercury (mm Hg), then the 110 and 70 can become evolved into information. While 110 and 70 may represent elements of a blood pressure measurement, it is knowledge that allows a practitioner to rationalize through the information, and promote the 110 and 70 in light of the correct context (i.e., systolic, diastolic measurements) and reasoning into knowledge. At this level, *knowledge* is "information that has been synthesized so

THEORY BOX

Sociotechnical Systems

Theory/Contributor	Key Idea	Application to Practice
Berg et al., (2003); Sittig and Singh (2010)	Technology can influence human social systems; conversely, humans and social systems can influence the roles and use of technology. Examining this dynamic relationship uncovers new insights.	As new technologies are introduced into practice, they affect how nurses perform and that performance can affect or alter the technology. Moxi, as an example, has learned to interact with patients in socially intelligent ways due to its self-learning abilities.

that relationships are identified and formalized" (p. 8). In this way, practitioners are able to use both tacit and explicit ways of interpreting knowledge to appreciate that these two numbers represent a blood pressure reading of 110/70 mm Hg—which, in many clinical situations, would represent a normal blood pressure reading of a healthy individual. While knowledge is one of the higher levels of insight that a practitioner can possess, the extension to wisdom takes actualized knowledge and uses this insight to "manage and solve human problems" (p. 8). Therefore, knowing a blood pressure of 110/70 mm Hg was within a normal range would allow a clinician to execute wisdom traits and actions to manage the care of a patient—including continuing clinical treatment and interventions for a patient presentation in which a blood pressure of 110/70 mmHg is deemed normal. See Table 18.1 for a summary.

This cascading continuum of data-information-knowledge-wisdom, while appearing logical, is

TABLE 18.1 Data, Information, Knowledge and Wisdom

Term	Meaning	Example
Data	Smallest unit of insight	The number 150
Information	Data plus meaning	150 mm Hg
Knowledge	Synthesized information so that relationships are identified and formalized	Potentially elevated systolic blood pressure value for this patient
Wisdom	Uses knowledge to manage and solve human problems	Further assessment is needed and additional information should be gathered related to the past presence of hypertension, its etiology, and other patient-specific factors and context that may be important for consideration

extremely important when exploring digital health technology, especially with some of the modern technologies present today. Unfortunately, many of the digital health technologies used by nurses today lack sensitivity to various elements of nursing knowledge and wisdom. Because knowledge and wisdom are extremely difficult attributes to automate, health technology systems commonly attempt to utilize information-level attributes in their programming and logic. For instance, the use of a BCMA technology assists in the automation and process control of *information* elements, such as compliance rates related to medication/barcode scanning, time of medication administration, and dosage of medication. While BCMA systems can assist in preventing certain types of information-related errors from occurring (e.g., various types of medication contraindications; incorrect route, time, dosages; or allergies), these types of systems are generally unable to fully synthesize information with other types of information not contained within the BCMA system. This inability to merge different and relevant types of disparate information (e.g., other clinical assessment data, patient presentation, and vital signs) can prevent the generation of higher-order knowledge attributes related to the medication administration process. Because many digital health technologies currently lack the ability to functionally replicate or mimic the knowledge and/or wisdom abilities of human nurses, these technologies focus almost purely on automating *information* elements of a patient's care and situation. Because information-level insights commonly lack higher fidelity, they are unable to relate one finding with the whole of a patient's situation. The Research Perspective illustrates an example of this.

While it may be easy to fault the programmers, developers, and vendors of health technology for generating systems that fail to endorse or amplify aspects of nursing knowledge and wisdom, this type of critique would be unfairly labelled. The types of knowledge and wisdom brought by nurses is extremely difficult to functionally replicate within technology. To date, there are increasing examples of published prototypical digital health technologies can *think* or *generate decisions* like a human clinician for isolated or specific situations (e.g., decision support related to sepsis prediction and treatment) (Muralitharan et al., 2021; Nemati et al., 2018; Vargo et al., 2020; Wang et al., 2020). While still relatively rare in healthcare, other sectors of society have been using intelligent technological systems to generate knowledge- and wisdom-level decisions. For instance, the nearly

RESEARCH PERSPECTIVE

Resource: Hong, J. Y., Ivory, C. H., VanHouten, C. B., Simpson, C. L., & Novak, L. L. (2021). Disappearing expertise in clinical automation: Barcode medication administration and nurse autonomy. *Journal of the American Medical Informatics Association, 28*(2), 232–238.

This study examined nurses' administration of medications using a BCMA system. Using a qualitative observation method, the researchers conducted 20 hours of observation on an inpatient clinical unit, 9 interviews with nurses working on the observed inpatient unit, and 18 additional interviews with nurses from a variety of other clinical settings. After qualitative data coding and analysis, the researchers uncovered a variety of thematic interpretations of nursing process as related to BCMA technology. For instance, the authors determined that the BCMA system viewed nurses as "doers" rather than "knowledge workers" (p. 236). Thus, aspects of the nurses' expertise and process autonomy related to medication administration were compromised by the various functions of the BCMA technology that enforced strict and inflexible workflow requirements.

Implications for Practice

Since much of nurses' knowledge translates into actions they take (i.e., such as administration of medications, dressing changes, suctioning, and more), clinical technology that seeks to automate various aspects of nursing processes may not capture the complexity of the knowledge that precedes or accompanies those acts, and acknowledge only the tasks themselves. This reinforces the need to better understand aspects related to the complexity of the nursing role, including what nurses do within practice from both social and technical perspectives; the professional and legal implications of practice, mediated through the use of healthcare technology; and other contextually based interpretations of the role (e.g., health system, culture, region of the world). Nurses have to be prepared to advocate for the complexity of their roles and the care they provide to patients.

---

omnipresent use of Internet personalization technologies that operate in the background of virtually all social media and eCommerce platforms could be conceived as exemplars of technological systems that can generate knowledge-level decisions and recommendations (Kumar et al., 2019). Although these types of technology are still in early development within many healthcare settings, these forms of innovations are expected to become more robust and present in the coming years. This understanding of moving from data to information to knowledge to wisdom is consistent with the American Association of Colleges of Nursing (AACN) *Essentials* competency of using information and communication technology to gather data, create information, and generate knowledge (AACN, 2021).

DATA, INFORMATION, KNOWLEDGE, AND WISDOM—IN THE FUTURE

Contemporary digital health technologies used in nursing practice commonly seek to automate various information-level attributes of clinical processes and nursing tasks. The current inability of these systems to embrace or replicate knowledge attributes (let alone wisdom) is a significant limitation of many current-day health technologies. Regardless, moving into the future,

a growing repertoire of emergent digital technologies will reshape how the profession views the generation of knowledge and wisdom to support practice. For instance, the increasing omnipresence of artificial intelligence (AI) and other process automation technologies (e.g., robotics) are innovations that will become more prevalent in healthcare environments over the next few decades (Pepito & Locsin, 2019). Nurses need to prepare for the eventual infusion of systems that possess knowledge-generating capabilities such as those found with AI. Significant thought leadership and preliminary evidence generated in the academic literature suggest that the wider-scale adoption of these kinds of intelligent systems is in the not-too-distant future (Archibald & Barnard, 2018; Booth et al., 2021; Buchanan et al., 2020, 2021; Pepito & Locsin, 2019; Strudwick et al., 2020)

EXERCISE 18.1 Consider some complex task you did most recently in the clinical area. Hypothesize what part(s) of the task might be changed, augmented, or replaced by AI. What are those elements? How will that help you in delivering care if some element of AI aided, augmented, or replaced those parts of the care? Could the whole task be replaced by AI? If so, what would the role of the nurse be related to the task?

WHAT IS ARTIFICIAL INTELLIGENCE?

AI is defined as "different forms of machines or digital systems that mimic the cognitive functions of a human, including actions like problem-solving, decision-making, and learning" (Booth et al., 2021, p. 402). Commonly, AI has also been used as a monolithic term to describe a variety of different types of intelligent systems and their related processes, including the subfields of machine learning, cognitive computing, and deep learning (Booth et al., 2021). Due to the ability of various applications that contain AI to self-learn or complete cognitive tasks once only possible by humans, excitement within the healthcare sector to leverage these technologies to assist in insight generation and other decision-support functions to support care is growing.

In general, AI possesses great potential to assist nurses in a variety of cognitive and decision-making tasks. To date, various publications and media reports show the promise of these kinds of cognitive technologies (Yu et al., 2018). Regardless, as described in the preceding sections, technology of all types can influence social systems and, reciprocally, all social systems can influence technological actors. Due to the relative newness of AI in modern healthcare settings, it is still too early to fully understand how emergent technology containing AI will influence the profession, patient care, or other elements related to the nursing role. One recently identified consequence of AI is the potential to reinforce aspects of inequity in the insights generated by these kinds of intelligent systems. Known as the automation of inequities, this turn of phrase has become a term used by both researchers and the media to denote the occurrence of when a self-learning technology unintentionally reinforces systematic biases or other types of inequity during its insight generation (Bullock, 2019; Eubanks, 2018). In a seminal report by Obermeyer et al. (2019), an AI-enabled care management system used in an American healthcare context systematically underestimated the healthcare needs of predominantly Black patients, as the Research Perspective shows. Further details of the Obermeyer et al. (2019) analysis can be found in the Research Perspective.

While these sorts of unintended algorithmic amplifications are beginning to be recognized, the potential to reinforce inequities and other systemic biases through the use of self-learning technologies is a concerning realization. Because it is sometimes impossible to reverse-engineer the decision-making logic of some AI technologies, bias infused in the outputs and insights generated by these systems have the potential to spread latently or go undiscovered (Gianfrancesco et al., 2018). With the increasing use of self-learning technologies driven by various AI processes, the nursing profession

RESEARCH PERSPECTIVE

Resource: Obermeyer, Z., Powers, B., Vogeli, C., & Mullainathan, S. (2019). Dissecting racial bias in an algorithm used to manage the health of populations. *Science*, *366*(6464), 447–453.

Obermeyer et al. (2019) discovered that allowing the AI system to use a patient's total *health care costs* as a proxy variable of a patient's *overall health status* resulted in unintended consequences related to the accuracy insights generated by the system. Originally, the developers of the AI system had made the assumption that individuals who had higher healthcare costs would also be high-risk patients from a care management perspective, requiring more intensive case management. However, due to the unequal access to treatment and affordability of healthcare in the United States, Black patients were discovered to be less likely to have a history of health/ medical interventions. Subsequently, their overall healthcare costs were lower, which may misrepresent certain patients' overall health status. The researchers were able to correct this algorithmic bias that was reflective of the systemic biases in the data sources.

Implications for Practice
Future technology developers must recognize the systemic biases contained within data sources in an effort to avoid unintentionally automating systems that ignore or diminish other determinants of health and contextual factors. This area of research is still very much in its infancy. How to manage this at an organizational level has yet to be determined. As a profession that prides itself on social justice and consideration of equity, the implications for practice from a nursing perspective are significant.

must become more adept at understanding the fluid interrelationship between the social and technical aspects of the nursing role and the potential future convergence points with AI systems.

EXERCISE 18.2 As described earlier, emergent digital technology with the ability to generate human-like knowledge-level decisions through data and information is beginning to appear in the healthcare system. As this technology becomes more popular and diffused throughout healthcare systems, what type of relationship will nurses have with these nonhuman, intelligent agents? Will nurses work with these emergent digital technologies in a collaborative fashion, using the best parts of human and nonhuman elements to generate clinical decisions to guide practice? Will there be a subtle shift of certain knowledge elements to AI (e.g., treatment and prognosis delineation and resource allocation)? Or will humans resist the encroaching presence of these types of technologies and begin to actively refuse or work around their use? Hold a discussion with at least three of your colleagues and discuss what you hypothesize the future will hold.

While a range of social- and nursing-centric implications may arise from the further development of AI, a variety of emergent technical consequences impacting aspects of privacy, security, ethics, regulations, and policy also need to be analyzed. As described earlier, the nursing profession has historically focused on *humans* when discussing its action, presence, and value structures. Although this humanistic position is warranted given nursing's philosophical underpinning, future technologies that contain self-learning abilities might challenge these traditional interpretations of action and behavior. Subsequently, when exploring the relationship that nurses currently have with technology, the blurring between human actions and those spread by technology can be at times difficult to separate. For example, a nurse using an EMR likely benefits from the system's ability to draw preexisting metadata and information about a patient (e.g., name, admission and discharge dates, transfer information, and past medical records), its ability to populate various data fields based on other previous entered data, and its ability to provide the environment to digitally document various care records. While at face value this interaction seems simplistic, exploring the nuance between the nurse and the EMR reveals a much more interrelated and complex relationship. If the EMR system were to become disabled or not accessible, many of the processes that were established through its use also become compromised (e.g., electronic documentation and the entering and reviewing of orders). Although the users of EMRs in clinical contexts generally have training related to downtime procedures, the complex and interwoven nature of an EMR system becomes highlighted in situations like this. Various roles of the nurse can be compromised or delayed when an EMR system goes down. Taken one step further, certain aspects of nursing work could be unable to be fully functional until the EMR is brought back online—after all, various actions and functions of the nurse are contingent on the EMR system (and vice versa). Moving into the future, the blurring of human and nonhuman roles will likely become even muddier than the example of a nurse's use of an EMR. With the embedding of AI and other self-learning technologies into clinical technology, it is unclear how essential certain technologies will become to the nursing role and how execution of the role will occur in various clinical contexts. For instance, in future healthcare systems that leverage AI technologies to help amplify or augment aspects of the nursing role, how much of care delivery will be exclusively conducted by humans versus how much of this care will potentially be augmented by technologies in conjunction with human labor?

WHAT IS PROCESS AUTOMATION?

While the word *automation* may seem antithetical to the essence of nursing, nursing has benefited from various aspects of automation over its entire existence as a profession. The word *automation* refers to a substitute for human labor or functions as a term to denote any form of innovation that helps to streamline, control, and make more predictable a given outcome(s) (Booth et al., 2021). The term *process automation technologies* has come to be defined as an innovation that seeks to re-engineer large-scale business operations (Khodambashi, 2013; Martinho et al., 2015). In nursing, many processes (as described earlier) are currently augmented in one fashion or another through elements of automation. Reflecting on nursing's practice over the decades, we can easily identify various apparatuses, processes, or systems that have experienced some form of automation. In fact, all contemporary digital health technologies—including EMR, BCMA, and point-of-care devices—introduce some level of automation on tasks and processes undertaken by nurses. Automation sometimes also occurs in imperceivable or unseen ways—for instance, the placement of supplies and equipment in strategic places on a hospital unit to assist the efficiency and work processes of clinicians; the processing of laboratory specimens; process optimization through Lean/Six Sigma methodologies; and clinician scheduling and patient assignment/triage processes. Aspects of automation have likely always existed across society in an effort to reduce human labor required to complete various tasks and procedures. Like the previous discussion of AI, the use of process automation technologies also presents a range of evolving existential questions for the profession to consider, including (1) how much automation will be tolerated by clinicians and patients?; (2) what types of activities, knowledge, and behaviors can or should be automated?; and (3) what are the intended and unintended consequences of amplifying automation of nursing-centric activities and knowledge? Few concrete answers exist; however, automation that will likely influence the nursing role over the coming decades is listed in Box 18.1. Each is important and will exert influence on the role of nurses in the future.

Task Automation

While the term *task* is sometimes viewed negatively, it would be disingenuous to suggest that nurses do not complete *tasks* in their role and delivery of care to patients. As knowledge workers, nurses need to possess adequate levels of both knowledge and wisdom to execute tasks appropriately, safely, and within acceptable ethical parameters. Many of the tasks completed by nurses are extremely nuanced, requiring skill, judgment, fine motor control, and other types of expertise

---

BOX 18.1 Three Types of Automation Influencing the Nursing Role

1. Task automation
2. Knowledge automation
3. Task–knowledge automation

---

that are difficult to replicate mechanically. For instance, wound care is an extremely knowledge-intense task due to the complexity of wound healing, patient complexity, dressing products, treatment trajectory, and a host of other important clinical and contextual factors. That said, many other tasks that nurses complete likely could be conceived as being of lesser knowledge density but were historically captured by the profession due to necessity, preference, or convenience. Nurses in direct patient care roles can likely identify a range of tasks completed in the care of patients that are not knowledge dense, including the collection of materials and supplies from central supplies, repeated transcription of data and information from various record systems, and other time-consuming activities such as contacting members of the care team and locating missing clinical records or notes. These tasks are not beneath a nurse, nor do they lack intrinsic value. However, in light of emergent digital health technologies containing AI and automation functionalities, contemporary tasks undertaken by nurses that do not add value to the profession or patient care should be thoroughly examined. Additionally, as we learned during the pandemic, these tasks are an extreme cost for expensive personnel to be performing. We know, too, that AI has become an integral part of screening applicants for open positions with positive results in terms of quicker decisions to hire times.

Current examples of robotics within healthcare environments can conceivably be described as task automating systems. Moxi is a healthcare *cobot* (collaborative robot) that has been described as "a socially intelligent robot that can aid nurses without making humans feel uncomfortable" (Nicholas, 2018). The Moxi robot that can assist nurses with a variety of lower-knowledge tasks, including the collection of supplies, delivering lab samples, distribution of personal protective equipment, and couriering of medications. Moxi, featured in the opening photograph of this chapter, can interact socially with patients and staff and often is seen as a fun feature rather than something that is threatening. Other service drone robots, such as TUG, also boast similar functionalities in terms of being able to ferry equipment and supplies around a healthcare environment autonomously (UNC Health Care, 2018) (see Fig. 18.1). Numerous other task automation robotics and systems exist or

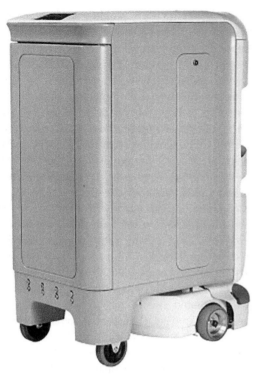

Fig. 18.1 The TUG robot delivers supplies to units to assist nurses in providing timely care.

are being designed for healthcare applications (Carter-Templeton et al., 2018; Maalouf et al., 2018). While he nursing profession is at no immediate risk of being replaced by robotic nurses, the increasing presence of task automation technologies such as Moxi and TUG speaks to an emergent reality that the nursing profession must reflect on, including (1) *what* tasks should be allocated or provided to nonhuman service drones; (2) *who* should decide the tasks that nonhuman service drones will adopt; and (3) *how* should service drone robots and other task automation technologies be factored into the clinical processes, care models, and health system delivery attributes of the future. At this point, many task automation robots are limited in functionality (e.g., completing low-knowledge tasks that are either repetitive or predictable). Therefore, the nursing profession must begin to consider the participation of nonhuman robotics and other task automation innovations in all future strategic planning, as their presence and functional abilities will likely only increase in the coming years.

Knowledge Automation

The augmentation of human knowledge through and with AI technology is already reality. In the future, the seamless integration of various emergent digital health technologies containing AI is almost guaranteed in clinical environments. Therefore, much like task automation, exploring the future implications of nursing knowledge automation is a needed activity within the profession. Currently, numerous prototypical emergent digital health technologies contain AI. These technologies use self-learning capabilities to help generate recommendations or insights from large datasets for human-level review. For instance, advanced clinical decision support (CDS) tools can be enhanced. Unlike other legacy CDS, which uses predetermined and static decision logic to generate insights for users, the CDS described by Cato et al. (2020) leveraged AI to provide clinicians with sepsis alerts and prompts related to a patient's risk for clinical deterioration. Although the CDS was able to functionally replicate aspects of clinician knowledge in the way the system processed and presented risk factors related to sepsis, the authors clearly state that the system was "designed to augment clinical expertise instead of replacing it" (p. 28). Subsequently, a human clinician using the CDS is free to ignore, qualify, or accept the advice provided by the system.

Knowledge automation can occur in very subtle and innocuous ways. Thus, the profession needs to remain vigilant to the intended and unintended consequences of such technology. Since AI-supported CDS has the ability to sway or influence the decision-making of humans, an entire cascade of previously established ways of knowing related to how nurses enact clinical decision-making may need to be reconceptualized. Emerging research has demonstrated that intelligent systems containing AI can actively shape and influence decision-making of humans (Araujo et al., 2020). Historically, nursing discourse exploring clinical decision-making has viewed technological actors as largely static and nonparticipatory in the decision-making process (Melin-Johansson et al., 2017; Nibbelink & Brewer, 2018). As demonstrated by the Cato et al. (2020) example, newer AI-driven CDS technology is *far* from neutral in the process of clinical decision-making and may unintentionally sway human behavior and actions. To date, work exploring how AI-powered devices automate aspects of knowledge generation and their influence on clinician decision-making has yet to be generated en masse. Regardless, with the inevitable scaling of technologies like the CDS described by Cato et al. (2020), conversation within the profession must occur regarding how humans work with various technologies that automate aspects of knowledge generation used to inform and guide practice decisions. This type of exploration of the intended and unintended consequences of knowledge automation systems should be an immediate priority for the profession.

Task-Knowledge Automation

Various process automation activities currently exist within the profession and are likely going to increase in both complexity and embeddedness in the coming decades. Therefore, the profession must undertake philosophical reflections about what will be the important attributes of nursing in the future. The automation of various nursing tasks and knowledge is probable. What remains less clear is *how* the profession will be involved in guiding and stewarding changes to leverage, or refute, various aspects of intelligent process automation technologies. Insights drawn from other disciplines can be useful in this regard. For instance, as described by Gutelius and Theodore (2019), automation used within warehouse and industrial settings had promised to alleviate arduous activities performed by workers in these environments. However, they suggest that productivity gains derived from automation will likely be coupled with corresponding work intensification in other tasks and activities. Although significant differences in complexity, knowledge requirements, and context exist between warehouse and healthcare settings, the nursing profession must remain cognizant of the various intended and unintended consequences of automation of both tasks and knowledge. Further, while *task* and *knowledge* automation elements were purposefully divided into two sections earlier in this chapter, in likelihood, *emergent digital technology of the future will potentially seamlessly blur together task completion and knowledge attributes*. Emergent exemplars of this combination can already be seen through the use of out-of-the-loop/on-the-loop autonomous drone technology and self-driving vehicles that seamlessly execute the completion of both tasks and knowledge generation (Agrawal et al., 2020; Goodall, 2016). Other more subtle task-knowledge-enabling technologies such as automated speech recognition systems that can execute tasks (e.g., clinical chart queries, clinical documentation, and voice transcription for emails or clinical records) and certain knowledge activities (e.g., parsing medical terminology from the voice record and generating basic notes for the clinical record) have begun to emerge in specific clinical domains where nurses work (Tims et al., 2020). Subsequently, the growing body of literature exploring the synergistic relationships between task and knowledge automation processes using artificial intelligence is an area of growing importance for a variety of industries, including healthcare (Coombs et al., 2020; Esmaeilzadeh et al., 2021). Fig. 18.2 provides a conceptual taxonomy depiction of activities and processes completed by nurses that involve various levels of task and knowledge complexities.

When contemplating future implications of automation of tasks and knowledge by emergent digital technologies, the authors recommend thinking about how the process of executing a task is driven by the insight of various knowledge structures. Knowledge is required to complete tasks and tasks require knowledge to be completed successfully. Future emergent digital technology that is able to juggle aspects of both task and knowledge attributes in their operations will require completely new interpretations of how nursing practice, healthcare delivery, liability, and ethics (among others) are actualized and interpreted.

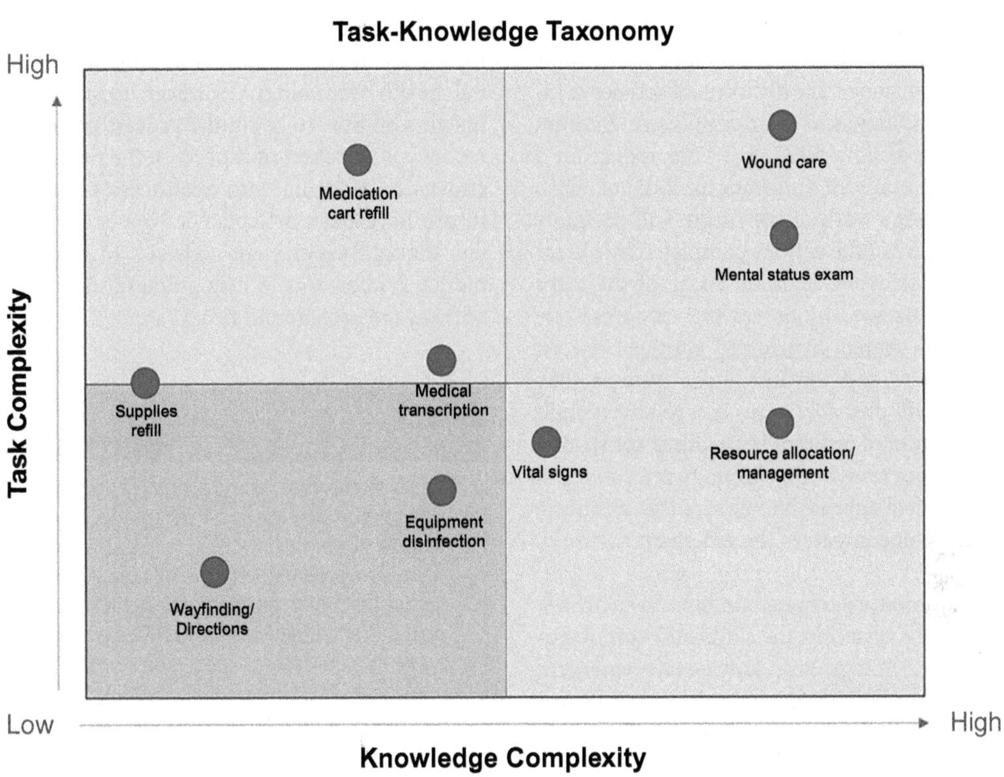

Task-Knowledge Taxonomy

Fig. 18.2 A Conceptual Taxonomy. This diagram is a conceptual overview that invites practitioners to consider and discuss the potential interconnectedness between task and knowledge and how future emergent healthcare technology with both task and knowledge abilities may influence certain nursing activities and processes. Note that this diagram should be viewed as an *oversimplification* of various activities that require both tasks and knowledge. It is recommended to be a conversation starter regarding the potential automation of various task and knowledge activities commonly undertaken by nurses and should not be interpreted in absolute or generalizable terms.

WHAT WILL NURSING LEADERSHIP NEED TO LOOK LIKE IN AN AUTOMATED AND AI-INFUSED WORK ENVIRONMENT?

All nurses will need to consider what aspects of knowledge work and tasks will be augmented by AI and process automation technologies if we want to be prepared for the future. The question is not *if* these forms of innovations will start to emerge en masse within healthcare settings but *when*. Therefore, we must begin to lay the foundational blueprints of the structure, processes, and operations of healthcare systems of the future. As practitioners who exist within all facets of the healthcare systems, nurses are ideally positioned to consult on

numerous elements related to patient care, population health, and wellness.

To do this, nurses need to develop their own personal conceptual framework from which to scaffold the increasing presence and power of AI and process automation technologies. Using past informatics project implementations (e.g., EMR systems/modules, point-of-care technology, and BCMA) as a template, it is probable that the growing diffusion of emergent digital technologies will occur over a decade or two and be filled with similar issues related to cumbersome project and change management, delays, and numerous unintended consequences. Even with the potential challenges that will be faced during implementation and stabilization, the subtle and fluid nature from which these innovations can invest themselves into processes and action is worth noting. For instance, the diffusion of self-serve kiosks, mobile technology, and the omnipresent Internet serve as examples of how difficult it is to reflect on a time when those kinds of innovations did *not* exist. Therefore, knowledge work of the future will probably look similar to many of the actions completed by nurses today, but with a sizable exception. Some of the tasks and knowledge possessed by nurses may progressively become viewed as shared, hybridized entities between human practitioners and the intelligent systems they use. This change will probably occur in a relatively fluid and nonconfrontational fashion. If anything, remaining cognizant that these forms of technology are *coming* is likely the best tactical approach to ensure that all future strategic planning encompasses the emergent nature of these systems.

Beyond situational awareness, we also need to become more actively versed in the skills and competencies related to technology and future-state emergent digital technologies. Unfortunately, we do not all possess the appropriate knowledge, skill sets, and comfort to engage in these important discussions in meaningful ways (Strudwick et al., 2019a). This could have negative consequences for the nursing profession and patient care. All levels of nursing education and continuing education programs, in which nurses often enroll, will require deeper focus on traditional informatics competencies (e.g., current state health technology such as EMR and BCMA). Nursing education must also provide insight on future healthcare systems that contain nonhuman actors with the ability to independently or semi-independently complete tasks and generate knowledge.

Drawing from experiences of other industries and sectors (Marr, 2018; Pichler et al., 2017), nurses will need to conceptualize and plan for a future that increasingly includes the everyday use and embeddedness of AI and process automation technologies. Nurses will need to ensure that any types of AI and process automation technology adopted for use in the nursing role and patient care has been thoroughly inspected for compatibility with how the nursing profession wishes to exist in the future. Further, the nursing profession will require leaders who possess the knowledge, skills, and expertise to consult on the development and implementation of various emergent digital health technologies. As outlined by Buchanan et al. (2020, 2021), the nursing profession has an important leadership role in transforming healthcare systems that will be utilizing emergent digital health technology. However, to date, few guiding insights on how to begin the process of acceptance and reconceptualization of aspects of the nursing profession and its relationship with healthcare ecosystems of the future have been articulated. Nurses can undertake a few thought-experiment activities to begin generating mental frameworks to help guide future practice. Some of these are provided in Box 18.2.

BOX 18.2   Thought-Experiment Activities to Guide Future Practice

1. Explore, examine, and deconstruct your current practice from a perspective that appreciates the roles of socially driven actors (i.e., clinicians, staff, patients, policy, governance, and so on) and those of technical actors (i.e., inhouse technical systems, societal technology trends, and so forth). While doing this, identify areas of convergence between human and technical roles, and where future synergy might occur related to the use or augmentation of previous work processes and practices through AI and automation technology.

2. Reflect on the task and knowledge attributes brought by nurses in modern day. Seek to identify tasks that are lower knowledge density in nature to execute. After identification of these tasks, consider whether removal or augmentation of these tasks to others or nonhuman technical actors would result in significant unintended consequences. For instance, even the most mundane clinical process may possess a host of latent protective forces that are never visible or immediately transparent. By tracing action and activity through human and technical actors in a given process, clearer interpretations of how processes are completed can be accomplished and insight into various hidden protective factors, opportunities for synergy, and other efficiencies may be discovered.

3. Reconceptualize what future nursing leadership roles may look like in the not-too-distant future. Will span of control and governance models require retrofitting to include nonhuman agents that are intelligent and/or requisite in critical operations? How should these technical actors be identified, labelled, and described in policy and governance materials? What sorts of liability, ethics, sustainability, and other aspects need to be revised in light of emergent digital technology that has the ability to generate knowledge and complete tasks?

CONCLUSION

Nurses need to reflect on their practice and how they conceptualize the forecast impacts of emergent digital technologies on healthcare system structures and processes. Remaining cognizant that these types of technology are quickly approaching (and, in some situations, already present) is the first and most important requirement. The onus will be placed on us to generate our own interpretations of the role that AI and process automation technologies will play within all aspects of healthcare delivery. A future healthcare system utilizing various types of emergent digital technologies will require not only knowledge of the technical systems but, more importantly, also require a deeper understanding of the social impacts of these systems. Leading change will require a robust set of skills to steward the safe and ethical use of these emergent technologies. Given that a future-state healthcare system will likely blur various social and technical aspects of care together in sometimes subtle and innocuous ways, leaders in this environment will be required to support staff through these changes.

In many ways, the coming advances in AI and process automation technology will challenge the nursing profession and its leadership to consider what the nursing role should be now and into the future. While nursing discourse has spent considerable time exploring the knowledge, roles, and abilities of nursing, the need for nurses and leadership to become versed in data science, artificial intelligence, and other robotic/process automation sciences is an area of immediate need (Buchanan et al., 2020, 2021; Remus, 2016; Risling, 2017). Without recasting the role and position of nursing for future practice *with* and *within* emergent digital health technologies, the profession will miss an important opportunity to steward and develop future-state healthcare practices and systems. What this may look like in the future is currently unclear. The development of new nursing leadership and practice roles that leverage the powers brought about by emergent digital technology, while retaining the historically fixed importance of nursing's ideas regarding patient-centered and compassionate care, will be the immediate challenge brought by this new human–technology dynamic. We are optimistic that the profession will rise to meet this need.

THE SOLUTION

The Director of Clinical Informatics, the Chief Nursing Executive, myself, project team members, and members of the quality and patient safety team convened to discuss how we would rectify the medication errors that were still occurring even with the BCMA system in place. It appeared that most medication errors occurred after the BCMA system was overridden by a nurse. We also examined the barriers and facilitators to using the system from social and technical dimensions (i.e., people, processes, technology). To help with this quality improvement process, nurses from across the organization were engaged in this project to both learn from their experiences but also gain their insights regarding various reasons and issues faced day to day when using the BCMA system. For instance, we found wireless Internet dead zones in some areas of the organization where the BCMA system needed to be used. Due to the BCMA system's reliance on an Internet connection, we found that during this type of eventuality, nurses sometimes opted to override the system.

We also found that we did not have enough barcode scanners during busy medication administration times and many patients didn't always wear their barcoded wristbands. So, once again, the nurses sometimes overrode the BCMA system.

When we shared the data with the clinical managers and other leadership, approaches were taken to attempt to address the challenges noted in the BCMA system's usage. This allowed us to improve our education, secure more equipment, provide better labeling, and decrease the number of overrides. All of that helped to reduce medication errors.

Would this be a suitable approach for you? Why?

Gillian Strudwick

REFLECTION

This chapter poses many ideas, some not yet borne out by reality because much of AI remains to be developed. We may simply be limited by our imagination! Because nursing relies so heavily on many complexities in the knowledge and wisdom realms, we have to ask ourselves whether the profession could be *left out* altogether as digital health technology evolves. Consider what nurses must do to ensure that we are included in the expansion of digital technology and how we can convince colleagues of AI's benefits to patients. How do you feel about AI yourself? Are you comfortable sharing your thinking with a device? Can you conceive of being less involved with patients? Record your reflection for future consideration.

BEST PRACTICES

While the evidence related to the influence of AI in healthcare processes and nursing is still being generated, sufficient insights exist from other industries to help generate recommendations for nursing moving into the future. What should nurses do? Consider the following:

Reflect on tasks that you do on a daily basis and what portions of them could be augmented or improved through the addition of an AI-enabled technology.

Using devices such as TUG or Moxi can improve nurses' efficiency by reducing the number of retrieval trips to various areas when supplies on a unit are inadequate. Determining high usage times and areas for such equipment is critical to determining where such devices have priority usage. Having at least a core of nurses engaged in the work that leads to improvement of AI-related devices ensures that the thinking of nurses is a part of the developmental process.

TIPS TO PREPARE FOR THE COMING OF ARTIFICIAL INTELLIGENCE IN NURSING

- Remain cognizant of various forms of technology containing AI and other automation elements to come or already functional within some of the systems you use both at work and home.
- Monitor what AI and related technologies are continuing to be embedded into a variety of processes and activities, sometimes in innocuous ways.

- Be involved in the design, use, and leveraging of various types of AI and other automation technologies to fully participate in the digital healthcare ecosystems of the future.
- Seek out the AI displays at conferences to learn what the new developments are.

REFERENCES

Agrawal, A., Abraham, S., Burger, B., Christine, C., Fraser, L., Hoeksema, J., & Cox, S. (2020). The next generation of human-drone partnerships: Co-designing an emergency response system. *ArXiv*, 1–13. https://arxiv.org/abs/2001.03849.

American Association of Colleges of Nursing (AACN). (2021). *The essentials: Core competencies for professional nursing education*. Washington, DC: Author.

Araujo, T., Helberger, N., Kruikemeier, S., & de Vreese, C. H. (2020). In AI we trust? Perceptions about automated decision-making by artificial intelligence. *AI and Society*, 35(3), 611–623. https://doi.org/10.1007/s00146-019-00931-w.

Archibald, M. M., & Barnard, A. (2018). Futurism in nursing: Technology, robotics and the fundamentals of care. *Journal of Clinical Nursing*, 27(11–12), 2473–2480. https://doi.org/10.1111/jocn.14081.

Ash, J. S., Sittig, D. F., Dykstra, R. H., Guappone, K., Carpenter, J. D., & Seshadri, V. (2007). Categorizing the unintended sociotechnical consequences of computerized provider order entry. *International Journal of Medical Informatics*, 76(Suppl 1), S21–S27. https://doi.org/10.1016/j.ijmedinf.2006.05.017.

Barnard, A. (1997). A critical review of the belief that technology is a neutral object and nurses are its master. *Journal of Advanced Nursing*, 26(1), 126–131.

Barnard, A., & Sandelowski, M. (2001). Technology and humane nursing care: (Ir)reconcilable or invented difference? *Journal of Advanced Nursing*, 34(3), 367–375. https://doi.org/10.1046/j.1365-2648.2001.01768.x.

Barnard, A. (2016). Radical nursing and the emergence of technique as healthcare technology. *Nursing Philosophy*, 17(1), 8–18. https://doi.org/10.1111/nup.12103.

Berg, M., Aarts, J., & Van der Lei, J. (2003). ICT in health care: Sociotechnical approaches. *Methods of Information in Medicine*, 42(4), 297–301.

Booth, R. G., Andrusyszyn, M., Iwasiw, C., Donelle, L., & Compeau, D. (2016). Actor-Network Theory as a socio-technical lens to explore the relationship of nurses and technology in practice: Methodological considerations for nursing research. *Nursing Inquiry*, 23(2), 109–120. https://doi.org/10.1111/nin.12118.

Booth, R., Strudwick, G., McMurray, J., Chan, R., Cotton, K., & Cooke, S. (2021). The future of nursing informatics in a digitally-enabled world. In P. Hussey, & M. Kennedy (Eds.), *Introduction to nursing informatics. health informatics* (pp. 395–417). Springer. https://doi.org/10.1007/978-3-030-58740-6_16.

Buchanan, C., Howitt, M. L., Wilson, R., Booth, R. G., Risling, T., & Bamford, M. (2020). Predicted influences of artificial intelligence on the domains of nursing: Scoping Review. *JMIR Nursing*, 3(1). https://doi.org/10.2196/23939, e23939.

Buchanan, C., Howitt, M. L., Wilson, R., Booth, R. G., Risling, T., & Bamford, M. (2021). Predicted influences of artificial intelligence on nursing education: Scoping Review. *JMIR Nursing*, 4(1), e23933. https://doi.org/10.2196/23933.

Bullock, J. B. (2019). Artificial intelligence, discretion, and bureaucracy. *American Review of Public Administration*, 49(7), 751–761. https://doi.org/10.1177/0275074019856123.

Carter-Templeton, H., Frazier, R. M., Wu, L., Wyatt, H., & T. (2018). Robotics in nursing: A bibliometric analysis. *Journal of Nursing Scholarship*, 50(6), 582–589. https://doi.org/10.1111/jnu.12399.

Cato, K. D., McGrow, K., & Rossetti, S. C. (2020). Transforming clinical data into wisdom. *Nursing Management*, 51(11), 24–30. https://doi.org/10.1097/01.NUMA.0000719396.83518.d6.

Collins, S., Phllips, A., Yen, P.-Y., & Kennedy, M. K. (2017). Nursing informatics competency assessment for the nurse leader: The Delphi study. *JONA: The Journal of Nursing Administration*, 47(4), 212–218. https://doi.org/10.1097/NNA.0000000000000467.

Coombs, C., Hislop, D., Taneva, S. K., & Barnard, S. (2020). The strategic impacts of Intelligent Automation for knowledge and service work: An interdisciplinary review. *Journal of Strategic Information Systems*, 29(4). https://doi.org/10.1016/j.jsis.2020.101600, 101600.

Emanuel, E. J., & Wachter, R. M. (2019). Artificial Intelligence in health care: Will the value match the hype? *JAMA*, 321(23), 2281. https://doi.org/10.1001/jama.2019.4914.

Esmaeilzadeh, P., Mirzaei, T., & Dharanikota, S. (2021). Patients' perceptions toward human–artificial intelligence interaction in health care: Experimental study. *Journal of Medical Internet Research*, 23(11). https://doi.org/10.2196/25856.

Eubanks, V. (2018). *Automating inequality: How high-tech tools profile, police, and punish the poor*. New York: St. Martin's Press.

Fagerhaugh, S., Strauss, A., Suczek, B., & Wiener, C. (1980). The impact of technology on patients, providers, and care patterns. *Nursing Outlook*, 28(11), 666–672.

Gephart, S., Carrington, J. M., & Finley, B. (2015). A systematic review of nurses' experiences with unintended consequences when using the electronic health record. *Nursing Administration Quarterly*, 39(4), 345–356. https://doi.org/10.1097/NAQ.0000000000000119.

Gianfrancesco, M. A., Tamang, S., Yazdany, J., & Schmajuk, G. (2018). Potential biases in machine learning algorithms using electronic health record data. *JAMA Internal Medicine*, 178(11), 1544–1547. https://doi.org/10.1001/jamainternmed.2018.3763.

Goodall, N. J. (2016). When driverless cars kill, it's the code (and the coders) that will be put on trial. *IEEE Spectrum*, 53(6), 28–58.

Gutelius, B., & Theodore, N. (2019). *The future of warehouse work: Technological change in the U.S. logistics industry*. Retrieved from http://laborcenter.berkeley.edu/future-of-warehouse-work.

Henderson, V. A. (1985). The essence of nursing in high technology. *Nursing Administration Quarterly*, 9(4), 1–9. https://doi.org/10.1097/00006216-198500940-00003.

Hong, J. Y., Ivory, C. H., VanHouten, C. B., Simpson, C. L., & Novak, L. L. (2021). Disappearing expertise in clinical automation: Barcode medication administration and nurse autonomy. *Journal of the American Medical Informatics Association*, 28(2), 232–238. https://doi.org/10.1093/jamia/ocaa135.

Khodambashi, S. (2013). Business process re-engineering application in healthcare in a relation to health information systems. *Procedia Technology*, 9(2212), 949–957. https://doi.org/10.1016/j.protcy.2013.12.106.

Koppel, R., Metlay, J. P., Cohen, A., Abaluck, B., Localio, R., Kimmel, S. E., & Strom, B. L. (2005). Role of computerized physician order entry systems in facilitating medication errors. *JAMA: The Journal of the American Medical Association*, 293(10), 1197–1203. https://doi.org/10.1001/jama.293.10.1197.

Kumar, V., Rajan, B., Venkatesan, R., & Lecinski, J. (2019). Understanding the role of artificial intelligence in personalized engagement marketing. *California Management Review*, 61(4), 135–155. https://doi.org/10.1177/0008125619859317.

Maalouf, N., Sidaoui, A., Elhajj, I. H., & Asmar, D. (2018). Robotics in nursing: A Scoping Review. *Journal of Nursing Scholarship*, 50(6), 590–600. https://doi.org/10.1111/jnu.12424.

Marr, B. (2018, August 29). The future of work: Are you ready for smart cobots? *Forbes*. Retrieved from https://www.forbes.com/sites/bernardmarr/2018/08/29/the-future-of-work-are-you-ready-for-smart-cobots.

Martinho, R., Rijo, R., & Nunes, A. (2015). Complexity analysis of a business process automation: Case study on a healthcare organization. *Procedia Computer Science*, 64, 1226–1231. https://doi.org/10.1016/j.procs.2015.08.510.

Matney, S., Brewster, P. J., Sward, K. A., Cloyes, K. G., & Staggers, N. (2011). Philosophical approaches to the nursing informatics data-information-knowledge-wisdom framework. *ANS. Advances in Nursing Science, 34*(1), 6–18. https://doi.org/10.1097/ANS.0b013e3182071813.

McGrow, K. (2019). Artificial intelligence: Essentials for nursing. *Nursing, 49*(9), 46–49. https://doi.org/10.1097/01.NURSE.0000577716.57052.8d.

Melin-Johansson, C., Palmqvist, R., & Rönnberg, L. (2017). Clinical intuition in the nursing process and decision-making—A mixed-studies review. *Journal of Clinical Nursing, 26*(23–24), 3936–3949. https://doi.org/10.1111/jocn.13814.

Muralitharan, S., Nelson, W., Di, S., McGillion, M., Devereaux, P. J., Barr, N. G., & Petch, J. (2021). Machine learning–based early warning systems for clinical deterioration: Systematic scoping review. *Journal of Medical Internet Research, 23*(2). https://doi.org/10.2196/25187.

Nemati, S., Holder, A., Razmi, F., Stanley, M. D., Clifford, G. D., & Buchman, T. G. (2018). An interpretable machine learning model for accurate prediction of sepsis in the ICU. *Critical Care Medicine, 46*(4), 547–553. https://doi.org/10.1097/CCM.0000000000002936.

Nibbelink, C. W., & Brewer, B. B. (2018). Decision-making in nursing practice: An integrative literature review. *Journal of Clinical Nursing, 27*(5–6), 917–928. https://doi.org/10.1111/jocn.14151.

Nicholas, G. (2018, December 17). Nurse robot Moxi gets schooled by Texas nurses. In *ZDNet*. Retrieved from https://www.zdnet.com/article/nurse-robot-moxi-gets-schooled-by-texas-nurses/.

Obermeyer, Z., Powers, B., Vogeli, C., & Mullainathan, S. (2019). Dissecting racial bias in an algorithm used to manage the health of populations. *Science, 366*(6464), 447–453. https://doi.org/10.1126/science.aax2342.

Orlikowski, W. J. (2010). The sociomateriality of organisational life: Considering technology in management research. *Cambridge Journal of Economics, 34*(1), 125–141. https://doi.org/10.1093/cje/bep058.

Pepito, J. A., & Locsin, R. (2019). Can nurses remain relevant in a technologically advanced future? *International Journal of Nursing Sciences, 6*(1), 106–110. https://doi.org/10.1016/j.ijnss.2018.09.013.

Pichler, A., Akkaladevi, S. C., Ikeda, M., Hofmann, M., Plasch, M., Wögerer, C., & Fritz, G. (2017). Towards shared autonomy for robotic tasks in manufacturing. *Procedia Manufacturing, 11*(June), 72–82. https://doi.org/10.1016/j.promfg.2017.07.139.

Remus, S. (2016). The Big Data revolution: Opportunities for Chief Nurse Executives. *Canadian Journal of Nursing Leadership, 28*(4), 18–28.

Risling, T. (2017). Educating the nurses of 2025: Technology trends of the next decade. *Nurse Education in Practice, 22*, 89–92. https://doi.org/10.1016/j.nepr.2016.12.007.

Robert, N. (2019). How artificial intelligence is changing nursing. *Nursing Management (Springhouse), 50*(9), 30–39. https://doi.org/10.1097/01.NUMA.0000578988.56622.21.

Saba, V. (2001). Nursing informatics: Yesterday, today and tomorrow. *International Nursing Review, 48*, 177–187.

Sandelowski, M. (2000). *Devices & desires: Gender, technology, and American nursing*. UNC Press Books.

Sittig, D. F., & Singh, H. (2010). A new sociotechnical model for studying health information technology in complex adaptive healthcare systems. *Quality & Safety in Health Care, 19*, i68–i74. https://doi.org/10.1136/qshc.2010.042085. *Suppl 3*(1).

Snowden, A., & Kolb, H. (2016). Two years of unintended consequences: Introducing an electronic health record system in a hospice in Scotland. *Journal of Clinical Nursing, 26*(9-10), 1414–1427. https://doi.org/10.1111/jocn.13576.

Strudwick, G., & McGillis Hall, L. (2015). Nurse acceptance of electronic health record technology: A literature review. *Journal of Research in Nursing, 20*(7), 596–607. https://doi.org/10.1177/1744987115615658.

Strudwick, G., Nagle, L., Kassam, I., Pahwa, M., & Sequeira, L. (2019a). Informatics competencies for nurse leaders. *JONA: The Journal of Nursing Administration, 49*(6), 323–330. https://doi.org/10.1097/NNA.0000000000000760.

Strudwick, G., Nagle, L. M., Morgan, A., Kennedy, M. A., Currie, L. M., Lo, B., & White, P. (2019b). Adapting and validating informatics competencies for senior nurse leaders in the Canadian context: Results of a Delphi study. *International Journal of Medical Informatics, 129*(June), 211–218. https://doi.org/10.1016/j.ijmedinf.2019.06.012.

Strudwick, G., Wiljer, D., & Inglis, F. (2020). *Nursing and compassionate care in a technological world: A discussion paper*. Toronto, Canada: AMS Healthcare.

Tims, C., Warwick, B., & Burge, T. (2020). *Creating a hands-free voice assistant at Houston Methodist with AWS*. Retrieved from https://aws.amazon.com/blogs/industries/creating-a-hands-free-voice-assistant-at-houston-methodist-with-aws/.

Trist, E. (1981). *The evolution of socio-technical systems: A conceptual framework an an action research program*. Toronto: Ontario Quality of Working Life Centre.

UNC Health Care. (2018). *The TUG robots are coming*. Retrieved from https://news.unchealthcare.org/2018/01/the-tug-robots-are-coming/.

Vargo, D., Zhu, L., Benwell, B., & Yan, Z. (2020). Digital technology use during COVID-19 pandemic: A rapid review. *Human Behavior and Emerging Technologies, 3*(1), 13–24. https://doi.org/10.1002/hbe2.242.

Wang, E., Brenn, B. R., & Matava, C. T. (2020). State of the art in clinical decision support applications in pediatric perioperative medicine. *Current Opinion in Anaesthesiology*, *33*(3), 388–394. https://doi.org/10.1097/ACO.0000000000000850.

Webster, P. (2020). Virtual health care in the era of COVID-19. *The Lancet*, *395*(10231), 1180–1181. https://doi.org/10.1016/S0140-6736(20)30818-7.

Wosik, J., Fudim, M., Cameron, B., Gellad, Z. F., Cho, A., Phinney, D., … Tcheng, J. (2020). Telehealth transformation: COVID-19 and the rise of virtual care. *Journal of the American Medical Informatics Association*, *27*(6), 957–962. https://doi.org/10.1093/jamia/ocaa067.

Yu, K. H., Beam, A. L., & Kohane, I. S. (2018). Artificial intelligence in healthcare. *Nature Biomedical Engineering*, *2*(10), 719–731. https://doi.org/10.1038/s41551-018-0305-z.

19

Managing Costs and Budgets

Sylvain Trepanier

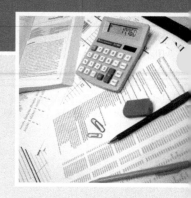

ANTICIPATED LEARNING OUTCOMES

- Evaluate significant factors escalating the costs of healthcare.
- Compare and contrast different reimbursement methods and their incentives to control costs.
- Differentiate costs, charges, and revenue concerning a specified unit of service, such as a visit, hospital stay, or procedure.
- Value why all healthcare organizations must make a profit.
- Give examples of cost considerations for nurses.
- Differentiate between the operating, cash, and capital budgets in terms of purpose and relationships.
- Explain the budgeting process.
- Identify variances on monthly expense reports.

KEY TERMS

budget
budgeting process
capital expenditure budget
capitation
case mix
cash budget
charges
contractual allowance
cost
cost-based reimbursement
cost-based system
cost center

diagnosis-related group (DRG)
fixed costs
full-time equivalent (FTE)
managed care
nonproductive hours
operating budget
organized delivery system (ODS)
payer mix
payers
price
productive hours
productivity

profit
prospective payment system
providers
revenue
unit of service
utilization
value-based purchasing
variable costs
variance
variance analysis

THE CHALLENGE

Flu season is a time when healthcare professionals across the nation prepare for immunizing their communities for the influenza (flu) virus. According to the Centers for Disease Control and Prevention (CDC), the overall burden of flu for the 2018 to 2019 season was estimated at 29 million flu illnesses, 13 million flu-related medical visits, 380,000 flu-related inpatient hospitalizations, and 28,000 flu-related deaths. Charge nurses, nurse managers, or nurse leaders are often asked months before the flu season for their estimated flu vaccine volume (based on historical

INTRODUCTION

Although many nurses will never need to create or manage a budget, all of us need to care about costs. While the public generally values the quality of healthcare, they are concerned about the costs. In our everyday work lives, we seldom pause to consider less expensive ways of enacting care.

Healthcare costs in the United States continue to rise at a rate greater than general inflation. In 2019, for example, Americans spent $3.8 trillion on health care—approximately 17.7% of the gross domestic product (GDP) (Centers for Medicare & Medicaid Services [CMS], 2021).

Despite our vast expenditures, major indicators reveal significant health problems in the United States as well as large disparities in health status related to gender, race, and socioeconomic status (U.S. Department of Health and Human Services, 2021). Our infant mortality rate is among the highest of all industrialized nations, and Black infants die at more than twice the rate of White infants. The average life expectancy is lower than in most developed countries, and men have a life expectancy that is six years less than that of women. One in eight women will develop breast cancer during her lifetime, with Black and Native American women experiencing a much higher death rate than White women. Violence-related injuries are on the rise and unintentional injuries, such as motor vehicle accidents, are a leading cause of death. We are not receiving a high-value return on our healthcare dollar.

The large portion of the GDP spent on healthcare poses problems to the economy in other ways. Funds are diverted from needed social programs such as childcare, housing, education, transportation, and the environment. The price of goods and services is increased; therefore, the country's ability to compete in the international marketplace is compromised. As the amount of the GDP devoted to healthcare expenses rises, the healthcare industry becomes more vulnerable to external influences. This creates a significant concern for a sector that already expresses concerns about being overregulated. Nurses must fully understand the cost of healthcare to ensure the fiscal viability of our healthcare system.

WHAT ESCALATES HEALTHCARE COSTS

Total healthcare costs are a function of the prices and utilization rates of healthcare services (Costs = Price × Utilization; Table 19.1). Price is the rate that healthcare providers set for the services they deliver, such as the hospital rate or physician fee. *Utilization* refers to the quantity or volume of services provided, such as diagnostic tests provided or the number of patient visits.

Price inflation and administrative inefficiency are leading contributors to increased prices for healthcare services. In recent decades, rises in healthcare prices have dramatically outpaced general inflation. Examples of factors that stimulate price inflation are insurance premiums, medical technology, drug costs, health plan administration, and waste. Administrative inefficiency or waste is primarily due to the large numbers of clerical personnel whom organizations use to process reimbursement forms from multiple payers. Nearly $496

TABLE 19.1 Relationship of Price and Utilization Rates to Total Healthcare Costs

Price	× Utilization Rate	= Total Cost	% Change
$1.00	100	$100.00	0%
$1.08[a]	100	$108.00	8.0%
$1.08	105[b]	$113.40	13.4%
$1.08	110[c]	$118.80	18.8%

[a] 8% increase for inflation.
[b] 5% more procedures done.
[c] 10% more procedures done.

billion is spent annually on administrative costs in the U.S. healthcare system (Gee & Spiro, 2019). This single fact indicates why some hospital administrators advocate for the elimination of multiple payers.

Several interrelated factors contribute to the increased use of medical services. These include unnecessary care, consumer attitudes, healthcare financing, pharmaceutical usage, increased cost of drugs, and changing population demographics and disease patterns. *Unnecessary care* is defined as care prescribed that does not contribute to the well-being of a patient. An example is additional laboratory tests that are unrelated to the plan of care.

Our attitudes and behaviors as consumers of healthcare also contribute to rising costs. In general, we prefer to "be fixed" when something goes wrong rather than practice prevention. When we need "fixing," expensive high-tech services typically are perceived as the best care. Many of us still believe that the physician knows best. Thus, we do not seek much information about the costs and effectiveness of different healthcare options. When we do seek knowledge, it is not readily available or understandable. We are also not accustomed to using other, less costly healthcare providers, such as nurse practitioners.

The way healthcare is financed contributes to rising costs. When third-party payers reimburse healthcare, consumers are somewhat insulated from personally experiencing the direct effects of high healthcare costs. However, in most instances, consumers do not have many incentives to consider charges when choosing among providers or using services. Also, the various methods of reimbursement have implications for how providers price and use services.

Evidence of pharmaceutical usage can be seen in advertisements in magazines and on television. No longer do pharmaceutical companies attempt to influence only the prescribers. They go directly to the consumer, who then goes to the prescriber. Because of some specific drug benefit programs, the consumer often is unaware of the total cost of a medication, which may be a "quick fix" (described previously) or a lifestyle enhancement, such as sexual enhancers or skin conditioning.

Changing population demographics also are increasing the volume of health services needed. For example, chronic health problems increase with age, and the number of older adults in America continues to rise. The fastest-growing population is the group aged 85 years and older. The growing societal problems of obesity, heart disease, homelessness, drug addiction, and violence have increased health services. In addition, the COVID-19 pandemic not only impacted healthcare costs but also undermined or closed some businesses in communities around the United States.

HOW HEALTH CARE IS FINANCED

On March 23, 2010, historic healthcare reform was signed into law—the Patient Protection and Affordable Care Act (ACA). This phased-in legislation includes some features that take effect quickly and others that were delayed for several years. Furthermore, the ACA has been questioned since signed into law and may remain as is, be revised, or be eliminated. However, knowing the essence of the ACA helps us understand what the public views as healthcare support. One of the significant benefits of the ACA is access to coverage regardless of the presence of any preexisting conditions. Although the ACA does not cover the entire population, a significant majority can be covered. The ACA reduced the total number of the uninsured and ensured access to care for more people, especially low-income individuals and people of color (Blumenthal et al., 2020). This coverage changes how individuals are insured and, thus, how they are viewed within the system. Multiple demands for nurses, especially those in advanced practice roles, will continue to emerge over the next several years. As all of these changes—including subsequent legislation—unfold, opportunities and challenges exist for how healthcare will be delivered and paid for. Those changes will alter what nursing does.

Healthcare is paid for by three primary sources: government (Medicare and Medicaid), private health insurance, and out-of-pocket (Tikkanen et al., 2020). Three-fourths of the government funding is at the federal level. Federal programs include Medicare and health services for military members, veterans, Native Americans, and federal prisoners. Medicare, the most extensive federal program, was established in 1965 and pays for care provided to people 65 years of age and older and some disabled individuals. Medicare coverage is separated into Medicare Parts A, B, C, and D. Medicare Part A is an insurance plan for the hospital, hospice, home health, and skilled nursing care paid for through Social Security taxes. Nursing home care that is mainly custodial is not covered. Medicare Part B is optional insurance that covers physician services, medical equipment, and diagnostic tests. Part B is funded through federal taxes and monthly premiums paid by the recipients. Medicare Part C is not a separate benefit. Part C is the part that allows private health insurance companies to provide Medicare benefits. These are known as Medicare Advantage Plans. Medicare Part D is the part that offers outpatient drug prescriptions. These plans change frequently and can be reviewed on www.medicareinteractive.org.

Medicaid, a state-level program financed by federal and state funds, pays for services provided to persons who are medically indigent, blind, or disable and children with disabilities. Medicaid, which varies by state, covers one in five Americans (Rudowitz et al., 2019). The federal government pays between 50% and 83% of total Medicaid costs based on the state's per capita income. Services funded by Medicaid vary from state to state but must include hospitals, physicians, laboratories, and radiology departments; prenatal and preventive care; and nursing home and home healthcare services.

Private insurance is the second major source of financing for the healthcare system. Most Americans have private health insurance, which usually is provided by employers through group policies. Individuals can purchase health insurance, but typically the rates are higher and provide minimal coverage. Health insurance that is so intertwined with employment is problematic, contributing to the rolls of uninsured and underinsured Americans. Many uninsured workers are employed in part-time, seasonal, or service positions in small businesses that cannot afford group insurance.

Individuals also pay directly for health services when they do not have health insurance or when insurance does not cover the service. Costs paid by individuals are called *out-of-pocket expenses* and include deductibles, copayments, and coinsurance. Health insurance benefits often cover limited preventive care and typically do not cover cosmetic surgeries, alternative healthcare therapies, or items such as eyeglasses and nonprescription medications.

HEALTHCARE REIMBURSEMENT

Prices in healthcare are not set by the same economic equilibrium found in all major industries. For the most part, pricing is highly influenced by the government and reimbursement plans. For example, both Medicare and Medicaid impose pricing on hospitals, with no room for negotiation. Health services researchers disagree on the exact effects of these reimbursement methods on cost and quality. However, considering these effects is important because changes in payment systems have implications for how care is provided in healthcare organizations. The U.S. government has offered reimbursement payment from a cost-based system to prospective payment systems and now a system that pays on performance (pay-for-performance), otherwise known as *value-based purchasing.*

A cost-based system consists of the cost of providing a service plus a markup for profit or excess income. Third-party payers often limit what they will pay by establishing usual and customary charges by surveying all providers in a specific area. Usual and customary charges rise over time as providers continually increase their prices. In cost-based reimbursement, all allowable costs are calculated and used as the basis for payment. Each payer (government or insurance company) determines the allowable costs for each procedure, visit, or service. Charges and cost-based reimbursement are retrospective payment methods because payment is selected after services are delivered. When the reimbursed costs are less than the full charge for the service, a contractual allowance (or discount) exists. Charges and cost-based reimbursement were the predominant payment methods in the 1960s and 1970s but have been largely supplanted by payer fee schedules determined before service delivery.

The prospective payment system (PPS) is a method in which the third-party payer decides what and how much will be paid for a service or episode of care. If the costs of care are higher than the payment, the provider absorbs the loss. If the costs are less than the payment, the provider makes a profit. In 1983, Medicare implemented a PPS for hospital care that uses diagnosis-related groups (DRGs) as the basis for payment.

The DRG system is a classification system that groups patients into categories based on the average number of hospitalization days for specific medical diagnoses, considering factors such as the patient's age, complications, and other illnesses. Payment includes the expected costs for diagnostic tests, various therapies, surgery, and length of stay (LOS). The cost of nursing services is not explicitly calculated and is typically considered as part of the room rates. With a few exceptions, DRGs do not adequately reflect the variability of patient intensity or acuity within the DRG. This is problematic for nursing because the number of resources (nurses and supplies) used to care for patients is directly related to the patient acuity. Therefore, many nurses believe that DRGs are not good predictors of nursing care requirements. In past years, Medicare reimbursed home health agencies, nursing homes, and ambulatory care providers through a PPS.

In addition to Medicare, some state Medicaid programs and private insurance companies use a DRG payment system. Although DRGs are not currently used for specialty hospitals (pediatric, psychiatric, and oncology), they are a dominant hospital payment force. Implementation of a PPS with DRGs resulted in increased patient acuity and decreased LOS in hospitals, along with a greater demand for home care. The need for hospital and community-based nurses also increased.

The pay-for-performance system was introduced in the early 2000s. It used a system that reimbursed hospitals and providers based on performance and outcomes rather than the cost associated with providing the care. The premise of this payment system is based on quality outcomes. Also referred to as value-based purchasing, it offers rewards and incentives to high-performing organizations. This approach was first used to pass the Medicare Prescription Drug, Improvement, and Modernization Act of 2003. This law provided incentives to hospitals that voluntarily submitted data on ten quality measures.

The pay-for-performance system eventually evolved into the Hospital Value-Based Purchasing Program (HVBPP) established by the ACA, which went into effect in October 2012. The incentives are based on how well a hospital performs on each measure or how much a hospital improves its performance compared with its performance at baseline. The overall score includes the clinical process of care measures and patient experience of care measures. For example, the patient care dimension includes responsiveness of staff, pain management, communication about medicine, cleanliness, and quietness of hospital environment.

THE CHANGING HEALTHCARE ECONOMIC ENVIRONMENT

Healthcare is a primary public concern. Rapid changes have been occurring to reduce costs and improve the nation's health and wellness. As shown in Box 19.1,

BOX 19.1	Healthcare Delivery Reform Strategies	
Strategies	**Key Features**
Managed care	Health plan that includes both service and financial considerations
Organized delivery systems	Networks of organizations; providers and payers
Competition based on price, patient outcomes, and service quality	Basis of cost and quality

strategies shaping the evolving healthcare delivery system include managed care, organized delivery systems (ODSs), and competition based on price, patient outcomes, and service quality. These strategies affect both the pricing and use of health services.

Managed care, also known as *managed cost*, brings together the delivery and financing functions into one entity in an attempt to control costs, utilization, and quality (Medicaid.gov, 2021). A significant goal of managed care is to decrease unnecessary services, thereby reducing costs. Managed care also works to ensure timely and appropriate care. Health maintenance organizations (HMOs) are a type of managed care system in which the primary physician serves as a gatekeeper who determines what services the patient uses. Because HMOs are paid on a capitated basis, the HMO's procedure is to practice prevention and use ambulatory care rather than more expensive hospital care. *Capitation* means that the provider is paid a fixed amount per patient for a defined period of time. In other forms of managed care, a nonphysician case manager arranges and authorizes the services provided. Many insurance companies have used case managers for years. Nurses who work in home health and ambulatory settings often communicate with insurance company case managers to plan specific patients' care. Preferred provider organizations (PPOs) and point-of-service (POS) plans are other types of managed care plans that give the patient more options than traditional HMOs for selecting providers and services. In a PPO, for example, patients have access to a large network of providers and hospitals. However, this comes at a higher price for the patients.

Organized delivery systems comprise networks of healthcare organizations, providers, and payers.

Typically, this means hospitals, physicians, and insurance companies. Such joint ventures aim to develop and market collectively a comprehensive healthcare package that will meet the largest numbers of consumers. Hospitals, physicians, and payers share the financial risks of the enterprise. Although hospitals share some risk now with prospective payment, physicians have not generally shared the risk. This risk sharing is expected to provide incentives to eliminate unnecessary services, use resources more effectively, and improve service quality.

Competition among healthcare providers is increasingly based on cost and quality outcomes. Decision-making regarding price and utilization of services is shifting from physicians and hospitals to payers demanding significant discounts or lower fees. Scientific data that demonstrate positive health outcomes and high-quality services are required. Providers who cannot compete based on price, patient outcomes, and service quality will find it difficult to survive as the system evolves. These facts directly impact how attractive an organization is for both patients and the nurses.

EXERCISE 19.1 What is the contractual allowance when a hospital charges $800 per day to care for a ventilator-dependent patient and an insurance company reimburses the hospital $685 per day? What is the impact on hospital income **(revenue)** if this is the reimbursement for 2500 patient-days?

EXERCISE 19.2 Assume that Medicare reimburses a hospice $70 for home visits. For one particular group of patients, it costs the hospice an average of $98 per day to provide care. What are the implications for the hospice? What options should the hospice nurse manager and nurses consider?

EXERCISE 19.3 For each reimbursement method, think about the incentives for healthcare providers (individuals and organizations) regarding their practice patterns. What incentives could change the quantity of services used per patient or the number or types of patients served? Are these incentives efficient? List the incentives. How might each method affect overall healthcare costs? (Think in terms of effect on utilization and price.) What do you think the effect on quality of care might be with each payment method?

EXERCISE 19.4 Obtain a copy of an itemized patient bill from a healthcare organization and review the charges. What was the source and method of payment? How much of these charges was reimbursed? How much was charged for items you regularly use in clinical care?

The Healthcare Economic Environment and Nursing Practice

What does the healthcare economic environment mean for the practicing professional nurse? We must value ourselves as providers and think of our practice within a context of organizational viability and quality of care. To do this, we must always demonstrate and articulate the value contribution of our practice. In other words, we must determine and advertise the *value* of nursing care and stop referring to it as a cost. Services that add value are of high quality, affect health outcomes positively, and minimize costs. The following content helps develop financial thinking skills and ways to consider how nursing practice adds value for patients by reducing costs. We need to learn to use these concepts in all of our roles in healthcare.

Nursing Services as a Source of Revenue

According to Title XVIII of the Social Security Act, most recently updated in 2017, an inpatient hospital admission means that a patient was admitted for purposes of receiving care for a period of two midnights or more (CMS, 2017). Furthermore, nursing services resourced by the hospital for care and treatment of inpatients are covered under the law and included in the PPS. Hospitals use a "daily room charge" based on a relative value of the intensity of nursing services rendered. This revenue-generating daily charge should be viewed as the revenue source for nursing services provided on any given unit. This data source can establish the total value contribution of nursing services, including nursing's contribution to the bottom line.

EXERCISE 19.5 How was nursing care charged on the bill you obtained? What are the implications for nursing in being perceived as an expense rather than being associated with the revenue stream? Why will this perception be less important in a capitated environment?

WHY PROFIT IS NECESSARY

Private, nongovernmental healthcare organizations may be either for-profit (FP) or not-for-profit (NFP). This designation refers to the tax status of the organization and specifies how the profit can be used. Profit is the excess income left after all expenses have been paid (Revenues − Expenses = Profit), and many NFP organizations designate their "profit" as surplus income. This term helps to clarify whether the organization is meeting its designation as a not-for-profit. FP organizations pay taxes, and their profits can be distributed to investors and managers. NFP organizations, on the other hand, do not pay taxes and must reinvest all of their profits, commonly called *net income* or *income above expense*. The purpose of reinvestment in the organization is to better serve the public.

All private healthcare organizations must earn more than the costs to make a profit to survive. If expenses are more significant than revenues, the organization experiences a loss. If revenues equal expenses, the organization breaks even. In both cases, nothing is left over to replace facilities and equipment, expand services, or pay for inflation costs. Some healthcare organizations can survive in the short run without profit because they use the interest from investments to supplement revenues. The long-term viability of any private healthcare organization, however, depends on consistently making excess income. Box 19.2

BOX 19.2   Income Statement of Revenues and Expenses From a Neighborhood Nursing Center: Fiscal Year Ending December 31, 2010

Revenues		
Patient revenues	$283,200	
Grant income	$60,000	
Other operating revenues	$24,000	
TOTAL	**$367,200**	**$367,200**
Expenses		
Salary costs	$140,400	
Supplies	$64,400	
Other operating expenses (e.g., rent, utilities, administrative services)	$79,900	
TOTAL	**$284,700**	**$284,700**
Excess of revenues over expenses [profit][a]		$82,500

[a] Loss would be shown in parentheses ( ) or brackets [ ].

---

presents a simplified example of an income statement from a neighborhood NFP nursing center.

Nurses and nurse managers directly affect an organization's ability to make a profit. Profits can be achieved or improved by decreasing costs or increasing revenues. In tight economic times, many managers think only in terms of cutting costs. Although cost-cutting measures are essential, mostly to keep prices down so that the organization will be competitive, increasing revenues also needs to be explored. Nurses in all roles can contribute to thinking creatively about both aspects.

UNDERSTANDING WHAT IS REQUIRED TO REMAIN FINANCIALLY SOUND

Understanding what is required for a department or agency to remain financially sound requires that nurses move beyond thinking about costs for individual patients to thinking about income and expenses and numbers of patients needed to make a profit. For example, the 2021 *Essentials of Baccalaureate Education* developed by the American Association of Colleges of Nursing (AACN) requires that baccalaureate education incorporate consideration of the cost-effectiveness of care (AACN, 2021). In a fee-for-service environment, revenue is earned for every service provided. Therefore, increasing the volume of services, such as diagnostic tests and patient visits, increases revenues. In a capitated environment in which one fee is paid for all services provided, increasing the overall number of patients served and decreasing the volume of services used is desirable. With capitation, nurses must strive to accomplish more with each visit to reduce return visits and complications. In today's value-based purchasing environment and reimbursement methodology, nurses need to understand their organization's reimbursement environment, identify how they can influence patient outcomes—such as reducing or eliminating hospital-acquired conditions (HACs) and facilitating patient- and caregiver-centered experiences of care—and have a strategy for realizing a profit in a specific circumstance.

Knowing Costs and Reimbursement Practices

As direct caregivers and case managers, nurses are frequently involved in determining the type and quantity of resources used for patients. This includes supplies, personnel, and time. Nurses need to know what costs are generated by their decisions and actions. Nurses also need to know how much items cost and how they

BOX 19.3 Strategies for Cost-Conscious Nursing Practice

1. Understanding what is required to remain financially sound
2. Knowing costs and reimbursement practices
3. Capturing all possible charges in a timely fashion
4. Using time efficiently
5. Discussing the costs of care with patients
6. Partnering with case management in reaching organizational goals
7. Evaluating cost-effectiveness of new technologies
8. Predicting and using nursing resources efficiently
9. Using research to evaluate standard nursing practices

are paid for in an organization to make cost-effective decisions. For example, nurses need to know per-item costs for supplies to evaluate lower-cost substitutes appropriately. While one nurse typically cannot change a supply source, a group can. Box 19.3 outlines strategies for cost-conscious nursing practice.

Case management has become a crucial role for all acute care organizations. Nurses must partner with case management in reaching organizational goals. The ideal partnership includes the following contributions by the nursing staff:

- Knowledge of patient goals, expected outcomes, and anticipated discharge date
- Comprehensive assessment of the patient and family
- Appropriate and timely interventions when the patient is not progressing as expected
- Proper management of pain, activity, skin integrity, bowel and bladder integrity, and cognition
- Ongoing patient and family education regarding discharge planning and preventing readmission
- Identifying barriers to discharge

In ambulatory and home health settings, nurses must be familiar with the various insurance plans that reimburse the organization. Each plan has different contract rules regarding preauthorization, types of services covered, required vendors, and so forth. Although nurses must develop and implement their goals of care with full knowledge of these reimbursement practices, the payer does not drive the care. Nurses still advocate for patients in meaningful ways while also working within the cost and contractual constraints. Moreover, when nurses understand the reimbursement practices, they can help patients maximize the resources available to them.

In hospitals, the cost of nursing care usually is not calculated or billed separately to patients; instead, it is part of the general per-diem charge. One major problem with this method is the assumption that all patients consume the same amount of nursing care and the acuity of the patient is not considered. Another problem with bundling the charges for nursing care with the room rate is that nursing as a clinical service is not perceived by management as generating revenue for the hospital. Instead, nursing is perceived predominantly as an expense to the organization. Although this perception may not matter in a capitated setting, in which all provider services are considered a cost, accurate nursing care cost data are needed to negotiate managed care contracts. Also, patients do not see direct charges and have no way to understand the monetary value of the services they receive.

Capturing All Charges in a Timely Fashion

Nurses also help contain costs by ensuring that all possible charges are captured. Several large hospitals report more than $1 million a year lost from supplies that were not charged. In hospitals, nurses must know which supplies are charged to patients and which ones are charged to the unit. Also, the procedures and equipment used need to be accurately documented. In ambulatory and community settings, nurses often need to keep abreast of the codes used to bill services. These codes change yearly; sometimes items are bundled together under one charge and sometimes they are broken down into different charges. Turning in charges promptly is also essential because delayed billing negatively affects cash flow by extending the time before an organization is paid for services provided. This is particularly significant in smaller organizations.

> **EXERCISE 19.6** You used three intravenous (IV) catheters to do a particularly difficult venipuncture. Do you charge the patient for all three catheters? What if you accidentally contaminated one by touching the sheet? How is the catheter paid for if not charged to the patient? Who benefits and who loses when patients are not charged for supplies?

Using Time Efficiently

The adage that time is money is fitting in healthcare—it refers to both the nurse's time and the patient's time. When nurses are organized and efficient in their care delivery and scheduling and coordinating patients' care, the organization will save money. In a value-based purchasing environment, doing as much as possible during each care episode is particularly important to decrease repeat visits and unnecessary service utilization. Because LOS is the most important predictor of hospital costs, patients who stay extra days cost the hospital a considerable amount, which, in turn, affects the overall profit as a long-term expense. Decreasing LOS also makes room for other patients, thereby potentially increasing patient volume and hospital revenues. Besides, most patients want to be out of the hospital. Nurses can become more efficient and effective by evaluating their major work processes and eliminating redundancy and rework areas. Automated clinical information systems that support integrated practice at the point of care will also increase efficiency and improve patient outcomes.

EXERCISE 19.7 The Visiting Nurse Association (VNA) cannot file for reimbursement until all documentation of each visit has been completed. Typically, the paperwork is submitted a week after the visit. When the number of home visits increases rapidly, the paperwork often is not turned in for 2 weeks or more. What are the implications of this routine practice for the agency? Why would the VNA be very vulnerable financially during periods of heavy workload? What are some options for the nurse manager to consider to expedite the paperwork?

Discussing the Cost of Care with Patients

Talking with patients about the cost of care is essential, although it may be uncomfortable. Discovering during a clinic visit that a patient cannot afford a specific medication or intervention is preferable to finding out several days later in a follow-up call that the patient has not taken the medication, or worse, learning that on readmission. Such information compels the clinical management team to explore optional treatment plans or find resources to cover the costs. Talking with patients about costs is vital in other ways too. It involves the patients in the decision-making process and increases the likelihood that treatment plans will be followed. Patients can make informed choices and better use the resources available to them if they have appropriate information about costs.

EXERCISE 19.8 A new patient visits the clinic and is given prescriptions for three medications that will cost about $220 per month. You check her chart and discover that she has Medicare (but not Part D) and no supplemental insurance. How can you determine whether she has the resources to buy this medicine each month and whether she is willing to buy it? If she cannot afford the medications, what are some options?

Evaluating Cost-Effectiveness of New Technologies

Cost-effectiveness is defined as a method to achieve a specific outcome for the least possible cost. The advent of new technologies is presenting dilemmas in managing costs. In the past, if a new piece of equipment was more comfortable to use or benefited the patient in any way, nurses were apt to want to use it for everyone, no matter how much more it cost. Now, we are forced to decide which patients need the new equipment and which ones will have equally good outcomes with the current equipment. Essentially, nurses analyze the cost-effectiveness of the new equipment for different types of patients to allocate limited resources. This is a new and sometimes difficult way to think about patient care and may not feel like a caring way to make these decisions. However, such choices conserve resources without jeopardizing patients' health and, thus, create the possibility of providing additional healthcare services.

EXERCISE 19.9 Last year, a new positive-pressure, needleless system for administering intravenous (IV) antibiotics was introduced. Because the system was so easy to use and convenient for patients, the nurses in the home infusion company where you work ordered it for everyone. Typically, patients get their IV antibiotics four times each day. The minibags and tubing for the regular procedure cost the agency $22 a day. The new system costs $24 per medication administration, or $96 a day. The agency receives the same per-diem (daily) reimbursement for each patient. Discuss the financial implications for the agency if this practice is continued. Generate some optional courses of action for the nurses to consider. How should these options be evaluated? What secondary costs, such as the cost of treating fewer needlestick injuries, should be included?

Predicting and Using Nursing Resources Efficiently

Because healthcare organizations are service institutions, the largest part of their operating budget typically is for personnel. For hospitals, nurses are the largest group of employees and often account for most of the personnel budget. Staffing is the first area that nurse managers can affect concerning managing costs; supply management is the second area. To understand why, understanding the concepts of fixed and variable costs is essential.

The total fixed costs in a unit are those costs that do not change as the volume of patients changes. In other words, with either a high or a low patient census, expenses related to renting, utilities, loan payments, administrative salaries, and salaries of the minimum number of staff to keep a unit open must be paid. Variable costs are costs that vary in direct proportion to patient volume or acuity. Examples include nursing personnel, supplies, and medications. Break-even analysis (BEA) is a tool that uses fixed and variable costs for determining the specific volume of patients needed just to break even (Revenue = Expenses) or to realize a profit or loss. BEA can be calculated using this formula:

$$\text{Break} - \text{even Quantity (N)} = \frac{\text{Fixed Costs (FC)}}{\text{Price (P)} - \text{Variable Cost per Patient (VC)}}$$

In hospitals and community health agencies, patient acuity systems help managers predict nursing care requirements. These systems differentiate patients according to the acuity of illness, functional status, and resource needs. Some nurses do not like these systems because they believe that the essence of nursing is not captured. However, we need to remember that these are tools to help managers predict resource needs. Used appropriately, patient acuity systems can help evaluate changing practice patterns and patient acuity levels and can provide information for budgeting processes.

Managing staff and decreasing LOS can achieve the most immediate reductions in costs. Hospitals strive to lower costs to attract new contracts and to be attractive as partners in provider networks. Therefore, staffing methods and patient care delivery models are being closely scrutinized. Work redesign, a process for changing the way to think about and structure patient care, is the predominant strategy for developing systems that better utilize high-cost professionals and improve service quality. Increased staff retention, patient safety, and positive patient outcomes result from effective work redesign processes.

EXERCISE 19.10 Given the definitions for fixed and variable costs, why do you think nurse managers have the greatest influence over costs through management of staffing and supplies?

Using Research to Evaluate Standard Nursing Practices

Htay & Whitehead (2021) conducted a systematic review (using primary research evidence) aimed at evaluating the effectiveness of the role of advance practice nurses compared with usual or physician-led care. The review included 13 randomized controlled trials from high-income countries conducted in both primary and

---

RESEARCH PERSPECTIVE

Resource: Liu, H., Zhu, D., Song, B., Jin, J., Liu, Y., Wen, X., Cheng, S., Nicholas, S., & Wu, X. (2020). Cost-effectiveness of an intervention to improve the quality of nursing care among immobile patients with strokes in China: A multi-center study. *Physician Weekly*, August 2020. https://www.physiciansweekly.com/cost-effectiveness-of-an-intervention-to-improve-the-quality-of-nursing-care-among-immobile-patients-with-stroke-in-china-a-multicenter-study.

Liu et al. (2020) conducted a study to evaluate the cost-effectiveness of a nursing intervention program for immobile patients who suffered from a stroke in China. Participants came from 25 hospitals across six provinces of China. A total of 7653 patients with a stroke were included.

Two groups were created (routine care and interventional care). All patients obtained a follow-up three months after enrollment into the study. The total healthcare care cost was abstracted from the system along with health outcome effectiveness data, measured by the EuroQol five-dimensional questionnaire (EQ-5D). The interventional group demonstrated statistically significant quality-adjusted life years and a decrease in the total cost of care.

Implication for Practice
The findings from this analysis provide evidence that an intervention program for immobile patients who suffer from a stroke is cost-effective.

hospital care settings. They concluded that advance practice nurses offer a positive impact compared with physicians related to patient satisfaction, reduction in wait times, and control of chronic care, and are more cost-effective. The Research Perspective describes the need for a business case related to outcomes.

BUDGETS

In most healthcare organizations, the primary financial document is the budget—a detailed financial plan for carrying out the activities an organization wants to accomplish for a certain period. An organizational budget is a formal plan stated in terms of dollars and includes proposed income and expenditures. The budgeting process is an ongoing activity in which plans are made, and revenues and expenses are managed to meet or exceed the plan's goals. The management functions of planning and control are tied together through the budgeting process.

Changes in medical practices, reimbursement methods, competition, technology, demographics, and regulatory factors must be forecast to anticipate their effects on the organization. Planning encourages the evaluation of different options and assists in the more cost-effective use of resources.

EXERCISE 19.11 A community nursing organization performs an average of 36 intermittent catheterizations each day. A prepackaged catheterization kit that costs the organization $17 is used. The four items in the kit, when purchased individually, cost the organization a total of $5. What factors should be considered in evaluating the cost-effectiveness of the two sources of supplies?

Theoretical Frameworks for Budgeting

Budgeting is an area of social science for which there has been little theoretical work. In 1997, Neuby, describing a literature review of over 70 years of manuscripts in political science and public administration, noted that articles about budgeting were basically devoid of theoretical guidance. However, Davis et al. (1996) presented three models based on the way that budget requests are made—in the case of this article, in the federal budget process. These models can be applied in a variety of budget development processes in all fields and include the following.

1. Requests are based on previous year's appropriations.
2. Requests are based on the previous year's appropriations, as well as the difference between the agency request and previous year's request.
3. Requests are made based on previous year's request.

All three approaches also take into account unusual circumstances that may impact the availability of funds.

In 1986, Wildavsky updated his original theoretical approach in the book entitled *Budgeting: A Comparative Theory of Budgetary Processes, second edition*. The principles of this theory are outlined in the Theory Box.

Nursing Budgets

A budget requires managers to plan and to establish explicit program goals and expectations. An important component of this planning is to be able to address the cost-effectiveness of care as described by the new AACN *Baccalaureate Essentials* (AACN, 2021). Historically, first-level managers in nursing, selected on the merit of their strong interpersonal skills and clinical expertise, may not have the requisite business preparation necessary for the first-line manager role. The Literature Perspective provides content that is necessary for the first-time unit manager.

Types of Budgets

Well-managed organizations use several types of interrelated budgets. This chapter's major budgets include the operating budget, the capital budget, and the cash budget. The way these budgets complement and support one another is depicted in Fig. 19.1. Many organizations also use the program, product line, or particular purpose budgets. Long-range budgets are used to help managers plan for the future. Again, although the majority of nurses in any organization do not create or control these budgets, understanding them is very useful.

Operating Budget

The operating budget is the financial plan for the day-to-day activities of the organization. The expected revenues and expenses generated from daily operations, given a specified volume of patients, are stated. Preparing and monitoring the operating budget, particularly the expense portion, is often the most time-consuming financial function for nurse managers.

The operating budget expense consists of a personnel budget and a supply and expense budget for each cost center. A cost center is an organizational unit for which costs can be identified and managed. Typically,

THEORY BOX

Theory/Contributor	Key Ideas	Application to Practice
Wildavsky (1986)	Purpose of budgeting: The purpose of budgeting is translating financial resources into human purposes. It provides a way to apportion funds to competing people and purposes. Planning the budget: This can be accomplished in two ways. • A centralized budget is achieved from the top down to the various departments and units. • A decentralized or independent and competitive budget starts at the unit level and moves throughout the various levels until it reaches the top level of the organization. Cultural implications: Budgets are cultural constructs, expressing desired relationships among people, maintaining, increasing, or decreasing the difference among them. Communication: Budgets are predictive communication. Decision-making: In budgeting, an individual or a group must calculate which alternative to consider and choose. When a group with responsibilities in different segments of the organization participates in developing a budget, both competition and collaboration may result. Calculating alternatives: Human determination is required for calculating complex budgets. Resource allocation: The level of resources allocated matters, as does the unpredictability of the current and future circumstances. Finalizing a budget with a rising level of appropriation is much easier than finalizing one with no increase or with a decrease.	A substantial portion of a unit budget reflects the staffing required for the patient population on that unit. The chief nursing officer (or other administrator(s)) completes all of the nursing service budgets. The nurse manager, in collaboration with nurses on the unit, develops the budget. The differing budget amounts in equivalent size units may indicate their relative importance to the total organization. When nurses review the budget, they can see how many nurses are likely to be a part of the unit. For example, the staffing budget should list the number of full-time equivalents of RNs as well as other team members. Despite competition, nurse managers who are responsible for finalizing the nursing service budget must also collaborate. Nurse managers must determine what is relevant to preserve in the unit budget as part of the negotiation. This might involve unit staff who can help propose optional ways to meet patient care needs. The power of nurse managers is related to, in part, the level of resources they are able to negotiate in the budget process. Unexpected events, such as a pandemic, may cause havoc in the proposed budget.

LITERATURE PERSPECTIVE

Resource: Welch, T. D., & Smith, T. (2020). Understanding FTEs and nursing hours per patient day. *Nurse Leader*, 18(2), 157–162.

The largest line item on a hospital's general budget is personnel, which consumes most of an organization's needs. The first-line manager is the most knowledgeable person about departmental needs and is uniquely positioned to negotiate financial requirements for personnel to meet and maintain efficient and high-quality patient care. Thus, mentors for first-line managers must assist them in developing the necessary financial skills for this role.

This article discusses the salary budget, unit of service (UOS), average daily census, nursing workload and skill mix, the full-time equivalents (FTEs), and the definitions

and interrelationships among these variables. Knowledge of these elements allows the nurse manager to adapt and change staffing as needed, evaluate budgetary deficiencies, and seek opportunities to improve efficiencies in patient care.

Implications for Practice

Financial competency for the first-level nurse manager provides a measure of independence important for the successful nurse manager and subsequent leadership roles. Competence in finance, specifically personnel budgets, provides the front-line nurse manager with the tools to properly manage the unit while both promoting and defending excellence in patient-centered care.

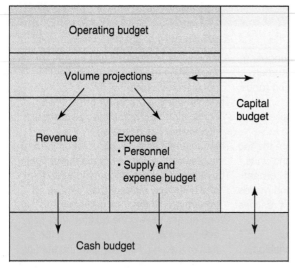

Fig. 19.1 Interrelationships of the operating, capital, and cash budgets.

TABLE 19.2   **Workload Calculation (Total Required Patient Care Hours)**

Patient Acuity Level[a]	Hours of Care Per Patient Day (HPPD)[b]	×	Patient Days[c]	=	Workload[d]
1	3.0		900		2700
2	5.2		3100		16,120
3	8.8		4000		35,200
4	13.0		1600		20,800
5	19.0		400		7600
Total			10,000		82,420

[a] 1, Low; 5, high.
[b] Number of hours of care needed based on acuity levels and numbers.
[c] Each day represents a unit of time. For example, 900 patients equals 900 patient-days.
[d] Total number of hours of care needed based on acuity levels and numbers of patient-days.

this is a clinical unit or division. The personnel budget is the largest part of the operating budget for most nursing units.

Before the personnel budget can be established, the volume of work predicted for the budget period must be calculated. A unit of service measure appropriate to the work of the unit is used. Units of service may be, for example, patient days, clinic or home visits, hours of service, admissions, deliveries, or treatments. Another factor needed to calculate the workload is the patient acuity mix. The formula for calculating the workload or the required patient care hours for inpatient units is as follows: Workload volume = Hours of care per patient day × Number of patient days (Table 19.2).

In some organizations, the workload is established by the financial office and given to the nurse manager. In other organizations, nurse managers forecast the volume. In both situations, nurse managers should inform administrators about any factors that might affect the forecast's accuracy, such as changes in physician practice patterns, new treatment modalities, inpatient versus outpatient treatment practices, and changes in technology or equipment. Being aware of rapid technological changes proves insightful for subsequent budget changes.

The next step in preparing the personnel budget is to determine how many staff members will be needed to provide the care. Because some people work full-time and others work part-time, full-time equivalents (FTEs) are used in this step rather than positions.

Generally, those costs do not change as the volume of patients changes. One-half of an FTE (0.5 FTE) equates to 20 hours per week. The number of hours to define an FTE may vary within an organization; therefore, knowing agency-specific meaning is critical.

Most organizations use 2080 hours per year to equal a full-time employee. The 2080 hours paid to an FTE i a year consists of both productive hours and nonpro ductive hours. Productive hours are paid time that is worked. Nonproductive hours are paid time that is not worked, such as vacation, holiday, orientation, and sick time. Education may be viewed as either depending on the organization's value for learning. Before the number of FTEs needed for the workload can be calculated, the number of productive hours per FTE is determined by subtracting the total number of nonproductive hours per FTE from total paid hours. Alternatively, payroll reports can be reviewed to determine the percentage of paid hours productive for each FTE. Finally, the total number of FTEs needed to provide the care is calculated by dividing the entire patient care hours required by the number of productive hours per FTE (Box 19.4).

The total number of FTEs calculated by this method represents the number needed to provide care each day of the year. The total FTEs do not reflect the number of positions or the number of people working each day. The number of positions may be much higher, mainly if

---

BOX 19.4 Productive Hours Calculation

Method 1: Add All Nonproductive Hours/FTE and Subtract from Paid Hours/FTE

	Example:	Vacation	15 days
		Holiday	7 days
		Average sick time	4 days
		Total	26 days

26×8^a hours = 208 nonproductive hours/FTE
2080 − 208 = 1872 productive hours/FTE

Method 2: Multiply Paid Hours/FTE by Percentage of Productive Hours/FTE

Example: Productive hours = 90%/FTE
(1872 productive hours of total 2080 = 90%)
$2080 \times 0.90 = 1872$ productive hours/FTE

Total FTE Calculation

Required Patient Care Hours	÷ Productive Hours Per FTE	= Total FTEs Needed
82,420	÷ 1872	= 44 FTEs

FTE, Full-time equivalent.
[a] Full-time equivalent. FTE pattern.

---

many part-time nurses are employed. Some nurses may be scheduled for their regular day off or vacation on any given day, and others may be out because of illness. Some positions that do not involve direct patient care, such as nurse managers or unit secretaries, may not be replaced during the nonproductive time. Only one FTE is budgeted for any position not covered with other staff when the employee is off.

> **EXERCISE 19.12** Change the number of patients at each acuity level listed in Table 19.2, but keep the total number of patients the same. Recalculate the required total workload. Discuss how changes in patient acuity affect nursing resource requirements.

The next step is to prepare a daily staffing plan and establish positions. Once the positions are established, the labor costs that comprise the personnel budget can be calculated. Factors that must be addressed include straight-time hours, overtime hours, differentials and premium pay, raises, and benefits. Differentials and premiums are extra pay for working specific times, such as evening or night shifts and holidays. Benefits usually include health and life insurance, Social Security payments, and retirement plans. Benefits often cost an additional 25% to 30% of a full-time employee's salary. In

other words, about one-third of an employee's expenses are related to benefits and have to be seriously considered when adding an FTE.

> **EXERCISE 19.13** If the percentage of productive hours per FTE is 80%, how many worked or productive hours are there per FTE? If total patient care hours are 82,420, how many FTEs will be needed?

The supply and expense budget is often called the *other-than-personnel services (OTPS) expense budget.* This budget includes various items used in daily unit activities, such as medical and office supplies, minor equipment, books, and journals. It also provides orientation, training, and travel. Although different methods are used to calculate the supply and expense budget, the previous year's expenses are commonly used as a baseline. This baseline is adjusted for projected patient volume and specific circumstances known to affect expenses, such as predictable personnel turnover, which increases orientation and training expenses. A percentage factor is also added to adjust for inflation.

The final component of the operating budget is the revenue budget. The revenue budget projects the income that the organization will receive for providing patient care. Historically, nurses have not been directly involved with developing the revenue budget, although this is changing. In most hospitals, the revenue budget is established by the financial office and given to nurse managers. The anticipated revenues are calculated according to the price per patient-day. Data about the volume and types of patients and reimbursement sources (i.e., the case mix and payer mix) are necessary to project revenues in any healthcare organization. Even when nurse managers do not develop the revenue budget, learning about its revenue base is essential for sound decision-making. Knowing this information also helps direct care nurses to know how they are paid.

Capital Expenditure Budget

The capital expenditure budget reflects expenses related to purchasing major capital items, such as equipment and the physical plant. The capital expenditure must have a useful life of more than one year and must exceed the organization's cost level. The minimum cost level requirement for capital items in healthcare organizations is usually $300 to $1000, although some organizations have a much higher level. Anything below that minimum is considered a typical operating cost.

Capital expenses are kept separate from the operating budget because their high cost would make the costs of providing patient care appear too high during the year of purchase. To account for capital expenses, the costs of capital items are depreciated. This means that each year, over the equipment's useful life, a portion of its cost is allocated to the operating budget as an expense. Therefore, capital expenditures are subtracted from revenues and, in turn, affect profits.

Organizations usually set aside a fixed amount of money for capital expenditures each year. Complete, well-documented justifications are needed because the competition for limited resources is stiff. Justifications should be developed using the principle of any business case and should include, at a minimum, the projected amount of use; services duplicated or replaced; safety considerations; the need for space, personnel, or building renovation; effect on operational revenues and expenses; and contribution to the strategic plan. Nurses play a major role in selecting equipment that best meets patients' needs.

Cash Budget

The cash budget is the operating plan for monthly cash receipts and disbursements. Organizational survival depends on paying bills on time. Organizations can be making a profit and still run out of cash. A profitable trend, such as a rapidly growing census, can induce a cash shortage because of increased expenses in the short run. Major capital expenditures can also cause a temporary cash crisis; thus, they must be staggered strategically. Because cash is the lifeblood of any organization, the cash budget is as important as the operating and capital budgets.

The financial officer prepares the cash budget in large organizations. Understanding the cash budget helps nurse managers discern (1) when constraints on spending are necessary, even when the expenditures are budgeted, and (2) the importance of carefully predicting when budgeted items will be needed.

The Budgeting Process

The budgeting process steps are similar in most healthcare organizations, although the budgeting period, budget timetable, manager level, and employee participation vary. Budgeting is done annually in relation to the organization's fiscal year. A fiscal year exists for financial purposes and can begin at any point on the calendar. In the title of some financial reports, a phrase similar to "FYE June 30, 2023" appears and means that this report is for the fiscal year ending on the date stated.

Significant steps in the budgeting process include gathering information and planning, developing unit budgets, developing the cash budget, negotiating and revising, and using feedback to control budget results and improve plans. Each organization sets a timetable with specific dates for implementing the budgeting process. The timetable may be anywhere from 3 to 9 months. The widespread use of computers for budgeting is reducing the time span for budgeting in many organizations. Box 19.5 provides nurse managers with data essential for developing their budgets. This step begins with an environmental assessment that helps the organization understand its position in regard to the entire community. The assessment includes, for example, the changing healthcare needs of the population, influential economic factors such as inflation and unemployment, differences in reimbursement patterns, and patient satisfaction.

Next, the organization's long-term goals and objectives are reassessed in light of its mission and the environmental analysis. This helps all managers situate the budgeting process for their units about the whole organization. At this point, programs are prioritized to allocate resources to programs that best support the organization in achieving its long-term goals.

BOX 19.5 Outline of Budgeting Process

1. Gathering information and planning
   - Environmental assessment
   - Mission, goals, and objectives
   - Program priorities
   - Financial objectives
   - Assumptions (employee raises, inflation, volume projections)
2. Developing unit and departmental budgets
   - Operating budgets
   - Capital budgets
3. Developing cash budgets
4. Negotiating and revising
5. Evaluating
   - Analysis of variance
   - Critical performance reports

Modified from Kovner, C., Finkler, S., Jones, C., & Mose, J. (2018). *Financial management for nurse managers and executives* (5th ed.). St. Louis, MO: Elsevier Saunders.

Specific, measurable objectives are then established; the budgets must meet these objectives. The financial goals might include limiting expenditure increases or making reductions in personnel costs by designated percentages. Nurse managers also set operational purposes for their units in concert with the rest of the organization. This is where units or departments interpret what effect the changes in operational activities will have on them. For instance, how will using case managers and care maps for selected patients affect a particular unit? Establishing the unit-level objectives is also the right place for involving direct care nurses in setting the unit's future direction.

Along with the specific organization- and unit-level operating objectives, managers need the organization-wide assumptions that underpin the budgeting process. Explicit assumptions regarding salary increases, inflation factors, and volume projections for the next fiscal year are essential. With this information in hand, nurse managers can develop the operating and capital budgets for their units. These are usually set in tandem because each affects the other. For instance, purchasing a new monitoring system will have implications for the supplies used, staffing, and staff training.

The cash budget is developed after unit and department operating and capital budgets. Then, the negotiation and revision process begins in earnest. This is a complex process because changes in one budget usually require changes in others. Learning to defend and negotiate budgets is an essential skill for nurse managers. Nurse managers who successfully negotiate budgets know how costs are allocated and are comfortable speaking about what resources are contained in each budget category. They can also clearly and specifically depict the effect of not having that resource on the patient, nurse, or organizational outcomes.

EXERCISE 19.14 If you can interview a nurse manager, ask to review the budgeting process. Ask specifically about the budget timetable, operating objectives, and organizational assumptions. What was the level of involvement for nurse managers and nurses in each step of budget preparation? Is there a budget manual?

The final and ongoing phase of the budgeting process relates to the control function of management. Feedback is obtained regularly so that organizational activities can be adjusted to maintain efficient operations. Variance analysis is the primary control process used. Variances are common because we don't control patients and their needs for care.

A variance is a difference between the projected budget and the actual performance for a particular account. For expenses, a favorable or positive variance means that the budgeted amount was more significant than the actual amount spent. An unfavorable, or negative, variance implies that the budgeted amount was less than the actual amount spent. Positive and negative variances cannot be interpreted as good or bad without further investigation. For example, if fewer supplies were used than were budgeted, this would appear as a positive variance and the unit would save money. This will be good news if supplies were used more efficiently and patient outcomes remained the same or improved. A problem might be suggested, however, if using fewer or less-expensive supplies led to poorer patient outcomes. Or it might mean that precisely the right amount of supplies was used but that the patient census was less than budgeted. To help managers interpret and use variance information better, some institutions use flexible budgets that automatically account for census variances.

Managing the Unit-Level Budget

How is a unit-based budget managed? At a minimum, nurse managers are responsible for meeting the fiscal goals related to the personnel and supply and expense part of the operations budget. Typically, monthly

TABLE 19.3   Statement of Operations Showing Profit and Loss From a Neighborhood Nursing Center: March 2018

CURRENT MONTH[a]				YEAR-TO-DATE[a]		
Budget	**Actual**	**Variance**	**Revenues**	**Budget**	**Actual**	**Variance**
Patient Revenues						
21,500	22,050	550	Insurance payment	64,500	66,150	1650
1500	1550	50	Donations	4500	4750	250
23,000	23,600	600	Net patient revenues	69,000	70,900	1900
Nonpatient Revenues						
5000	5000	0	Grant income (#138-FG)	15,000	15,000	0
500	500	0	Rent income	1500	1500	0
5500	5500	0	Net nonpatient revenues	16,500	16,500	0
28,500	29,100	600	**Net revenues**	85,500	87,400	1900
Expenses						
Personnel						
7750	8500	(750)	Managerial/professional	23,250	24,400	(1150)
2000	1800	200	Clerical/technical	6000	5800	200
9750	10,300	(550)	Net salaries and wages	29,250	30,200	(950)
1200	1400	(200)	Benefits	3600	4000	(400)
10,950	11,700	(750)	Net personnel	32,850	34,200	(1350)
Nonpersonnel						
2500	2500	0	Office operating expenses	7500	7500	0
2000	2100	(100)	Supplies and materials	3000	3050	(50)
300	450	(150)	Travel expenses	900	450	450
4800	5050	(250)	Net nonpersonnel	11,400	11,000	400
15,750	16,750	(1000)	**Net expenses**	44,250	45,200	(950)
Revenues Over/Under Expenses						
10,750	12,350	(400)	**Net income**	41,250	42,200	950

[a] Values expressed in 000s.

reports of operations (see Table 19.3) are sent to nurse managers. They want to review the big picture of the operation of the unit by reviewing patient and nonpatient revenues with the expenses of both personnel and nonpersonnel for the month. Although the month may show some variance, due to such factors as a conference or vacations, the year-to-date (right-hand side of the report) should be fairly reflective of the months-to-date in comparison to the year before. Obviously, when some major event such as the pandemic occurs, it is difficult to manage a budget because comparisons cannot be readily made and predictions will not likely be accurate.

The "bottom line" indicates whether the revenues for the unit are over or under those projected for the month and for the year to date and can provide some guidance to the manager about whether to control expenses more closely or whether the strategies the unit has implemented to reduce costs or lengths of stays are effective.

Nurse managers investigate and explain the underlying cause of variances more significant than 5%. Many factors can cause budget variances, including patient census, patient acuity, vacation and benefit time, illness, orientation, staff meetings, workshops, employee mix, salaries, and staffing levels. To accurately interpret budget variances, nurse managers need reliable data about the patient census, acuity, and LOS; payroll reports; and unit productivity reports.

Nurse managers can control *some* of the factors that cause variances, but not all. After the causes are determined and controllable by the nurse manager, steps are taken to prevent the variance from occurring in the future. However, even uncontrollable variances that increase expenses might require the actions of nurse managers. For example, if supply costs rise drastically because new technology is being used, the nurse manager might have to look for other areas where the budget can be cut. Information learned from analyzing variances also is used in future budget preparations and management activities.

Also, nurse managers monitor the productivity of their units. Productivity is the ratio of outputs to inputs; that is, productivity equals output/input. In nursing, outputs are nursing services measured by hours of care, number of home visits, and so forth. The inputs are the resources used to provide the services, such as personnel hours and supplies. Only decreasing the inputs or increasing the outputs can increase productivity. Hospitals often use hours per patient day (HPPD) as one measure of productivity. For example, if the standard of care in a critical care unit is 12 HPPD, then 360 hours of care are required for 30 patients for one day. When 320 hours of care are provided, the productivity rating is 113% (360/320 = 1.13), meaning that the unit was overproductive or very productive. However, we must consider the quality component of any productivity model related to care. In home healthcare, the number of visits per day per registered nurse is one measure of productivity. If the standard is five visits per day but the weekly average was 4.8 visits per day, productivity decreased. Variances in productivity are not inherently favorable or unfavorable and require investigation and explanation before judgments can be made about them. For example, a description of the variance (4.8 visits per day) might include the fact that one visit took twice the amount of time generally spent on a home visit because of patient needs, preventing the nurse from making the regular five visits per day. The extra time spent on one patient was productive time but not adequately accounted for by this productivity measure (visits per day).

Although they do not have direct accountability for the budget, direct care nurses play an essential role in

meeting budget expectations. Many nurse managers find that routinely sharing the budget and budget-monitoring activities with the whole team fosters an appreciation of the relationship between cost and the mission to deliver high-quality patient care. Providing the team with access to cost and utilization data allows them to identify patterns and select appropriate, cost-effective practice options that work for the staff and patients. Managers and staff who work in partnership to understand that cost versus care is a dilemma to manage rather than a problem to solve will develop innovative, cost-conscious nursing practices that produce good outcomes for patients, nurses, and the organization.

EXERCISE 19.15 Examine Table 19.3 and identify major budget variances for the current month. Are they favorable or unfavorable? What additional information would help you explain the variances? What are some possible causes for each variance? Are the causes you identified controllable by the nurse manager? Why or why not? Is a favorable variance on expenses always desirable? Why or why not?

CONCLUSION

Managing costs and understanding budgets are essential for nurses in all positions within the organization. The current emphasis on "value" makes knowing what costs are and how to control them necessary. Understanding the basics of a budget helps nurses at all levels in an organization cite the economic impact of decisions related to care. Considering the paramount influence that nurses have on establishing the value contribution, taking actions at the point of care (such as capturing charges promptly) are as important as actions in the manager's office (such as ensuring proper resource allocation) or actions in the executive suite (such as projecting patient volume or changes in delivery). To further develop the value proposition, the importance of engaging the entire team cannot be overstated. Planning significantly impacts the outcome, which puts nursing in a positive or limited perspective in an organization.

THE SOLUTION

Many factors contribute to which flu vaccine should be purchased for the unit and all were considered before a decision was made. First, I created and used my professional "network" to assist with my assessment of the volume needed for the clinic. Reaching out to neighboring clinics and their leadership gave me an approximate indication of the volume of flu vaccines needed. I also used data from the community assessment from my organization and talked to other nurse managers with similar clinics within the organization. Second, we had limited quality data to determine if there were any risks of nosocomial infection or any patients who had been cross contaminated using a MDV. This type of data is important in completing an accurate assessment of the use of an MDV versus an SDV. Third, we evaluated the cost of the MDV versus the SDV. According to several studies, the MDV costs approximately between $0.32 to $0.50

per dose administered. Lastly, we took into consideration the skill set of the nurses and the operational workflow of the clinic (waste, storage, drawing up the vaccines, and so on). Considering our limited budget, we decided on a hybrid approach. We ordered MDVs and SDVs. We asked for assistance from our quality department to assist with data collection as it relates to risk, infection, and performance improvement. We also completed time and motion studies regarding the operational workflows of using each type of vial. After a year of observation, we determined that the SDV would be used in our same-day clinics due to limited storage, fast-paced clinic setting, novice nursing staff, and minimal cost difference to overall clinic operations.

Would this solution be suitable for you? Why?

Jamie M. Hughes

REFLECTIONS

Consider a recent "typical" day in the clinical area. Did you consider costs as you provided care to a patient? Were you aware of that patient's financial resources as part of your decision-making process for discharge planning? What specific activities did you do that led to costs to the patient or organization? Could you have avoided any costs? Would value could you identify that nurses bring to health care?

BEST PRACTICES

Changes in the organization may affect the unit budgets. The nurse manager must be aware of planned changes that will take effect during the year for which the budget is being created and the impact on staff, supplies, or equipment. Close communication with upper management regarding potential changes is critical to developing an accurate budget. All nurses can benefit from understanding the basics of the organization's and unit's budgeting process and assuring their language conveys their care is a value and not an expense.

TIPS FOR MANAGING COSTS AND BUDGETS

- Know the significant changes in the organization and how they might affect the organization's budget.
- Analyze the supplies you use in providing care and what is commonly missing as one way to make recommendations about supply needs.
- Evaluate what your patients would find most helpful during the time you care for them.
- Decide which of your actions create costs for the patient or the organization.

- Be aware of how changes in patient acuity and patient census affect staffing requirements and the unit budget.
- Know how charges are generated and how the documentation systems relate to billing.
- Be knowledgeable about the anticipated discharge day and discharge plan, and include the patient and the family in the plan upon admission.
- Examine the upsides and downsides of the cost–care polarity thoughtfully.

REFERENCES

American Association of Colleges of Nursing (AACN). (2021). The essentials: Core competencies for professional nursing education. Retrieved on April 28, 2022 from https://www.aacnnursing.org/Portals/42/AcademicNursing/pdf/Essentials-2021.pdf.

Blumenthal, D., Collins, S. R., & Fowler, E. (2020). *The Affordable Care Act at 10 years: What's the effect on health care coverage and access?* The Commonwealth Fund. Retrieved from https://www.commonwealth-fund.org/publications/journal-article/2020/feb/aca-at-10-years-effect-health-care-coverage-access.

Centers for Medicare & Medicaid Services (CMS). (2017). *Medicare Benefit Policy Manual.* Retrieved from https://www.cms.gov/Regulations-and-Guidance/Guidance/Manuals/downloads/bp102c01.pdf.

Centers for Medicare & Medicaid Services (CMS). (2021). *Historical.* Retrieved from https://www.cms.gov/Research-Statistics-Data-and-Systems/Statistics-Trends-and-Reports/NationalHealthExpendData/NationalHealthAccountsHistorical.

Davis, O. A., Dempster, A. H., & Wildavsky, A. (1996). A theory of the budgetary process. *The American Political Science Review, 60*(3), 529–547. https://www.cmu.edu/dietrich/sds/docs/davis/A%20Theory%20of%20the%20Budgetary%20Process.pdf.

Gee, E., & Spiro, T. (2019). *Excess administrative costs burden the U.S. health care system.* Center for American Progress. Retrieved from https://www.americanprogress.org/issues/healthcare/reports/2019/04/08/468302/excess-administrative-costs-burden-u-s-health-care-system/.

Htay, M., & Whitehead, D. (2021). The effectiveness of the role of advanced nurse practitioners compared to physician-led or usual care: A systematic review. *International Journal of Nursing Studies Advances, 3,* 100034. Retrieved from https://www.sciencedirect.com/science/article/pii/S2666142X21000163.

Kovner, C., Finkler, S., Jones, C., & Mose, J. (2018). *Financial management for nurse managers and executives* (5th ed.). St. Louis, MO: Elsevier Saunders.

Liu, H., Zhu, D., Song, B., Jin, J., Liu, Y., Wen, X., Cheng, S., Nicholas, S., & Wu, X. (2020). Cost-effectiveness of an intervention to improve the quality of nursing care among immobile patients with strokes in China: A multicenter study. *Physician Weekly.* August 2020. Retrieved from https://www.physiciansweekly.com/cost-effectiveness-of-an-intervention-to-improve-the-quality-of-nursing-care-among-immobile-patients-with-stroke-in-china-a-multicenter-study.

Medicaid.gov. (2021). *Managed Care.* Retrieved from https://www.medicaid.gov/medicaid/managed-care/index.html.

Neuby, B. L. (1997). On the lack of a budget theory. *Public Administration Quarterly, 21,* 131.

Rudowitz, R., Garfield, R., & Hinton, E. (2019). *10 things to know about Medicaid: Setting the facts straight.* Kaiser Family Foundation. Retrieved from https://www.kff.org/medicaid/issue-brief/10-things-to-know-about-medicaid-setting-the-facts-straight/.

Tikkanen, R., Osborn, R., Mossialos, E., Djordjevic, A., & Wharton, G. A. (2020). *International Health Care System Profile: United States.* The Commonwealth Fund. Retrieved from https://www.commonwealth-fund.org/international-health-policy-center/countries/united-states.

U.S. Department of Health and Human Services. (2021). *History of Healthy People.* Retrieved from https://health.gov/our-work/healthy-people/about-healthy-people/history-healthy-people.

Welch, T. D., & Smith, T. (2020). Understanding FTEs and nursing hours per patient day. *Nurse Leader, 18*(2), 157–162.

Wildavsky, A. (1986). *Budgeting: A comparative theory of budgetary processes* (revised ed.). Budgeting. United States: Transaction.

20

Selecting, Developing, and Evaluating Staff

Diane M. Twedell

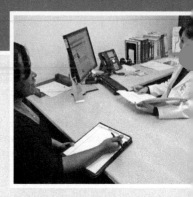

ANTICIPATED LEARNING OUTCOMES

- Compare and contrast the various methods of employee performance appraisal.
- Describe the principle that supports behavioral interviewing technique.
- Provide examples of appropriate and inappropriate performance feedback.
- Articulate the importance of a job description in the orientation of a new employee.

KEY TERMS

behavioral interviewing   empowerment   position description
coaching   performance appraisal

THE CHALLENGE

An important component of employee satisfaction is the ability for employees to be engaged in their work and involved in decision-making. In my first year as a nurse manager, I did a full assessment of the committee structure in the work unit, including function, membership, outcomes, and effectiveness. As expected, I found gaps, ones I felt I could influence. Many of the staff who were change agents on the unit were not on unit committees—not because it wasn't an option but because they thought the committees were not relevant. I needed to reengage the entire nursing team and help make a shift in the team's commitment to begin changing the culture.

What do you think you would do if you were this nurse?

Jolene Piper, MSN, BSN, RN
Nurse Manager, Mayo Clinic Health System, Albert Lea, Minnesota

INTRODUCTION

Nurse leaders are key individuals whose leadership can directly influence quality, safety, service, and satisfaction for patients and frontline nurses. Nurse leaders and managers are really the chief retention officers of a patient care area and have a huge impact on the environment for patient care. Nurse leaders and frontline nurses help shape the environment and learning milieu for new employees.

Nurses must clearly understand what is expected of their performance, including the ramifications of not meeting those expectations. This understanding can be achieved only when all members of the organization have clearly defined roles and overall objectives.

The ongoing development, mentoring, and coaching of staff is vital for a healthy and engaging work environment. Once nurse managers hire new frontline nurses, the ongoing support mentioned previously is essential. Think of a tree and how it needs ongoing care and feeding; you can't just dig a hole and put the tree in the ground. Similarly, you can't just hire and walk away from a new nurse who requires ongoing development, performance feedback, and coaching to reach optimal growth.

ROLES IN AN ORGANIZATION

All individuals within an organization play a role. Every role requires an individual to assume the personal as well as the formal expectations of a specified position. Employees must have clear role expectations and perceive that their contributions are valued. Employees who understand their roles and are empowered to succeed in those roles have been noted to demonstrate increased personal health, job satisfaction, and individual performance. They are then more likely to be committed to the organization and to provide a higher level of patient care. These principles are applicable to leaders, managers, and followers.

Nursing program graduates enter the profession with various levels of educational and life experiences. The unit nurse leader plays an integral role in assisting these individuals in the development and acquisition of the complex role as professional nurse. Role development evolves over time and may occur numerous times in a nurse's career. As an example, a registered nurse (RN) who is an expert medical-surgical nurse takes a new position in the operating room as a circulating RN; this is a new role for the nurse. Whenever such a change occurs, the nurse is likely to feel less confident and competent than before because, instead of typical functioning, the nurse is also focused on learning a new role. The Theory Box provides an overview on the complexity of taking on a new role.

> **BOX 20.1 Excerpts from an Ambulatory Care Nurse Job Description**
>
> - Assesses comprehensive data, including physical, psychosocial, emotional, and spiritual needs of the patient.
> - Involves patient, family, and healthcare team members in formulating a culturally appropriate plan of care.
> - Implements plan of care in partnership with patient, family, and healthcare team.

> **EXERCISE 20.1** Obtain a position description for a registered nurse from an ambulatory care setting and a hospital. Compare them and analyze the general categories. Are specific behaviors outlined? What competencies are different? What competencies are similar?
>
> The position description should reflect current practice guidelines and competency-based requirements. As nursing care models shift to the ambulatory setting, home, and community, nurses must have a clear understanding of the performance that is expected. The nurse is responsible for clearly understanding the roles of the patient care assistant to whom care is delegated. Clear and concise position descriptions for all employees provide the basis for roles in an organization.

Position descriptions provide written guidelines detailing the roles and responsibilities of a specific position within the organization. The position description reflects functions and requirements of specific roles in an institution. Box 20.1 demonstrates examples of expectations for a nurse in an ambulatory care environment.

THEORY BOX

Theory/Contributor	Key Ideas	Application to Practice
Dynamics in Organizations Kahn, Wolfe, Quinn, Snoek, & Rosenthal (1964) developed this theory.	Roles within organizations affect an individual's interactions with others. Acquisition of these roles is time dependent and varies based on individual experiences and value systems. For effective communication to take place, role expectations for performance must be understood by all individuals involved.	The role of the professional nurse is complex. Role acquisition, role clarity, and role performance are enhanced by the use of clear position descriptions and evaluation standards.

Adapted from Kahn, R. L., Wolfe, D. M., Quinn, R. P., Snoek, J. D., & Rosenthal, R. A. (1964). *Occupational stress: Studies in role conflict and ambiguity.* New York: Wiley.

SELECTION OF STAFF

The selection of staff is one of the most important functions that nurse managers complete in their daily routines. Nurse managers want the most qualified individual for the position who also fits the culture of the patient care environment and organization. If an applicant values that the needs of the patient come first, and this value is also articulated via the organization, the individual has similar values. Nurse managers must decide whether frontline nurses will be included in the process and provide appropriate preparation for the interview team (Meyer, 2020). Frontline nurse involvement provides diversity in points of view, which can be valuable to a broad view of healthcare.

Some organizations use contracted services to shorten the interview time and provide a more relevant applicant pool; others manage the process as a totally internal process. Either way, candidates for a position are eventually interviewed at the unit level by the nurse manager or that person's designee. Sometimes, a team of unit employees is involved, depending on the organization and availability.

A nurse manager and an applicant both must prepare for an interview to truly determine whether the individual is a good fit for the organization. The manager's focus before and during the interview is to create questions that are well thought out. Identification of the attributes wanted in a frontline nurse can help guide the selection of interview questions. Interview questions should be directed to evaluate values and critical thinking skills. The phrase "the best predictor of future behavior is past behavior" is the premise on which behavioral interviewing is based. Behavioral interviewing requires applicants to provide an example of a situation that they experienced that highlights how they have dealt with a particular issue. An example of a behavioral interview question could be: *Tell me about a time when you were working in a group and there were problems with other individuals who were not doing their fair share. What did you do to maintain a team environment?* If the manager opted to include fronline nurses, they too can contribute questions and set expectations for what responses should address. Another strong question to ask can relate to the organization's mission: Our mission is……; how does that relate to your personal values?

Interviews should be held in a private location where interruptions can be avoided. Providing applicants with information about the position through an e-mail and attaching a copy of the position description for the applicant to review before the interview can help shape the nature of the interview. Even during times of dire shortages, focusing on fit between the person and the organization is critical to prevent additional turnover.

Applicants appreciate the opportunity to tour the patient care area either before or after the actual interview. At the conclusion of the interview, the nurse manager should indicate when applicants will hear about their interview result, who will contact them, and how they will be notified. The shorter the response time, the more satisfying this is for the applicant. Applicants should be thanked for their time and interest in pursuing a position. Because people typically are on their best behavior during an interview, any concerns demonstrated during the entire interview process should be taken seriously. Those who are involved in interviews have the accountability for sharing such concerns and for answering questions applicants have in the most honest way possible.

Applicants also have responsibilities in the interview process. Applicants should arrive on time and alone and be appropriately dressed in business attire. They should be prepared to answer questions honestly and thoughtfully. The use of behavioral-based interviewing requires applicants to describe previous situations and how they were handled. They may also be asked to describe why they are interested in working in a specific work area. At the end of the interview, applicants should thank the nurse manager for the manager's time and provide any specific follow-up information the manager has requested. A formal note of appreciation for the interview may be sent by the applicant afterward. The wise manager always does the same. With the predicted shortage of registered nurses, small gestures such as this help influence competitive offers.

> **EXERCISE 20.2** You are applying for a position as a primary care registered nurse in a community-based outpatient clinic in a rural community and are invited to an interview. Outline how you will prepare for this interview and what questions you will ask.

DEVELOPING STAFF

Once the interview and offer are completed and an applicant has accepted the position, strategies are implemented to help the individual acclimate to the organization and new role. Organizations use a variety of approaches, including orientation to the organization, the department,

RESEARCH PERSPECTIVE

Resource: Owings, C. R., & Gaskins, S. W. (2020). Evaluation of a community-based nurse residency. *Journal for Nurses in Professional Development, 36*(4), 185–190.

This article focuses on the evaluation of the impact of a nurse residency program in a community-based hospital. The study was done using a secondary data analysis and a sample size of 121 participants in a Vizient nurse residency program. All participants were new graduates with less than one year of nursing experience. Study participants completed the Casey-Fink survey online through the Vizient database. Findings indicated that participants in the nurse residency program in a community hospital felt supported, experienced lower personal stress levels, and had increased comfort in communication skills and leadership capacity. Participants in the nurse residency program turnover rate was half the turnover rate of nurses not in the residency program.

Implications for Practice

Nurse residency programs have the ability to positively impact the transition for a new graduate nurse in a community hospital setting. The ability to recruit and retain nurses in rural and community settings is an ongoing challenge. A nurse residency program can provide a mechanism to increase staff engagement and successful onboarding.

---

and role or new graduate residency programs that may provide ongoing support and education for up to a year. Residency programs in hospitals have increased in numbers over recent years and other organizations, such as those that are community based, have taken on the task of creating such programs, as the Research Perspective illustrates. General orientation to the organization is usually a structured program for every new employee. It typically includes the mission, vision, values, benefits, safety programs, and other specific topics for the day-to-day operation of the organization. The orientation period must be used efficiently to benefit both the employee and the organization. Whether during orientation or later, new nurses would be wise to identify role models and mentors to support their professional growth. This proactive approach helps link the individual with the person most likely to be influential on the person's career.

Retention of new nursing personnel begins on the day of their hire because costs for replacement and turnover can be substantial. Costs for turnover for a bedside RN range from $40,038 per year to $51,700 for a medical-surgical hospital RN in 2021 per Nursing Solutions Inc. (2021). These costs can vary tremendously based on amount of specialty training required, such as for critical care, emergency department, and labor and delivery, along with the availability of nurses at any given time. Factors related to turnover cost include human resource expenses, temporary replacement costs, lost productivity, training, relocation expenses, and terminal pay cuts. Although the cost of turnover may be calculated differently, the cost of replacement is high. Nurse managers and educators can play a pivotal role in ongoing development of staff. A watchful eye and recognition of

talents displayed by nurses throughout their onboarding and ongoing employment can help retain nurses in an organization. As an example, a nurse educator may see that a direct care nurse is excellent at providing diabetic patient education in a primary care clinic. The nurse educator can recommend the idea of becoming a certified diabetic educator as a development goal.

Orientation is a time for new employees to learn the work environment and the staff. Many institutions use preceptors who are frontline nurses, because of their strength as role models, to help orient new staff. Bodine (2020) notes that the preceptor is an important integrating force for the new employee's transition and can impact the organization's retention rate. Despite the importance of preceptors in an effective orientation, preceptor preparation can be an ongoing challenge due to turnover and workload, as the Literature Perspective illustrates for one organization's approach.

Preceptors work with orientees to complete a needs assessment to direct and guide the orientation of new employees in the clinical setting. An important first step is to determine how new employees like to learn. Various learning style assessment tools are available for preceptors to use. When preceptors understand the learning style of new employees, a better focus for implementation of orientation goals is provided. New employees work with preceptors who understand specifically how to address the individualized learning needs. As an example, orientees may learn best by observing a complex dressing change before actually performing it on a patient. Preceptor preparation is an important component of successful onboarding of new nurses. During times of high turnover and hiring in a work unit, nurses who

LITERATURE PERSPECTIVE

Resource: Bagioni, D., Lucas-Breda K., & Eichar, S. (2020). Enhancing preceptor preparation with the 5-minute preceptor. *Nursing, 50*(12), 15–17.

This publication focuses on the importance of preceptor education and specifically how to build critical thinking skills in newly hired frontline nurses. While most healthcare organizations have preceptor preparation programs, constant change in personnel occurs and not all preceptors have participated in these programs. A 5-Minute Preceptor (5MP) strategy was utilized. A five-step process was built to reflect a nursing-specific focus to provide education and feedback from preceptors. The 5MP process includes the following: take a stand (e.g., deciding what to do), probe for supporting evidence, teach general rules, reinforce the positive, and correct misinterpretations and errors. Nurse preceptors believed the process was something that could be used easily, deployed quickly, and was usable.

Implications for Practice

Nurse preceptors need tools that are simple and applicable to practice that focus on critical thinking for the frontline nurse. Although providing formal professional development for nurse preceptors is important, tools that can be easily deployed for less experienced and prepared preceptors will always be needed in the constantly changing healthcare environment.

have not been formally trained as a preceptor may need to step into the role. The Literature Perspective speaks to how one organization helped prepare staff nurses to precept in these types of situations.

Continued development of the staff is a distinct role for the nurse leader. Every member of the nursing team has ongoing needs for continued growth and development. Nurse leaders get to know their employees and what their interests and career goals are. Formal meetings and everyday interactions with frontline nurses help a nurse leader learn what is important to employees. Specific individual development plans can be determined for each employee. The ongoing competency and staff development is critical for the professional development of the staff member. Ongoing competencies are required for many critical components of the frontline staff nurse position, including Basic Cardiac Life Support, Advanced Cardiac Life Support, ECG interpretation, and more. Specific education related to life safety, such as active shooter drills, fire, tornado, and mass casualty events, are all required on a yearly basis. Additionally, specialty areas have expectations for maintaining competencies that contribute to safe, quality patient care.

Empowerment strategies are useful for individual professional development and overall development of staff. Empowerment is a process that acknowledges the values and judgment of individuals and trusts that their decisions will be the correct ones. For individuals to feel empowered, the environment must be open and people must feel safe to explore and develop their own potential. The organizational environment must encourage individuals to use the freedom of making decisions while retaining the accountability for the consequences of those decisions. Organizations with a strong investment in a professional practice development model are more likely to support the development of expert nurses who will impact expert nursing care and patient outcomes (Creta & Gross, 2020). Positive feedback, achievement recognition, and support for new ideas enhance employees' feelings of empowerment and their ability to perform effectively. What is important to remember is this: empowerment is an internal sense. Nurse managers can create a climate in which others feel safe to speak up, but that doesn't mean they will. Sometimes, as Brene Brown says in her classic work, we feel anxious about being vulnerable (Brown, 2015).

> **EXERCISE 20.3** Think about a nurse leader and a nurse manager whom you interact with on a regular basis. What are the similarities and differences in the nurse leader's and nurse manager's behaviors that support empowerment?

PERFORMANCE APPRAISALS

Feedback to employees regarding their performance is one of the strongest rewards an organization can provide. Performance appraisals are individual evaluations of work performance. Ideally, appraisals are conducted on an ongoing basis, not just at the conclusion of a predetermined period. Performance appraisals are generally done annually and also may be required after a scheduled orientation period for new employees.

The intent of performance appraisals is to allow the individual to integrate comprehensive feedback to improve performance.

Performance appraisals can be formal or informal. An informal appraisal might be as simple as immediately praising the individual for performance recognized. A compliment from a family member or patient might be conveyed. Some work areas have a specific bulletin board for thank-you notes from patients and their families. Sometimes a simple "Thank you for all your hard work today!" can be extended from the nurse manager to the staff. The more specific the feedback can be, however, the more influential it is on reinforcing specific performances.

The formal performance appraisal involves written documentation according to specific organizational guidelines. The formal performance appraisal usually involves the use of a standard form or method developed by the organization to measure employee performance. Employees must have a clear understanding of their job description. Providing a new employee a position description is helpful because it can provide a basis for how the individual's performance will be measured. The example in Box 20.2 contains an excerpt from a performance appraisal form in which a nurse manager can evaluate a frontline nurse related to health teaching and promotion.

A performance appraisal is an opportunity for the employee and manager to have a dedicated time together to review how the employee is meeting the performance expectations outlined in the position description. It provides an opportunity to give the employee feedback related to not meeting, meeting, or exceeding expectations. Addressing strengths and areas for improvement related to the employee's performance is important. Although the most improvement can occur with capitalizing on a person's strengths, all expectations must be met at a satisfactory or better level.

If an employee is not meeting performance expectations, a performance improvement plan is put in place with specific, measurable, achievable goals outlined that is understood and articulated by both the manager and the employee. This allows each individual to understand one's role expectations and the ramifications when not meeting performance goals.

Specific behaviors by the nurse manager enhance the actual appraisal process. Box 20.3 provides key behaviors for the performance appraisal session.

Ongoing feedback is essential between the nurse manager and employees. An employee's regular performance appraisal should never be the first time a concern is identified. Feedback is best given as soon as a positive or negative occurrence with the employee happens. For example, if a frontline nurse demonstrates inappropriate behavior at a patient care area staff meeting, the manager should provide feedback about the behavior as soon as possible after that meeting.

Performance appraisals may include self and peer evaluations as well as managerial components. In sophisticated units, a 360 evaluation may be made. This

---

BOX 20.2 Performance Appraisal, Clinical Registered Nurse

Health Teaching and Health Promotion

___a. Uses teaching strategies appropriate to patient's condition and learning needs.

___b. Uses health promotion to support patients and families in developing skills for self-management.

___c. Maintains a safe, clean, and organized environment for patients, families, and staff.

Performance Levels (Enter code in blank)
AE: Achieves expectations
NFD: Needs further development
UTA/NA: Unable to assess/not applicable

BOX 20.3 Key Behaviors for the Performance Appraisal Session

- Provide a quiet, controlled environment, without interruptions.
- Maintain a relaxed but professional atmosphere.
- Put the employee at ease; the overall objective is for the best job to be done.
- Review specific examples for both positive and negative behavior.
- Allow the employee to express opinions, orally and in writing.
- Provide written future plans for learning needs and goals.
- Set follow-up dates as necessary to monitor improvements, if cited.
- Show the employee confidence in the employee's performance.
- Be sincere and constructive in both praise and criticism.

BOX 20.4   **Performance Appraisal Goal and Accomplishment Examples**

Examples of Goals

1. Obtain specialty certification as a Critical Care Registered Nurse (CCRN) from the American Association of Critical-Care Nurses by the end of next January.
2. Participate in shared governance committee as unit representative next year.

Accomplishments (12 Months Later Summary)

1. Successful completion of CCRN examination (see documentation submitted).
2. Participated in every unit council meeting (see attendance records for the unit council meeting) and chaired the documentation task force of the shared governance committee (see email asking me to chair this committee).

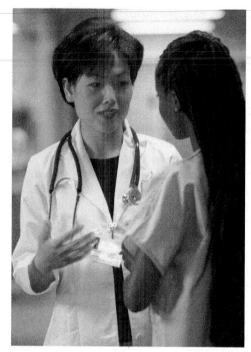

Fig. 20.1 Coaching can promote team building and optimal performance of the employees. (Copyright © Photodisc/iStock/Thinkstock.)

means that peers, subordinates, and unit nurse leaders all provide input so that an individual nurse has a full performance perspective. An advantage for an individual is seeing where relationships need to be strengthened; an advantage for a manager is being able to speak from a broad perspective about performance.

A critical part of the performance appraisal is the development of goals and career development for the upcoming year. The employee should come to the appraisal prepared to discuss goals to accomplish over the next year. Examples of goals that may be put into an individual nurse's appraisal are noted in Box 20.4.

COACHING

The overall evaluative process can be enhanced if the manager uses the technique of coaching. Coaching is the process that involves the development of individuals within an organization. This coaching process is a personal approach in which the manager and the employee interact on a frequent and regular basis with the ultimate outcome that the employee performs at an optimal level. Coaching can be by an individual or may involve a team approach (Fig. 20.1). When implemented in a planned and organized manner, coaching can promote team building and optimal performance of employees. Coaching is a learned behavior for the nurse manager, which takes time and effort to be developed.

Hancock and Meadows (2020) note that coaching provides the employee with ideas, support, and inspiration. The rewards for both the employee and the nurse leader are significant. Coaching involves asking questions, supporting forward movement and general guidance, rather than telling someone what to do. Coaching generally takes more time and has longer lasting effects.

CONCLUSION

Selecting new members of a team is critical to success for both the frontline nurse and the nurse manager. Nurse managers and their teams know their individual patient care areas best and are critical to the interview and orientation process. Selecting the right individual for the right reasons is key to successfully achieving positive outcomes for the individual, patient, and organization. Making certain that new employees are oriented in a comprehensive manner and providing ongoing feedback—including a regular, formal evaluation—helps people grow in their own right and contribute more effectively to the mission of the organization.

THE SOLUTION

My experiences as leader of a unit council on an inpatient medical surgical unit early in my career sparked my interest in change management, leadership, and engagement. A primary care unit council existed but it needed to be reenergized. I wanted a primary care unit council to be something staff wanted to be a part of. As the nurse manager, I wanted a group I could lean into to help me implement change. The unit council could help me identify gaps and support change management from a peer-to-peer model rather than a top-down implementation approach.

I was enthusiastic about developing this unit council and getting new members rotated in immediately. Developing nurses as a group is an important part of the development process.

First, the team decided to change the structure of the council to have co-leaders. Having an LPN and RN co-leading the group together was essential to support change. Traditionally, this council leadership role was only for RNs on the committee.

Reenergizing the committee didn't happen overnight. When issues or concerns were brought up, such as requesting a change in a workflow or process, the unit council was my first consideration for seeking feedback or input on the matter. It became a standing agenda item every month at staff meetings to highlight what things are being covered by the unit council. We shared the council meeting minutes with all staff, and a member of the council usually had a moment to talk or answer questions from the broader group. These actions allowed the staff to see that they had a voice and an impact on decisions.

During a difficult Minnesota winter, several clinic days were impacted due to weather, and we were faced with suddenly opening Saturday clinics for patient access. Very few individuals were volunteering to work on these Saturdays. Patient needs had to be be met; thus, a system to choose people to staff Saturday clinics had to be developed. Immediately, I engaged the unit council to discuss, brainstorm, analyze, and implement the plan for staffing. These were the subtle but important ways staff could be involved. Yes, staffing Saturday clinics was a temporary and unpopular project. However, staff representatives, through the primary care unit council, could choose how the staffing process was created, tracked, and implemented. The unit council and staff were able to establish parameters around how the process would be done. The patient needs were able to be met and clinic access was achieved. Working in shared leadership improves satisfaction, drives excellence, and cultivates leaders, who perhaps didn't know they had it in them or even wanted to be a part of it.

Would this be a suitable approach for you? Why?

Jolene Piper

REFLECTION

Have you gained a new perspective on the role of the nurse leader or manager while reading this chapter? Explain how you gained appreciation for how the nurse leader affects the environment in a patient care area. How would you help someone develop in that person's role if you were in charge of a unit?

BEST PRACTICES

Nurse leaders are pivotal in implementing positive work environments. Nurse leaders who provide a high frontline nurse engagement, robust orientation and professional development programs, and coaching are important to nurse recruitment and retention. Engaged frontline nurses lead to better patient outcomes and satisfaction.

TIPS FOR SELECTING, DEVELOPING, AND EVALUATING STAFF

- Value the role of the nurse leader in recruitment and retention of frontline nurses.
- Articulate the importance of the preceptor in influencing new orientees in their intention to stay at an organization.
- Identify how the new frontline nurse joining an organization can set goals for professional development in the first year.
- Expect that nurse leader ongoing feedback and coaching contributes to the success of an individual nurse and the organization.

REFERENCES

Bagioni, D., Lucas-Breda, K., & Eichar, S. (2020). Enhancing preceptor preparation with the 5-minute preceptor. *Nursing, 50*(12), 15–17.

Bodine, J. (2020). Preceptor selection: The first step to a successful orientation. *Journal for Nurses in Professional Development, 36*(6), 362–364.

Brown, B. (2015). *Rising strong: The reckoning, the rumble, the revolution.* New York: Spiegel & Grau.

Creta, A. M., & Gross, A. H. (2020). Components of an effective professional development strategy: The professional practice model, peer feedback, mentorship, sponsorship, and succession planning. *Seminars in Oncology Nursing, 36*(3), 151024.

Hancock, B., & Meadows, M. T. (2020). The nurse manager and professional governance: Catalysts for leadership development. *Nurse Leader, 18*(3), 265–268.

Kahn, R. L., Wolfe, D. M., Quinn, R. P., Snoek, J. D., & Rosenthal, R. A. (1964). *Occupational stress: Studies in role conflict and ambiguity.* New York: Wiley.

Meyer, S. (2020). Hiring 101. *Nursing Management, 51*(1), 51–53.

Nursing Solutions Inc. (2021). *2021 NSI National Health Care Retention and RN Staffing Report.* East Petersburg, PA: Author.

Owings, C. R., & Gaskins, S. W. (2020). Evaluation of a community-based nurse residency. *Journal for Nurses in Professional Development, 36*(4), 185–190.

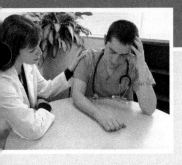

21

Managing Personal and Personnel Problems

Karren Kowalski

ANTICIPATED LEARNING OUTCOMES

- Differentiate common personal/personnel problems.
- Relate role concepts to clarification of personnel problems.
- Examine strategies useful for approaching specific personnel problems.

- Prepare specific guidelines for documenting performance problems.
- Value the leadership aspects of the role of the novice nurse.

KEY TERMS

absenteeism	nonpunitive discipline	role strain
chemically dependent	progressive discipline	role stress

THE CHALLENGE

I work in a hospital that uses a float pool of well-prepared staff who are ready to be assigned to various areas so that the appropriate level of care can be provided. As you might expect, these nurses, especially when new to the hospital, are not always familiar with all of the aspects of every unit. One of the nurses employed at the hospital in the resource float pool was floated one day to the surgical unit. During her shift, she cared for a patient, who, while unattended, fell out of bed. The nurse manager of the float pool was asked to determine what happened. *What would you do if you were this nurse?*

Kathleen Bradley, DNP, RN, NEA-BC
Associate Chief Nursing Officer (ACNO), Practice & Innovation, Informatics Liaison, Executive Director, Center for Professional Excellence & Inquiry, Stanford Children's Health

INTRODUCTION

Relatively new nurses often say, "As a new direct care nurse, I don't think of myself as a leader, so how is this information applicable?" In reality, even newly licensed registered nurses (NLRNs) with limited experiences are responsible for and, thus, lead assistive and support personnel. They often lead a team consisting of licensed practical nurses (LPNs)/licensed vocational nurses (LVNs) and unlicensed nursing personnel (UNP) who are responsible for a group of patients. Nurses may be responsible for including other team members such as housekeeping personnel and allied health professionals (e.g., respiratory therapists, pharmacists, dietitians, and physical therapists) in providing excellent quality care for patients. The NLRN must know how to handle difficult situations, including the decision to involve the unit leadership. Working effectively with people can be quite satisfying. On the other hand, working with people presents some of the greatest challenges in the workplace. Problems such as absenteeism, uncooperative or unproductive employees, clinical incompetence, employees with emotional problems, and employees with substance use issues are only a few. If a nurse or a new leader wants to be successful, these problems must be dealt with in ways that minimize their effects on patient care and on staff morale. Just as documentation of patient care is critical, documentation of performance problems is critical. Overall goals are to assist the employee in the improvement of performance, to maintain the highest standards for the delivery of patient care, and to provide a supportive environment in which all staff members deliver the best care and attain work satisfaction. From this perspective, in this chapter we examine several specific employee problems, addressing the leader's role and options as well as the responsibilities of the NLRN and the other frontline nurses.

PERSONAL/PERSONNEL PROBLEMS

Absenteeism

One of the most troublesome personnel problems is that of absenteeism (van Vulpen, 2021). Inadequate staffing adversely affects patient care both directly and indirectly. When an absent caregiver is replaced by another who is unfamiliar with the routines, employee morale suffers and care may not meet established standards. Replacement of absent personnel by temporary personnel or overtime paid to other employees is very costly, and the cost of fringe benefits used by absent workers is quite high. Working with inadequate staffing or working overtime to cover for absent workers creates physical and mental stress. Replacement personnel can also be problematic because these employees need more supervision, which not only is costly but also may decrease productivity and the quality

of patient care. Indirectly, coworkers may become resentful about being forced to assume heavier workloads or being pressured to work extra hours. Chronic absenteeism may lead to increased staff conflicts, to decreased morale, and eventually to increased absenteeism among the entire staff. Given that nurses may prefer to avoid conflict and negative behavior and to accommodate or make excuses for these situations, one way to confront persistent absenteeism is to discuss the situation directly with the employee in person using the format in Table 21.1. Any frontline nurse can use this same approach to convey to a peer what the impact of absenteeism has on the rest of the team. This same communications format (columns 1 and 2) can be used for many other difficult situations.

If a unit, clinic, or area has consistent excessive absenteeism, leaders in that area need to become involved. We know that some leaders have a style that may be offensive to employees, which could exacerbate absenteeism and other issues, such as decreaed job satisfaction. This can lead to decreased patient satisfaction. Even an NLRN who is leading a team, especially in clinic areas with fewer RNs, must pay attention to the style of leadership employed. Many positive concepts of leadership are found in transformational leadership, servant leadership, or authentic leadership styles. The most important aspect is to avoid any behaviors that alienate staff or prove to be toxic (see the Research Perspective).

Absenteeism also has a deleterious effect on the financial management of a nursing unit. When employee costs are excessive, they compromise the ability to support other creative efforts of the unit, such as staff education and new equipment, and may affect staff–patient ratios. Also, as care delivery systems become more complex and technically oriented, successful nurse leaders realize that technology is not a replacement for human caregivers. Absent caregivers cannot be replaced with machines.

TABLE 21.1   Confronting Persistent Absenteeism

Beginning Statement	Decoding the Statement	Statement in Full
"When I observe that……"	Action the person has/has not taken	"When I observe that you have been absent 3 days this month…….
"I feel…."	Your feeling or reaction	"….. I feel concerned and somewhat alarmed….."
"Because….."	Consequences for person, other team members, the unit/the facility	"Because absences have a negative impact on the team, which may have to work shorthanded, and this also can affect the quality of patient care…"
"Can you see how…."	The Tie Down: Seek agreement from the employee concerning outcomes or consequences of behavior	"Can you see how excessive absences affect the smooth functioning of the unit, the workload of other team members, and the safety of patients?"

RESEARCH PERSPECTIVE

Resource: Labrague, L., Nwafor, C., & Tsaras, K. (2020). Influence of toxic and transformational leadership practices on nurses' job satisfaction, job stress, absenteeism and turnover intention: A cross-sectional study. *Journal of Nursing Management, 28,* 1104–1113.

This study examined the influence of two types of leadership practices on nurses' job satisfaction, psychological distress, absenteeism, and intent to leave the organization or even the profession. The literature attributes favorable nurse retention factors to the implementation of transformational leadership practices. However, the literature is silent about the causal association between toxic leadership and job performance/outcomes.

This cross-sectional study involving 770 registered nurses from 15 Philippino hospitals focused on data collected using 7 self-report scales. When the leadership practice was described as toxic, registered nurses reported various negative attributes, such as greater absenteeism, job dissatisfaction, psychological distress, and the intent to leave the profession. Transformational leadership, on the other hand, was associated with greater job satisfaction and lower intents to leave the practice of nursing.

Implications for Practice

Clinical nurse retention strategies must include measures that grow and foster transformational leadership approaches and retrain or end toxic leadership practices through professional development. Some toxic leaders may need to find alternative employment.

Psychology Today (2021) identified burnout as another cause of absenteeism. Although the term "burnout" has been used since 1975, it is still not recognized as a diagnosis in the Diagnostic Manual of Mental Disorders (DSM-5), although, as of 2022, the World Health Organization recognizes it in its International Classification of Diseases (ICD-11). In general, burnout refers to workplace stress that results in feelings of exhaustion, negativism and a disconnect from one's work and colleagues for a prolonged period. During the COVID-19 pandemic, many nurses and other healthcare providers experienced an intensification of burnout due to such factors as staffing shortages (which continue), lack of equipment and supplies (which remains an issue at least sporadically), and disruptive relationships with patients and families (which have intensified in many situations). This lack of control in the situation and seeming unending conditions that feel unsupportive of many of the values nurses have continue to aggravate the potential for burnout. The cynicism, depression, and lethargy that are characteristic of burnout occur when a person is not in control of how a job is carried out, such as what we experienced during the pandemic. People also experience a sense of the stress being unending, resulting in feelings of emptiness and apathy, with no hope of amelioration.

We all remember photographs of nurses sitting on the floor in hallways with their heads in their hands, a picture of abject despair. Nurses were required to work in situations that conflicted with their professional values and sense of self.

Nurses who experienced the least amount of burnout were those in facilities where the leadership was present and seen by the staff. These leaders made frequent rounds, talked with nurses and communicated about the daily issues and shortages. They helped with care where possible and demonstrated caring and concern for the nurses.

Absenteeism cannot be totally eliminated. Unplanned illnesses, accidents, bad weather, sick family members, a death in the family, and even jury duty, which are legitimate reasons for missing work and beyond the control of management, will always occur. However, some portion of absenteeism is voluntary and preventable. Thus, the cause must be identified so that it may be addressed. These stressors lead to a poor work environment and lower the morale of fully engaged nurses. Other members of the team, including NLRNs, have an obligation to identify negative effects of absenteeism.

Absenteeism may also indicate poor work satisfaction. Dissatisfied staff may, in fact, be completely disengaged, which can lead to increased absences. If the leader believes that the issue is attributable to work dissatisfaction, unit-based discussions may lead to insight about the sources. Such discussions provide an excellent opportunity for the NLRN to listen, learn, and speak to issues. If the underlying cause can be identified, the loss of a dissatisfied employee may be preventable if retention is the goal. Some employees who convey that they are never happy with their jobs may continually disrupt the overall unit with their absenteeism and should be terminated.

Psychology Today (2021) addresses stress from a historical perspective as well as its impact today and describes stress from two perspectives, the psychological perception of pressure and the body's multisystem response to it from metabolism to muscles to memory. Although some stress is necessary, due to the need for appropriate responses to the challenges and uncertainties of our everyday existence, the automatic response to short-term "danger" or high stress is known as the *fight-or-flight response*, which prepares us to meet a threat or to flee.

Healthcare crises, the pace of modern life, and the constant increase in the rate of change, especially technological change, create feelings of inadequacy and an inability to cope. Physical symptoms associated with these stressors can include chest pain, headaches, indigestion (including nausea and loss of appetite), constipation or diarrhea, stomach cramps, muscle cramps, neck or back pain, or an increase in the frequency of flu and colds. Such symptoms can easily lead to absenteeism and can be problematic for the organization.

With role theory as a framework, absenteeism has been linked to role stress and role strain. Absence from work is a way of withdrawing from an undesirable situation short of actually leaving, and many employees increase their absenteeism just before submitting their resignation. If a healthcare worker is experiencing some form of role stress, absenteeism might be used as a strategy. Role strain may be reflected by (1) reduced involvement with colleagues and the organization, (2) decreased commitment to the mission and the team, and (3) job dissatisfaction. All of these could be manifested through absenteeism. With this framework, management of absenteeism is based on the belief that competent role performance requires interpersonal competence. Role competence is demonstrated through the ability of a person to act in a way that honors both the tasks and the interpersonal relationships. Role behavior occurs in a social context rather than in isolation. Consequently, NLRNs learn their role, both clinical and leading a team, from observing their peers functioning. They also learn adaptation to stress from their peers and could learn absenteeism as a coping strategy. In order to address such situations, the nurse leader needs to understand the existing situation, when the situation changed to its current status, when it needs to change further, and how to accomplish such change. People who are more satisfied in their work usually commit to "being there" for their team, which can enhance job satisfaction and may be an effective strategy toward reducing absenteeism. NLRNs can also learn this strategy from their peers and leaders.

One model for addressing issues in a nonpunitive way can be found in Fig. 21.1. This model demonstrates how undesirable behaviors, such as absenteeism, can be successfully altered. Box 21.1 identifies specific steps that are involved in nonpunitive discipline.

This model of nonpunitive discipline allows employees to free themselves from some role stress by clarification of role expectations and assumptions. Employees can receive

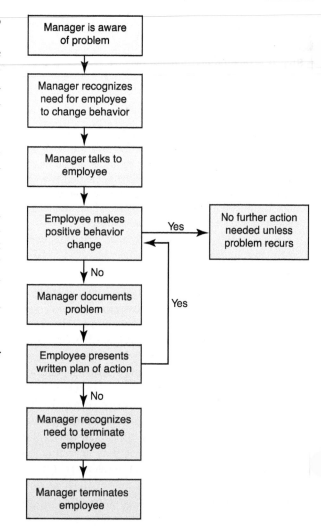

Fig. 21.1 Model for behavioral change.

satisfaction from the realization that a problem may not be inadequate performance caused by personal faults but rather a lack of clarification of role expectations within the organization. NLRNs may be called on to implement the process described in Box 21.1. For example, the NLRN may be involved with the nurse manager regarding an issue with assistive personnel or, in extenuating circumstances, may be initiating the process. For example, the NLRN might work with a UNP member who is absent or arrives late. On the other hand, a staff member who is actually quite ill, and even contagious to co-workers and patients, might come to work, infecting everyone. Remember, the focus is on the clear understanding of the situation, the growth of the individual, the smooth and effective functioning of the team, and the safety of the patients.

BOX 21.1 Steps to Clarify Role Expectations

Step 1: Remind the employee of the employment policies and procedures of the agency. Sometimes an employee does not know or has forgotten the existing standards, and a reminder with no threats or discipline is all that is needed. The employee must remain ultimately accountable to the organization's policies and procedures.

Step 2: When the oral reminder does not result in a behavior change, put the reminder in writing for the employee and cite the prior oral discussion. These oral and written reminders are simply statements of the problem and the goals to which both the manager and the employee agree. The employee must voluntarily agree with the manager that the behavior in question is not acceptable and must agree to change.

Step 3: If the written reminder fails, only then grant the employee a day of decision, which is a day off with pay, to arrive at a decision about future action. Pay is given for this day so that it is not interpreted as punishment. The employee must return to work with a written decision as to whether to accept the standards for work attendance. Remember that this is a voluntary decision on the employee's part. Emphasize to the employee that it is the employee's decision to adhere to the standards.

Step 4: If the employee decides not to adhere to standards, termination results. However, if the employee agrees to adhere to the standards and in the future does not, the employee, in essence, has terminated employment. Keep a copy of the written agreements and give the employee a copy. The manager should be clearly aware of the organization's policy for termination and request assistance from the human resources department as deemed necessary.

EXERCISE 21.1 Review the policy manual at a local healthcare organization to determine what constitutes excessive absenteeism. What are the identified consequences?

Uncooperative or Unproductive Employees

The problem of uncooperative or unproductive employees is another area of frustration for the nurse leader. Coker (2018) identified two major dimensions of job performance that relate to this problem: motivation and ability. The type and intensity of motivation vary among employees because of differing needs and goals that employees express. The leader can best handle employees with motivation problems by attempting to determine the cause of the problem and by working to provide an environment that is conducive to increased motivation for the employee. If the employee is uncooperative or unproductive because of a lack of ability, education and training are appropriate interventions.

The manager can determine lack of ability on the part of an employee in various ways. Frequent errors in judgment or techniques are often an indication of lack of knowledge, skill, or critical thinking. This illustrates the need for the nurse leader to document all variances or untoward events carefully after discussing them with the employee. When the nurse manager has thorough documentation, trends may be discovered that, in turn, suggest that a specific employee is having problems. The nurse manager can cite problem behaviors and perhaps even trends to the employee. Corrective action is easier to pursue and resolution is more effective with this strategy. When the problem is determined to result from a need for more education or training, the manager can work with the education department or the clinical specialist for the involved unit to help the employee improve one's skills. Most employees are extremely cooperative in situations such as this because they want to do a good job but sometimes do not know how. Employees may deny that they need help or may be too embarrassed to ask for help. When the manager can show an employee concrete evidence of a problem area, cooperation is enhanced. Frontline nurses may wish to keep personal notes about major performance issues because they may be indicators of larger issues than simply being uncooperative. We know that some of our colleagues may act out in an effort to seek help prior to deciding to end their lives. With the increased concern for mental wellness, we certainly wouldn't want to ignore someone's behavior that could be interpreted as an issue requiring an intervention. In other words, in today's work world anywhere, our alertness of others likely needs to be greater than it once was.

Immature Employees

Sometimes, an unproductive employee simply lacks maturity. This lack of maturity may be described as *emotional intelligence underdevelopment* that results in such problems as being socially inept or unable to control one's impulses. These employees are commonly defensive and emotional or tearful. They lack self-insight into their behavior. On occasion, immaturity in an employee may not be readily apparent to the leader but may be manifested in any of the following actions: defiance, testing of workplace guidelines, passivity or hostility, or little appreciation for any management decisions. The challenge for the nurse leader is not to react in kind but rather to relate to this employee in a positive and mature manner. A sense of humor and the ability to ease the employee into a more receptive mood can be helpful. However, the leader needs to determine whether the undesirable behaviors are reflecting a state of being uncomfortable or incompetent. For example, if an employee states, "Administration is always making decisions to make our jobs harder," rather than making a hostile or defensive comment in reply, the manager could take the employee aside and say, "I notice that you seem to be angry about this new policy. Let's talk about it some more." Immature employees either act immaturely all of the time or regress to an immature level when stressed. The nurse leader must recognize immaturity in an employee and react calmly and without anger. The leader must keep in mind that this employee may be displaying dynamics rooted in unresolved personal issues and that the behavior is not a personal attack on the leader. The best way to deal with this behavior is to hold a direct conversation with the employee about the specific problem and define realistic limits of acceptable behavior with consequences for nonadherence. Generally, employees comply with specific limits but will test management in other areas. As this testing occurs, the leader must continue the same limit-setting technique. Remember that the immature employee usually has problems because of a lack of self-worth, power, and self-control. Praise and affirmation are valuable tools that the leader can use to help these employees feel better about themselves.

> **EXERCISE 21.2** A nurse comes to you, the nurse leader, and states that one of the other nurses is tying a knot in the air vent (pigtail) of nasogastric tubes. This nurse does not know how to approach the employee to discuss the problem. What would you do?

Clinical Incompetence

Clinical incompetence is possibly one of the most frustrating problems that the nurse manager and team mates face, although it may be entirely correctable. To understand this problem, we must first understand what constitutes clinical competence, which is defined as the combination of knowledge, skill, attitude, and ability to provide safe and effective care without the need for supervision (Schrimmer et al., 2019). Knowledge is usually achieved through education and clinical experience, which is considered the basis for the skills and attitudes (see Literature Perspective). Skill is the ability to use knowledge and to continually learn and grow in clinical practice (Nabizadeh-Gharghozar et al., 2020).

LITERATURE PERSPECTIVE

Resource: Nabizadeh-Gharghozar, Z., Alavi, N., & Ajorpaz, N. (2020). Clinical competence in nursing: A hybrid concept analysis. *Nurse Education Today, 97*(2020), 104738.

Clinical competence (CC) in nursing is central to the functioning of the profession and to safe patient care. Yet some controversies exist that deserve further investigation, such as those involving the very definition of competence and the association between limited competency and an increase in errors and mortality rates. Most definitions have a common interstanding of clinical competency as a complex and multidimensional concept that many describe as a state but these authors view as a growth process. This hybrid concept analysis showed that it consists of a series of attributes and traits that form a basis for professional practice, many aspects of which may not be objective or measurable. Methodologically, this analysis is divided into three phases: (1) a theoretical phase that consisted of an extensive review of the literature; (2) the field work phase in which a qualitative study was done to explore participant experiences (four university lecturers, four clinical instructors, 4 students, and 6 hospital nurses were interviewed); and (3) the analysis phase in which the findings of the two previous phases were combined. The results determined that competence is a holistic term that refers to a person's overall capacity to do something successfully. Therefore, in nursing, competence is the ability to do a job successfully by meeting desired outcomes in differing conditions in the real world. Organizational factors that impact CC include staff and resource shortages; job burnout leading to low morale, negative attitudes, and lack of support; low salaries and poor social status; as well as an ethical atmosphere and sense of empowerment of staff. Personal factors include patience, anger management, effective coping skills, serenity, morale conscience, punctuality, physical and mental health, and discipline.

Implications for Practice
By considering these results, nurse managers and nurse educators will be able to design and implement activities for clinical nurses that will increase the knowledge, skills, attitudes, and abilities to provide safe, quality care to patients and families. The NLRNs will have an appreciation for these factors and can work toward identified individual goals.

The American Association of Colleges of Nursing's Essentials (2021) identifies 10 domains upon which competencies are based that form the practice of nursing. NLRN typically meet the entry level competencies at a generalist's level. Frontline nurses with varying educational and experiential backgrounds can range from competent in one area and expert in another to expert in multiple areas. Assigning nurses to areas where they normally do not work disadvantages them and the organization—and most of all the patient. This is not a case of clinical incompetence; it is a case of misassignment. When a nurse or UNP is missing a specific skill set or has an inability to master skills, we sometimes describe the person as clinically incompetent.

A problem with clinical competence may surface immediately in a new employee. Despite an effective interview process, a lack of fit may exist between the NLRN's strengths or skill set and the needs of the unit. Such a nurse can be coached and supported to gain competence or to find a different position, one that fully utilizes the individual's strengths and skills. At other times, clinical incompetence comes as a surprise when coworkers "cover" for another employee. Some nurses are unwilling to report instances of clinical incompetence because they do not want to feel responsible for getting one of their peers in trouble or because they, too, may sometimes feel inadequate. When other employees are engaged in enabling behavior by covering for the mistakes of one of their peers, the nurse manager may be surprised to discover that the employee does not know or cannot do what is expected of that employee. Sadly, the employee in question has been able to cover incompetence by hiding behind the performance of another employee. The nurse manager must remind employees that part of professional responsibility is to maintain quality care and, thus, they are obligated to report instances of clinical incompetence, even when it means reporting a coworker. Ignoring violations of a safety rule or poor practice is unprofessional and cannot be tolerated. Additionally, some state nursing practice acts make failure to report a violation of a rule or regulation a disciplinary offense.

Most healthcare agencies use skills checklists or a competency evaluation program to ascertain that their employees have and maintain essential skills for the job they are expected to do. A skills checklist is one way to determine basic clinical competency. Box 21.2 presents an example related to a specific competency. A clinical competency checklist typically contains a number of basic skills along with ones that are essential for safe functioning in the specific area of employment (Woten &

Karakashian, 2018). Any type of skills review should be directly linked to quality improvement indicators. The employee may be asked to do a self-assessment of the listed skills or competencies and then have performance of the skills validated by a peer or coworker. This is a very effective method for the manager to assess the skill level of employees and to determine where additional education and training may be necessary. In addition, if the manager discovers that an employee cannot perform a skill adequately, the skills list can easily be checked and directly observed behaviors can be assessed to determine at what level the employee is functioning. At the completion of the assessment, a specific plan for remediation can be developed. Sometimes, an employee may be able to perform all of the tasks on a skills checklist but still cannot manage overall patient care effectively. In questioning the employee or in evaluating the employee's performance, if the manager determines that a lack of knowledge or problems with time management exist, formal education may be the proper course of action. In either event, the manager must establish a written contract containing a plan of action that sets time limits within which certain expectations must be achieved. This ensures compliance on the part of the employee and simultaneously sets a time frame for the manager's action. A more comprehensive program for competency evaluation might include not only the skills checklist but also unit-specific objectives, an overall framework for evaluation, and critical-thinking exercises that are interactive in nature—for example, a complex patient situation such as an assessment in which the nurse is unclear as to what the next step might be. The role of the NLRN leader, particularly with ancillary personnel, is to support the nurse manager as well as to be helpful and supportive of the team members who are striving to improve, learn, and grow as healthcare workers.

EXERCISE 21.3 A nurse manager began hearing complaints from patients about a nurse named Nancy. Patients were saying that Nancy was abrupt and uncaring with them. The manager had not received any complaints about Nancy before this time. Thus, she questioned Nancy about why this was occurring. Nancy reported that her mother was very ill, and she was so worried about her and so upset that she could not sleep and was tired all of the time. She went on to say that she was having trouble being sympathetic with complaining patients when they did not seem to be as sick as her mother. How would you respond as the nurse manager?

BOX 21.2 Example of a Skills Checklist

Purpose

1. The clinical skills inventory is a three-phase tool to enable the newly hired registered nurse (RN) and the nurse manager to determine individual learning needs, verify competency, and plan performance goals.
2. The RN will complete the self-assessment of clinical skills during the first week of employment. The RN will use the appropriate scale to document current knowledge of clinical skills.
3. The nurse manager will document observed competency of the orientee or delegate this to a peer. All columns must be completed on the inventory level.
4. At the end of orientation, the new RN and the manager will use the inventory to identify performance goals on the plan sheet. The skills inventory will be in a specified place on the nursing unit so that it is available to the manager and other RNs. It should be updated at appropriate intervals as specified by the manager.

Scale for Self-Assessment

1 = Unfamiliar/never done
2 = Able to perform with assistance
3 = Can perform with minimal supervision
4 = Independent performance/proficient

Score for Validation of Competency

1 = Unable to perform at present
2 = Able to perform with assistance
3 = Progressing/repeat performance necessary
4 = Able to perform independently

Clinical Skills (Examples)	Self- Assessment			Validation			
	Scale	Date	Comment	Score	Date	Initials	Comment
Epidural catheter care							
NG/Dobhoff							
Insertion							
Management							
Preoperative care/teaching							
Postoperative care/teaching							

Plan Sheet for Skills Inventory

Name _____

Date _____

Goals	Date to Be Completed
_____	_____
_____	_____
_____	_____
_____	_____
_____	_____
_____	_____

Orientee's signature _____

Manager's signature _____

Date _____

When an employee's behavior changes significantly, personal problems with which the employee cannot cope may be the cause. The nurse manager is not and should not be a therapist but must intercede, not only to help the individual with the problems but also to maintain proper functioning of the unit. In dealing with the employee who exhibits behaviors that indicate emotional problems, the manager (and sometimes a peer who could be a NLRN) assists the individual to obtain professional help to cope with the problem. The individual's work setting and schedule may need to be adjusted. This may require support from other staff members so that no negative patient care results. The manager acknowledges to the employee that the employee is experiencing emotional difficulties and yet the standards of patient care cannot be compromised. Staff are reassured to witness the care and concern shown a fellow staff member who is in great difficulty. They can interpret that similar support would be given to them if they were in a difficult situation.

The most important approach that the manager can take with an emotionally troubled employee is to provide support and encouragement and to assist the individual to obtain appropriate help. Many organizations have some kind of employee assistance program (EAP) to which the manager should refer any troubled employee. During this process, the manager must remember to check with the human resources department about any implications that may occur because of the Americans with Disabilities Act (ADA). If an employee has a documented mental illness, the employing organization may be under certain legal constraints as specified in the ADA. The nurse manager should always remember that many resources are available to assist with personnel problems, including—in some states—services through the professional association. The manager should never feel required to know all of the legal implications regarding employment policies. Rather, the manager must know that help is available and how to access it.

Emotional Problems

Emotional problems among nursing personnel may affect not only the involved individual but also coworkers and, ultimately, the delivery of patient care. The nurse manager must be aware that certain behaviors, such as poor judgment, increased errors, increased absenteeism, decreased productivity, and a negative attitude, may be manifestations of emotional problems in employees.

> **EXERCISE 21.4** As a nurse manager in a community health agency, you have just had a meeting that was called by several of your direct care nurses. They expressed concern regarding another nurse colleague who has come to work angry and spiteful during the past week. They state she has made cutting and spiteful remarks to coworkers. Staff are beginning to turn away from her and not help her. She has refused to discuss her distress with her colleagues. These nurses express concern and want you to resolve the situation. What is your response? What would you do?

Substance Use

Substance use, or chemical dependency, among nursing personnel places patients and the organization at risk. Such an employee adversely affects staff morale by increasing stress on other staff members when they have to assume heavier workloads to cover for the chemically dependent employee who is not performing at full capacity or who is often absent. As a result, patient care may be jeopardized because staff are focusing more on the problems of a coworker than on those of the patients. NLRNs must be aware of the professional responsibilities of reporting incidents in which peers or team members exhibit signs of chemical dependency.

The manager is responsible for early recognition of chemical dependency and referral for treatment when appropriate (National Council of State Boards of Nursing, 2018). State laws vary as to the reportability of chemical dependency. As is true for all nurses, a nurse manager is responsible for upholding the nurse practice act and should be familiar with the legal aspects of chemical dependency in the state of employment. As with the employee with emotional problems, the nurse manager should be aware of ADA issues and check with the human resource department for help with how to handle the employment of a chemically dependent employee. Most states and agencies have reporting requirements regarding substance use. The state board of nursing is a key place to determine specific details required by a given state. All nurse managers should familiarize themselves with the nurse practice act in the state in which they are employed and with the personnel policies relating to substance use in their employing agency. Furthermore, nurse managers should ensure that staff are familiar with legal requirements.

In the present social climate, more interest exists in helping affected individuals than in punishing them; showing empathy and understanding also facilitates their work. Identification of an employee with a chemical dependency is usually difficult, especially because one of the primary symptoms is denial. The primary clue to chemical dependency is any behavioral change in an employee. This change could be any deviation from the behaviors the employee normally exhibits. Some specific behaviors that the nurse manager should note are mood swings, a change from a tidy appearance to an untidy one, an unusual interest in patients' pain control, frequent changes in jobs and shifts, or an increase in absenteeism and tardiness.

When a manager suspects that an employee may be chemically dependent, the manager must intervene because patient care may be jeopardized. A manager facing a problem with an impaired nurse must be compassionate yet therapeutic. Knowing that denial may be one of the primary signs of substance use, the manager must focus on performance problems that the nurse is exhibiting and urge the nurse to seek counseling or treatment voluntarily. EAPs always protect the employee's privacy and are usually available free or at a minimal charge to the employee. The manager should strive to refer any troubled employee to the EAP and/or to the state's peer assistance program. This removes the manager from the counseling role and helps employees get the professional help they need without fear of a breach in confidentiality. If a nurse refuses to seek help voluntarily for a substance use problem, the manager is responsible for following the established policy and laws for such employees. The manager must remember that if the employee who uses substances is terminated and not reported to the State Board of Nursing, the manager not only may be violating a law but also may be enabling this employee to obtain employment in another organization and potentially be in a position to harm patients and coworkers.

Many states have rehabilitation programs for chemically impaired nurses so that they may return to nursing if rehabilitated. Nurse managers are sometimes asked to assist with monitoring the progress of a chemically impaired nurse. Specific guidelines are established through the rehabilitation program with the cooperation of the employee, the organization, and the manager. The manager is typically asked to provide feedback about the employee's progress to the employee and to the state or rehabilitation program involved. These programs vary. However, for example, a nurse who has been an admitted user of opioids may be allowed to work in a setting in which this drug is never used or the nurse may not be permitted to administer any controlled substances to patients. This, of course, puts an added burden on other staff members. Nonetheless, it can be a positive experience for all because nurses face some of their professional responsibility by helping another nurse while upholding patient care. Often, as a part of their therapy, these nurses are required to share openly with other staff members what their problem is and what they are doing to control it. When handled in a positive, professional way, the nurse manager can turn a potentially destructive situation into a positive, constructive one. Regardless of the type of personnel issue, the manager needs to have a plan in place for ongoing monitoring and follow-up of issues and problems.

Most health professionals are aware of the national opioid situation in the United States because it has been emphasized politically. Considerable federal funding is available to address this health crisis.

EXERCISE 21.5 Review your state's nurse practice act and rules and regulations. What are you required to do if you believe a nurse has a problem with chemical dependency?

Incivility

Incivility or lateral violence in the workplace is disruptive behavior or communication that creates a negative work environment, thus interfering with quality patient care and safety (AACN, 2016). Such behavior is often nurse to nurse or provider to provider. These behaviors include nonverbal innuendo such as eye rolling or eyebrow raising, verbal affronts, undermining activities, withholding information, sabotage, infighting, scapegoating, backstabbing, failure to respect privacy, and broken confidences. Uncivil behavior must be addressed. The first step by the manager, or any nurse for that matter, when observing the unwanted behavior may be a discussion with the offending nurse. The next step, after a formal discussion by the manager, is written documentation in the personnel file if the behaviors do not abate. This is followed by a stepwise disciplinary action in association with the human resources department. New nurses need to be cognizant of behaviors of incivility and to understand the guidelines and rules relevant to such behavior in the facility. Also, they need to support increased teamwork by behaving in a positive, upbeat manner and to not become enmeshed in negative behavior on the unit.

From a study of 79 respondents to an electronic survey of newly licensed nurses, Smith et al. (2020) identified four strategies to stop bullying behavior. They were:
1. Discuss the incident with peers or the manager or seek support.
2. Use a de-escalation strategy such as agreeing how everyone will respond when one of you is attacked.
3. Exhibit Upstanding behaviors such as intervening in a situation you observe or calling out the inappropriate behavior.
4. Responding with aggression, which includes such activities as "talking over" the bullying person or calling out the inappropriate behavior.

Each of these behaviors is an assertive approach to bullying behaviors and requires the commitment of the team to be effective. While an individual can call out behavior and stand up to a bully, it is always more effective if that message is delivered by more than one sender. However, it is better to be delivered by one than not at all. Documenting each of the encounters is important–both the observations you made of the incivility and the actions you took, including to whom you reported the event. In addition to organizational policies, federal policy may also be a part of substantive backing of your situation. Title VII of the Civil Rights Act of 1964 makes it illegal for an employer, manager, or supervisor to take certain actions against employees based on their sex, religion, race, national origin, or color. Businesses can be held responsible for the actions of their management, supervisory staff, and employees. Bullying rises to the level of harassment when any reasonable employee would consider the behavior uncomfortable, offensive, or hostile.

Since the pandemic, we have seen that some patients and their families have more difficulty controlling their personal behavior than they did before. Because frontline nurses are the ones with greatest contact with patients and families, we all need to be sure that we know the safety policies and deescalation techniques to best manage situations we might encounter. While administration is concerned with the safety of patients, they also are concerned with the safety of their employees. If they are not, they could lose employees and their reputation. Harassment becomes illegal when tolerating it becomes a condition of your employment—you either put up with it or you're out of a job. Nurses can choose how they respond or react to uncivil or bullying behavior. These choices can mean the difference between thriving and merely surviving.

DOCUMENTATION

Documentation of personnel problems is unquestionably one of the most important but also one of the most onerous aspects of the nurse manager's job (Fig. 21.2). As much as some managers may want to wish them away, personnel problems probably will not "disappear" and, therefore, will eventually have to be resolved. Through careful, ongoing documentation of problems, the manager makes the task of identifying and correcting problems much less burdensome.

Documentation cannot be left to memory! At the time that an employee is involved in a problem situation or receives a compliment or does something extremely well, a brief notation to this effect must be placed in the personnel file. This entry includes the date, time, and a brief description of the incident. Adding a short notation as to what was done about a problem when it occurred is also helpful. Along with this, the nurse manager should keep a log or summary sheet of all reported errors, unusual incidents, and accidents. These extremely important data should include the date, time, and names of involved individuals and should be tallied monthly for analysis by

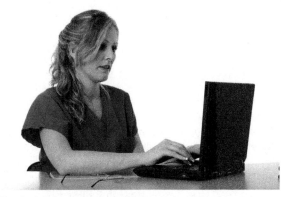

Fig. 21.2 Documentation of personnel problems is an important aspect of the nurse manager's job. (Copyright © geotrac/iStock/Thinkstock.)

the manager. The few extra minutes each day that the manager spends tracking these data provide invaluable information about organizational and individual functioning. This tracking can then be used to pinpoint an individual's problem areas, areas of excellence in individual performance, and overall organizational problem areas. The manager who keeps careful records about organizational functioning has greater control in the management of personal and personnel problems. Box 21.3 describes content and format for such documentation and provides an example as an illustration.

BOX 21.3 Documentation of Problems

- Description of incident: An objective statement of the facts related to the incident
- Actions: Statements describing the plan to correct or prevent future problems
- Follow-up: Dates and times that the plan is to be carried out, including required meeting with the employee

Several patients reported that Becky Smith (night-shift RN) was "curt" and "gruff" and seemed uncaring with them. I called Becky into my office and reiterated the complaints that I had received, including the specifics of times and incidents. I reminded Becky about what my expectations were relating to patient care, emphasizing the importance of a caring attitude with all patients. We discussed what the possible cause of Becky's behavior might be, such as problems at home or lack of sleep. Becky denied being curt or gruff but agreed that some of her mannerisms might be misinterpreted. I suggested to Becky that perhaps she needed to be particularly aware of her body language and to soften her tone of voice. After discussing this incident and reminding Becky of the importance of caring in nursing, I cited the policy regarding behavior and told Becky that this behavior would not be tolerated. I told Becky we needed to meet every Friday morning at the end of Becky's shift to discuss how the week had gone and to determine how she was interacting with the patients assigned to her. I also told Becky I would be checking with patients to see what they had thought of Becky, pointing out that I do this routinely.

These weekly meetings are to be conducted for 6 weeks, followed by monthly meetings for a 3-month period. If problems do not recur, the meetings will be discontinued after this time.

Joseph P. Riley, RN, MSN
Nurse Manager, Hanson Way Hospital

It can also be valuable for the nurse who is the recipient of uncivil behavior to keep personal notes similar to those described here. This documentation can then be used if the nurse is asked to recall specific incidences. These can be kept privately in a journal or in an electronic file.

PROGRESSIVE DISCIPLINE

When an employee's performance falls below the acceptable standard despite corrective measures that have been taken, some form of discipline must be enacted. Most organizations use some form of progressive discipline to correct problem behaviors. When the nurse leader suspects that specific behaviors may lead to progressive discipline, all interactions must be documented and the human resources department must be involved in the process to ensure accurate adherence to all policies. Progressive discipline consists of evaluating performance and providing feedback within a specified structure of increasing sanctions. These sanctions, progressing from least severe to most severe, are described in Box 21.4. Examples of the kind of workplace behavior that usually involves progressive discipline and could even result in immediate termination are harassment and chemical use.

BOX 21.4 Steps in Progressive Discipline

1. Counsel the employee regarding the problem.
2. Reprimand the employee. A verbal reprimand usually precedes a written one, but some organizations issue both a verbal and a written reprimand simultaneously. When the documentation is written, the employee must sign to verify that the problem was discussed. This does not mean that the employee agrees with the reprimand. It means only that the employee is aware of a written reprimand that is to be placed in the employee's personnel file. The employee always receives a copy of a written reprimand.
3. Suspend the employee if the problem persists. The individual will be suspended without pay for a specified period, usually several days or longer according to the agency policy. During this time, the employee may realize the seriousness of the problem based on the resulting discipline.
4. Allow the employee to return to work with written stipulations regarding problem behavior.
5. Terminate the employee if the problem recurs.

TERMINATION

At times, even though the manager has done everything possible to gain the cooperation of a problem employee, the problems may persist. In such cases, termination is the only choice. Termination is one of the most difficult things a manager does; thus, guidelines are needed to be certain that a manager can perform this task without contributing to further distress for either party. Additionally, an organization may require that a representative from human resources or security (or both) be present. Specific guidelines should be followed (Box 21.5).

The nurse manager needs to be confident in the knowledge that all policies regarding termination have been followed before having an actual termination meeting with the employee. It is almost always preferable to err on the side of caution when proceeding with termination of an employee. Remember that termination is something that the employee has caused as a result of persistent problem behaviors or certain behaviors for which the organization has zero tolerance. Termination is not done at the whim of management; it results from failure on the part of the employee to change a problem behavior.

Situations that may warrant immediate dismissal include theft, violence in the workplace, and willful abuse of a patient, to name a few. Again, the manager should use the assistance of the human resource department to ensure that all of the organization's policies are being upheld correctly. The following example illustrates that a manager needs to anticipate a termination to ensure ongoing standards:

Michael has gone through all of the steps in the progressive discipline process as a result of his abusive behavior toward his coworkers. He returned to work and seemed to be doing well until about 6 weeks later, when he slammed down his clipboard during report and angrily accused the charge nurse of always giving him the worst assignments. The nurse manager was present and asked Michael to come into her office. At this point, she told Michael she was relieving him of his assignment that day and asked him to go home to cool off. The manager told him that she would call him the following day about what would be done. Michael went home, and the manager reviewed the incident with her nurse administrator. They both agreed that Michael's behavior not only was intolerable but also violated the terms of his probation and, therefore, he should be terminated. The manager called Michael the following day, as she had agreed to do, and asked him to come and meet with her. The manager and administrator met with Michael and reviewed the incidents and the disciplinary measures leading up to this incident. The nurse manager asked the administrator to be present at the scheduled meeting because it is a good practice to have a witness in a confrontational situation such as termination. The manager stated to Michael that she regretted it had come to this but pointed out to him that his behavior had violated all of the agreed-upon stipulations and, as a result, he would be terminated immediately. Michael seemed embarrassed and anxious and had numerous excuses, but the manager remained firm and merely repeated that Michael, in not fulfilling the agreement, had chosen to end his employment.

BOX 21.5 Guidelines to Effective Termination

1. The manager must be confident that everything possible has been done to help the employee correct the problem behaviors.
2. The manager must recognize that if employment continues, this employee will have a deleterious effect on overall organizational functioning and, more important, on nursing care.
3. The employee must have been made fully aware of the problem performance and of the fact that all of the correct disciplinary steps have been followed.
4. The nurse manager should check with the human resources and legal departments before proceeding to ensure that termination is justifiable legally and that proper steps have been followed.

EXERCISE 21.6 Review a healthcare organization's policies regarding termination. What are the conditions—such as stealing, violence, or coming to work under the influence of alcohol or drugs—that are described as cause for immediate dismissal? Is using substances at work one of those conditions? Consider how you would intervene with a colleague who exhibited one of these behaviors or conditions.

CONCLUSION

Managing personal and personnel issues is a challenge for every manager. The process is time-consuming and detail oriented and does not always result in a positive outcome. All employees share a role with managers to prevent and control personal/personnel problems in their work setting. Everyone must be willing to refuse to allow unethical behavior from coworkers and to speak out and act appropriately when problems occur. The focus of all action is the protection of others: patients and employees.

THE SOLUTION

The nurse manager in charge of the resource float pool wanted to assess the float pool nurses' critical-thinking skills and did this through weekly rounding. The charge nurses of each unit also completed a peer assessment form whenever a nurse floated to the unit so that the nurse who floated there could receive feedback. In this manner, if a pattern emerged from either the rounding assessment or the peer reviews, the float nurse could receive immediate coaching. Finally, the nurse manager decided to have the staff review published information about hourly rounding and review the patient fall protocols from the various units where the float nurse worked.

Would this be a suitable approach for you? Why?

Kathleen Bradley

REFLECTIONS

Think about a time when you were "bullied," humiliated, or publicly berated. How did it make you feel? What was your response? How well did your response work? Now that you have read this chapter, what might you do differently versus what you did before reading this chapter?

BEST PRACTICES

Although most of us don't like paper work, personnel problems is one area where keeping detailed records is really important. When a problem exists, intervening early is usually beneficial for the person and the organization. Trying to determine if the problem is transient or not is worthwhile for the manager. Frontline nurses have a critical role to play in this area too, even though it may feel uncomfortable.

TIPS IN THE DOCUMENTATION OF PROBLEMS

- Identify the incident and related facts.
- Describe actions taken by the manager when the problem was identified.
- Develop an action plan for everyone involved.
- Schedule a follow-up meeting to evaluate progress of the action plan.
- Remember to document everything objectively and completely!

REFERENCES

American Association of Colleges of Nursing. (2021). The essentials: Core competencies for professional nursing education. Retrieved from https://www.aacnnursing.org/Portals/42/AcademicNursing/pdf/Essentials-2021.pdf.

American Association of Critical Care Nurses (AACN). (2016). *AACN standards for establishing and sustaining health work environments: A journey to excellence* (2nd ed.). Aliso Viejo, CA: Author.

Coker, D. (2018). *Foolproof ways to deal with unproductive employees.* Retrieved from https://theHRdigest.com/foolproof-ways-to-deal-with-unproductive-employees.

Labrague, L., Nwafor, C., & Tsaras, K. (2020). Influence of toxic and transformational leadership practices on nurses' job satisfaction, job stress, absenteeism and turnover intention: A cross-sectional study. *Journal of Nursing Management, 28,* 1104–1113.

Nabizadeh-Gharghozar, Z., Alavi, N., & Ajorpaz, N. (2020). Clinical competence in nursing: A hybrid concept analysis. *Nurse Education Today*, 97(2021), 104738.

National Council of State Boards of Nursing (NCSBN). (2018). *A nurse manager's guide to substance use disorder in nursing.* Chicago: Author.

Psychology Today. (2021). *Burnout.* Retrieved from https://www.psychologytoday.com/us/basics/burnout.

Psychology Today. (2021). Stress. Retrieved from https://www.psychologytoday.com/us/basics/stress#:~:text=Stress%20generally%20refers%20to%20two%20things%3A%20the%20psychological,multiple%20systems%2C%20from%20metabolism%20to%20muscles%20to%20memory.

Schrimmer, K., Williams, N., Mercado, S., & Polancich, S. (2019). Workforce competencies for healthcare quality professionals: Leading quality-driven healthcare. *Journal for Healthcare Quality*, 41(4), 259–265.

Smith, C. R., Palazzo, S. J., Grubb, P. L., & Gillespie, G. L. (2020). Standing up against workplace bullying behavior: Recommendations from newly licensed nurses. *Journal of Nursing Education and Practice*, 10(7), 35. https://doi.org/10.5430/jnep.v10n7p35.

van Vulpen, E. (2021). *Absenteeism in the workplace: A full guide.* Retrieved from https://digitalhrtech.com/absenteeism/.

Woten, M., & Karakashian, A. (2018). *Precepting: Building a competency-based orientation program.* Glendale, CA: Cinahl Information Systems.

22

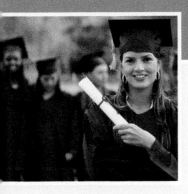

Role Transition

Diane M. Twedell

ANTICIPATED LEARNING OUTCOMES

- Delineate strategies that will assist nurses through a successful role transition.
- Construct the full scope of a manager role by outlining responsibilities, opportunities, lines of communication, expectations, and support.
- Describe the importance of a mentor–mentee relationship in professional development of a new manager.
- Describe the phases of role transition by using a life experience.

KEY TERMS

mentor	role negotiation	role stress
role internalization	role strain	role transition

THE CHALLENGE

I was in school obtaining my master's degree with a young growing family at home. I had a job I loved but I couldn't shake the inner craving for something more. A position for nurse manager of primary care came open in the largest ambulatory unit at my organization. I took the risk, applied for the position, an offer was extended, and I accepted it. The department was rich with a culture of teamwork, allegiance, strong personalities, and many long-tenured nurses. These nurses were some of the best in the building and handled high-demand workloads. I had been a staff nurse in another area that shared a break room with many of these nurses; now, I was expected to lead them. How was I going to be accepted? Would they trust me, and how would they look to me for guidance when they have two to three times more years of nursing experience as I do?

What would you do if you were this nurse?

Jolene D. Piper, MSN, BSN, RN
Nurse Manager, Mayo Clinic Health System, Albert Lea, Minnesota

INTRODUCTION

Role transition involves transforming one's professional identity. A new graduate makes a transition from the student role to the nurse role. The new graduate nurse faces the first of several professional transitions, some of which will be easier than others. These transitions continue with career growth and development. Consider the frontline nurse who becomes a nurse manager—the individual must transition into the new role as a generalist, orchestrating diverse tasks and getting work done through others. Much of role transition depends on reflection on the feedback received from performance appraisals, mentors, and others. Proactive nurses inquire about their potential career options within an organization and actively seek transitions that fit their clinical and role expertise.

Organizations play a key role in assisting employees through role transitions. Changes in roles can be either painful or exciting, depending largely on the work culture and support provided.

Knowing what to expect during this transformation can reduce the stress of role transition and lead to highly engaged nursing staff and quality patient outcomes.

TYPES OF ROLES

Accepting a management or formal leadership position dictates accepting three roles that involve complex processes. The roles of leader, manager, and follower are complex because they involve working through and with unique individuals in a rapidly changing environment. Additionally, in any situation, a nurse can perform all three roles. Examples of the people with whom you interact and the processes involved in each role are shown in Table 22.1.

Leader

This is a person who demonstrates and exercises influence over others. In the evolving healthcare environment, the nurse leader providing direct patient care also must function as a leader, manager, and follower. Depending on the unit size and structure, the leader may act as charge nurse on the unit for the day, assigning patients to nursing staff and working in concert with the team to provide direct care. As *leader*, the nurse leader recognizes the uniqueness of each patient and provides feedback on clinical progress. The nurse leader also serves as a manager working with the staff as a team to manage all needs on the unit. In addition, the nurse leader will act as a follower in providing care following the appropriate orders and carrying out the directions of care team members.

TABLE 22.1 Leader, Manager, and Follower Roles: Interactions and Processes Involved in Each Role

Role	People With Whom Interactions Occur	Processes Involved in the Role
Leader	Persons being led Peers "Boss" Regulating agencies	Listening Encouraging Inspiring Motivating Organizing Problem solving (high level) Developing Supporting
Manager	Persons being supervised Administrators Supervisors Regulating agencies	Organizing Budgeting Hiring Evaluating Reporting Disseminating Listening Influencing Problem solving (unit level)
Follower	Supervisor Peers	Conforming Implementing Contributing Completing assignments Alerting Listening Influencing Problem solving (patient and team level) Questioning

Manager

This is a person with accountability for a group of people. As a manager, the nurse links the patient to the resources to achieve clinical outcomes. Medical information is translated into a format that the patient can use to make informed decisions about treatment and self-care. Through referrals, the nurse manager facilitates continuity of care within the larger system. The nurse manager serves in a planned manner as the conduit of information for the various other departments in the organization to facilitate the timely and safe care for patients. On a day-to-day basis, this co-ordination is typically implemented by the direct care staff by virtue of the plans developed by the managers of the services.

Follower

This is a person who contributes to a group's outcomes by implementing activities and providing appropriate feedback. As a *follower*, the nurse is accountable to the team and the supervisor for completing the work that is assigned. The nurse as a follower practices within the policies and procedures of the organization and the standards of the profession.

The daily work of a nurse transitions seamlessly through the three roles, and although this may feel very different during role transition, it occurs during that same time. The nurse is assigned to a preceptor whom the nurse follows and learns the cultural norms and practices of a patient care unit; the nurse is also a manager in helping patients navigate a complex system of care and a leader in providing individualized assessment and care to every patient. That same nurse may also lead a change that is needed to improve the care of patients. Similarly, the chief nursing officer (CNO) leads the nursing function of the organization, manages the executive offices of the nursing department, and follows the chief executive officer and board directives. As is true of followership in any role, the CNO also challenges decisions and intervenes when seeing issues that concern patient care or staff safety or well-being.

ROLES: THE ABC'S OF UNDERSTANDING ROLES

Another approach to the complexity of role transition is the acronym ROLES, in which each letter represents a component common to roles (Box 22.1).

- **R** stands for responsibilities. What are the specified duties in the position description for the new position? What tasks are to be completed? What decisions must the person in this position make?

BOX 22.1 **Roles Acronym**
Responsibilities
Opportunities
Lines of communication
Expectations
Support

- **O** stands for opportunities, which are untapped aspects of the position.
- **L** represents lines of communication, which are the heart of every leadership role. No matter what role an individual is in, multiple relationships exist with supervisors, staff, and peers.
- **E** stands for expectations. Expectations can vary depending on your goals. Colleagues may expect a nurse anesthetist to be on call every weekend. Frontline nurses have specific expectations of their nurse leader. Learning as much about the expectations others hold for a position and for you provides greater clarity about your fit in the role.
- **S** stands for support, which is closely tied to expectations about performance. All roles are shaped to some degree by the support and services others provide. The frontline nurse has peers available when a second opinion is needed. The same nurse may feel lost when confronted with questionable findings during a home visit.

ROLE TRANSITION PROCESS

Some individuals may find it helpful to think about role transition in a common social context. The process of developing an intimate relationship with another person provides a familiar framework for considering role transition. This approach is explained in Box 22.2 in detail.

Patricia Benner's historic work, "From Novice to Expert" (1982), provides a framework for the ongoing development of nurses. It is based on five different levels of practice: novice, advanced beginner, competent, proficient, and expert. Even very experienced nurses become novices again when introduced into a new role. For example, a very savvy and experienced intensive care unit (ICU) nurse becomes an ICU nurse manager—the individual may be expert in the clinical ICU skills and assessment techniques, but the new world of management may be overwhelming. Therefore, the individual would now be a novice or advanced beginner again in the new role of nurse manager.

Becoming a manager or assuming a new role requires a transformation—a profound change in identity. Such a transformation invokes stress as the person changes roles to learn the management role. Several strategies can be helpful in easing the strain and speeding the process of role transition (Box 22.3). No matter what the transition is, this movement involves the development of a capacity for leadership.

EXERCISE 22.1 You have been a frontline nurse on a busy medical-surgical unit for 3 years. You have been successful in both the clinical practice and in being involved with the shared decision-making committee. A full-time assistant nurse manager position has opened on the evening shift, and you are considering applying for the position. As you begin to contemplate this position, what thoughts do you have related to moving from a frontline registered nurse (RN) to a leadership position? Detail what you would do to prepare yourself for this question at the interview: "How will you prepare to transition from a peer to a supervisor on this patient care area?" Develop two to three interview questions you might anticipate being asked during the interview about your values and how you work with others. Develop two to three interview questions you want to ask about the position and the support you will have.

BOX 22.2   Role Transition Process

Moving out of old roles while learning new roles requires an identity adjustment over time. The persons involved must invest themselves in the process. In this way, role transition can be compared with developing a relationship. The process of developing an intimate relationship with another person provides a familiar framework for considering role transition. Relationships typically move through the phases of dating, commitment, honeymoon, disillusionment, resolution, and maturity.

Role Preview
During the dating phase, the interested persons spend structured time together. Both parties present their best characteristics and dedicate much energy to developing the relationship. Although both parties present their best characteristics, both also are alert to clues that the other party cannot meet their expectations. For example, you may consider the financial and emotional resources that the other person would bring to the relationship. The individuals might spend time with each other's families to get a feel for the emotional climate in which the other person grew up.

Interviewing for a management position is similar to dating. An interview involves touring the unit, visiting with people, and attempting to make a good impression. The potential employer is also attempting to make a favorable impression. Interviewees want to determine whether an organization will support their growth as they support the growth of the organization. Questions are asked about the role of the manager, and the potential manager mentally evaluates whether the described role matches personal expectations about management. Both of these examples represent the phase "role preview."

Role Acceptance
Through the dating process, two people may decide that they want to spend the rest of their lives together and commit to the relationship, or one or both people may decide that they do not want to establish a long-term relationship. In a similar way, after the role preview of the interview process, both parties may agree to establish a relationship as employee and employer. Or one or both of the parties may decide not to establish the relationship. In dating, the public decision to leave other similar relationships and establish this new relationship represents a formal commitment. In role transition, the formal commitment of the employment contract implies acceptance of the management role, or "role acceptance."

Role Exploration
In new relationships, a time of dating and commitment is usually followed by a honeymoon. More than a trip to a vacation spot, the honeymoon has become synonymous with excitement, happiness, and confidence. In a new work role, people also experience a honeymoon phase. The new graduate may be relieved that the educational program was successfully completed and now a salary can be earned. When a new manager is hired, the employer is excited that the search is over. The staff is happy to have a leader, especially if staff members had input into the hiring decision. The new manager is happy, excited, and, most of all, confident in exploring the new roles involved in the management position.

Role Discrepancy
Whether by a gradual process or as the result of a particular event that serves as the turning point, the honeymoon is eventually over and disillusionment about the relationship occurs. For example, one person may make an expensive purchase without consulting the partner. An argument is followed by a period of painful silence. Similarly, the honeymoon phase in a new employment position can be followed by a period of disillusionment.

BOX 22.2   Role Transition Process—cont'd

Role discrepancy, a gap between role expectations and role performance, causes discomfort and frustration. Role discrepancy can be resolved by either dissolving the relationship or by changing expectations and performance. The importance of the relationship and the perceived differences between performance and expectations, the basis of role discrepancy, must be considered in light of personal values. When the relationship is valued and the differences are seen as correctable, the decision is made to stay in the relationship. This decision requires the couple or the manager to develop the role.

Role Development

Choosing to change either role expectations or role performance or to change both is the process of role development. In an intimate relationship, open communication can clarify expectations. Negotiation may result in reasonable expectations. Certain behaviors may be changed to improve role performance. For example, one person in the relationship learns to call home to let the other know about the possibility of being late.

To reduce role discrepancy in a new management position, the same open communication and negotiation must occur. Expectations need to be clarified and stipulated by both parties. New managers evaluate management styles and techniques to determine which ones best fit them and the situation. The personal management style evolves as the individuals develop the management roles in their own unique ways. If role discrepancy can be reduced and the role developed to be satisfactory to both parties, the new manager can focus on developing the roles of the position and proceed to the phase of role internalization.

Role Internalization

Role internalization occurs in relationships as they mature. No longer do the persons in the relationship consciously consider their roles. They have learned the behaviors that maintain and nurture the relationship. The behaviors become second nature. The energy spent on establishing and developing the relationship can be redirected toward achieving mutual goals. In the same way, managers who have been in management positions for several years have internalized their roles. Usually, they do not consciously consider their roles. Managers know they have reached the stage of role internalization when they focus on accomplishing mutual goals instead of contemplating whether their role performance matches their role expectations. Managers who have internalized their roles have developed their own unique personal style of management. Table 22.2 summarizes the comparison between the phases of developing an intimate relationship and the phases of role transition to a nurse manager.

Unexpected Role Transition

Not every relationship is successful. Some relationships end in an argument, divorce, or death. When a relationship ends unexpectedly, a person goes through a grieving process. In a similar way, when a person is fired, a position is eliminated, or a job description changes dramatically, the person may have to grieve before being able to engage in role transition. Healthcare is in a tumultuous state. Mergers, acquisitions, and reductions in workforce are commonplace. To be successful, workplace restructuring must be undertaken with the same sensitivity afforded a person who has lost a relationship through death or divorce. Role transition takes time, even in reverse.

The initial response to a change in role can be shock and disbelief. The person may feel numb and unable to function. As the numbness wears off, the person may become angry. The anger fuels resistance to the change and may be directed toward those who initiated the role change. The anger may be directed internally, leading to depression. If the person is unable to acknowledge and talk about the loss, the period of grief may be extended, or emotional baggage may be created that is carried into the next role. Grieving can eventually resolve in acceptance. Lessons learned from the experience are identified and internalized. A new role is sought, and the "dating" begins again.

When a relationship is dissolved in the case of death or divorce, a legal document is prepared to formally dissolve the financial and social obligations between the persons involved. The loss of a position as a result of restructuring or a buyout should involve a similar process. The employer may offer the nurse a severance package that includes financial compensation and outplacement services. If the employer does not offer a written agreement, the nurse should formally request and negotiate reasonable compensation and assistance. Similar to signing a prenuptial agreement, a nurse may have signed a contract with the employer when hired. The terms of that agreement may require the employer to buy out (pay the salary and benefits) for the time remaining on the contract.

Jennifer Jackson Gray

TABLE 22.2 Comparison of Phases in Developing an Intimate Relationship and Undergoing Role Transition as a Nurse Manager

Phase in Developing an Intimate Relationship	Phase in Role Transition as a Nurse Manager	Characteristics of Phase
Dating	Role preview	Presentation of best characteristics to make favorable impression; both parties evaluate each other to determine likelihood of the other being able to fulfill one's expectations
Commitment to relationship	Role acceptance	Public announcement of mutual decision to initiate contract
Honeymoon	Role exploration	Experience of excitement, confidence, and mutual appreciation
Disillusionment	Role discrepancy	Awareness of difference between role expectations and role performance; reconsideration of whether to continue with contract
Resolution	Role development	Negotiation of role expectations; adjustment of role performance to approximate expectations and to find one's own unique style
Maturation of relationship	Role internalization	Performance of role congruent with one's own beliefs and individual style; achievement of mutual goals

---

BOX 22.3 Strategies to Promote Role Transition

Strengthen internal resources.
Assess the organization's resources, culture, and group dynamics.
Negotiate the role.
Grow with a mentor.
Develop management knowledge and skills.

STRATEGIES TO PROMOTE ROLE TRANSITION

When a transition is likely, nurses can employ specific strategies to enhance the success of that transition.

Internal Resources

A key strategy in promoting role transition is to recognize, use, and strengthen one's values and beliefs. Behavior is influenced by values and beliefs. New leaders need to keep sight of their own values and beliefs. The role of manager is not for everyone. You must consider whether personal goals and professional fulfillment can best be achieved through management. One's commitment to the challenges of managing can provide the desire to persevere during the process of role transition.

Individuals in transition who understand their own personal values are best equipped to respond to situations and relationships. A person's value does not depend on the quality or quickness of the adjustment to the management role. An exercise such as writing down short statements of belief or self-affirmations and posting this information may be helpful as a visual reminder.

Changing circumstances in healthcare raise the need for flexibility. The effective leader must be able to learn and master new skills, translate information for staff, and adapt behavior to the situation. The new leader should also not expect too much of oneself all at once; understanding that this transition takes time will help with flexibility.

Organizational Assessment

A new manager is much like an immigrant in a new country. An immigrant learns how to access the available resources to acclimate to the new environment. Cultural practices of the new country may seem strange or odd. Such differences can be analyzed and decisions made about which aspects to incorporate into one's own culture. Added subtle differences in communication patterns or group dynamics can also be identified. Understanding the nuances of social interactions is often the most difficult aspect of acclimating to a new country. The transition is smoother for immigrants who understand themselves, assess the new environment, and learn how to communicate within groups.

The new manager must also learn how to access resources in the organization. Approaching the organization as a foreign culture, the new manager can keenly observe the rituals, accepted practices, and patterns of communication within the organization. This ongoing assessment promotes a speedier transition into the role of manager. An immigrant who spends energy bemoaning the difficulties of the new country may fail to enjoy the advantages that were the attractions to the country in the first place. In the same way, the manager who focuses on the weaknesses of the organization may lack the energy to internalize the new role, a step that is critical to being an effective leader. A new manager who feels out of place in the new role may feel similar to the immigrant who wants to go home. The new manager may forget the reasons for taking the new position and just want to return to a frontline nurse role to be comfortable again.

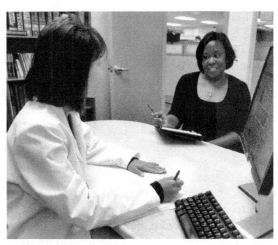

Fig. 22.1 Negotiating a role can create new opportunities for both parties to the negotiation. A written addendum may be all that is necessary to recreate a new understanding of what the new expectations are.

> **EXERCISE 22.2** You have successfully obtained the position as a nurse manager in a busy ambulatory care clinic in a business park setting. You are encountering many situations that you have never dealt with before and are feeling a bit lost. What strategies could you use to help you negotiate these situations more successfully?

Role Negotiation

A strategy that is helpful during conflicting role expectations is role negotiation. The priority of different role expectations may also require role negotiation with the person above you in the line of command. Ask for input as to which expectations have the highest priorities. Explain personal and family expectations and clearly state the priority that meeting those expectations has. The process may have to be repeated several times before agreement on the expectations related to roles and the priority of each expectation is determined (Fig. 22.1). Each person's role contributes to the result. All individuals must understand their roles or the team may fail. The Theory Box provides an overview of role theory as applied to healthcare professionals and can be helpful as an overarching conceptual framework.

THEORY BOX

Theory/Contributor	Key Ideas	Application to Practice
Hardy (1978) is credited with applying role theory to healthcare professionals. A role is the expected and actual behaviors associated with a position. Role expectations are the attitudes and behaviors others anticipate that a person in the role will possess or demonstrate. **Role stress** is a social condition in which role demands are conflicting, irritating, difficult, or impossible to fulfill. **Role strain** is the subjective feeling of discomfort experienced as the result of role stress.	Role stress is a precursor to role strain. Role stress is associated with low productivity and performance. Role stress and role strain can lead a person to withdraw psychologically from the role. Clear, realistic role expectations can decrease the role stress for a new nurse manager.	Clear, realistic role expectations can increase productivity.

Data from Hardy, M. E. (1978). Role stress and role strain. In M. E. Hardy & M. E. Conway (Eds.), *Role theory: Perspectives for health professionals*. New York: Appleton-Century-Crofts.

The best time to negotiate is before accepting a position. Consider what kind of support you believe is critical to your new role, such as conferences, certification, an executive coach, or consultation. Even if you are in the position, you can negotiate support, for example, by describing what you have tried and found dissatisfactory.

Mentors

The process of mentoring is not a new concept. This concept has been alive since Homer's *Odyssey*. Odysseus leaves Ithaca to fight in the Trojan War. Before leaving, he entrusts his son to Mentor. Mentor was to develop and prepare this son for his life and duties. Mentors are a tremendous source of guidance and support for frontline nurses and managers, serving both career functions and psychosocial functions. Hahn et al. (2021) noted that "nurse leaders appreciated being mentored and when it was a solid relationship, the actual experience of being mentored brought them joy" (p. 19). A manager who mentors frontline nurses also noted the following: "I think what's been meaningful in my practice is the opportunity to mentor other nurses that are young in their career and to be able to help guide their career" (p. 19).

Mentors need training and feedback to become valuable and effective to mentees. Skills such as assessing competence, providing constructive feedback, and goal development are critical to a mentor's success in guiding a mentee. Career functions are possible because the mentor has sufficient professional experience and organizational authority to facilitate the career of the mentee. The mentor may suggest that the mentee be appointed to a key nursing committee or volunteer for a special assignment.

The mentor can help provide exposure or opportunities for the mentee to build a reputation of competence. With exposure, the mentor provides protection by absorbing negative feedback, sharing responsibility for controversial decisions, and teaching the unwritten rules about "how things are done around here." These unwritten rules may be more important to job success than the written rules. The Literature Perspective highlights an organizational mentoring program for critical care nurses.

Mentors provide information about how to improve performance, including feedback on current performance. Mentoring requires frequent contact and willingness on the part of the mentee to accept feedback. Challenging assignments are given to the mentee that will stretch the limits of knowledge and skill. The mentor helps the mentee learn the technical and management skills necessary to accomplish the task, such as which numbers on the budget printout are added to achieve the total expenditures.

Having a blend of complementary personalities between mentor and mentee is essential. The personal and professional connection between the mentor and mentee is powerful; thus, having similar interests and motivations is important. The interpersonal relationship between the mentor and mentee involves mutual positive regard. The mentee identifies with the mentor's example because the mentee respects the career accomplishments of the mentor. This role modeling is both conscious and unconscious. The mentee with character and self-respect will evaluate the behaviors of the mentor and select those behaviors worthy of being emulated.

Counseling, another psychosocial function of the mentor, allows the mentee to explore personal concerns.

LITERATURE PERSPECTIVE

Resource: Dirks, J. L. (2021). Alternative approaches to mentoring. *Critical Care Nurse, 41*(1), e9–e16.

This article provides an overview of the components of building a successful mentoring program within an organization for critical care nurses. Mentoring can be utilized for new graduate and experienced critical care nurses. Nurses at all phases of their career can benefit from having mentors. An organization must approach a mentoring program with appropriate fiscal and human resource supports for it to be truly successful. Effective mentoring programs benefit the organization, staff, and, most of all, the patients.

Important components of a mentoring program include mentor selection; mentor–mentee matching for optimal compatibility; setting goals and expectations with regularly scheduled touchpoints; and periodic evaluation with outcomes, goals, and objectives.

Implications for Practice

Nurse mentoring programs are an effective way to increase nurse engagement and drive satisfaction for retention in an organization. Nurse executives and leaders proposing mentorship programs within their organization need to ensure adequate resources for them to be successful in the long term.

Confidentiality is a prerequisite to sharing personal information. The best mentors can provide guidance while recognizing that the mentee may choose to disregard the advice. Mentors rely heavily on two strategies: asking questions and telling stories. The latter is designed to illustrate a point, and the former is designed to help the mentee explore personal thoughts to reach a decision.

Admiration for a mentor and recognition of the mentee's commitment to self-success can provide an environment of trust in which a mentor–mentee relationship begins. Both persons develop positive expectations of the relationship, and both take the initiative to nurture the new relationship. As more of the mentor functions are experienced, the bond between the mentor and mentee grows stronger. Mijares and Radovich (2020) note that "nursing has always embodied the image of compassionate healing and teaching for patients, the act of mentorship is the application of those same principles of compassion, but this time, for one another" (p. 280).

EXERCISE 22.3 Provide an example of how a new frontline nurse in a rural hospital can benefit from a mentor–mentee relationship.

Management Education

Management performance can be hindered by a specific knowledge deficit. For example, the nurse manager may lack business skills or knowledge about legal aspects of supervision. Leadership support is pivotal for charge nurses and nurses new to leadership positions to be successful. Lawson (2020) noted that the significance of competency for nurse leader orientation and development should be the same as when a new graduate nurse begins in an organization. Refer to the Research Perspective to read about more specific nurse manager role transition practices.

Leadership Certification

Experience and education provide a firm basis for seeking additional credentials. A nurse holding an administrative position at the nurse executive level with a baccalaureate preparation and 24 months of experience can take an examination to become a certified nurse executive (NE-BC). Nursing administrators with master's degrees and experience at the executive level can take an examination to become a certified nurse executive, advanced (NEA-BC). The website of the American Nurses Credentialing Center (ANCC, 2021) has detailed information about these certification examinations (https://www.nursingworld.org/our-certifications/nurse-executive/).

A certification credential also was developed by the American Organization for Nursing Leadership (AONL, 2021) exclusively for the nurse executive and the certified nurse manager leader, the Certification in Executive Nursing Practice (CENP) and Certified Nurse Manager Leader (CNML; https://www.aonl.org/initiatives/certification). These credentials are recognized in the profession as designating someone whose knowledge and experience are credible.

RESEARCH PERSPECTIVE

Resource: Warshawsky, N. E., Caramanica, L., & Cramer, E. (2020). Organizational support for nurse manager role transition and onboarding: Strategies for success. *Journal of Nursing Administration, 50*(5), 254–260.

This study focuses on what processes and practices are supportive to the transition of a nurse into the nurse manager role. A mixed-method design was utilized to describe transition practices from a broad spectrum of nurse managers across the United States at an American Organization for Nursing Leadership (AONL) conference. Paper surveys and focus group interviews were completed related to current role transition support and an ideal role transition.

Results ranged from no planned organized transitions to 30-, 60-, 90-day road maps to the position. A bootcamp program with a capstone and a nurse manager fellowship were noted as exemplars. There were multiple others that provided toolkits, nurse manager competency checklists, and AONL tools.

Nurse managers indicated that an ideal role transition program would coalesce around the following themes: structured onboarding with specialized processes, mentorship and coaching, knowledge development courses, and program evaluation.

Implications for Practice
Appropriate graduate education preparation is needed for nurse managers and formal onboarding programs are needed. Organizational support for a culture of ongoing mentoring, coaching, and ongoing tuition reimbursement for further education is required.

CONCLUSION

Transitions from a frontline nurse position to charge nurse or nurse manager pose new challenges. Nurses who make these transitions with minimal discomfort are reflective of role theory in action. Although nurses today are better prepared to take on more formal leadership roles, the roles themselves are more challenging. Charge nurses and managers are responsible for mentoring and coaching new staff as they transition to their new roles. These transition activities take time and effort to achieve the best results possible.

THE SOLUTION

When I started my journey as the nurse manager, I knew most of the staff if not all of them already. I knew how many children they had, and what they had done for their last family vacation. The foundational work was already laid in terms of getting to know the team, and, in turn, they knew me. This was a blessing and a curse. It allowed some staff to immediately accept me because they had a level of trust in me and my character. Others took quite a bit of time because they doubted my abilities to do the work and assumed I was in over my head. They were right, partially. I was new to primary care and I needed them. I needed them to teach me their role, to allow me time to understand their department, while also gaining my footing as a nurse leader. My overarching goal was not to be their leader in a singular all knowing, all powerful sense; I needed to be a part of their team first. I was the leader with a high level of responsibility, but I was a member of their team also.

I leaned in hard on my leaders and mentors whom I sought feedback from regularly. My graduate schoolwork became laser focused on the concept that a highly engaged nurse manager led to highly satisfied nurses, which yielded excellent patient care. I sought out leadership opportunities through my employer. While feeling passionate professionally over that first year and cultivating a level of trust with the team, I had to work hard to sustain a work and home life balance that worked for me. This effort laid a foundation for my success as a nurse leader and cultivated a strong working relationship with the team I was a part of, not in front of.

Would this be a suitable approach for you? Why?

Jolene Piper, MSN, BSN, RN
Nurse Manager, Mayo Clinic Health System, Albert Lea, MN,
United States

REFLECTIONS

Consider various role transitions you have experienced personally. What valuable lessons did you learn? What do you wish you had known before or during a role transition? If you were offered your ideal position tomorrow, do you know what lessons you would carry forward and why and how you would use those?

BEST PRACTICES

All individuals experience role transition in their daily lives—you can utilize a variety of resources to successfully navigate the transition. Mentoring can serve as a powerful tool in personal and professional role development. Ongoing professional development, leadership support, and professional certification all assist in providing advanced credibility and knowledge in the specialty field of nursing and nursing leadership.

TIPS FOR ROLE TRANSITION

Anticipate and prepare for role changes.
- Identify the responsibilities, opportunities, lines of communication, expectations, and support for a role.
- Use your internal resources to negotiate a role that is consistent with your values and life commitments.

REFERENCES

American Nurses Credentialing Center (ANCC). (2021). *Nurse executive certification (NE-BC®)*. Retrieved from https://www.nursingworld.org/our-certifications/nurse-executive/.

American Organization for Nursing Leadership (AONL). (2021). *AONL credentialing center certification programs*. https://www.aonl.org/initiatives/certification.

Benner, P. (1982). From novice to expert. *American Journal of Nursing, 82*(3), 402–407.

Hahn, J., Galuska, L., Polifroni, E. C., & Dunnack, H. (2021). Joy and meaning in nurse manager practice: A narrative analysis. *Journal of Nursing Administration, 51*(1), 38–42.

Hardy, M. E. (1978). Role stress and role strain. In M. E. Hardy, & M. E. Conway (Eds.), *Role theory: Perspectives for health professionals*. New York: Appleton-Century-Crofts.

Lawson, C. (2020). Strengthening new nurse manager leadership skills through a transition-to-practice program. *Journal of Nursing Administration, 50*(12), 618–622.

Mijares, A. H., & Radovich, P. (2020). Structured mentorship and the nursing clinical ladder. *Clinical Nurse Specialist: The Journal for Advanced Nursing Practice, 34*(6), 276–281.

23

Managing Your Career

M. Margaret Calacci and Debra Hagler

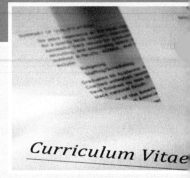

Curriculum Vitae

ANTICIPATED LEARNING OUTCOMES

1. Apply key concepts of holistic career construction.
2. Appraise academic programs, continuing education activities, certifications, and organizational involvement for career development.
3. Design professional documents for a specific career opportunity.

KEY TERMS

career construction
certification
continuing education
curriculum vitae

licensure
mentor
portfolio

professional association
   (organization)
professional brand
résumé

THE CHALLENGE

Unbridled passion. That's how I would describe my start in nursing. I had such a desire to "help others" and "make a difference" but found it challenging to identify how those aspirations could impact a productive and fulfilling career. At the start of my undergraduate nursing program, I was convinced that I was destined to be a pediatric or obstetric nurse and was hard pressed to consider other options. However, the vision of my ideal career began to change during my final semester of nursing school. This shift can be credited to several different facets of growth throughout my program. But the main influence was my experience

volunteering in both the police and fire departments as a member of their grief support team. I was exposed to many connections and experiences I had not previously considered. Therefore, frontline critical care quickly became my passion, and at the completion of my nursing program, I knew this was the area of nursing where I would begin my career. This was a new direction and required rethinking!
What would you do if you were this nurse?

Rachel Breslauer, RN, BSN
Critical Care Travel Nurse, Aya Health, Phoenix, AZ

INTRODUCTION

Whether positions are plentiful or not, nurses have the opportunity to manage their careers. We can succumb to desperate please or explain what our career goals are and negotiate conditions beneficial tot he organization and to

ourselves. Demonstrating professionalism allows us to continue to convey our value to the organization and to society.

The nursing profession offers hundreds of career opportunities. Some of these career options are the traditional roles that nurses have performed for centuries—providing frontline care, public health, community-based health, leading teams or organizations, or teaching. According to the U.S. Bureau of Labor Statistics (2021), a 7% growth rate is projected for registered nurses from 2019 to 2029. The combination of population growth and soaring public interest in wellness and disease prevention, chronic disease management, regenerative or restorative care, and palliative and hospice care will provide new opportunities for nurse professionals (American Association of Colleges of Nursing [AACN], 2021). Expansion of technology and globalization of work allows for additional possibilities where flexible and adaptive professionals can craft career success. Professionals can leverage these expanding roles in managing a primary care portfolio or influencing behavior as a health coach. Nurses who adopt a growth mindset can find innovative work as entrepreneurs, telehealth practitioners, informatics specialists, business leaders, or legislative policy experts.

Having so many career options creates challenges in deciding how to design or manage professional opportunities. An effective playbook or a helpful mentor could help guide your path toward the next step in your career. For example, you might identify a new assignment or process improvement project to best prepare for advancement in a specific field or role. Thinking broadly about your career in the rapidly changing field of healthcare is critical to remaining competent, adaptable, and relevant.

WHAT IS A CAREER?

A career is defined as progress throughout an individual's professional life, which develops as the individual selects positions that contribute to professional goals and growth. A nursing career extends beyond employment opportunities to include how an individual engages in organizing activities for person-centered care. This may consist of coordination of care, individual or family teaching for that care, supporting the providers of that care, studying care delivery, or engaging in the broader perspective of professional and community service.

A work situation is composed of two elements—person and opportunity—interacting in a complex environment. A good career fit is built on values, similar goals, and tolerable (or growth-producing) differences. Analyzing position statements and the required skills in light of individual talents can help determine positions that fit your strengths. If gaps occur between the requirements of a "dream" position and your skills, consider whether professional development or other non-work activities might help improve the match between your current and desired future qualifications. Knowing the structure of the job, the organization's mission and vision, and how they are interpreted through various roles provides a sense of the organization's direction to understand a position's potential fit. Career success refers to a positive outcome over time, beyond a single employment position. Your achievements can be subjective, measuring whether you have met your own goals, or objectively from an external focus on how your outcomes compare with others on tangible measures such as salary, promotions, and occupational status (Xin, 2020).

CAREER FRAMEWORK

The four components that make up the Whole-Life Career Counseling Intervention Framework (see Theory Box) include goal clarification, mapping resources or barriers, developing an action strategy, and consistently assessing and monitoring your adaptability (Hirschi, 2020). The framework also encourages career counseling utilizing a circular self-directed career management strategy integrating feedback loops to meet work/life/career balance. A nurse can use the framework as a foundation for making decisions related to common career transitions, such as an initial career choice; changing positions, employers, or roles; seeking promotion; recruiting to a different work setting; involuntary job loss; retirement; and, for many, an encore role following a traditional retirement.

Individuals influence most aspects of their career management, whereas their employing organizations influence other elements. Choosing an employment setting and organization is an important decision that goes far beyond the immediate position: Employers who promote professional advancement opportunities for their team members support many more possibilities for individuals throughout their careers (Bagdadli & Gianecchini, 2019). For example, a new graduate nurse who is supported through a formal residency program may have increased confidence and be retained in the organization. The results of a study surveying 51 hospital organizations with an active nurse residency program suggests that the transition from residency to independent work is influenced by the correlation between self-efficacy and performance (McMillen, 2020). Thus, if you have confidence in your ability and a sense of belonging within the organization, you will most likely positively affect patient care and success in your work. Maintain a positive career focus by regularly meeting

THEORY BOX
Whole-Life Career Counseling Intervention Framework

Theory/Contributor	Key Ideas	Application to Practice
Andreas Hirschi	Goal clarification across work and nonwork goals	Define the relationships between work and nonwork goals and their effects on personal values and choosing life directions.
	Map resources and barriers related to goal attainment	Resources can be positive emotions, education, *competencies*, or expertise required for nursing practice in a particular setting. Licensure is designed to ensure the baseline competencies (i.e., the minimum expectations). However, many additional competencies are essential in a prosperous professional career.
		Barriers may be feelings of low self-esteem, lack of confidence, or misaligned organizational culture that decreases career success.
	Develop action strategies for goal attainment	Prioritize larger goals into small steps or chunks that can more easily be attained.
	Monitor and adapt goals	Personal reflective assessment of work through feedback loops that will help determine if they are achieving the plan or if adaptations need to be made to reach the dream role.

From Hirschi, A. (2020). Whole-life career management: A counseling intervention framework. *The Career Development Quarterly*, *68*(1), 2–17.

with your manager to consider your manager's respective and cooperative roles in career development. These meetings can yield useful conversations about how to reach your personal goals and the organization's goals.

CAREER CONSTRUCTION

Nurses can engage in active, holistic career construction by establishing personal objectives and seeking growth opportunities to enhance their professional portfolio (Goodrich Mitts, 2020). Additionally, the connection of opportunities to personal values, such as a focus on equity and inclusion, may generate well-being through integration of life/work success (see Literature Perspective).

Knowing Yourself

The best opportunity for nurses to construct their careers and for a manager to help nurses gain meaningful experiences is for individuals to know themselves. Understanding your motivation, values, and commitment forms the basis for understanding your authentic self. Whether positions are plentiful or scarce, knowing yourself can focus the available work or selection process toward capitalizing on your strengths. Not everyone has access to a career coach, but you can look to your educational organization to find a career

counseling or resource center. As an alternative, you may consider assessing your strengths through a formal avenue, for example, the Clifton Strengths Assessment (*https://www.gallup.com/cliftonstrengths/en/253868/popular-cliftonstrengths-assessment-products.aspx*) or the Myers Briggs Inventory (myersbriggs.org).

Throughout school and initial nursing experiences, awareness begins to evolve, helping each of us determine our preferences for our work. Therefore, the beginning of creating a person–position fit is in understanding the person involved. Some positions add more to what we want to be able to achieve in the long term than other positions do. For example, an opportunity that offers educational compensation or flexible scheduling might be preferable when the goal is to return to school and complete advanced education for a specialized role.

Being able to describe yourself from various perspectives is useful. First, knowing your strengths and growth areas tells you what you bring to a position and what you can rely on. When you know your competencies, you better understand how they can influence your work behavior. You can then use competencies as a filter in reading position descriptions to find your fit in an organization. Analyzing the AACN *Essentials* (AACN, 2021) for either the entry level or advanced level provides a comparison with your current competencies to show what work

LITERATURE PERSPECTIVE

Resource: De Vos, A., Van der Heijden, B., & Akkermans, J. (2020). Sustainable careers: Towards a conceptual model. *Journal of Vocational Behavior*, 117, 103196. https://doi.org/10.1016/j.jvb.2018.06.011.

Sustaining a career requires the capacity to adapt because most professionals will experience numerous changes in their work over the course of a career. An individual is the focus of a career, but systemic factors and the passage of time can have a major impact on an individual's ability to adapt. The system around the individual that may be changing includes family and peers, supervisors, employers, educational systems, and society. Factors within and outside an individual also change the context and meaning of the career over time. Experiences and events provide opportunities for dynamic learning and reassessment of the person–career fit.

Sustainable careers are characterized by mutually beneficial consequences for people and for their surrounding context over the long term. In other words, a good person–career fit when viewed over an extended time must exist. People have a major impact on the sustainability of their career by proactively making choices and taking the initiative to develop and maintain competency, plus adapting to career events and system changes. In order to have a career characterized by happiness, health, and productivity, it is essential that people be mindful about who and what matters to them.

Implications for Practice

The work you choose to do now likely will not look the same in the future. Periodically reassess what is important and meaningful to you in your work and your career. Make plans to maintain key competencies and develop new skills to support adapting to a constantly changing health role and environment.

---

needs to be done to meet required or desired standards. Finally, entering into such analyses can help you see the bigger picture of what you can glean from a particular position that might contribute to your overall goals. All of this work helps you to know yourself well to pursue a job or career path that fits you and your strengths.

Consideration of a career path such as advanced practice registered nurse, nurse leader, or educational simulationist includes reflection on prior work's most rewarding aspects. For example, the nurse who determines that teaching patients, families, and students is the most personally satisfying aspect of practice might plan to develop a career as a nurse educator. In contrast, someone who finds data fascinating and enjoys seeking answers may pursue a research or nursing informatics career.

Core career development strategies are important to success. One fundamental approach for career development is planning to obtain the right education and experience to meet future goals. Another critical strategy is selecting professional peers and mentors to provide useful advice. Having a few well-chosen peers, mentors, and role models who respond openly from various perspectives can enrich career planning and development (Fig. 23.1). Mentoring can take on different forms, such as group mentoring, following a mentor on social media, or speed mentoring, where you spend a short time asking focused questions. These actions can inspire new thinking and new opportunities and steer you toward

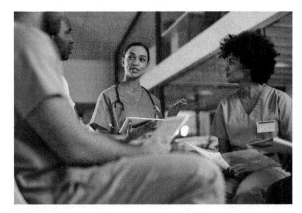

Fig. 23.1 A mentor can inspire new thinking and new opportunities to steer you toward various roles and clinical areas. (Copyright © LumiNola/istock.)

multiple roles and clinical areas. A mentor person can create connections for you and help guide decisions related to timing and context. Mentors might even be able to create opportunities for you to test new approaches to clinical care or to unique aspects of a position (see the Research Perspective).

EXERCISE 23.1 Think about an experienced nurse whom you consider as a role model. Would you want that person as a mentor? If so, how would you enlist that person's assistance in guiding your career?

RESEARCH PERSPECTIVE

Resource: Greco, K., & Kraimer, M. (2020). Goal-setting in the career management process: An identity theory perspective. *Journal of Applied Psychology, 105*(1), 40–57.

Goal setting is often recommended as a route to career success. Surveys of 312 early career professionals from a wide range of professional disciplines provided information about career goals at three points in time. Researchers assessed the quality and content of career-related goals in reference to participants' identification with their professions and their relationships with mentors in the professions. Two categories of mentoring relationships were studied: career mentoring and psychosocial mentoring. Career mentoring was defined as career development support and enhanced advancement through sponsorship, exposure and visibility, coaching, protection, and providing challenging assignments. Psychosocial mentoring was defined as addressing interpersonal aspects and belonging, including serving as a role model and providing counseling, friendship, and advice.

Survey analysis indicated that psychosocial mentoring was positively related to professional identification. However, when psychosocial mentoring was not present in a mentoring relationship, career mentoring was positively related to professional identification. Mentoring relationships that support the belonging aspect of socialization to a career role through psychosocial mentoring provided support for the development of professional identification and higher-quality career goals. When psychosocial mentoring was not present, career mentoring provided some level of support for developing an identity in the professional role.

Implications for Practice
Think about the type of relationship you hope to have with a mentor and discuss the expectations that each of you has for that relationship. If you and your mentor are both comfortable with the process of psychosocial mentoring, that process may provide more support for developing your professional identity and vital career goals.

Knowing the Position

Few people, including nurses, hold the same employment position forever. Rapid changes in healthcare require an evaluation of each employment opportunity and assessment of risk. Ask yourself whether the work contributes to increasing your skills and competencies. Does the position have the potential to recast your professional profile so that others see your potential for more significant contributions? Do the benefits offset the limitations of the job? Is the professional practice environment diverse and inclusionary? Is the organization a safe and collaborative setting for healthcare professionals and patients?

Position assessment begins with understanding the vision, purpose, and values of the organization. A thorough evaluation requires finding out specifics of the position, which may be available only through an interview. Many nurse managers look within the organization to hire by transferring someone from a different role across the organization. Thus, one key strategy to use is selecting an organization where you want to work, even if the initial position available is not exactly the best fit for your goals. The potential for inside connections and networking, in addition to knowledge about management styles in the organization and future position openings, can lead you to the position that is the right fit for you. You may find a job that is a good fit for

you at one point, but over the course of a career, it may no longer be suitable. The work may have changed as much as you did. If the movement was in harmony, the fit remains; if the position changes one way and the person in another, the fit devolves.

> **EXERCISE 23.2** Review your dream job requirements to see how your competencies and experience prepare you for the role. What do you still need to work on?

CAREER ADVANCEMENT

One of the keys to maintaining competence and adaptability is continuing to learn. The 2021 AACN *Essentials* emphasize "the ability to demonstrate a spirit of inquiry that fosters flexibility and professional maturity" (AACN, 2021).

Nursing professional development is a vital phase of lifelong learning in which nurses engage to develop and maintain competence, enhance professional nursing practice, and support achievement of career goals" (American Nurses Association [ANA], 2019). Active involvement in education, service, and scholarship opportunities can help prepare you to deal with new roles and challenges. Engaging in service activities (both community and professional organizations) and sharing your knowledge through research, writing, and speaking (scholarship) allow you to influence others in the profession and through the profession. When positions are scarce or when you are competing for a very desirable position, community and professional service experience and scholarly contributions to nursing may give you the advantage over other candidates. Learning also can occur through informal means: in a conversation with colleagues, by observing leaders in the workplace, through reading an article, or in reflective thought. One way to maximize this learning is to share ideas with others, giving credit to the original source as needed.

Academic Progression

Although prior experience can enrich the learning process, completing an advanced degree early in your career may enhance your career opportunities. Before you make a significant investment in time and money to earn an advanced degree, think carefully about your career goals and how the degree will create value. Admission to graduate programs may require taking a test such as the Graduate Record Examination (GRE), having an above-average

grade point average (GPA), and graduating from a professionally accredited nursing school. Box 23.1 lists some of the factors to consider in selecting a graduate program.

If you dream of conducting clinical research, earning a PhD will likely be the best preparation for the role. If you want to be a primary care provider in advanced practice, consider earning a DNP. Suppose you're going to teach future healthcare professionals. In that case, you may be able to prepare for that role in a variety of ways: a master's degree or doctoral degree in nursing or education or a graduate degree in a related field such as public health, sociology, genetics, or informatics. Remember, however, most teaching positions in nursing require a master's degree or higher in nursing. In addition, the increasing complexity of healthcare leads to a need for nurses who are also experts in areas outside nursing. Earning a graduate degree in another field may put you in the position of translating advanced knowledge from other disciplines to improve healthcare. When combined with a graduate degree in nursing, a transdisciplinary skill set may make you highly desirable in a growing organization. Think what potential exists with a dual doctorate!

BOX 23.1 Factors to Consider in Selecting a Graduate Program

Accreditation
- Does the program have a national nursing accreditation (master's/doctoral level)?
- Is the institution regionally accredited (e.g., North Central Association of Colleges and Schools)?

Role Preparation
- How closely does the program of study meet your career goals?

Credits
- How many graduate credits are required to complete the degree?
- How many are devoted to clinical or practicum experiences?
- How many relate to classroom experiences?

Thesis/Research
- Is a thesis/dissertation/applied project required?

Faculty
- What credentials do faculty members hold?
- Are they in leadership positions in the state/national/international scenes?
- Are they competent in your field of interest?

Current Research
- What are the current research, practice, and policy strengths of the institution?

Flexibility
- Do these strengths fit with your interests, or is there flexibility to create your own direction?
- Is flexibility present in scheduling and progressing through the program?
- Is classroom attendance required, or is online or blended attendance an option?

Admission
- What is required?
- Is the GRE used?
- What is the minimum undergraduate GPA expected?
- Is experience required? What kind? How much?

Costs
- What are the total projected costs? What financial aid is available?

Working while attending a graduate program may be difficult, but it is common among graduate students in nursing. Consider how you learn best. Do you thrive in person-to-person discussions? Do you need to be face-to-face, or are you comfortable with learning via a virtual connection? Do you want some "intense" interactions with others combined with individual activities? Each of these preferences has a solution. For example, remote learning provides an additional option for earning an advanced degree. Flexible scheduling and the convenience of online courses permit many individuals to participate who would not be able to attend traditional programs because of class times or geographic distance. Programs with a combined approach capture the strengths of both approaches. If you prefer to learn in interaction with others, actual physical immersion with others may be a driving force.

Consider the following example of seeking out a graduate program that fits. You know you want to work with older adult patients. You review the most recent year's online issues of the *Journal of Gerontological Nursing* and *Geriatric Nursing* and scan the articles. Are some articles particularly intriguing? Where are those authors affiliated? You can also search online using terms such as "geriatric center of excellence" to find related graduate programs. Do you know any experts in gerontology or geriatrics in your own workplace? Ask those experts for suggestions about academic programs. Review professional organization websites related to gerontology and consider joining to network with other members. These are good starting places for connecting with others with similar interests and knowing firsthand about available programs.

As one of today's nursing leaders said after earning a doctoral degree: Doors opened up that I didn't even know existed—that is what education can do for you The point is that we often don't know what we don't know until we learn more. And then, we realize we must commit to lifelong learning.

Licensure

Requirements for demonstrating continued nursing competency in the United States vary by state. Licensure carries certain expectations about maintaining competence and reflecting professional standards. Consumers, insurers, regulatory agencies, and employers expect that nurses will meet professional and legal standards. Changing geographic locations during a career may entail meeting different regulatory requirements for continuing professional development.

Certification

Consumers, nurses, managers, and administrators value certification as evidence of specific expertise. Certification signifies the completion of requirements in a particular field beyond preparation for licensure. Nurses earn certification as recognition of competence in one or more specialty areas as an expectation in some employment settings for career advancement; in the field of advanced practice nursing, it is a requirement for practice and reimbursement. In many states, certification in advanced practice is the mechanism to achieve recognition as an advanced practice registered nurse from the board of nursing.

Obtaining certification may require testing, continued education, and documented time in a specific practice area. Certification renewal is a process of continued recognition of competence within a defined practice area and may require ongoing participation in continuing education. Certification plays an important part in the advancement of a career and the profession. In some fields, more than one examination exists; others use an examination in the broad field and numerous options for subspecialties. The American Nurses Credentialing Center (ANCC) (*https://www.nursingworld.org/ancc/*) offers numerous certification examinations for nurse generalists, nurse practitioners, clinical specialists, nurse administrators, nurse case managers, ambulatory nurses, and informatics nurses. In addition, nursing specialty organizations offer many other certifications through their credentialing organizations.

EXERCISE 23.3 Assume you are interested in graduate education.

- Search the Internet to locate information about three graduate education programs that align with your interests.
- Determine what specialties exist that fit your interests at the master's/doctoral level.
- Consider doctoral programs permitting entrance from the baccalaureate level.
- Evaluate the clinical interest within the programs of study.
- Decide whether the diverse roles of the advanced practice registered nurse are appealing.
- Determine the location of programs nearby and access to distance programs.

Continuing Education

Lifelong learning is a professional attribute that also contributes to professional growth. As you assess career construction benchmarks, additional education will be needed. Selecting among the numerous opportunities to pursue continuing education may be difficult. Continuing education is defined as "systematic professional learning experiences designed to augment nurses' knowledge, skill, and attitudes, thereby enriching the nurses' contributions to quality health care and their pursuit of professional career goals" (ANA, 2019).

Depending on your particular goal, you may consider programs that offer micro-credentials, badges, or stackable credentials toward a more extensive certificate or degree. Box 23.2 lists factors to consider in selecting a continuing education offering. For example, if the cost is a significant factor, program length and speaker credentials may be less influential factors.

In addition to increasing your knowledge base, continuing education provides professional networking opportunities, contributes to meeting certification and licensure requirements, and documents additional efforts to maintain or develop leadership or clinical expertise. Sponsors of continuing education include employers, professional associations, schools, and entrepreneurs.

Professional Associations

The nursing profession embraces the expectation that nurses will belong to professional associations and provide leadership in improving communities. The challenge, of course, is how to incorporate these activities into a busy, committed life!

Belonging to a professional association demonstrates leadership and provides opportunities to meet other leaders, participate in policy formation, continue specialized education, and shape the future. Professional associations (organizations) are groups

---

BOX 23.2   Factors to Consider in Selecting a Continuing Education Offering

Accreditation/Approval
- Is the course accredited and approved? If so, by whom?
- Is that recognition accepted by a certification entity and by the nursing board (if continuing education is required for reregistration of licensure)?

Credit
- Is the amount of credit appropriate in terms of the expected outcomes?

Course Title
- Does it suggest the type of learner to be involved (e.g., advanced)?
- Does it reflect the expected outcomes?

Speaker(s)
- Is the speaker known as an expert in the field?

Objectives
- Are the objectives logical and attainable?
- Do they reflect knowledge, skills, attitudes, or a combination of these?
- Do they fit a learner's needs?

Content
- Is the content reflective of the objectives?
- Is the content at an appropriate level?

Audience
- Is the audience designed as a general or specific one (e.g., all registered nurses or experienced nurses in state health positions)?

Cost
- What is the direct expense for an individual to attend? Is it affordable?
- Is the cost equitable with that of similar nursing conferences?
- Is travel required?
- Is the program offered online?

Length
- Is the total time frame logical in terms of objectives, personal needs, and time away from work?
- Does the time frame permit a break from intense learning?

Provider
- Does the provider have an established reputation for quality programs?

of people who share professional values and join their colleagues to effect change. Many nursing associations set standards and objectives to guide the profession and specialty practice. Although associations may have very different agendas and goals related to their specialty areas, many nursing organizations share the long-term goal of uniting and advancing the profession. Those "additional" activities and interests enrich a career and provide invaluable insight into clinical and professional issues.

Associations represent nurses in particular areas of the profession. Some are clinically focused, such as the American Association of Critical-Care Nurses, the Oncology Nurses Association, and the American Association of Neuroscience Nurses. Others are role focused, such as the American Organization for Nursing Leadership and the National League for Nursing, or represent specific groups of nurses, such as the American Assembly for Men in Nursing and the National Black Nurses Association. Many specialty organizations offer networking opportunities, informative publications, and discounts on conference rates and liability insurance to attract future members.

The "umbrella organization" representing all nurses throughout the United States and its territories is the ANA (*www.ana.org*). The ANA provides guidance on nursing and health policy issues as well as advancing the nursing profession by directing standards of best practice, advocating for safe, ethical work settings while ensuring health and wellness for all (ANA, 2020).

The Honor Society of Nursing, Sigma Theta Tau International, established in 1922, is an example of an invitational association. The organization's mission is to create a global community of nurses who lead in using scholarship, knowledge, and technology to improve the health of the world's people (*www.nursingsociety.org*). Membership is available to nurses enrolled in baccalaureate, master's, and doctoral education programs and to community leaders through a nomination process. This organization provides small grants to aid in beginning research and disseminates research and leadership information through various publications and international meetings.

Connecting With an Organization

An organization's size is not as important as how the group is structured and who leads it. Read about the officers and membership composition of the organization before making a commitment through membership. Most associations have a website that lists biographical information about the leaders, locations of upcoming local and national meetings or activities, current policy issues and their positions, election information, and other valuable resource links. Many organizations send regular email newsletters.

Upon joining a nursing organization, you may receive information on the organization's history, future meetings and current activities, officer contact information, and local contacts. Contact the local office of the organization if one exists so that you can immediately begin networking. Most associations are composed of volunteers who have different motivations for becoming involved. Taking time to talk to an officer or attend a local meeting and observe the group and the dynamics before making service commitments will help ensure that you make an informed decision. Research the organization, talk to the members, determine the sense of the group dynamics, and assess what you want to derive from the experience and how you can contribute to the organization. Look at your strengths and talents to determine whether there is a need or a fit within the organization for your particular talents. Examples of tangible benefits of professional association membership are in Box 23.3.

Reasons for Involvement

Nurses who define themselves as leaders and want to influence beyond their workplaces should join at least one professional association. Some reasons for joining

---

BOX 23.3   Tangible Benefits from Organizational Involvement

- Substantial discounts on continuing education and professional journals
- Professional standards beyond the individual's workplace
- Resources and discounts for certification
- Quick access to staff experts
- News on legal, legislative, and educational issues
- Group insurance plans for professional liability, healthcare, and disability
- Travel services, such as auto rentals, hotel stays, and restaurant visits
- Discounted retail services
- A personal sense of advancing the organization's work

organizations include feeling a sense of responsibility to the profession, contributing to the profession's greater good, enhancing your résumé and marketability, supporting particular legislative interests, and social networking. Organizations need both active and passive participants to carry out their missions and conduct activities and business. Organizational involvement is a socialization process that can improve morale—being around others who take pride in and celebrate the nursing profession is contagious. Whatever your preferred level of involvement, you can contribute significantly to your profession by becoming a member of a professional association; progressing to active involvement guarantees a world of opportunities.

Some nurses choose to belong to the nurses' association in their state of employment, whereas others are required to do so. Employment contracts may require nurses to join a union and pay dues to receive employment in some locations. In other localities, the nurses' associations may also be a collective bargaining organization.

Personal and Professional Benefits

Networking and exposure to different nursing profession opportunities are two of the most valuable benefits of belonging to an organization. Some nurses may stop working for a time because of changing priorities. Organizational membership can help you stay connected to professional issues and colleagues through meetings and publications, smoothing the transition back into practice. In addition to networking, the professional organization can serve as a training ground to build skills and gain leadership experience. Box 23.4 lists examples of competencies gained in professional organizations.

BOX 23.4 Competencies Developed Through Organizational Involvement

- Conflict management
- Interpersonal communication
- Public speaking
- Mentoring
- Meeting management
- Agenda development
- Facilitation
- Delegation
- Consensus building
- Strategic thinking
- Team building
- Political advocacy
- Legislative work or lobbying
- Problem-solving

All nurses encounter ethical dilemmas and professional challenges. The *Nurses Code of Ethics* (ANA, 2015) provides a foundation for discussion of values such as diversity, equity, and inclusion of professional practice and person-centered care. In addition, membership in nursing organizations can provide a continuous source of professional colleagues to draw on for advice and support in those concerns. Members of a nurses' professional association can be nonbiased, safe colleagues to ask for advice about your situation, especially when you may not want to discuss it with coworkers who could be directly involved. Members may be able to help you connect to the experts in the field.

CONTRIBUTING TO SCHOLARLY ACTIVITIES AND RESEARCH

Nurses and others have contributed over many years to developing the art and science of nursing. Now may be your turn to contribute to improving care. Seek opportunities to learn about particular interest areas and contribute to healthcare knowledge beyond your own daily assignment. Discuss your areas of interest in health topics with leaders in the workplace. For instance, perhaps you notice that patient falls are increasing on your unit or that you are seeing more patients who have fallen at home—thus, you are interested in preventing falls. As a starting point, you could review information about falls prevention on health-related or government websites such as the Quality Safety Education for Nurses (QSEN) site (*https://qsen.org/using-a-fishbone-rca-diagram-to-problem-solve-falls/*); the Centers for Disease Control and Prevention site (CDC, *https://www.cdc.gov/homeandrecreationalsafety/falls/community_preventfalls.html*); or The Joint Commission (TJC, https://www.jointcommission.org/). You might join your organization's practice council or interprofessional safety committee to collaborate on solutions. Your team might seek help from a health information specialist to obtain the most pertinent research and other evidence and ask for support from a clinical nurse specialist or health researcher to appraise the evidence about falls and falls prevention. Experienced researchers and leaders can help the team access or collect baseline data for comparison over time and plan how to pilot an intervention on your unit or in your organization. Those resource persons can also help the team manage the steps for administrative approval and facilitate the process to try out the intervention.

Whether or not you feel the project was successful, knowing what did or did not work builds knowledge that others can use. Through professional presentations, your team can share the outcomes and lessons learned with other professionals in or beyond the organization. Through publication in a professional journal, your team can share the knowledge you have gained with professionals worldwide. It may sound daunting at first to think of yourself as a team member doing a presentation at a professional conference or submitting a manuscript for publication. The satisfaction of developing nursing knowledge to improve health begins with taking those first steps to get involved in the issues most important to you and your patients.

EXERCISE 23.4 Imagine you have decided to earn a master's or doctoral degree in nursing. Develop a strategic plan to meet your graduate education goal.
- Appraise your core strengths, experience, and values that influence your plan.
- Where are your priority interests?
- Identify a target date for completion of the program.
- What barriers do you perceive that would interfere with beginning or completing your strategic plan?

CAREER MARKETING STRATEGIES

Whether you are an experienced nurse or in the transition to a practice area for the first time, being strategic in crafting and promoting your professional brand is essential in controlling the narrative of your positive contributions to the profession. A professional brand is a marketing construct of how you project your individual strengths, values, and communication to show your value.

This section aims to help you design a systematic strategy for documenting your professional activities and marketing your brand throughout your career. The process begins with personal reflection and self-assessment on how you wish to convey your professional identity. Perhaps you could begin by writing a personal mission statement. Like an organization, telling your authentic story may set you apart from other candidates by leveraging your passions, values, experiences, and your unique individual strengths. As your career grows, so

too will the ensuing conversations that help positively identify your distinctive contributions defining your professional persona over the long term.

EXERCISE 23.5 Construct an outline of your professional brand. What do you want your image/brand to represent? How will you exemplify it through your curriculum vitae/résumé/interview?

Beyond the résumé, curriculum vitae (CV), or digital portfolio, building relationships and networking through social media outlets can either enhance or harm your branding package during the job search process. For many years running, nursing remains the most admired profession for honesty and ethics (Reinhart, 2020). With this reputation, your "digital footprint," the evidence available about you through online searches, should not contain unflattering information that would detract from your marketing goals. Use one or more search engines to discover associations to your name and review the information you find. Remove information that detracts from your professional message on social interaction sites that you can edit. For example, potential employers may interpret a photograph of you drinking what appears to be alcohol in a party setting as evidence of risky health behaviors. Currently, few laws limit cyber vetting by hiring managers. Even if you have a clean digital footprint, you should consider asking about the prospective organization's legal and ethical policy during the hiring process. Some companies may volunteer to disclose a policy: "as a proactive step towards self-regulation, employers should clearly declare if they engage in cyber vetting and specifically outline what social media platforms will be examined during the hiring process" (Jacobson, 2020). Furthermore, it may be beneficial to review the National Council of State Boards of Nursing (NCSBN) (2018) or your local nursing board to evaluate what constitutes problematic posts. The important lesson here is that you need to put your best foot forward and present your professional brand's realistic portrait.

Data Collection

The reflective task of data collection is to develop a comprehensive view of your professional attributes for your résumé, CV, and portfolio. Together, the three documents present the accomplishments that led to your current professional identity as a nurse. One way to maintain these important documents is to have a digital file containing references, awards, recognitions, copies of evaluations, and documents reflecting your successes. Although this information will take some time to develop and maintain, having it will be of benefit as you prepare for an evaluation, seeking a promotion, or applying for a new opportunity.

Some organizations provide electronic portfolios for your professional records so that you can readily access and convert the information into marketing documents as you need them. For example, the National Student Nurses Association, the American Association of Colleges of Nursing (AACN), and The Honor Society of Nursing Sigma Theta Tau International (Sigma) each

provide such a digital approach. The list in Table 23.1 identifies suggested documents to create or update a CV, résumé, or portfolio. If you do not have any documentation for a specific category, retain the heading as a reminder and think about what you would like to be able to list there in the future.

The extent of data collection depends on your unique background. If you are new in the profession, analyze any electives, organizational positions, special assignments, or honors you received during school. If you are a second-career nurse, consider relating your previous paid or volunteer work to include relevant skills that demonstrate leadership, financial responsibility, political astuteness, or communication proficiency. If you have a long history as a nurse or a prior relevant career, start with your most recent employment and work backward.

TABLE 23.1   Data Collection for Professional Brand/Profile Documents

Topics	Data
Education	Name of school, address, phone numbers, website, years of attendance, date of graduation, the title of degree(s) conferred, minor(s) earned, honors received (e.g., Dean's List)
Experience	Dates of employment, position title, name of the organization, location, and phone numbers, website, typical duties (role description), salary range, immediate supervisor
Career Development	Dates attended, topics and any notable outcomes, type and amount of credit earned (e.g., CEUs or contact hours), certificates, badges
Community/Organizational Service	Dates of service, name of committee/task force and the parent organization (e.g., name of the hospital or professional organization), your role on the committee (e.g., chairperson, secretary, member), general description of committee's functions, any distinctive accomplishments
Publications	Articles: author(s), year of publication, title, journal, volume, issue, pages; books: author(s), year of publication, title, location, name of the publisher, and doi or ISBN number
Honors	Date, description of the award, unique factors related to recognition (e.g., competitive, community-wide, national)
Research	Date, title of the research, institutional review board number (or statement of exemption from consideration), role in research (e.g., principal investigator, co-investigator, team member), funded/unfunded
Speeches/Presentations/ Posters	Date, title of speech or presentation given, place, name of sponsoring organization, nature of the engagement (e.g., keynote, concurrent session), note if refereed
Workshops/Conferences	Date, title of workshop/conference, place, name of sponsoring group, nature of the presentation, and a brief description of the activity
Certification	Initial date of certification, expiration date, certifying body, area/type of certification
Teaching responsibilities	Date, course title, number of students, ratings if available. Include mentoring and precepting responsibilities.

Curriculum Vitae

A curriculum vitae (CV) is an all-inclusive but superficial record of one's professional life. Typically, it begins with your name prominently displayed and centered in boldface font, followed by the contact information in separate lines below. Include applicable contact information such as address with zip code, phone number (identify a cellphone, work, and, if relevant, a landline), email address, website address, and handles for Twitter, Facebook, or LinkedIn. Avoid casual or personal usernames to ensure that you appear professional in your communication. Present information in the body of the CV using reverse chronological order (most recent information first) with categories such as professional experience, academic and professional preparation, certifications, teaching responsibilities, research, publications, papers/presentations/posters, other creative works, honors, awards, grants, memberships in professional organizations and societies, service, and professional development.

Résumé

A résumé helps the potential employer create an image of a candidate outlining previous education and work that brings value to the new organization. Résumés are concise, customized documents with examples focused on the qualifications tailored to the position you seek. Unlike the CV, a résumé provides details. It is presented in sentences or phrases (not both) to share the value of the information. For example, rather than listing years of service in a position by title and organization, a résumé might include information that you served as the only nurse to provide some exceptional service. For the experienced nurse, a résumé could be used to reflect increasing skills, certifications, and abilities. For the new nurse, it could focus on specific "extra" skills or competencies that are not generally expected of a recent graduate. The résumé is a better choice than a CV for advertising your skills and talents to a prospective employer. Details and action verbs help the reader view you as accomplishing meaningful work. Verbs related to outcomes (produced, created, led) are more powerful in conveying your achievements than process words (participated, attended).

Basically, résumés can be produced in two ways: conventional and functional. The conventional approach provides chronological information about positions and activities. The functional approach combines multiple positions into role areas you want to highlight as an area of strength that matches a particular position option. Although a conventional résumé emphasizes experience as a heading, the functional résumé headings may relate to implementing evidence-based practice or client education and describe how you achieved results across several positions. A functional approach is best if you plan a sharp departure from your present position or have considerable experience outside of nursing. Be sure to include lessons learned regarding critical thinking, teamwork, conflict management, and communication. Focus on your experience in diverse roles or positions rather than the specific positions held.

As with the CV, your résumé should be current, error-free, grammatically correct, accurate, and logical. Documents should be printed on high-quality paper. Electronic résumés are sent as a pdf file so that no distortion in the design or layout occurs. Bringing a résumé to an interview is especially useful if you previously provided a CV. In fact, bringing copies of what you already submitted may help a prospective employer who may not have had ready access to your materials earlier.

Professional Letters

During your career, you will need to communicate effectively through digital or printed correspondence. Every well-designed letter markets you as a professional. The commonly used correspondence includes a cover letter, thank-you letter, and resignation letter. You may also write an email declining positions that you have been offered or recommending others for positions.

Professional letters have a similar format, usually three paragraphs: the introduction, body, and conclusion. Just as with the résumé and CV, letters should be error-free, grammatically correct, accurate, and logical. Use business formatting on a single page with classic typeface (e.g., Times New Roman), a 10- or 12-point font, and high-quality paper. If sending the letter digitally, create a pdf file so that the layout will not be distorted. Match your name and contact information as presented on your résumé and CV. This is especially important for the cover letter because it accompanies another document. See Table 23.2 for the format and content of professional marketing correspondence.

TABLE 23.2 Professional Letters

Type of Communication	General Content
General Business Format: Making a good first impression	Date and inside address the name and credentials of the addressee, the person's title, the name of the organization, the street address, city, state, and zip code, email, and website if available.
	The typical greeting (e.g., "Dear Ms. Smith") is followed by a colon or comma.
	Between the greeting and the closing are paragraphs conveying the letter's main message.
	The end of the letter (closing) allows several line spaces between the word (e.g., *Sincerely*) and your printed name followed by your credentials. If your address and other contact information did not appear at the top of the letter, it should appear below your typed name. The space between the closing and your name should allow enough room for your signature.
	Proofread for layout, typographical errors, spelling, and content.
Digital Cover Letter: The key to getting your résumé or curriculum vitae read and entry to the interview process	The first paragraph is a brief description of your interest in a specific position and how you learned about it.
	The second paragraph emphasizes 2 to 3 unique experiences or strengths on the résumé or CV supporting your "fit" to both the position and organization.
	The closing paragraph conveys enthusiasm about an interview and when you will follow up.
Thank You Email: Creating a positive impression for present and future interactions	Expresses an appreciation for the time and opportunity to interview.
	The first paragraph identifies what position you interviewed for and a key statement about your discussion to help the interviewer recall the interview. If multiple positions are available, prioritize your choices.
	The middle paragraph reiterates a strength or experience pertinent to the job. You can add a topic you found interesting during the discussion or the reply to an unanswered question in the interview. If you indicated you would provide something to the interviewer, you should reference it here, even if it is an attachment.
	The third paragraph references specific expectations about the outcome and when you will follow up.
Resignation Letter: Closure and future reference	Request a meeting with your manager to communicate your resignation in person.
	A letter should follow your meeting outlining the discussion with the manager to include the following:
	• Date and whether it is negotiable with employment terms
	• Reason for resignation
	• Outline of ongoing projects and plan to transfer duties
	• Aspects of the employment experience that enhanced your career development
	• Major contributions you made to the organization and those the organization helped you gain

The Interview

When your career marketing strategy attracts an employer's interest, the next step is preparation for the interview (Table 23.3). Your position research strategy includes looking up the organization's website, reviewing press articles, checking out social media, or finding someone in the organization to speak with informally.

Interviewing is a two-way proposition; the interviewee should be gathering as much information as the interviewer. Both sides should be making judgments throughout the process so that if a position is offered, the interviewee will be prepared to accept, decline, or explore further. Often, applicants are interviewed by a panel or participate in a series of interviews that allow

TABLE 23.3   Interview Goals

Preparation	Review the organization's mission, vision, and values statements before the interview. Obtain statistics and facts.
	Have 3 to 5 questions rehearsed and ready to ask about the company or position.
	Recheck your résumé and curriculum vitae for emphasis and new information.
	Print additional copies of your résumé and curriculum vitae to bring to the interview.
	Practice using "action" words as you describe your experience.
	Have a story ready that illustrates your brand.
	Plan your transportation, clothing, and accessories, including portfolio and pen.
Appearance	Arrive on time and alone.
	Wear comfortable clothing one step up from usual office attire. If jeans are the norm, wear dress slacks. If business casual is the norm, then wear a suit.
	Make a memorable entrance, make eye contact, shake hands, and smile.
	Greet everyone you meet, including the receptionist, security guard, or cleaning staff. Say, "Hello, I'm [name]."
	Position yourself with the interviewer so that you are not at "odds" or having to sit in an uncomfortable position to talk.
Personal characteristics	Accentuate the positive! Appear interested—project competence, confidence, and energy.
	Describe who you are from your mission statement, including personality traits. Be expected to cite examples of when these traits helped or hindered you in previous situations.
	Describe how your education and experience prepared you for this position.
	Describe your skills as a member and leader of a team.
	Describe situations that characterize your energy, initiative, drive, ambition, enthusiasm, and professional values.
	Answer questions directly but know when not to or ask for clarification.
	Say only positive and honest things about your present employer.
The work itself	Discuss the primary position responsibilities.
	Ask about new program directions.
	Prepare to address hypothetical situations that display your problem-solving, reasoning, self-confidence, knowledge, and critical thinking. (Creates opportunity to evaluate you in action and under some stress.)
	Ask to speak to current employees.
Organizational fit	Ask intelligent questions that suggest you have prepared for this interview.
	Be clear about what you believe to be distinctive about this organization and how it meets your expectations for a position. Ask hypothetical questions that allow you to learn how the people with whom you speak live out the organization's values.
	Articulate your "fit" with the organization's philosophy, mission, and vision.
Professional opportunities	Keep in mind key points that summarize your experience and its value to the potential employer.
	Inquire about opportunities, educational support, and work-life balance.
	Be clear about what you expect to obtain from any position you consider, including advancement opportunities.
	Secure a time frame for notification of an offer.
Follow-up	Write a thank-you email message.
	Evaluate your performance: Focus on your strengths and weaknesses during the interview and how to manage them in the future.

fellow employees more say in the hiring process. Many prospective employers administer basic skills tests for the application process in business and healthcare settings. You might ask what to anticipate and, if you have already completed such appraisals, bring the results with you to share with your interviewer.

To feel more at ease, wear professional but comfortable clothing to the interview. Rehearse possible answers, questions to ask, and points to make so that you are prepared for the interview. Be ready to describe why you want the job, what you know about the organization, then connect to your values, skills, and experience alignment with the position. Have examples ready that set you apart from the other candidates, such as your ability to problem solve, team skills, or work habits.

INTERVIEW TOPICS AND QUESTIONS

Interviews have many stages, beginning with your initial contact. Be mindful of any interaction you make with a parking attendant, administrative personnel, and conversations in the elevator or hallway. This information can often give you clues about the culture of the organization. During interviews, employers should ask the same questions of all applicants for a given position. In addition to providing comparable information as the basis for a decision, the applicant's expectation for equal treatment is upheld. Employers often use behavioral interviewing techniques and ask clinically focused questions to identify the most appropriate applicant for the vacant position. Most likely, the first question will be, "tell me a little about yourself." The answer should focus on your knowledge, skills, and abilities that make you the best fit for the job. If you have done your homework, you will know what the employer is looking for in your answer. Be prepared to cite how you have faced challenges and dilemmas because those types of questions are likely to be asked. Rather than being asked, "What are your weaknesses?" you may be asked, "Tell me how you handled the last mistake you made" or "How did your educational program prepare you for critical care nursing?"

Only questions related to the position and its description are legitimate. Employers should not ask unrelated questions, and applicants should decline to answer if asked inappropriate questions, samples of which are provided in Table 23.4 (U.S. Equal Employment

TABLE 23.4 Inappropriate and Appropriate Interview Questions

Sample of Inappropriate Questions	Sample of Appropriate and Legal Questions
How old are you?	Do you know that this position requires someone at least 21 years old?
What does your husband (wife) do?	This position requires that no one in your immediate family be in the healthcare field or own interests or shares in any healthcare facility. Does this pose a problem?
Who takes care of your children?	Attendance is important. Are you able to meet this expectation?
Are you working "just to help out"?	What are your short-term and long-term goals?
Do you have any disabilities?	Is there anything that would prevent you from performing this work as described?
Where were you born?	This position requires U.S. citizenship. May I assume you meet this criterion?
What are the names of all of the organizations to which you belong?	To which professional organizations do you belong?
What is your religious preference?	We subscribe to a specific religious philosophy and mission. Do you understand that all employees are expected to promote this philosophy, and are you able to do so?

Opportunity Commission, https://www.eeoc.gov/prohibited-employment-policiespractices#recruitment). If the interviewer asks an inappropriate question, the applicant can choose not to answer the direct question by addressing the content area. For example, if asked about your spouse's employment, you might say, "I believe what you are asking is how long I will be able to be in this position. Let me assure you that I intend to be here for at least two years." Each of the content areas may be acceptable for an employer to ask, but the questions in column one of Table 23.4 are phrased inappropriately. The second column identifies approaches that are both appropriate and legal. The key to ensuring a fair interviewing process is being prepared, knowing what can be asked legitimately, and knowing how to respond to inappropriate questions.

EXERCISE 23.6 Select a partner and role-play an interview for a professional nursing position. The potential employer (manager) should focus on the competencies of the prospective employee. Include questions and scenarios about common conflicts and challenges seen in the clinical setting. The interviewee (prospective employee) should highlight competencies, decision-making abilities, and critical-thinking abilities when responding to the situation-based questions. Reflect on the process and discuss what learning you can apply to future interviews.

You may consider the following questions:
1. Why did you choose to go into nursing? (motivation)
2. Give me an example of a time where you disagreed with a coworker. (conflict management)
3. What was the most useful criticism you ever received? (reflective practice)
4. Please give an example of a time when you had to address an angry client. What was the problem, and what was the outcome? (customer service)
5. Everyone has made some poor decisions or has done something that just did not turn out right. Has this happened to you? What happened? What would you do differently in the future? (decision-making)

Questions to ask the interviewer:
1. How can someone measure success in this role? What are the expectations for the first six months? (focus)
2. Why is the position open? Was there a promotion? (upward mobility)
3. What are some of the day-to-day responsibilities of this position? (actual work)
4. Can you tell me a little more about the team I will be working with? (teamwork)
5. Can you describe the culture of the organization? (leadership)

If you are well prepared, you will know the organization's stated values and beliefs and whether they are compatible with your own. An interview challenge is to determine whether those stated beliefs are lived or are merely printed words. If numerous people in the organization can communicate how the mission is translated into a specific role, the beliefs are likely lived ones.

EVALUATE AND NEGOTIATE AN OFFER

Now that you have successfully found a new opportunity, attended the interview, have made a favorable impression, and subsequently received an offer, you have the opportunity to evaluate it against your personal values and career construction goals. Maybe you are in the fortunate position of multiple offers. Either way, you should start by knowing your value in both monetary terms and experience. You can search websites or talk with current employees you know to better understand the expected pay scales. Though many organizations have a set salary for the position, you may negotiate other areas of the package, such as vacation, flex time, and shift differential, or other benefits. It is important to go in knowing your value and what you are willing to accept in the offer so that you can keep it brief. Be appreciative as you start the negotiation. Remember to get the offer in writing at the end of your negotiation (Acosta, 2021).

CONCLUSION

A successful career requires leadership and management strategies designed to systematically move you toward your desired goals. Finding a good fit in a position and a career is important for personal and professional satisfaction. Whether through graduate education, continuing education, certification, service in professional or nonwork associations, or scholarship, your continuous professional development is a crucial component of your success as a nurse. Involvement in professional associations or mentoring can open doors to opportunities and skill development. Documenting and representing qualifications through marketing documents such as résumés, CVs, and professional letters support your professional brand to secure meaningful employment opportunities and far-reaching career success.

THE SOLUTION

Looking for my first job was more uncertain than I had expected it to be. I wanted to expand upon what I had learned in nursing school by working for an organization that would provide dynamic learning opportunities and push me to embrace this complex area of frontline nursing. I decided to remove all limitations and expanded my job search to include the entire country, not just Arizona, my home state, and my comfort zone. My dream job was out there; I just needed to search for it. The process took longer than anticipated, and after countless interviews and multiple job offers, I had found the perfect fit as a nurse resident at the University of Kentucky. Thus, I began my year-long ICU nurse residency program, where I would kickstart my career and build a critical care foundation that has since served me well.

After completing my residency, I returned to Arizona and began working as a frontline nurse in an emergency department to grow and learn within the critical care field. While I loved being a frontline critical care nurse, I realized a part of me still felt unfulfilled. Teaching has always been a dream and passion, and I try very hard to integrate it into my practice. I sought out every opportunity to teach and educate in addition to using best practices for myself. I was the first on my unit to volunteer for precepting both nursing students and new graduate nurses. I signed up for every possible education course I found interesting that my hospital offered and would contribute to furthering my field knowledge. I took on the role of the educator within the emergency department when that opportunity presented itself. This was done while preparing to begin a master's program with a nursing education concentration. This was made possible by combining my love for nursing and a passion for teaching to help support and inspire future nurses to find a path they love.

When the COVID-19 pandemic began and quickly grasped the state of New York, I knew I could be doing more with my prior nursing experience. At that point, I transitioned to my crisis nursing journey. I spent the better part of the year traveling to "hotspots," starting in New York, Miami, Phoenix, Guam, and, later, San Francisco. I was able to provide relief and support to areas that were affected hardest. This allowed me to grow as a nurse, fuel my passion for teaching, and solidify my commitment to becoming a nursing instructor.

A career as a nurse does not have to be a linear progression. As I've learned over the last few years, taking every opportunity to grow in my knowledge, skills, and experience will suit me. Our profession allows space to explore and grow within your passions, which makes nursing so spectacular. Everybody has a different journey, and I can't wait to see where mine is heading next.

Would this be a suitable approach for you? Why?

Rachel Breslauer

REFLECTIONS

Think about what you have done in your professional work in nursing and beyond. Consider the most meaningful examples of your caring. What was your most challenging experience? What did you learn today that helps you be a better nurse and person?

What are your career goals? What actions do you need to do in the next three to five years to progress toward those goals? Write a one-paragraph summary.

BEST PRACTICES

Consider that anything on the Internet is traceable to you and what message those postings convey. If you are trying to establish a specific professional image, how you create your communications everywhere reflects—or contradicts—your image. Establishing a system for maintaining information about your achievements and general employment history is easier earlier in your career rather than later.

TIPS FOR SUCCESSFUL CAREER MANAGEMENT

Leader

1. Update your CV at least every six months so that you always have an accurate, current set of accomplishments and qualifications to share when a special opportunity appears.
2. Join two or more professional organizations: a broad professional group and a specialty.
3. Volunteer in your profession and your community.

Manager

1. Find a mentor and be a mentor.
2. Attend at least one professional meeting each year to network with colleagues. When possible, travel outside of your geographic area.
3. Think about what you need to be employable in the face of health system changes.

Follower

1. Focus on your strengths and build them into spectacular performances; hone the basics so that you are always prepared.
2. Create an individual mission statement.
3. Keep digital versions of documents related to your accomplishments filed together in a folder.

REFERENCES

Acosta, D. (2021). How to negotiate salary for a new job: Dos and don'ts. *Wall Street Journal*. https://www.wsj.com/articles/how-to-negotiate-a-job-offer-the-dos-and-donts-11607553703.

American Association of Colleges of Nursing (AACN). (2021). *AACN essentials*. https://www.aacnnursing.org/Portals/42/AcademicNursing/pdf/Essentials-2021.pdf.

American Nurse Association (ANA). (2019). *Career and professional development*. https://www.nursingworld.org/resources/individual/.

American Nurses Association (ANA). (2015). *Code of ethics for nurses with interpretive statements*. https://www.nursingworld.org/practice-policy/nursing-excellence/official-position-statements/.

Bagdadli, S., & Gianecchini, M. (2019). Organizational career management practices and objective career success: A systematic review and framework. *Human Resource Management Review, 29*(3) 353–370. https://doi.org/10.1016/j.hrmr.2018.08.001.

Goodrich Mitts, N. (2020). Crafting a career narrative: A comparison of career construction and traditional career counseling. *ProQuest Dissertations Publishing*. Retrieved from https://www.proquest.com/openview/1b1e1306b2f6e1dbb0bf9a626c4f4011/1.pdf?pq-origsite=gscholar&cbl=51922&diss=y.

Hirschi, A. (2020). Whole-life career management: A counseling intervention framework. *The Career Development Quarterly, 68*(1), 2–17. https://doi.org/10.1002/cdq.12209.

Jacobson, G. (2020). Cybervetting job applicants on social media: The new normal? *Ethics and Information Technology, 22*(2), 175–195. https://doi.org/10.1007/s10676-020-09526-2.

McMillen, J. E. (2020). *The impact of nurse residency programs on recruitment and retention of new graduate nurses* (Order No. 28000799). ProQuest Dissertations & Theses Global. (242150012).

National Council of State Boards of Nursing (NCSBN). (2018). *A nurse's guide to the use of social media*. Retrieved from https://www.ncsbn.org/NCSBN_SocialMedia.pdf.

Reinhart, R. J. (2020). *Nurses continue to rate highest in honesty, ethics*. Gallup Inc. Retrieved from https://news.gallup.com/poll/274673/nurses-continue-rate-highest-honesty-ethics.aspx.

U.S. Bureau of Labor Statistics. (2021). *Office of Occupational Statistics and Employment Projections*. https://www.bls.gov/ooh/healthcare/registered-nurses.

Xin, Z., Zhou, W., Li, M., & Tang, F. (2020). Career success criteria clarity as a predictor of employment outcomes. *Frontiers in Psychology, 11*, 1–11. https://doi.org/10.3389/fpsyg.2020.00540.

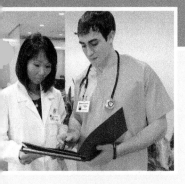

24

Developing Leaders, Managers, and Followers

Jacqueline L. Gonzalez

ANTICIPATED LEARNING OUTCOMES

- Analyze the roles of followers, managers, leaders, and staff in creating a satisfying and healthy working environment for frontline nurses, yielding positive patient outcomes.
- Evaluate transactional, transformational, authentic, and other leadership styles for effectiveness and their correlational potential for positive outcomes.
- Ascertain leadership challenges and successes in balancing generational differences, including mentoring and professional development.
- Discover and recognize leadership opportunities and development strategies and how leadership skills acquisition can be applied.
- Identify skills and tools to navigate complex systems, such as emotional intelligence and maximizing resources, along with the use of technology.

KEY TERMS

authentic leadership
budgets
bullying
case management
follower
healthy work environment

incivility
intergenerational nurse workforce
leader
leadership
managed care
management

Maslow's Hierarchy of Needs
mentor
nurse manager
organizational culture
transactional leadership
transformational leadership

THE CHALLENGE

Nurse managers as leaders are faced with daily conflict that arises when there is a difference in perspective or opinion between team members. In today's complex work environment, there are intraprofessional teams that work collaboratively with nursing. Therefore, sometimes individual opinions or perspectives regarding patient care may vary based on each person's experiences and biases. However, conflict among groups can be healthy and beneficial, as it generates conversation from opposing views, developing approaches that can be agreed on by the team. When discussion becomes unhealthy, such as being too personal, chaos can result.

The important competencies of a strong leader include the ability to develop a shared vision, to resolve and manage conflict, and to build team cohesion while ensuring

(Continued)

INTRODUCTION

Leadership is a complex, highly essential, and challenging skill expected of all nurses. *Leader* performance is not a formal position but rather an attribute. Nightingale (2020) summarized leadership as "the action of influencing others" by shaping professional and personal skills, including the use of interpersonal abilities, positive behaviors, and positive qualities. Leading occurs through every role in an organization, from follower to formal leadership roles. Leading is demonstrating courage when a patient needs an advocate or support with an intervention. An organized group of colleagues addressing a departmental or corporate concern is leading in order to find a solution. When a leader is formally placed in charge of a project or promoted to a specific management position, the decision is primarily based on leader readiness.

Nurses must possess leadership skills to lead others and to make positive contributions in society and in healthcare. In fact, one of the competencies for BSN-prepared nurses outlined in the American Association of Colleges of Nursing *Baccalaureate Essentials* (AACN, 2021) is to develop the capacity for leadership. Within work organizations, certain nurses are designated as managers. Those that are followers may be asked to step into charge nurse roles, leading teams of people on a unit through their shift of work. These individuals are all important to ensuring that care is delivered in a safe, efficient manner. Nurse leaders are also vital in the workplace to elicit input from others and to formulate a shared vision for the preferred future.

Management can be viewed from different perspectives. The core of role theory began with

management theory, a science that has undergone numerous changes in the past century. Frederick Winslow Taylor's early principles of scientific management (see Theory Box) were developed in the era of manufacturing (Kukreja, 2020). In the mid-1900s, change theory was developed by Kurt Lewin; Peter Drucker established the principle of management by objectives. All of these theories are based on differing principles designed to depict the management of personnel in achieving organizational goals and objectives. Practice in the 1930s through the 1970s was dominated by participative, humanistic management theories. Although changes in healthcare delivery no doubt are affecting the roles of nurse leaders, managers, and followers, the relevance of social role theory continues. Newman & Newman (2016) describe social role theory as the linkage between social development and personal development. Behaviors include role expectations, the assumption of social roles, and the expected norms of those roles

Role expectations are the behavioral expectations that are shared or related to each person's role. When a new nurse manager enacts a new role, expected behaviors are associated with attaining and delivering results within the role. Importantly, as a nurse manager assumes the social role, the enactment of this role includes the anticipated and predictable qualities of social behavior of the role, such as demonstrating leadership, creating a safe and positive culture within the work environment, and managing budgets and financial resources.

The evolutionary process of management theories has affected how managers address workers' concerns and needs. The beginning management theories

THEORY BOX
Principles of Scientific Management

Principle	Application to Practice
1. Replace everyday work methods with those based on a scientific review of the tasks at hand.	Study and quantify underlying reasons for delays in the operating room for first case starts to improve efficiency.
2. Select, develop, and train each person working rather than to leave it to them to do it themselves.	When hiring new nurses, build a standardized RN residency or orientation program to build reliability and consistency into practice.
3. Work together with workers to make sure that the scientific methods that have been implemented are being followed.	Collaborate with colleagues utilizing process improvement methods such as observing central line dressing changes, ensuring adherence to established practice norms and to achieve optimal outcomes.
4. Make sure the work is divided scientifically into those who are planning the work and those that actually perform the tasks.	When performing patient assignments, review patient acuity/intensity and the skill sets of the nursing team before assigning. Do not assign just by dividing the number of patients by the number of staff on duty without considering patient needs/staff competencies.

From Kukreja, S. (2020). *4 principles of scientific management.* Retrieved from https://www.managementstudyhq.com/taylor-principles-of-scientific-management.html

discounted concern for workers' psychological needs and focused on productivity and efficiency. In utilizing theories relating to human relations and working conditions, the workers' social needs and motivations became focal points for the nurse manager. McLeod (2020) uses Maslow's groundbreaking work to describe the motivational model of the human Hierarchy of Needs that reflects the need for human satisfaction at the most basic level (physiologic, safety) before reaching higher levels (love and self-esteem) and, finally, achieving full potential or self-actualization. McLeod (2020) discussed Maslow's hierarchy in relationship to the employee's purpose, belongingness, esteem, and self-actualization. Leaders have a duty of care to help employees feel that they develop purpose at work; organizations that commit to a career ladder build toward developing their employees' self-potential.

THE DEFINITION OF MANAGEMENT

Management is a generic function that includes focusing on completing the work that must be done. Thus, almost every nurse has a vested interest in management. Nurses must manage the care of their patients; they must also self-manage and manage others for whom they are accountable, even when their titles do not reflect a formal management role (Fig. 24.1).

Although managers must manage personnel, they must also lead people and view them as resources in accomplishing today's work. For example, the American Organization of Nurse Executives (AONE) (2016), now known as the American Organization for Nursing Leadership, offers the Nurse Manager Learning Domain Framework representing three separate domains for the development and learning framework of the nurse manager. These domains are reviewed here and include the following:

- The science: Managing the business
- The art: Leading the people
- The leader within: Creating the leader in yourself

Nurses are responsible for fostering and managing relationships with those they report to, their peers, and frontline staff for whom they are accountable. Skilled managers have competency in human relations, technical skills, and organizational skills. Nurse managers use such skills as problem solving, motivating, controlling, following through, aligning, and inspiring people.

THE NURSE MANAGER

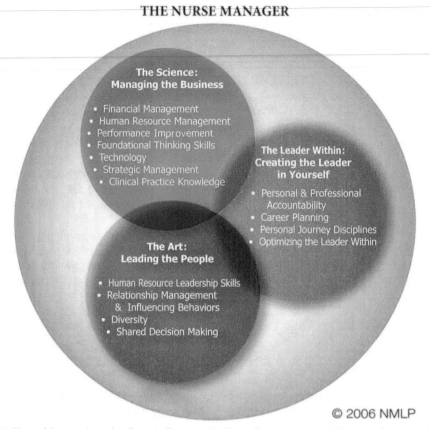

The Science:
Managing the Business

- Financial Management
- Human Resource Management
- Performance Improvement
- Foundational Thinking Skills
- Technology
- Strategic Management
- Clinical Practice Knowledge

The Leader Within:
Creating the Leader
in Yourself

- Personal & Professional
  Accountability
- Career Planning
- Personal Journey Disciplines
- Optimizing the Leader Within

The Art:
Leading the People

- Human Resource Leadership Skills
- Relationship Management
  & Influencing Behaviors
- Diversity
- Shared Decision Making

© 2006 NMLP

Fig. 24.1 Nurse Manager Learning Domain Framework. (From Development and Learning Framework of the Nurse Manager. Copyright © 2016, by the American Organization of Nurse Executives [AONE]. All rights reserved.)

WHAT IS A LEADER?

A leader is an individual who works with others to develop and set a clear vision of the preferred future and articulate a pathway to attain goals to that aim. According to Raso et al. (2020, p. 489), "leadership is not necessarily tied to a position of authority." However, caring in leadership is a very important and influential concept—great leaders have emerged and have been responsible for helping society to move forward by articulating and carrying out caring visions throughout time. Dr. Martin Luther King, Jr., called his vision a *dream*, which was developed because of the input and lived experiences of countless others. Mother Teresa called her vision a *calling*, which was developed out of the suffering of others. Florence Nightingale called her vision *nursing*, developed because people were experiencing a void that was a barrier to their ability to regain or establish health.

She was able to push through a new practice vision that saved lives. A leader is an individual who works with others to develop a clear vision of the preferred future and to make that vision happen. An individual can have an impressive title; however, that title does not make that person a leader. No matter what the person with a title does, that individual can never be successful without having the ability to inspire others to follow. The leader must be able to inspire the commitment of followers.

Leaders Have Followers

Leaders are involved with formulating and shaping ideas. Covey (1992), in his classic work, identified eight characteristics of effective, principle-centered leaders (Exercise 24.1). Effective leaders are continually engaging themselves in lifelong learning. They are service oriented and concerned with the common good. They radiate positive energy. For people to be inspired and motivated, they must have a positive leader. Effective leaders believe in other people who may be their followers. They lead balanced lives and see life as an adventure. Effective leaders are synergistic; that is, they see things as greater than the sum of their parts and they engage themselves in self-renewal.

EXERCISE 24.1 Covey's Eight Characteristics of Effective, Principle-Centered Leaders

List Covey's eight characteristics of effective leaders on the left side of a piece of paper or a word processing document. Next to each characteristic, list any examples of your activities or attributes that reflect the characteristic. Some areas may be blank; others may be full. Think about what this means for you personally.

1. Engages in lifelong learning
2. Service oriented
3. Concerned with the common good
4. Radiates positive energy and enthusiasm
5. Believes in other people
6. Leads balanced life and sees life as an adventure
7. Synergistic, that is, sees things as greater than the sum of their parts
8. Engages in self-renewal

Leader's Role in Leading Change—The Nurse Manager as Change Leader

Leadership is key for nursing as a profession to move forward with changes in healthcare and society. Abbott (2020, p. 27) states that changes in healthcare are more about how leaders guide through uncertainty rather than necessarily organizational direction. The public depends on nurses to advocate for the public's needs and interests. Nurses must step forward into leadership roles in their workplace, in their professional associations, and in legislative and policy-making arenas to effect the changes that are needed. Nurses as leaders set goals for the future and the pace for achieving them. The public depends on nurse leaders to move the consumer advocacy health agenda forward.

Moreover, within healthcare or other organizations, certain nurses are designated as managers. These individuals are important to ensuring that care is delivered in a safe, efficient manner. Nurse leaders are also vital in the workplace to elicit input from others and to formulate a collective vision for the preferred future. Developing frontline staff today is critical to helping them reach their potential and work as a team. Nurse managers often begin their leader experience as a charge nurse. Organizations offering foundational leader education for charge nurses have improved resiliency and transformational and transactional skills, yielding more positive outcomes (Spiva et al., 2020). Continued leadership development education is essential for nursing leadership progression and success.

Leadership as a Primary Determinant of Workplace Satisfaction

Nurse satisfaction within the workplace is an important construct in nursing and healthcare administration. Turnover is extremely costly to any work organization in terms of money, skill, talent, knowledge, and quality of care. Thus, being mindful of frontline nurse satisfaction is both an economic and a professional concern. The role of the nurse manager is pivotal in ensuring nurse satisfaction and that followers have expectations of their manager in creating a milieu that encourages collaboration and positive outcomes for patients and staff.

In a small convenience study of charge nurse effectiveness, leadership style development and leader resiliency showed additional correlations. Improvement was demonstrated in leadership outcomes, transactional and transformational leadership, and resiliency for all subjects (Spiva et al., 2020).

EXERCISE 24.2 Follower Behavior

Follower behavior nurtures and supports—or deteriorates—leader behavior. Identify the behavior you exhibited during your most recent clinical experience. What was supportive? What did not support the leader? What could you have done differently?

Emotionally Intelligent Leadership Style

Emotionally intelligent (EI) leadership has been found to be significantly associated with the implicit rationing of nursing care. When rationing important elements of care occurs by clinical nurses (due to a lack of time, inadequate staffing, or skill mix) patient outcomes suffer and higher patient mortality and poor patient outcomes follow (Blizzard & Woods, 2020). Emotional intelligence leadership presence or empathy has been reported to build a positive work environment contributing to a higher quality of care as well as positive outcomes for patients (Blizzard & Woods, 2020).

RESEARCH PERSPECTIVE

Resource: Blizzard, L., & Woods, S. (2020). The relationship between the implicit rationing of nursing care and emotionally intelligent leadership style. *Journal of Nursing Administration, 50*(12), 623–628.

A cross-sectional randomly sampled survey study of 35,039 direct-care RNs from acute care hospitals in Oregon from September 2017 to March 2018 determined the relationship between the nursing work environment, leadership styles, and nurses' perceptions of implicit rationing of nursing care. One of the study's outcomes noted an association between lower amounts of implicit rationing of nursing care and positive RN perceptions of emotionally intelligent leadership style presence. Nurse satisfaction with nursing care increased in an environment of teamwork, communication, recognition, and support.

Implications for Practice

Nurse faculty and nurse leaders are encouraged to provide education and development related to the assimilation of leadership skills fostering emotional intelligence. Pairing new nurse leaders with mentors who demonstrate elements of emotional intelligence is essential for creating optimal safe, healthy work environments with positive patient outcomes.

Leaders Create a Healthy Work Environment

A healthy work environment is one that is good for nurses, patients, and the organization. Leaders must be committed to creating and maintaining an environment of positivity. Nurse managers and nurse educators (Wunnenberg, 2020) may need education and assistance to manage bullying, discourage intent to leave, and address issues as they present themselves or become enculturated in the environment (Hartin et al., 2020). Disruptive behaviors such as bullying and incivility are incongruent with a healthy work environment. A strategic plan to change/create the culture requires vision and prioritization.

Key standards are discussed regarding leading change for a healthy work environment in Table 24.1 (Sarik et al., 2020, p. 30; Grant et al., 2020). The nurse leader also plays an important role in supporting new nurses and encouraging them through their transition from novice nurses to expert nurse. It is through this support that the leader can achieve positive patient outcomes enhancing the organization to achieve its safety, quality, and financial goals (Matter & Wolgast, 2020).

Nurse Managers Advocate for a Patient Safety Culture and Departmental Excellence

In a descriptive, correlational study of 34,514 nurses from 535 hospitals regarding characteristics of a culture of patient safety, staffing adequacy was found to be a strong predictor along with support from management and the creation of a learning and improvement culture (Lee & Dahinten, 2020). In the process, considerable learning can occur. When staff feel respected by their leader, they genuinely feel recognized and appreciated. As a result,

they practice in a culture oriented toward positive patient outcomes and safety. When nurse managers use good listening skills and advocate for staff ideas and suggestions, the staff feels cared for by their leader.

Nurse managers must be able to focus on both the individual and the larger goals and outcomes of the department and organization. The manager's aim is to enable people to develop their abilities and strengths to the fullest and to achieve excellence, thus contributing to the department's overall success. Managers must help people develop realistic, attainable goals that provide an avenue of individual growth that also contributes to the organization's well-being. Active participation, encouragement, and guidance from the manager and the organization are needed for the individual's developmental efforts to be fully actualized. Nurse managers who are successful in motivating staff often provide an inclusive environment that facilitates clearly set, achievable goals that can result in both team and personal satisfaction. Nurse managers must possess qualities of a good leader: knowledge, integrity, ambition, good judgment, courage, stamina, enthusiasm, communication skills, planning skills, and administrative abilities. Similarities exist between managers and leaders; these same skills, applied differently, are equally important for followers.

From Follower to Nurse Manager and Leadership Development

Managers address complex issues at the front line by organizing, planning, budgeting, and setting target goals. They meet their goals by planning, organizing, staffing, controlling, following up, and problem solving. By contrast, official leaders "an organizational culture" of teamwork, setting a broad direction, developing a shared vision, and communicating that direction to staff. Followers collaborate and communicate to translate that direction into action, sharing perceptions about successes and barriers to achieving the vision and demonstrating willingness to take on leadership roles as situations arise. Managers address complexity and change, whereas senior leaders primarily set vision and address change. Followers implement patient care change and provide input into organizational change. Successful organizations embrace manager, senior leader, and follower traits that are relationship based. This drives change and positive outcomes, ensuring a healthy and effective work environment.

Porter O'Grady and Clavelle (2020) advocate that structural empowerment is the framework for building shared governance and impacting positive patient outcomes. Role expectations are the behavioral expectations that are shared or related to each person's role. When a new nurse manager enacts a new role, expected behaviors are associated with delivering results within the role. Importantly, as a nurse manager assumes the social role, the enactment of this role includes the anticipated and predictable qualities of social behavior of the role, such as demonstrating leadership, managing budgets and financial resources, and creating a positive culture within the work environment.

> **EXERCISE 24.3** In a small group, discuss the staffing needs of a very busy neurology unit for a particular night shift. The patient care staffing needs of this unit are very high, including three new postoperative patients. Today, the unit has extra staff on duty. However, over the last few days, the department had been very busy and short-staffed. Everyone worked together as a team to provide excellent care on these challenging days. Hospital resources are scarce, and if extra staff are left on duty, the unit will be over budget. How does the manager motivate the staff? Starting a critical conversation that will engage them in understanding the need to contribute to unit cost-effectiveness is needed—how would you want to hear this conversation? What might concern the nurses? What approach might engage the nurses more to work together through this shift? What is the most effective leadership approach in this situation?

The evolutionary process of management theories has affected how managers address workers' concerns and needs. The beginning management theories discounted concern for workers' psychological needs and focused on productivity and efficiency. When theories concerning human relations evolved from the Hawthorne Corporation's studies of working conditions, workers' social needs and motivations became focal points for the nurse manager. Perhaps often used in nursing, Maslow's (McLeod, 2020) groundbreaking work describing the human Hierarchy of Needs reflects on the needs of human beings that must be satisfied at their most basic level (physiologic, safety) before reaching higher levels (love and self-esteem) to achieve self-actualization.

THE PRACTICE OF LEADERSHIP

Leadership Approaches

How one approaches leadership depends on experience and expectations. Many leadership theories and styles have been described. Three of the most popular theory-based approaches are transactional leadership, transformational leadership, and authentic leadership (see the Theory Box).

Transactional Leadership

Transactional leadership includes the historical "boss" image as evidenced by a study based in Jordan (Sullman et al., 2020). In this study, transactional leadership based on contingent reward allocation appears to be among the most common style demonstrated by nurse leaders. This includes being collaborative and goal directed, and offering rewards. Passive-avoidant leaders are more reactive, avoid interventions or conflict, and generally do not communicate clearly with their followers (Sullman et al., 2020). In this descriptive cross-sectional study by Sullman et al. (2020), nurse retention is clearly correlated with the presence of transformational leadership. Transactional leadership relies on formal authority and the power of organizational position to reward and punish performance. Followers are fairly secure about what will happen next and how to "play the game" to get where they want to be. A transactional leader uses a *quid pro quo* approach to accomplish work (Richards, 2020). Transactional leaders value and reward followers for high performance and penalize others for poor performance, motivating followers by offering external rewards that generate compliance with expectations.

In a transactional leadership environment, employees understand that decisions are generally made with little or no input from team members.

Transformational Leadership

Transformational leadership is based on an inspiring vision that changes the framework of the organization for employees. This style of leadership involves communication that connects with employees' ideals in a way that causes emotional engagement. The transformational leader can motivate employees by the articulation of an inspirational vision; by encouragement of creative, innovative thinking; and by individualized consideration of each employee, thus, accounting for individual needs and abilities. Bringing people together around an inspiring vision and yet valuing individuals as distinct beings suggests a finely tuned, mindful approach to the role of leader. The most important outcome is the correlation between transformational leadership and positive patient and staff outcomes and nurse retention. When employees are connected and empowered in caring for their patients, they feel a sense of ownership and responsibility. Robbins and Davidhizar (2020) argue that when these outcomes are positive, organizational profitability increases.

The historic work by Covey (1992) says, "The goal of transformational leadership is to transform people and organizations in a literal sense, to change them in mind and heart; enlarge vision, insight, and understanding; clarify purposes; make behavior congruent with beliefs, principles, or values; and bring about changes that are permanent, self-perpetuating, and momentum-building" (p. 287). A transformative leader creates a vision of what quality could look like and then provides specific actions that create a sense of community, which supports satisfaction, retention, communication, and interprofessional work. This type of leader listens to the views of others, finds ways to remove barriers, fosters creativity and innovation, and serves as an advocate for those who care for patients.

A transformative leadership style seems particularly suited to the nursing environment. For example, the American Nurses Credentialing Center's Magnet Recognition Program® places great emphasis on this type of leadership to move an organization to high levels of quality. The Program® focuses on structural empowerment values, shared governance, and its impact on care, which is a model that has been built under the transformational leadership umbrella. Structural empowerment is optimized when there is a transformational leader who supports innovation and empowerment in a professional practice environment.

A transformational leadership style has proven to be a significant contributor in forecasting nurse turnover. Therefore, nurse leaders who are inspirational, influential, and encourage followers' personal growth and development, have a positive impact on lessening turnover.

AUTHENTIC LEADERSHIP

Long (2020), in her summary review, finds that authentic leadership is defined by having deep values and beliefs as well as a strong sense of self-awareness. These attributes can positively impact the experience of new nurses and yield a positive work environment and enhanced well-being at work. This leadership style can have a positive effect on building competence and confidence and new graduate nurse retention.

Wei et al. (2020) performed a comprehensive review of nurse leader styles and suggested that transformational and authentic leadership styles had a positive impact in reducing nurse burnout and create an inspirational work environment that supports nurse engagement. Transformational leadership is hard work. Investment of time and energy is required to bring out the best in people. However, a leader does not have to be good at everything. A good leader seeks to create a common vision and achieve the whole from the contributions of the various members of a team.

EXERCISE 24.4 Define a clinical or management issue that sparks your passion. Assume that you have 6 weeks to make a difference. Create a plan identifying your leadership tasks, the support required from others, and the time frame to effect change. Move the issue toward resolution. Think about what you would do if no one was responsive to your issue. Consider why the issue is more important for you but not for others.

THEORY BOX

Comparison of Outcomes in Transactional, Transformational and Authentic Leadership

Transactional Leadership (Richards, 2020)	Transformational Leadership (Pearson, 2020; Robbins & Davidhizar, 2020)	Authentic Leadership (Raso, 2019; Long, 2020; Doherty & Revell, 2020; Pearson, 2020)
Leader Behaviors		
• Good for completing tasks and achieving short-term goals • Task driven • Contingent reward (*quid pro quo*) • Punitive less than expected performance • Management by exception (active)—monitors performance and takes action to correct • Management by exception (passive)—intervenes only when problems exist • Inspirational and motivational • Intellectually stimulating • Individualized consideration	• Translates vision to action • Sets clear goals • Works well with interprofessional teams • Displays confidence • Inspires and motivates others • Can advocate for nurse-led research • Develops a professional practice environment • Communicates well and empowers others	• Based on strong sense of self, values, and beliefs (guides from the heart) • Ability to influence others to achieve a shared vision • Stands for issues leader knows are important • Caring • Shared decision-making respected • Integrity • Resilient
Effect on Follower		
• Fulfills the contract or gets punished • Does the work and gets paid • Corrects errors in a reactive manner • A shared vision • Increased self-worth • Challenging and meaningful work • Coaching and mentoring can happen • A sense of being valued	• Motivates and inspires • Fosters innovation and creativity • Engaged • Assists in meeting greatest potential • Grows in professional practice • May provide certainty in times of environmental change • Stirs emotions to strive for the best	• Builds respect and loyalty • Fosters a healthy work environment • Empowers workforce • Motivational • Hopeful • Achieves shared vision with support • Encourages optimism
Organizational Outcomes		
• Work is supervised and completed according to the rules. • Deadlines are met. • Low to stable levels of commitment are typical. • May see lower profitability, patient/staff dissatisfaction, noncommitted	• Increased commitment • Increased job satisfaction • Increased morale • Long-term organizational strategy and vision collectively achieved with engaged workforce • Engagement of staff with purposeful increased performance	• Can advance nursing's professional role in the organization • Creates an environment of hopefulness and optimism

BARRIERS TO LEADERSHIP AND FALSE ASSUMPTIONS

Leadership demands a commitment of effort and time. Many barriers exist to both leading and following. Good leadership and good followership go hand in hand, and both strengthen the mission of the organization.

Becoming more proficient in leadership skills allows leaders, managers, and followers to approach problems from new perspectives, breaking down barriers to success, and positive outcomes. Some people have false assumptions about leaders and leadership. For example, some believe that position and title are equivalent to leadership.

RESEARCH PERSPECTIVE

Authentic Leadership

Resource: Spiva, L., Davis, S., Case-Wirth, J., Hedenstrom, L., Hogue, V., Box, M, Berrier, E., ... Ahlers, L. (2020). The effectiveness of charge nurse training on leadership style and resiliency. *Journal of Nursing Administration, 50* (2):95-103.
This pre-post study design was conducted at an integrated health system with comparison and intervention groups. The objective was to study the effectiveness of an evidenced-based pilot education program for charge nurses that measures improvement in resiliency and leadership style. A random sample of charge nurses participated, including 22 who received intervention and 19 who were in the control group. Two questionnaires were used to measure leadership style and resiliency. An evidence-based curriculum was used, including an instructor-led classroom mode along with interactive WebEx training. Class courses included critical thinking and supervisory skills. Course objectives were based on the American Organization for Nursing Leadership's Nurse Manager Competencies.

Study findings indicated a statistically significant median increase in transformational, transactional, and leadership outcomes in the postintervention phase. A similar increase in resiliency scores was reported. The charge nurses in the study demonstrated higher satisfaction with behavior in leadership followed by effectiveness and, then, the ability to motivate. Those charge nurses in attendance demonstrated higher resilience at postintervention.

Implications for Practice

The role of the charge nurse is integral in any healthcare organization due to its complexity and multifaceted demands. Preparing and supporting these leaders for future development and succession is important. By providing professional development for the charge nurse or leader role, these nurses gain confidence and essential skills that benefit them and their department as well as achieving improved outcomes.

Having the title of Chief Executive Officer or Chief Nursing Officer does not guarantee that a person will be a good leader. Consequently, a good executive is not necessarily also a good leader. Furthermore, assuming a management or administrative role may confer the title of leader on an individual, yet the skills required may not be evident. Inspired and forward-moving organizations often select these executives specifically because of their ability to build a vision and lead others toward it. Leadership is an earned honor and an action-oriented responsibility.

Others believe that workers who do not hold official management positions cannot be leaders. Some nursing units are managed by the nurse manager and clearly led by the unit clerk or the expert frontline nurse. Leaders are those who do the best job of sharing their vision of where the followers want to be and how to get there. Many new nurse managers make the mistake of assuming that along with their new job comes the mantle of leadership. Leadership is an earned right and privilege.

MENTORING AND COACHING

Mentoring

Mentoring is an important aspect of development. It is important to find a mentor or more than one mentor to develop personally or professionally. Leaders, managers, and followers may identify opportunities to grow; finding a mentor who can assist and reflect is essential to learning. Mentoring occurs in all styles of leadership but is perhaps most powerful in transformational and authentic leadership. A mentor is someone who models behavior, offers advice and criticism, and coaches the novice to develop a personal leadership style. A mentor is a confidante and coach as well as a cheerleader and teacher. In other words, a mentor is knowledgeable and skilled.

Where do you find a mentor? Usually, a mentor is someone who has experience and some success in the leadership realm of interest, such as in a clinical setting or in an organization. A respected faculty member; a nurse manager, director, or clinician; or an organizational officer or active member may be a mentor. Mentorship is a two-way street. The mentor must agree to work with the novice leader and must have some interest in the novice's future development. A mentor can be close enough geographically to allow both observation and practice of leadership behaviors, as well as timely feedback. A mentor may also be geographically remote yet remain well connected to the mentee. A mentor should provide advice, feedback, and role modeling. In addition, the mentor has a right to expect assistance with projects, respect, loyalty, and confidentiality. In a mentoring relationship, aspiring leaders soak up knowledge and experience and should expect to pay it forward by serving as a mentor to a young, aspiring leader in the future.

Using Benner's model of moving from novice to expert is the framework identified by Quinn (2020) as very pertinent to grow leadership skills. Most managers were mentored, formally or informally, at one time in their career by someone of high regard or influence. In turn, a manager should focus attention on preparing future successors. The mentor does not insist on his or her own way, but rather the relationship allows for a commitment to a specific purpose. This notion is especially important in terms of nurse manager growth, particularly in the development of moral courage and clinical leadership to manage complex situations and personnel challenges. Having a solid mentor when faced with these situations allows nurse managers to explore options and role-play situations to achieve the best professional outcome. The role of mentor is a significant one that leaders, including managers and followers, must embrace (Kennedy et al., 2020). Mentoring is viewed as an interactive, multifaceted role that assists frontline staff, especially novice nurses, with setting realistic, attainable goals. Through mentoring their staff, nurse managers can help boost staff self-confidence, thereby helping them gain professional satisfaction as they reach their goals.

Coaching

Preparation for nursing practice challenges requires planning, education, and coaching to enable nurses to build confidence and experience in practice. Mentorship includes ongoing coaching and critique of what elements were and were not successful in problem-solving a situation. Being prepared for unprecedented or stressful situations can help to build confidence and self-awareness. Coaching is often associated with authentic leadership, including building cooperation, successful communication, and effective decision-making (Reiser & Gonzalez, 2021). Benner's model includes coaching and mentoring as the underpinning for career growth and development.

BUILDING A HEALTHY WORK ENVIRONMENT

Creating a positive work environment includes promoting teamwork and strong collaboration among nurse managers and the frontline staff. Nurses know and appreciate the nurse manager's attention and supportive leadership when the leader's focus is on improving areas that can affect patient care and patient safety. Grant et al,

(2020) discussed stressors that frontline nurses experience contributing to burnout, turnover, dissatisfaction, and, importantly, impacting the nurses' wellness and patient safety. Additionally, as healthy work environments are created and sustained, successful outcomes of the Quintuple Aim will be embedded in the culture. In order to achieve positive results, leaders must stress the importance of building desirable and collaborative unit-level work environments that result in the delivery of high-quality care and frontline staff retention. Nurse managers can create winning situations by building and engaging productive teams as they work toward accomplishing departmental and organizational goals and objectives. They can also motivate their teams by ensuring opportunities for continued growth and development that are directly correlated to a more knowledgeable workforce.

Standards for creating and maintaining a healthy work environment (Table 24.1) demonstrate the necessary domains of a healthy work environment as classically defined by several leading professional nursing organizations. Nurse managers today must serve as leaders who embrace uncertainty, can lead through change, and who seek to understand behaviors and relationships before attempting to change them. Now, when new nurses enter the workforce with enormous technological demands for their knowledge and skills, nurse managers need to help support their growth and their comfort while being flexible in managing the unknown.

Bullying, Incivility, and Workplace Violence

One of the greatest ongoing challenges a nurse manager faces is preventing bullying and supporting staff who may be exposed to bullying, incivility, or actual violence in the workplace. Hartin et al. (2020) described the covert tactics, disrespectful attitudes, and dysfunctional relationships that occur with bullying, stressing the importance of manager identification and action for prevention. With teamwork described as essential for providing high-quality care, other characteristics are critical to teamwork, including leadership, trust, and communication. Nurse managers must create positive work environments in which staff feel empowered and encouraged (Wunnenberg, 2020). As a Magnet® organization, one hospital identified some disruptive and bullying behaviors among the frontline staff. The positive outcomes achieved from this organization yielded national recognition from Sigma Theta Tau International (Sarik et al., 2020). Frontline leader development was

Domains of a Healthy Work Environment	American Organization of Nurse Executives (2004)	American Association of Colleges of Nursing (2005)	Association of periOperative Registered Nurses (2015)
TABLE 24.1	**Standards for Creating and Maintaining Healthy Work Environments**		
Collaboration	A culture that promotes collaboration through trust, diversity, and team orientation	True collaboration encouraged	Collaborative practice culture: All team members are treated respectfully; disruptive behaviors not tolerated
Communication	A culture with clear, respectful, open, and trusting communication	Skilled communication: Communication skills equal to clinical skills	Communication-rich culture: clear, respectful, inclusive, timely, open, and trusting communication
Decision-making	A structure for participation in shared decision-making	Effective decision-making: Nurses feeling valued in directing and leading care and operations of the organization	Shared decision-making: nurses participating in decision-making and policy development; responsible for their practice
Staffing	Adequate numbers of qualified staff to meet patient expectations and provide balance to the work and home life of staff	Appropriate staffing: Effectively meeting patient needs with matched nurse competencies	Presence of adequate numbers of qualified perioperative registered nurse staff: work and on-call schedules that promote positive work–life balance; quality care provided by adequate staffing
Recognition	Recognition of contributions of nursing staff and recognition by nurses of the contributions they provide to practice	Meaningful recognition: Recognize value that every nurse brings to workplace	Recognition of contributions from nursing and their value: recognized by peers and team members for performance; growth options available
Leadership	Presence of a leader who serves as an advocate for nursing, supports empowerment of nurses, and ensures availability of resources	Authentic leadership: Authentically embrace healthy work environment and engage team in achieving	Presence of expert, visible, and believable nursing leadership: leadership skills at all levels; nurses as advocates; share decision-making
Accountability	A culture in which everyone is accountable and knows what is expected		Accountable for professional practice and to team members: clear role expectations and definitions
Self-actualization	Ongoing education and professional development		Encouragement of professional practice and growth/development: ongoing education, certification and development encouraged and promoted

Data from American Association of Critical-Care Nurses (AACN). (2005). *AACN standards for establishing and sustaining healthy work environments.* https://www.aacn.org/nursing-excellence/healthy-work-environments; American Organization of Nurse Executives (AONE). (2004). *Nursing Organizations Alliance™ principles & elements of a healthful practice/work environment.* https://www.aonl.org/elements-healthy-practice-environment and Association of periOperative Registered Nurses (AORN). (2015). *AORN position statement on a healthy perioperative practice environment.* https://www.aorn.org/guidelines/clinical-resources/position-statements.

aimed at holding employees responsible for professional behavior and setting behavioral expectations. Leaders received coaching as well as tools and resources. The departments developed heightened recognition and awareness of negative behaviors, and communicated expectations to employees. Each unit developed a vision to eliminate disruptive behaviors. Upon reassessment, outcomes of the unit previously recognized for bullying were improved—for example, staff engagement and satisfaction rose from Tier 3 to Tier 1 (the best performance) and there were significant improvements in nursing care from the patients' perspective.

NURSE MANAGER ROLE AND THE INTERGENERATIONAL WORKFORCE

Nurse managers face many complexities in everyday work as they lead their staff. Managing an intergenerational nurse workforce while continuing to ensure the establishment and maintenance of a positive and harmonious workplace environment is certainly a challenge. In a study by Hisel (2019), a quantitative nonexperimental comparative study of 95 nurses measuring work engagement of generational nurses was implemented. The study found that veteran generational nurses were most engaged, followed by the Baby Boomers, Gen Xers, and Millennials.

Dols et al. (2019) identified the intent to stay in the job in a study of Hispanic and non-Hispanic nurses and found that there was no significant difference in staff satisfaction. The preferred traits of nurse leaders were tested; all 3 generations of nurses wanted similar professionalism and advocacy for nurses. Gen Xers and Boomers desired a leader with good judgment. Millennials appreciate clinical competence in their leader. Gen X nurses liked mentors, and Boomers and Millennials prefer to be empowered. Nurse managers must understand what motivates the different generations and use that knowledge to bring together teams to achieve departmental goals. One example is with technology implementation—Millennial nurses may support the learning needs of Baby Boomers. In contrast, the Baby Boomers may provide education, encouragement, and mentorship as the frontline staff gain confidence and learn new skills.

Results of the Nurse Wellbeing at Risk 2020 National Survey (Emergingrnleader.com, 2020) illustrated the need for and the importance of support and coaching for the youngest nursing cohort, Generation Z (nurses born between 1997 and 2015) (Sherman, 2021; Nurse Wellbeing at risk: A national survey, 2020). Generation Z nurses reflected substantially lower baseline data of exceptional or very sound mental well-being (American Psychological Association [APA], 2018). Managing the different groups may require different strategies and words, but the core for all is about safety and quality. While these generational differences serve as useful guidelines, no one should be stereotyped based on the group to which that person belongs generationally.

QUALITY INDICATORS

The nurse manager and staff are consistently concerned with the quality of care that is being delivered on their unit. The National Database of Nursing Quality Indicators (NDNQI), developed by the American Nurses Association (ANA) and now managed by Press Ganey, is an excellent resource for the nurse manager. The NDNQI measures are specifically concerned with patient safety and aspects of quality of care that may be affected by changes in the delivery of care and personnel or staffing resources. The quality indicators address staffing mix and nursing hours for acute-care settings as well as other care components, such as nurse satisfaction. The NDNQI is designed to assist healthcare organizations in identifying links between nursing care and patient outcomes.

Hospitals are compared across the nation in these measurements and others, such as core measures developed by The Joint Commission (2022), and the Centers for Medicare & Medicaid (CMS). Core quality measures typically evaluated include care associated with acute myocardial infarctions, congestive heart failure, the treatment of pneumonia, and patient satisfaction. As with the NDNQI measures, the core measures are concerned with level of quality of care and outcomes of care. Organizations may also benchmark within their system or within groups of other organizations to compare outcomes and practices.

MANAGED CARE AND CASE MANAGEMENT

The goal of managed care is to provide needed healthcare services efficiently and at an appropriate cost. In essence, this requires nurse managers to know and incorporate business principles into patient-care practices. Nurse managers who know business principles become conduits for ensuring safe, effective, affordable care. Reimbursement changes include the pressure on providers working with private and public payers to take on more risk or to expect a lower payment structure. Value-based purchasing links provider payments to enhanced performance, with the intent of eliminating adverse events; utilizing evidence-based standards of care; increasing transparency; incentivizing for improved patient experience, and recognizing hospitals that deliver lower costs and higher quality of care. The CMS can withhold payments by law at a percentage (2%) (CMS, 2021). Market consolidations will be driven by cost reduction and market competition as mergers may become more common. Finally, consumer changes include more expectations of receiving care and services on demand, streamlining scheduling and registration for a positive patient experience, and continued focus on engaging consumers and the customer experience. Nurse managers need to be aware of the continued review of healthcare costs and the organizational drive toward cost reduction with improvements in quality of care.

Case management is a method used to provide care for patients in inpatient and outpatient service areas. Increasingly, more traditional acute inpatient care is moving to outpatient service areas. The key to effective case management is proactive care coordination from the point of admission, with identified time frames throughout the patient stay in accomplishing appropriate care outcomes. The nurse manager often provides oversight of or essential collaboration with case managers. In some settings, the nurse manager is the immediate supervisor of the case managers. Case management involves components of case selection, multidisciplinary assessment, collective planning, coordination of events, negotiation and collaboration, and evaluation and documentation of the outcomes of patient status in measures of cost and quality. Case managers are employed in acute care settings, rehabilitation facilities, subacute care facilities, community-based programs, home care, and insurance companies. These managers must possess a broad range of personal, interpersonal, and management skills.

BUDGETING AND FINANCE

Financial skills, including knowledge of the budget process as well as the components that comprise the nursing or departmental budget, are essential for nurse managers and nurse leaders. Budgetary allocations, whether they are related to the number of dollars available to manage a unit or related to full-time equivalent employee formulas, are the direct responsibility of nurse managers. Nursing salaries are a large portion of an organization's personnel budget. For highly centralized organizations, only the administrative leaders at the executive level decide on the budgetary allocations. "Flat" organizational structures encourage the allocation of decentralized responsibilities to nurse managers in the patient care areas; the nurse managers must understand, determine, and allocate fiscal resources for their designated unit. In the decentralized organizational model, nurse managers must have the business and financial skills to be able to prepare, justify, and present a detailed budget that reflects the short-term and long-term needs of the unit. Nurse managers need to be highly conversant with several key budgetary concepts, especially in those areas that are driven by their units of service (e.g., hours and tests). Productivity measurement is common and essential for controlling labor expenses (e.g., overtime or contract labor). Supply costs are intense in critical care and other areas, thus, must be closely monitored, along with overall costs versus revenues, validation of charge capture, and, importantly, the overall contribution margin (net revenue minus variable costs). Historical data should be reviewed for trends. New technologies, surgeries, and procedures that may change departmental budget requirements should be reviewed as well. It is up to the nurse manager or nurse leader to utilize data to present a compelling argument and a logical position. The nurse leader must be able to successfully operate the department while gaining the respect of and credibility from financial and operational leaders. Perhaps the most important aspect of a budget is the provision for a mechanism that allows some self-control, such as decision-making at the point of service, which does not require previous hierarchical approval and a rationale for budgetary spending. Self-scheduling is one way of allowing staff control. However, the nurse manager must set parameters to guide scheduling so that the department remains within the budget.

FOLLOWER AS NURSE LEADER

Followers as nurse leaders create an environment in which others can experience satisfaction and have ideas for increasing the level of workplace satisfaction

BOX 24.1 **What Followers Expect from their Leaders**

- Respect
- A future-focused palpable direction
- A safe and positive healthy work environment
- Control of and engagement with decisions that affect them
- Recognition and rewards for good work
- A work–life balance
- Professional development and guidance

BOX 24.2 **Key Concepts Managers Consider**

- Hire the right people.
- Create, support, and develop active followers and emerging leaders.
- Secure and manage resources (fiscal, physical, and personnel) to support the provision of quality of care.
- Develop people to their full potential based on talent and qualifications.
- Support decisions made closest to the point of care delivery.
- Manage and share data to measure productivity and quality to provide optimal outcomes.
- Foster an environment of collaborative relationships with all disciplines.
- Hold yourself and others accountable.

for nurses on the team (Box 24.1). Leaders are those who creatively pose solutions to problems and capitalize on opportunities in the workplace. Furthermore, they support others who offer numerous ideas about various issues, including patient safety. Nurses who believe that they have good ideas for future improvements should volunteer for opportunities to lead, such as participating in practice councils, clinical unit standards committees, or legislative committees to pose new solutions. If the hospital, ambulatory clinic, or other workplace has no formalized mechanism for nurse input into organizational decision-making, nurses find informal avenues for influence, including asking thought-provoking questions, filing official complaints, creating unit campaigns, or holding informal discussions.

Leadership can be developed, and direct care nurse leaders can help establish workplaces that are satisfying and rewarding. Magnet® facilities, for example, depend on direct care nurse leadership to create and innovate, improving the quality of work and enhancing patient safety.

Novice leadership skills that contribute to future leadership success involve learning how to work in groups, dealing with difficult people, managing conflict, reaching consensus on an action, and evaluating actions and outcomes objectively, to create life skills that could transfer to subsequent practice.

Nurse Leader Development Within the Workplace

Nurses in numerous positions and various organizations serve as leaders. Because every nurse has the opportunity to serve as a leader, every nurse can exercise the right to lead. Leadership effectiveness depends on

mastering the art of persuasion and communication. Success depends on persuading followers to accept a vision by using convincing communication techniques and making it possible for the followers to achieve the shared goals. Several important leadership tasks, when performed effectively, will help ensure the expectations of success from followers (Box 24.2).

NURSE MANAGER AS LEADER

Management and leadership, although different constructs, can be a strong combination for success. The nurse in the role of manager ensures that the day-to-day procedures of the workplace are performed consistently and correctly, yielding positive patient outcomes. Just as the effective manager pays attention to employee selection, hiring, orientation, continuing employee development, and financial accountability, in the role of leader, the manager raises the level of expectations and helps employees reach their highest level of potential excellence.

A primary role of the leader is to inspire. The nurse manager may be seen as the embodiment of leadership in nursing. That person is the "face of leadership" to those in direct care, often balancing the needs of the patient with interdisciplinary input. Developing a shared vision of the preferred future is a goal of the nurse manager in the role of leader of direct care nurses. The nurse manager inspires staff by involving them in changing the workplace to make it more satisfying. In so doing, the nurse manager also develops personal leadership skills (Box 24.3).

In order to help frontline nurses adapt when they resist change, it is important that the manager be able to inspire them to address the change that is thrust on them. When nurses are active participants in change from its inception, they are far more likely to be invested in outcomes. Their contributions can enhance their organizational commitment and create a sense of pride in successful outcomes.

NURSE EXECUTIVE AS LEADER

Leader is a term often used interchangeably with the term *nurse executive*. However, many others may lead in any organization and can be, and *are*, seen as nurse leaders, not just the nurse executive. A primary goal of the nurse executive is leadership within the workplace. The nurse executive is responsible for the practice of nursing, staffing resources, evidence-based policies and procedures, patient quality and safety, and collaborating with others in the environment. They can create opportunities for direct care nurses and managers to have optimal input into organizational decision-making related to operations and strategic planning for the future, thus creating a shared vision of the preferred future.

The concept of empowerment is important to the role of leadership for the nurse executive. It suggests that power must be given away or shared with others in a work organization. Direct care nurses may be encouraged to have input into decisions or they may be given considerable information about how decisions are made. The ability to make or influence changes in the organization is a powerful tool and followers can provide valuable input for change. Nurses must believe that their input and ideas are considered when change occurs. Having input in decisions, having some control over the environment, and receiving feedback about actions taken or not taken all contribute to a feeling of being empowered to have control over one's practice and one's life.

The fact is that both management and leadership skills in the nurse executive are foundational. The ability to balance the day-to-day operating systems with the ability to lead and influence a nursing service organization into the future is a winning combination (Box 24.4).

Developing true leadership expertise takes place over time and should not be expected during the first year or two of nursing practice. Movement toward increasingly complex leadership experience allows the new nurse to move from leading and planning with an individual to working with groups, such as families or communities. With increasing educational achievement and career experience comes increasing complexity of leadership capabilities.

LEADERSHIP WITHIN PROFESSIONAL ORGANIZATIONS

In the United States, the best and most important step to take in becoming a leader within the nursing profession is to join a professional organization. Many nurses today take part in several organizations. These associations may be general and broad (e.g., the ANA), role based (e.g., the AONL), or clinically focused (e.g., the American Association of Critical-Care Nurses [AACN]). Volunteering for local committee memberships is a valued, foundational, and useful way to learn and to grow within the association. Many of the professional specialty organizations maintain a national or regional presence rather than having state or local chapters. Some have local chapters (e.g., the Association of periOperative Registered Nurses [AORN]), especially in the larger, more populated areas across the country. The major impact of the professional specialty organization is sharing and dissemination of information, advocacy and discussion of mutual clinical or role concerns, and education regarding the latest innovations in the field. Leadership opportunities are available to present posters or papers at local, regional, or national conferences, as well as to serve on committees and boards.

After becoming established in a local association, running for elected office in the local district or chapter association is a way that many leaders within professional associations start their leadership careers. It is not unusual to be unsuccessful in the first attempt at running for an elective office in a professional association. However, persistence can do three things: (1) it can help with name recognition, (2) it can let members know your abilities and that you are serious about being an association leader, and (3) it can allow for mentoring from those in office.

Leaders from local levels often hold office at the state level later. Volunteering for committee assignments and running for elected office in a state-level association establishes leadership interest within a professional association. This pathway of professional involvement and leadership may seem like a linear progression to more global opportunities for leadership in the profession. On occasion, well-known leaders who have held high offices at the national or state level may choose to utilize their expertise by returning to serve in local or regional offices.

LEADERSHIP IN THE COMMUNITY

Nurses as Community Opinion Leaders

Nurses are valued and respected members of their communities. As such, they are viewed as trusted professionals and have an opportunity to serve as catalysts in community leadership roles. In partnership with others in the community, nurses can help build a more just, more peaceful, and healthier society. Many avenues are available for nurses to serve as community opinion leaders, including attendance at civic gatherings such as city commission and school board meetings. These are excellent ways to be aware of what is happening in the community and to offer input as a nurse and advocate. For instance, when the school board begins deliberating on whether the budget will accommodate a registered nurse for every school or whether to replace a registered nurse with a trained clerk who can record vaccinations, a nursing voice in the audience could clarify the importance of school nurses to a school population. Writing letters to the editor of a newspaper and participating in public forums give the nurse an avenue to share expertise and mold community opinion.

Nurses as Community Volunteers

Many opportunities exist for volunteer participation in the community. Nurses bring a unique leadership skill set to community activities. The ability to understand complex systems, as well as to understand interpersonal dynamics and communication techniques, constitutes knowledge that is valuable in community volunteer opportunities. Leadership in mobilizing volunteers for health fairs, screening activities, and educational events is a community need that nurses can and do fill. Such activities promote health and advance the health of the entire community in important ways. Nurses can also lead efforts to engage others in the community in volunteer activities. In addition, nurses can organize individuals in the community to help develop a vision for the future of the community's health, healthcare opportunities, and healthcare delivery.

From the perspective of the nurse as a community leader, a unique opportunity exists to work with schools, city or county governments, and other community entities to formulate a vision for improving the health of the community through disease prevention and health promotion. The nurse can be a catalyst for a community to recognize present problems and to develop a plan to reach a preferred future.

LEADERSHIP THROUGH APPOINTED AND ELECTED OFFICE

Nurses are valuable leaders in elected and appointed offices at the local, state, and national levels. Because of the trustworthiness of nurses in general by the public, nurses are able to mobilize resources to raise monies, develop support, and to be elected to office. The potential for nurses in offices at all three levels of government is great. However, the number is small in relation to the percentage of the population that nursing represents. In addition to typical sources of campaign support, various healthcare-related political action committees provide assistance to nurses who want to run for office. Nurses who are elected members of governmental bodies can exert their leadership to shape the vision of the government to help meet the health and societal needs of citizens. At all levels, nurse leaders may be asked by a legislator to provide information on a particular policy position. Local government opportunities include school boards, city councils, and community boards dealing with various community initiatives. At the state level, opportunities include serving in the state legislatures; being appointed to state boards, such as the state board of nursing or the state board of health; or serving on special task forces such as those created by the legislature, a state board, or the governor. At the national level, opportunities include being elected as a U.S. representative (nurses are few, but present), being elected as a U.S. senator (no nurse has served in this capacity as of this writing), being appointed to a federal commission or board, or serving as an expert for a legislator or legislative body.

CONCLUSION

The nurse is in a trusted role as knowledge-based advocate, nurturer, and provider of care to the most vulnerable in our society. Nurses who choose leadership roles have many of the needed talents to serve their followers and their profession. Visionary and responsible leadership is vital to the future success of nursing as an art and a science. Professional nursing has been blessed with excellent leaders and will continue to be led by the visionary nurse leaders of tomorrow. Nurse managers have a responsibility to the patients they serve by supporting a healthy work environment that promotes advocacy for the health and healing of patients. By setting the example of professionalism, the nurse manager leads by influence and models the behaviors that the followers (direct care nurses) can follow. The manager plays a pivotal role in the well-being of a unit: the manager must encourage ethical practice, guiding direct care staff in delivering excellent and safe care to achieve the desired results and outcomes. Coaching and mentoring are essential skills for self-development and for leading others.

THE SOLUTION

The patient under discussion had many complex care needs, often requiring tests and procedures, and needed teaching to be able to understand the risks, benefits, and potential outcomes. In the day following the conflict, I investigated the concerns and perspectives brought by both the frontline nurse and the APRN in the care of this patient. I then asked to meet with both of them to explore their concerns by allowing each one an opportunity to explain their point of view. I acknowledged their concerns and their standpoints. When both sides were heard, I used this time as an opportunity to engage in coaching and conflict resolution to raise awareness as well as to gain respect for each other's ideas. Using this time, we began to build a common vision for what the patient may need that would be shared and discussed with other team members and the patient.

As leaders in healthcare, it is important that we prepare to provide reflective learning, removing frustration and resolving disputes more readily. I was steadfast in mentioning the organization's policies and guidelines that facilitate a healthy work environment that serves as an underpinning of successfully working together on behalf of the patient. After coaching, I scheduled individual meetings to provide feedback and assess their progress, avoiding the need for a formal disciplinary process and reinforcing team cohesion. If the behaviors had continued, I would have involved the support of human resources to assist; however, coaching and debriefing with staff leads to trust, openness, and conflict resolution.

Would this be a suitable approach for you? Why?

Peggy Townsend

REFLECTIONS

Consider the various leadership opportunities available to nurses. Ponder what makes sense to you in terms of your involvement to make yourself better, the profession better, and healthcare better. What will you do?

What specific activities must you engage in? What specific groups must you align with to achieve your expectation of involvement?

Think about the role of the nurse manager from your observations and experience. What do you identify as your opportunities in the roles of a follower or nurse manager and how would you proceed in your own development to prepare for leadership opportunities?

What is your personal leadership style and how would you strengthen your "tool kit" to successfully manage challenges you may face?

Picture a leader whom you admire and reflect on the person's style of leadership. How does it compare with your own? What skills do you need to further develop to be a more effective leader?

THE EVIDENCE

Effective leadership requires self-development, coaching, and mentoring to master skills such as effective communication, interprofessional collaboration, and workplace challenges. Numerous studies support the importance of skills that lead change, encourage teamwork, motivate colleagues, and transform and innovate practice. Generational groups and cultures have different values that may influence how nursing practice is performed. It is the role of the nurse leader to bring teams together with authenticity and a positive attitude that values all team members.

Having both management and leadership skills is important in the effectiveness of a leader in order to execute well. The leader must be open to learning and lead by taking risks in the best interest of the patient and team.

TIPS FOR GROWTH AS A FOLLOWER

- Followers will provide input regarding organizational change if requested.
- Follower growth is enabled when working in an organization that fosters structural empowerment underpinned from the ANCC Magnet Recognition Program® (2022).
- Followers will need support and mentoring when moving into a manager or leadership role.

TIPS FOR A NEW MANAGER

- As a new manager, take an assessment of your opportunities that are not your strength or get in your way of developing leadership skills, such as finance, communication (verbal or written), or public speaking.
- Take a look at those people you most admire or see as having these skills as attributes.
- Take one skill at a time and ask them to mentor and coach you as to how to improve and learn.

TIPS FOR BECOMING A LEADER

- Take advantage of leadership opportunities and practice your leadership skills.
- Expect to stumble occasionally but learn from your mistakes and continue.
- Get help; for example, identify a strong mentor who will give you feedback and insights into growing your skills in order to develop leadership abilities.
- Take risks to gain more experience and to test growth in your abilities.

REFERENCES

Abbott, K. (2020). Strong and sure leadership guides the way to lasting change. *Frontiers of Health Services Management, 36*(3), 27–33.

American Association of Colleges of Nursing (AACN). (2021). *AACN essentials.* Retrieved from https://www.aacnnursing.org/Portals/42/AcademicNursing/pdf/Essentials-2021.pdf.

American Nurses Credentialing Center Magnet Recognition Program®. (2022). https://www.nursingworld.org/organizational-programs/magnet/magnet-model/.

American Organization of Nurse Executives [AONE]. (2016). *Nurse Manager Learning Domain Framework. From Development and Learning Framework of the Nurse.* https://www.aonl.org/system/files/media/file/2019/04/nurse-manager-competencies.pdf.

American Organization of Nurse Executives (AONE). (2004). *Nursing Organizations Alliance™ Principles & elements of a healthful practice/work environment.* Retrieved from https://www.aonl.org/system/files/media/file/2020/02/elements-healthy-practice-environment_1.pdf.

American Psychological Association (APA). (2018). *Stress in America: Generation Z.* Retrieved from https://www.apa.org/news/press/releases/stress/2018/stress-gen-z.pdf.

Association of periOperative Registered Nurses (AORN). (2015). *AORN position statement on a healthy perioperative practice environment.* Retrieved from https://www.aorn.org/guidelines/clinical-resources/position-statements.

Blizzard, L., & Woods, S. (2020). The relationship between the implicit rationing of nursing care and emotionally intelligent leadership style. *Journal of Nursing Administration, 50*(12), 623–628.

Centers for Medicare & Medicaid Services. (2021). *The hospital value-based purchasing (VBP) program. Centers for Medicare & Medicaid.* Retrieved from https://www.cms.gov/Medicare/Quality-Initiatives-Patient-Assessment-Instruments/Value-Based-Programs/HVBP/Hospital-Value-Based-Purchasing.

Covey, S. R. (1992). *Principle-centered leadership.* New York: Simon & Schuster.

Doherty, D. P., & Revell, S. M. H. (2020). Developing nurse leaders: Toward a theory of authentic leadership empowerment. *Nursing Forum, 55,* 416–424.

Dols, J. D., Chargualaf, K. A., & Martinez, K. S. (2019). Cultural and generational considerations in RN retention. *Journal of Nursing Administration, 49*(4), 201–207.

Nurse Wellbeing at risk: A national survey. (2020). By *NurseGrid, Keener & HealthStream,* 1–11. Retrieved from https://assets.website-files.com/5f0fb8b3fe05ad6a00a17225/5f7169c-761f2643379ea9f50_NurseWellbeingAtRisk-Final2020-web.pdf.

Grant, S., Davidson, J., Manges, K., Dermenchyan, A., Wilson, E., & Dowdell, E. (2020). Creating healthful work environments to deliver on the Quadruple Aim: A call to action. *Journal of Nursing Administration, 50*(6), 314–321.

Hartin, P., Birks, M., & Lindsay, D. (2020). Bullying in nursing: How has it changed over 4 decades? *Journal of Nursing Management, 28,* 1619–1626.

Hisel, M. E. (2019). Measuring work engagement in a multigenerational workforce. *Journal of Nursing Management,* 1–12.

Nightingale, A. (2020). Implementing collective leadership in healthcare organisations. *Nursing Standard, 35*(5), 53–57. https://doi.org/10.7748/ns.2020.e11448.

Kennedy, J. A., Jenkins, S. H., Novotny, N. L., Astroth, K. M., & Woith, W. M. (2020). Lessons learned in implementation of an expert nurse mentor program. *Journal for Nurses in Professional Development, 36*(3), 141–145.

Kukreja, S. (2020). *4 principles of scientific management.* Retrieved from https://www.managementstudyhq.com/taylor-principles-of-scientific-management.html.

Lee, S. E., & Dahinten, V. S. (2020). The enabling, enacting, and elaborating factors of safety culture associated with patient safety: A multilevel analysis. *Journal of Nursing Scholarship, 52*(5), 544–552.

Long, T. (2020). Effect of authentic leadership on newly qualified nurses: A scoping review. *Nursing Management, 27*(3), 28–34.

Matter, S., & Wolgast, K. A. (2020). Making good use of your limited time: Supporting novice nurses. *Nursing Clinics of North America, 55,* 39–49.

McLeod, S. A. (2020). *Maslow's hierarchy of needs. Simply Psychology.* Retrieved from. https://www.simplypsychology.org/maslow.html.

Newman, B. M., & Newman, P. R. (2016). Chapter 6: Social role theory. In Taylor & Francis (Eds.), *Theories of human development* (pp. 167–172). Psychology Press.

Pearson, M. M. (2020). Transformational leadership principles and tactics for the nurse executive to shift nursing culture. *Journal of Nursing Administration, 50*(3), 142–151.

Porter-O'Grady, T., & Clavelle, J. T. (2020). The structural framework for nursing professional governance: Foundation for empowerment. *Nurse Leader, 18*(2), 181–189.

Quinn, B. (2020). Using Benner's model of clinical competency to promote nursing leadership. *Nursing Management, 27*(2), 33–41.

Raso, R., Fitzpatrick, J., & Masick, K. (2020). Clinical nurses' perceptions of authentic nurse leadership and healthy work environment. *Journal of Nursing Administration, 50*(9), 489–494.

Raso, R. (2019). Be you! Authentic leadership. *Nursing Management, 50*(5), 18–25.

Reiser, L. V., & Gonzalez, J. F. Z. (2021). Coaching and mentoring: Leveling up preceptorship. In Presented at the Sigma Theta Tau International: Creating Healthy Work Environments Conference, Virtual Event, March 12, 2021, Presentation E03.

Richards, A. (2020). Exploring the benefits and limitations of transactional leadership in healthcare. *Nursing Standard*, *35*(12), 46–50.

Robbins, B., & Davidhizar, R. (2020). Transformational leadership in healthcare today. *The Health Care Manager*, *39*(3), 117–121.

Rundio, A. (2022). The Nurse Manager's Guide to Budgeting & Finance (3rd ed.). Indianapolis, Indiana, USA: Sigma Theta Tau International Honor Society of Nursing.

Sarik, D., Thompson, R., Cordo, J., Roldan, I., & Gonzalez, J. (2020). Good for nurses, good for patients: Creating a healthy work environment in a pediatric acute care setting. *Nurse Leader*, *18*(1), 30–34.

Sherman, R. (2021). Keeping an eye on Generation Z nurses. *Nurse Leader*, *19*(1), 6–7.

Spiva, L., Davis, S., Case-Wirth, J., Hedenstrom, L., Hogue, V., Box, M., Berrier, E., & Ahlers, L. (2020). The effectiveness of charge nurse training on leadership style and resiliency. *Journal of Nursing Administration*, *50*(2), 95–103.

Sullman, M., Aljezawi, M., Almansi, S., Musa, A., Alazam, M., & Ta'an, W. (2020). Effect of nurse managers' leadership styles on predicted nurse turn-over. *Nursing Management*, *27*(5), 20–25.

The Joint Commission. (2022). https://www.jointcommission.org/measurement/measures/#da5c13bca86a4ca0ba58d-7feff614849_df8bd6b2c5e04894b59d75e0418940cd.

Wei, H., King, A., Jiang, Y., Sewell, K. A., & Lake, D. (2020). The impact of nurse leadership styles on nurse burnout: A systematic literature review. *Nurse Leader*, *18*(5), 439–450.

Wunnenberg, M. (2020). Psychosocial bullying among nurse educators: Exploring coping strategies and intent to leave. *Journal of Nursing Scholarship*, *52*(5), 574–582.

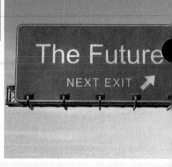

Thriving for the Future

Patricia S. Yoder-Wise

ANTICIPATED LEARNING OUTCOMES

- Value the need to think about the future while meeting current expectations.

- Ponder at least two projections for the future and what they mean to the practice of nursing.

KEY TERMS

chaos	innovation	vision
complexity compression	shared vision	VUCA
forecasting		

THE CHALLENGE

The future of nursing relies on nurses to work across the healthcare system in roles beyond traditional roles of patient care.

I know that most of us are not aware of, or exposed to, roles beyond patient care and the traditional operational leadership track. Most of us have been encouraged to do one of two things: (1) go back to school and get an advance practice degree or (2) follow the leadership path from charge nurse to CNO. In order for healthcare to evolve to meet the needs of a changing population, I thought we need nurses to take the path less travelled and embed nursing care into other parts of the healthcare systems. I particularly thought we all need to find our own joy in our professional journey, to follow our heart, not necessarily the path others prescribe for us.

My faculty said start in Med Surg: I chose ED. My clinical leaders said go into operations; I chose education and innovation. My friends said why get a PhD: I chose to follow my passion for leadership knowledge. Each time, I went against conventional advice to follow my passion to lead me to what I thought would be the future.

Then, I left normal healthcare and decided to join a start-up tech company, which was life changing and very scary!

What would you do if you were this nurse?

Dan Weberg, PhD, MHI, RN
Clinical Professor and Innovation Executive
The Ohio State University College of Nursing and Simovative
Solutions LLC
Alameda, CA, United States

INTRODUCTION

If you were old enough in 1999, you may remember the frantic activity surrounding the advent of the year 2000 when computer dates would switch to a new century. At that time, the year was represented digitally by two digits, and people were concerned that electronic records could not decipher 1999 from 2099—frenzy ensued. Imagine the relief when a tiny Pacific island-nation transitioned without a glitch! If that island could do it, so could we! This situation was totally predictable and we threw energy into averting the problem.

Think now to 2015 and someone has asked you, "What do you envision doing in 5 years?" Not one of us likely said we would be responding in one way or another to a worldwide pandemic. And yet, that is where we were in 2020. That, too, was predictable, although less so. Thus, because it was not as tangible as a visually evident computer programming problem, we did not have the same orchestrated worldwide response to the pandemic that we had to the computer issue.

Both of these are examples from the past of being able to thrive in the future. Some might argue that the impact of the pandemic was all negative. Yet, if we examine the benefits, we can see that even out of tragedies we find new ways to do things that make the future better. In some ways, many of the changes that occurred were already planned and simply implemented sooner and in greater quantity or intensity than originally planned. For example, as Clipper (2020) points out, the pandemic accelerated what was already in development and in many cases has created a view of necessity for the change. The Literature Perspective identifies areas of impact. Yes, it was available before, but not as an expectation as a part of service. The flexibility to change from what we were *planning* to do to what we *needed* to do is a strength of humanity's ability to survive. That also is a part of the obligation of being a nurse—making the future better in healthcare by being responsive to what is happening in the moment and improving on the best options at the time.

If during this time you did not feel you were being pulled in many directions, you were fortunate. We usually like having a name for what we are living through and there is one: VUCA, which stands for Volatility, Uncertainty, Complexity, and Ambiguity. This term was originally attributed to the U.S. Army War College (Garras, 2010) and later made popular by Bob Johansen (2012). It is the perfect term to describe the aspects of both personal and professional lives. What is likely amazing is that in 2012, which seems relatively calm in terms of life today, Johansen could activate this term! What we often do not reference as frequently, however, was the second VUCA Johansen discussed, perhaps VUCA 2.0, as Table 25.1 illustrates. That VUCA stands for Vison, Understanding, Clarity, and Agility. In other words, out of chaos (VUCA) comes great hope (VUCA 2.0). Chaos can be viewed as a state of complete disarray or confusion. Our obligation for the future is to focus on bringing VUCA 2.0 into perspective and to use all of our talents and tools we have at our disposal to do so.

The dichotomies of today pose challenges in healthcare. Think, for example, when patients are told to "log in" to their "patient portal" to create their "electronic record." Some people alive today have cellphones for the sole purpose of being able to push numbers to call someone to speak to them. They have no computer; they have no idea what "log in" means. The only portal they know is that round hole in rooms on ships.

TABLE 25.1	**From VUCA to VUCA 2.0**
Volatility	**Vision**
Uncertainty	Understanding
Complexity	Clarity
Ambiguity	Agility

Source: Johansen, B. (2012). *Leaders make the future: Ten new leadership skills for an uncertain world.* Oakland, CA: Berrett-Koehler, Inc.

LITERATURE PERSPECTIVE

Resource: Clipper, B. (2020). The influence of the COVID-19 pandemic on technology: Adoption in health care. *Nurse Leader, 18*(5), 500–503.

Clipper identifies three areas of healthcare technology in which growth accelerated during the pandemic. They are telehealth/virtual care, artificial intelligence (AI), and robotics. In part, one of the key attractions of technology was the lower potential for exposure to the virus. Telehealth/virtual care allowed people to limit their exposure to clinics and the requirements of processing to be seen in person. AI, as an example, provided more rapid and accurate diagnoses related to the virus and robots were readily accepted in various activities, such as room cleaning.

Implications for Practice

Although many of these technologies were in place prior to the pandemic, they were used less intensely. The pandemic increased the timeline and intensity of use; the results are that healthcare personnel now rely on these technologies as a part of routine care. This success likely will lead to easier adoption of additional new technologies in the future.

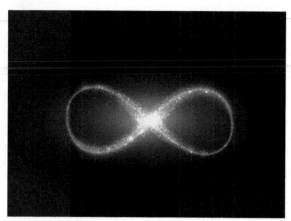

Fig. 25.1 The infinity symbol represents the never-ending cycle of change. (Copyright © Tatianazaets/iStock/Thinkstock.)

Two people can be speaking two different languages even though they are both speaking the same language and using the same words. How can that be. We just read an example of that with the "log in" and "portal" examples. We went through periods where the word "cool" meant "hot", until it didn't anymore.

Some of our older citizens recall that families took care of their family members at home. This often occurred because they didn't trust hospitals or couldn't afford the care offered in one. Today we are returning to care in the home with the expansion of the hospital at home concept often supplemented with devices to assist with monitor care remotely.

These never-ending changes affect us as nurses, too, just as patients are affected by them. The symbol for infinity (Fig. 25.1) has no beginning or ending. That is how change is—never ending.

2021, A YEAR OF REDIRECTION

Several reports were issued in 2021, two of which were delayed because of the outbreak of the COVID-19 pandemic, and all of which have major implications for the future of nursing and how the profession might thrive. In order of their release, we will look first at the Tri-Council for Nursing's *Transforming Together: Implications and Opportunities from the COVID-19 Pandemic for Nursing Education, Practice, and Regulation* (2021). This document was the outgrowth of an invitational conference held virtually to discuss valuable lessons learned as a result of the response that nurses provided during the

TABLE 25.2 **Key Themes from the Tri-Council Summit**
• Equity and health equity
• Ethics
• Nursing workforce
• Innovation
• Interprofessional emergency planning and response
• Mental health and well-being

Source: Tri-Council on Nursing. (2021). *Transforming together: Implications and opportunities from the COVID-19 pandemic for nursing education, practice, and regulation*. Author.

pandemic. The Tri-Council comprises the following organizations: the American Association of Colleges of Nursing, the American Nurses Association, the American Organization for Nursing Leadership, the National Council of State Boards of Nursing, and the National League for Nursing. It focuses on education, practice, and regulation. Without going into great detail, the key themes of the report (Table 25.2) provide nurses with guidelines for prioritizing concerns for improving healthcare.

If we look at the list for a moment, we can readily see that some of those issues are topics that have been addressed before, perhaps not in a fully intense manner. Now they have become major issues. As an example, mental health services have historically been woefully lacking in the United States and the pandemic precipitated the need for even more services. An underfunded, understaffed system has now been asked to do even more.

EXERCISE 25.1 Select a topic, such as nurse suicide, and determine its prevalence in the population. Compare nurse suicide with physician suicide and with suicide in the general population. Now, go immediately to Exercise 25.2.

EXERCISE 25.2 Select a clinical facility where you are able to see benefits that employees are able to access. What support is available specifically for mental health? What is available for employee well-being? Are you able to assess the culture of support for employee well-being, including mental health, in this organization? Does it support or hinder nurses seeking support of such services?

An example of a specific concern identified in this work was the supply chain challenges. We all heard about healthcare workers being asked to reuse personal protective equipment that was never intended to be reused because there was a national—and worldwide—shortage. In addition to causing angst among those who were forced to reuse their equipment, this problem pointed to the fact that we needed a national plan that could deploy supplies to areas where they were needed in a timely manner and to secure replacements in an equally timely manner. What this also did was raise the question of rationing care for patients with less survivability odds in order to conserve the supplies we had. Few of us have lived through such a time in civilian life, which produced further ethical dilemmas.

One outcome of all of this was clear, which was repeated in other reports: No organization can do the work alone. Too much needs to be done! The "take away" from the meeting sponsored by the Tri-Council was that this was an opportunity to engage people with nurses to address nurses' concerns so that patients may benefit. Each of us has a passion for something we would like to see happen in the profession. We often consider only the avenues within nursing to achieve our dream. As well, consider who external to the profession could help us advance what we want to see happen. What groups are critical to advancing our cause?

Next is the *Essentials* work of the American Association of Colleges of Nursing (AACN, 2021): *The Essentials: Core Competencies for Professional Nursing Education, 2021*. Although the AACN addresses only the education of nurses prepared at baccalaureate and higher degree levels, these competencies often form the basis for all aspects of nursing education in terms of points of comparison. This set of revisions is fairly dramatic as it moves to one of competencies and addresses two levels while not specifying degrees. The AACN identified 10 domains (broad areas of performance) that, taken together, form professional nursing (Table 25.3). A competency-focused expectation means that learning might look very different from one learner to the next and may take differing amounts of time to achieve the expectation of a competent level of performance. This has major implications for all sorts of educational endeavors that have been built around time and achievements (semesters and grades).

TABLE 25.3 The Ten Domains of Professional Nursing
• Knowledge for nursing practice
• Person-centered care
• Population health
• Scholarship of nursing practice
• Quality and safety
• Interprofessional partnerships
• Systems-based practice
• Information and healthcare technologies
• Professionalism
• Personal, professional, and leadership development

Source: American Association of Colleges of Nursing. (2021). *The essentials: Core competencies for professional nursing education*. Author.

EXERCISE 25.3 Consider some content or concept that was challenging for you to learn. Recall how you felt about "deadlines" for testing. Assuming that this content or concept is important to your practice today, how would you structure a learning experience that focused on developing competency? Consider how the traditional objectives (by the end of the…) would change.

An example of a major point throughout this document is the need to focus on communication. Unlike a topic such as anatomy, in which we can point to structures and rely on rules for remembering how various elements are structured and relate to each other, communication is more nebulous and requires the integration of numerous sciences, some of which are in early development. In addition to language sciences, we know that culture influences communication. We also know that vision and hearing capabilities influence what people understand in communicating with others. More recently, we know that being emotionally intelligent is critically important to communicating—and living—effectively. Communication becomes even more important when we consider how often it is the "designated blame" (meaning the root cause of an error or misunderstanding) between patients and care providers, between care providers themselves, and between care providers and managers. Communication is so complex that any inaccuracies can create problems. Yet, for the most part, we survive those misunderstandings and move on. However, we can do better! That is why communication in healthcare is so critical. To illustrate how communication relates to our ability to thrive in the future, consider the subcompetency 6.4c: *Engage in constructive communication to facilitate conflict management.* Because the future is unknown, conflict should be expected. Not everyone will agree that some particular event or product will be part of our future. If people are really adamant about their views, conflict is likely to ensue. How we are able to hold discussions that allow for diverse viewpoints about the unknown takes talent to avoid conflicts that could ruin an otherwise productive group. The competency of engaging in constructive communication is critical to the success of future work. Further, to be an effective member of a group willing to think about the future requires being able to address subcompetency 3.2c: *Use culturally and linguistically responsive communication strategies to relate to issues related to various populations that nurses will be engaged with in new ways in the future.*

The third major report, as you might suspect, was the National Academy of Medicine's *The future of nursing (FON) 2020–2030: Charting a Path to Achieve Health Equity* (2021). Designed as a follow-up to the original *Future of Nursing* report, which focused on nurses, this report focuses on what we do as a profession. Note that all three of the reports addressed the issue of health equity. The reason for this, of course, is that not enough has been done to ensure equitable care across populations. For example, although we have stopped excluding female subjects from participation in appropriate research studies, we still find that the care of women lags behind that of men in certain disease categories.

EXERCISE 25.4 Select a medical diagnosis commonly associated with a unit where you have clinical experience. Determine whether treatment differences occur based on gender. Are treatment options as aggressive irrespective of gender? What about race? Are there differences among Whites, Blacks, Native Americans or Asians? If such differences exist, is a rationale presented?

Each of these reports requires intense attention, yet most of us will likely devote little time to them. We are consumed with other aspects of our professional lives.

So, what can we do? Organizations, authors, and journals often synthesize such reports in order to distill the messages to strategies applicable to our roles or clinical areas. Find those distillations and consider the implications of what your role and clinical expertise suggest. Adopt one or two strategies that speak most strongly to you and address those religiously. Few of us can take on a full range of strategies in addition to our regular work. However, we can enhance our work by adopting new ideas into our required performance.

LEADERSHIP DEMANDS FOR THE FUTURE

Nurse leaders consistently say that the characteristic they are most seeking in today's professional nurse is leadership. In probing what that means, we often find themes relating to our activities that may have both direct and serendipitous outcomes. Leaders want professional nurses to take charge of situations in which safety is at stake or time must be conserved. Further, they see that we shape the public's view of the profession, the organization in which we work, and healthcare in general. We influence interprofessional views of what it is to be a professional, and we create the expectations of the nursing profession's potential. Being able to take action when we suspect "something isn't right"—whether with the patient or the organization—means that we have different expectations than we did several years ago. All of those examples shape the leadership potential that exists for the future. In short, however, this means that we must develop the capacity for leadership throughout our careers beginning in our prelicensure programs and increasing our competencies through ongoing professional development.

If we think about the world as a loose web, we know that every element has the potential to influence every other element. This connectivity, whether within our profession or within the team, means that we influence others all of the time just as others influence us. This influence molds our practices and beliefs as we move healthcare forward and subsequently changes how we influence others. Thus, positions without formal leadership titles contain expectations for leadership, and we must all be prepared and willing to lead whenever the need arises. As an example, this response is exhibited every time a mass casualty occurs. Consider how nurses led discoveries and care during the COVID-19 pandemic. Why did they do this? They were the best prepared to do so. The ability to be bicultural—both leading and following—is crucial to quality care, especially in crisis situations.

LEADERSHIP STRENGTHS FOR THE FUTURE

Because so much of nursing's work is accomplished in teams, we have considerable strength in inclusivity (the politics of commonalities). We tend, as do most people, to face our everyday work not capitalizing on thinking long term because we are typically consumed with work focused on the short term. Many change efforts are slow and cumbersome; the structure of change (the layers in the organization) may be overwhelming and the process detailed. That is the basis of the Institute for Healthcare Improvement (www.ihi.org), which supports small changes and encourages failing fast to determine whether a given small change is worthwhile pursuing. The IHI has short-circuited that drawn-out process of formal research studies in an attempt to bring quicker solutions to today's care. Although this rapid change (known as *rapid cycle improvement)* has produced positive results, we may see activities associated with this process as something "layered on" the already full schedule most of us experience at work. However, this emphasis, which is focused on improved care, is critical for safe patient care. The opportunity to engage in a rapid cycle improvement not only has the potential to enhance patient care but also helps you develop new skills that are useful for the future. So much change today happens in the VUCA format rather than in the planned, drawn-out approach. Thus, learning to fail fast and move on becomes a valuable skill. This also means we need to become competent at dealing with ambiguity and to be able to move forward through it to a clearer point of practice. A great place to start is always with the things we call the *work-arounds*. However, as Dr. Dan Weberg points out, sometimes the work-around is the answer. The rapid change then becomes focused on how to convert the policy to match the work-around process.

When we are faced with the pressures of providing care to a patient versus changing the system, we often remain focused on the patient. Thus, we lose the opportunity to change how we deal with an issue for many patients. To be effective in the future, we must embrace the opportunities to think longer term and more broadly so that more people are affected by our actions. This is the foundation of population health work—affect many. Moving from micromanaging to focusing on establishing expectations for a population may make us feel uncomfortable. However, that movement reinforces our ability to deal with longer-term, larger issues. In addition, the quest for meaning suggests that our actions today create the foundation on which future leaders will build. If we fail to capitalize on today's opportunities, we are diminishing the place at which future leaders will start their careers. Our goal should be to raise expectations about what comprises good, safe, quality care and determine how nurses should contribute to those expectations. This potential is especially critical in times of dramatic, chaotic changes.

How, then, do today's practitioners know what will be expected in the future? At the leadership level, Pesut says that we must "monitor industry trends, forecasts, and disruptions" (2019, p. 202). For all of us, the answer may seem trite: Continue to learn and to practice! Each of the reports mentioned at the beginning of this chapter identified the importance of lifelong learning. Without it, we become irrelevant (and unsafe!) and so does our profession. Our foundation begins with our concern for and advocacy about patient care. That foundation is fairly well ingrained in professional nurses' beliefs. The movement from focusing on the nurse–patient relationship to the big picture of nursing (politics and public or health policy activities) may take several years, but the foundation is there. Fagin, in her classic work (2000), identified that we all move from a focus on the nurse–patient relationship over time and, with additional preparation, move to the higher levels of leadership that focus on larger group changes and policy development. What we do in our professional lives is the legacy we leave for future generations. As Yoder-Wise, Kowalski, and Sportsman (2021, p. 5) say, "Legacies take time to build and take the commitment of more than one leader…The ability to maintain commitment and persist in tending seeds (the people we influence) leads to a legacy."

EXERCISE 25.5 Consider that many years have passed and you are at a time in your life when you might logically die. Rather than being sad that your life is ending, consider all of the good you have accomplished in life and in nursing. Your next of kin is asked to say what your nursing legacy is. What one or two sentences would you want to have said about your contributions to nursing?

Building a legacy requires taking risks. No organization wants all of its employees feeling free to do whatever they think should be done. On the other hand, even if an organization's official stance is that everyone must follow the policies and procedures, no responsible organization wants everyone to abide by the exact rule. Why? If we all did that all of the time, we would never change practice. We have to be willing to make sound judgments in knowing what risks to take and to what extent and what our tolerance is for lacking evidence. Realistically, though, progress is not made by "sticking to the rules." The question, then, is how do we know when it is safe to innovate?

VISIONING, FORECASTING, AND INNOVATING

Whether you are a leader, a follower, or a manager, being able to visualize in your mind what the ideal future is becomes a critical strategy.

A vision can involve one person or a group or whole organization. No matter how we engage in a visioning activity, we must be open and honest about what we think for the future. Finding those who do not necessarily think as we do, but who are creative thinkers, allows us to test ideas so that we enhance our own thinking and performance to higher levels. In the classic book, *The fifth discipline: The art and practice of the learning organization* (2006), Senge said that leadership is really about people working at their best to create the future. And that, in reality, is what we do every day. Creating a vision often requires believing that conditions could be improved, or seeing that a process from a totally unrelated discipline could relate to ours, or that the way in which we think we must deliver care is no longer practical even though it is viewed as the best method. Most people are excellent at identifying problems, but as many have asserted: We understand the problems—what we need are the *solutions*. That is what a vision is about. While leaders shoulder the responsibility for creating a vision, think about how useful we all can be if we have a visionary mindset rather than a problem mindset as we think about the future.

Forecasting is a specific process whereby we take in information that is current and focused on the future. The Projections for the Future Section illustrates some of the current and futuristic thinking that we should consider as we think about the future. Forecasting is most commonly associated with weather and economics, although it can be applied to any aspect in society. It requires a degree of logic (e.g., can we afford to do this, is the technology available, will people agree to participate, and so forth) and a degree of considered risk-taking or willingness to speculate about the consequences of actions taken.

Innovation is focused on taking current ideas and resources to create a better way to provide care, to move a strategy forward more rapidly, or to use something for a totally different purpose than intended. An example of what is currently innovative is the creation of MakerNurse (makernurse.com). Another example is using Voice Vibes (https://www.myvoicevibes.com), an artificial intelligence feedback system designed to improve communication. A third example is Mursion (https://www.mursion.com), a virtual-reality trainer. Each of these is a totally different answer to innovation and each is moving the practice of the profession forward.

Those are examples of major disruptive types of innovations. Zuber and Weberg (2020), however, advocate for a "calmer" view of innovation: "the ability of teams in an organization to adapt to changes in the environment" (p. 290). They identify three tensions that interfere with our being more innovative, as the Literature Perspective points out. Those tensions are:

1. Bad failure versus good—when bad failure causes harm, versus good failure, which simply shows that the current plan did not work.
2. Individual creativity versus organizational innovation—addressing local issues that may spread to the whole organization.
3. Top-down leadership versus innovation microclimate movements—innovation developed in a network, not a top-down approach.

LITERATURE PERSPECTIVE

Resource: Zuber, C., & Weber, D. (2020). Frameworks for leading frontline innovation in health care: failure, microclimates, and leadership. *Nurse Leader, 18*(3), 290–295.

Innovation is critical to the future of any organization. It takes solid leadership support to ensure that all nurses are able to engage in being innovative. Without a different view by leaders of what innovation is, an organization's ability to be innovative is limited. The word "failure" typically has a negative connotation—yet, it is often the act that advances our work. These authors identify ways to change from bad to good failures and, thus, be more productive. Additionally, viewing innovation in a network perspective is far more productive than thinking of it as a top-down activity.

Implications for Practice
Frontline nurses can readily engage in innovative practices with the support of leaders. Leaders need to consider what passion individuals have for solving specific problems in clinical areas so that microclimate changes can result in success.

EXERCISE 25.6 Select a group of three or four peers and brainstorm about what you think the future of nursing will be. Consider how technology will affect what we do; consider where our primary place of service will be and how we will deliver care. Determine how you will address the problem of healthcare inequity. Think about the changes in society and the political pressures for effective healthcare and what those might mean for nursing. Think about how you would reform healthcare. Create a list of ideas to share with others.

Although no one knows the future for certain, many groups are engaging in formal discussions and predictions. At the least, we do know that we are preparing for another pandemic. These groups range from structured groups, such as the World Future Society (www.wfs.org) *and the Future Today Institute* (https://futuretodayinstitute.com/) to ones that produce routine and special reports and books. Most of us are not futurists, yet we can use a simple technique to remain current with what the future could hold. We all can commit to being open to new information from atypical sources that we don't usually access and to consider what that information might offer us in benefitting us and the people we serve. The view of "what if" creates a view of potential for the future.

THE WISE FORECAST MODEL©

A useful and accessible model for thinking about the future is the Wise Forecast Model© (Yoder-Wise, 2011). Box 25.1 contains its three steps.

This three-step model emphasizes what each of us must do proactively to create our own future rather than to passively react to changes as they occur. Our careers can either happen to us or we can prepare for them.

The first step, *learn widely*, means that we must extend our sources of knowledge beyond our role and

BOX 25.1   The Three Steps to The Wise Forecast Model©

1. Learn widely
2. Think wildly
3. Act wisely

Source: Yoder-Wise, P. S. (2011). Creating wise forecasts for nursing: The Wise Forecast Model©. *The Journal of Continuing Education in Nursing: Continuing Competence for the Future*, 42(9), 387.

clinical areas of interest. In fact, we must extend our learning beyond nursing and healthcare. *Widely* might encompass another discipline, such as architecture or engineering. This extension does not mean that someone has to seek a degree in a new field. Learning about the field and how its professionals think might create new ways to think about issues affecting nursing. Just-in-time learning occasionally may feel stressful, yet it provides new information when needed. We experienced this type of learning during the early months of the pandemic when knowledge was changing so rapidly. Thinking about what that learning means beyond the original intent can also create new ways of thinking about an issue. *Widely* might also include works related to future-based or general publications, such as *FastCompany* or *Wired*. Subscribing to Ted Talks' science newsletter, as an example, also provides new ideas (http://ted.us1.list-manage.com/subscribe?u=07487d1456302a286cf9c4ccc&id=83c20124eb).

Initially, this kind of learning may need to be deliberate. In other words, you might need to set aside specified times to seek this diverse information. After a few such sessions, however, information from other fields can pique your interest to the point that you can create a file of "tidbits" of information.

The second step is to *think wildly*. Now we are limited only by our imagination. For example, from the beginning of the invention of computers, users have not been content with their size and function. Thus, computers evolved from one or two room-sized mainframes to hardware we could have in our homes, to a laptop computer we could carry in our backpacks, to a smartphone we could hold in our hands. Step two is designed to create connections among disparate thoughts. Thinking wildly includes creating wild questions. Sometimes, they are what leads to a wild idea that just might lead to innovation.

Step three, *act wisely*, is designed to draw us back to the reality of what is possible within the organization in which we work, with the funding we have available, and with the amount of time we have to invest in an activity. Acting wisely is, in a sense, a recovery phase to help us balance the wild thinking with the reality of resources and possibilities.

Because the future is about teams and group work, many implications exist for nursing. Developing or strengthening skills related to working with others along with facilitating their work and being effective in making decisions about practice and the workplace will be crucial. If the work is team based, how will evaluations and compensation be structured in the future? Will you receive favorable reviews because the team you work with is productive? Will a team receive a bonus or merit salary increase? If you are not a team player, will you be useful to the organization at all? How will the role of the nurse as a frontline leader and the role of the nurse leader change? These are examples of how to rethink the future.

Consider the differences among the nurses. For example, some people are interested in being able to see the world. That used to mean traveling abroad for a vacation. A smart, trendy employer might create an international collaborative that allows nurses to retain their home organization benefits while practicing throughout their home country and the world.

SHARED VISION

The concept of shared vision suggests that several of us buy into a particular view. We might all agree that nurses should manage the entire healthcare system. If we all agree on that view, it is a shared vision. We also might agree, perhaps more realistically, that having more than one theory of nursing allows for creativity in nursing, which creates groups of nurses with shared visions of how they view nursing as a profession.

Stability and total chaos are the opposite ends of a continuum. Moving in some way between those two ends suggests that we live in a constant state of disequilibrium in which we strive toward stability while recognizing we experience chaos (VUCA). In times of great stability, society makes little progress and life may seem serene. In contrast, society may transform itself during times of great chaos, and life may seem uncontrollable. Thus, thinking about the projections for the future becomes more important. For example, consider what people were doing, thinking, believing, and valuing in November of 2019. Then, think about each in relation to May of 2020. We moved from some point on that continuum closer to chaos, no matter where we were in the world or what we were doing.

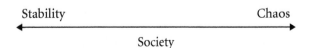

As we continue to move from "traditional" practices to evidence-based ones and from a heavy focus on tertiary care to one that values primary care, we can assume

that we might experience more chaos. The comfort of the known is gone; rather, practices are evaluated on a regular basis and changes are incorporated so that we are all doing the latest "best" for patients. Again, we saw this in practice during the pandemic. Practices changed so rapidly, we had difficulty remembering what the current practice was. Some practices changed during the shift. In our efforts to do the best we can as soon as we can, we have experienced the phenomenon of complexity compression, a term that means many changes are happening almost simultaneously and that before one practice can be firmly implanted in our minds, we are already addressing some other new change. This compression can be distracting or useful. Complexity compression is what most of us experienced in our roles during 2020 as a result of the impact of the pandemic. When too many things happen at once or too quickly, we have difficulty processing any of them completely.

PROJECTIONS FOR THE FUTURE

If you read *Trend Letter* or *The Futurist* (The World Society publication) or books by classic authors such as Isaac Asimov, Arthur C. Clarke, Aldous Huxley, George Orwell, and H. G. Wells, you will find comparable themes about the future. Some ideas that were developed over the past decade have transformed what we do and how we behave. For example:

- Adjustable glasses (creating sharp vision as a person's visual acuity changes), originally created for emerging economies, are available worldwide.
- 3D printers create internal organs that might not normally be available to those who need them.
- Devices such as the Oculus Rift would allow us to observe simulated events we might not want to experience in real life (e.g., this could be a way to learn to interact with highly emotionally unstable people).
- Through molecular analysis, researchers can swab your mobile phone to determine what you eat and drink, what you wear (clothing and makeup) and what medications you take.
- Temporary tattoos can monitor your health.

The following are some forecasts for the future that will affect nursing. Some are clearly related to healthcare; others have a tangential impact. In all cases, it is possible to ask the "what if" questions with each (e.g., what if this happens? Or what if more can happen?).

- Knowledge will continue to change dramatically, requiring that we all be dedicated learners. With or without state law, continuing education will be mandatory and essential if we intend to be relevant.
- Knowledge will evolve from the intensity of the current information evolution so that we will access content with meaning and applicability for our work.
- As the healthcare system continues to evolve and as employers limit healthcare coverage and genetics allows us to know more about how an individual would respond to treatment, a shift toward eliminating the current disparities is more likely. Healthcare also seems to invade one's rights to privacy and choice because, as an example, everyone will have an electronic health record.
- Technology will continue to revolutionize healthcare. (Robots will provide care and monitor our health; and because they can be "empathetic," people may interact with them in a very personal way. Search for Romotive and Kodomora.)
- Creating a tricorder, the handheld device from the television series *Star Trek* to assess people's health status, has been a goal that will allow any of us to quickly access data and determine certain health conditions (http://tricorderproject.org/index.html).
- The following elements of demographic diversity will all have major implications for healthcare delivery:
  - More people who are older
  - More people moving to different parts of the country or the world
  - A greater need for speaking two or three languages
  - A view of the "glocal" community (worldwide diversity in our local communities)
- People will feel the need to be satisfied with an experience, not simply service.
- Dichotomies will intensify. For example, increased violence and simultaneously an increased expectation for civility will exist.
- Stores will be either very small or huge, and the expansion of those existing only online will continue.
- Macromarketing (targeting masses) will be out; micromarketing (targeting specific populations) will be in. This trend will continue to intensify and it will intensify applications to healthcare.
- In most communities, the emergency department will be the primary source of care for persons with mental health disorders.
- We could become narrower in our views of the world because we can be catered to based on our distinctive interests. As an example, consider micromarketing,

in which retailers know what brands and sizes of clothing you prefer and send you only information about those products on a regular basis. The danger of this, of course, is that narrow views often lead to intolerance of broader or diverse views.
- Job security will be out; career options will be in.
- Mobile electrocardiograms will allow individuals to run their own EKGs and will allow nurses to have more data in any emergent situation. (Consider what smartwatches already do!)
- Breathalyzers will diagnose disease.
- Competition will be out; cooperation will be in.
- Work will be sporadic.
- More people will be living with chronic diseases.
- A focus on prevention/wellness care will include patient accountability expectations, with higher insurance rates for those who continue to engage in unhealthy behaviors.
- Water, not oil, will be the scare resource, according to the World Future Society.
- Robotics will change how chronic diseases can be managed. Being able to have them provide care and monitor specific health indicators will extend nurses' reach.
- Bioengineering will make possible interventions that currently do not exist.
- Emphasis on prevention will redirect care efforts and create new services.
- Work will be accomplished by teams.
- Everyone will need to be a leader. The future explodes with potential.

EXERCISE 25.7 Review the list of projections and consider how each might affect what you envision as your career. Evaluate each of the items to determine which ones you believe will be most important to you. Rank in order the top five. Compare your list with two or three colleagues' lists and offer your rationale for your selection. After you hear other viewpoints, consider whether you would change your own rankings.

In nursing, we have issues we can consider in the more narrowed scope of the world, for example:
- How will shared governance continue to enhance the role of clinical nurses?
- How will Magnet™ and Pathways to Excellence™ (ANCC) designations affect where nurses seek employment? (Think wildly!)
- How will continuing competence be measured in the future?

- How will healthcare emerge over the next several years as a desirable field in which to work and as a source of help for health-related needs?
- How will the increasing number of men in nursing change the "profile" of the profession?
- Will our profession's ethnic diversity reflect that of the population we serve?
- What can healthcare organizations learn from business and vice versa?
- Will increasing concern about terrorism affect the flow of nurses across borders?

HOW DO WE PREPARE FOR THE FUTURE?

In addition to reading, thinking, and acting differently (The Wise Forecast Model; see Box 25.1), Weberg proposes a simple approach: it just takes one. He suggests that we can focus on one collaboration, one change, one behavior or one connection (Weberg, 2021, p.77). In other words, we do not need to make the future a complex challenge that seems insurmountable. Rather, we can look at the numerous possibilities, select one, and decide what we want to do about that one thing. The profession, however, must address the bigger picture in order to advance to where it needs to be in the future because, as Weberg points out, the various structures, politics and fragmentations in nursing's leadership might limit our potential. While major organizations address the big-picture issues, we each can move the future forward by grasping the "one" idea or task we choose to take on to bring about change. If we each do that, we can bring about millions of changes and the future will allow nurses and the profession to thrive.

CONCLUSION

Numerous changes will occur throughout our lifetimes. How soon will we say (if we haven't already), "When I was young . . . ."? Our remembrance might be of something that today is considered fairly advanced. For those who want to thrive, the future forecasts are like the gold ring on the merry-go-round. If you risk and reach far enough, you can grasp it! Lead on … ¡Adelánte!

THE SOLUTION

In my own path, I followed the path less travelled and tried to impact the profession. From simulation nurse educator, to continuing education director, to nursing technology and innovation leader, to building a new medical school and, most recently, Vice President for Transformation in Nursing, I never did pure operational roles or advanced practice. My experience in small organizations, academia, large academic medical centers, and start-up companies prepared me to see across the health system—and beyond—and understand the entire landscape of where nurses add value and where our profession can go in the future.

Working throughout the system allowed me to grow as a nurse and as a leader and understand different viewpoints in order to lead innovation. If I would have stayed in a traditional route, I would not be as effective as a future innovation-focused leader. Each nontraditional role added to my perspective and skill as an influencer and leader. From influencing my undergraduate faculty to adopt simulation, to influencing physicians in building a medical school, to supporting tech experts in building a nursing-focused start-up—each experience gave me a set of skills that rounded out my executive leadership capabilities. Each also allowed me to see things differently and challenge teams differently than if I would have been in operations or advance practice alone. Look to the future and imagine what might be if you let yourself be! The worst part is being scared of being the first or having only a few people who get what you are doing! And think where you might be in the next decade!

Would this be a suitable approach for you? Why?

Dan Weberg

▮ REFLECTIONS

Learning widely, thinking wildly, and acting wisely (The Wise Forecast Model) is a simple process to consider the future. Consider how you can incorporate that into your professional practice. How will you learn outside of the profession and practice of healthcare? Do you have people in your life who encourage you to think wildly? If not, how will you be able to do so and still be accepted as a member of the team? What strategies are you most comfortable with when introducing ideas you want to advance in a situation? How will you get a group to commit to act with you on some different idea?

BEST PRACTICES

The key to remaining employable and successful is to remain relevant and engaged. That means we need to spend some of our time being strategic about our career and how nursing is changing. While we all get to help shape the future of nursing, we are also shaped by the changes that happen to the profession. Being proactive about what is happening allows us to be on the forefront of change and ready to assume new roles and expectations.

TIPS FOR THRIVING IN THE FUTURE

- Scan the general literature external to nursing and healthcare and "think wildly."
- Listen to divergent viewpoints from diverse sources about big issues that focus on policy and the future.
- Ask yourself "what if" questions.
- Remember that all the easy problems have already been solved—your opportunity lies in answering challenging ones!
- Look for practical, easily implemented, widely available solutions whenever possible.

REFERENCES

American Association of Colleges of Nursing (AACN). (2021). *The Essentials: Core Competencies for Professional Nursing Education*. Author.

Clipper, B. (2020). The influence of the COVID-19 pandemic on technology: Adoption in health care. *Nurse Leader, 18*(5), 500–503.

Fagin, C. (2000). *Essays on Nursing Leadership*. Springer.

Gerras, S. J. (Ed.). (2010). *Strategic leadership primer* (3rd ed.). Carlisle Barracks, PA: Department of Command, Leadership, and Management, United States War College. https://publications.armywarcollege.edu/pubs/3516.pdf.

Johansen, B. (2012). *Leaders make the future: ten new leadership skills for an uncertain world*. Oakland, CA: Berrett-Koehler, Inc.

National Academy of Medicine. (2021). *The future of nursing (FON) 2020–2030: Charting a path to achieve health equity*. Washington, DC: The National Academies Press.

Pesut, D. J. (2019). Anticipating disruptive innovations with foresight leadership. *Nursing Administrative Quarterly, 43*(3), 196–204.

Senge, P. (2006). *The fifth discipline: The art and practice of the learning organization*. New York: Doubleday Currency.

Tri-Council on Nursing. (2021). Transforming together: Implications and opportunities from the COVID-19 pandemic for nursing education, practice, and regulation. Author.

Weberg, D. (2021). Building the profession of the future: challenging assumptions. *Nursing Administration Quarterly, 45*(1), 71–78.

Yoder-Wise, P. S. (2011). Creating wise forecasts for nursing: The Wise Forecast Model©. *The Journal of Continuing Education in Nursing: Continuing Competence for the Future, 42*(9), 387.

Yoder-Wise, P. S., Kowalski, K., & Sportsman, S. (2021). *The leadership trajectory: Developing legacy leadership*. Elsevier.

Zuber, C., & Weber, D. (2020). Frameworks for leading frontline innovation in health care: failure, microclimates, and leadership. *Nurse Leader, 18*(3), 290–295.

INDEX

Note: Page numbers followed by *f* indicate figures, *t* indicate tables, and *b* indicate boxes.